AUTOIMMUNITY AND TOXICOLOGY

AUTOIMMUNITY AND TOXICOLOGY

Immune Disregulation Induced by Drugs and Chemicals

Editors

M.E. Kammüller, N. Bloksma and W. Seinen

Department of Basic Veterinary Sciences
Section of Immunotoxicology
Faculty of Veterinary Sciences
University of Utrecht
Yalelaan 2, NL-3508 TD Utrecht
The Netherlands

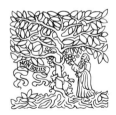

1989
ELSEVIER
AMSTERDAM · NEW YORK · OXFORD

ISBN 0-444-81023-4

Published by:

Elsevier Science Publishers B.V.
(Biomedical Division)
P.O. Box 211
1000 AE Amsterdam
The Netherlands

Sole distributors for the USA and Canada:

Elsevier Science Publishing Company. Inc.
655 Avenue of the Americas
New York, NY 10010
USA

Library of Congress Cataloging-in-Publication Data

Autoimmunity and toxicology: immune disregulation induced by drugs and chemicals/editors, M.E. Kammüller, N. Bloksma, and W. Seinen
   p.   cm.
   Includes bibliographies and index.
   ISBN 0-444-81023-4 (U.S.)
   1. Autoimmune diseases—Pathogenesis. 2. Immune system—Effect of drugs on. 3. Immune system-Effect of chemicals on.
4. Immunotoxicology. I. Kammüller, M.E. II. Bloksma, Marie Anna, 1949—. III. Seinen, W.
   [DNLM: 1. Autoimmune Diseases—chemically induced. 2. Immunity—drug effects. 3. Toxicology. WD 305 A9392]
RC600.A847   1989
616.97'071—dcl9
DNLM/DLC
for Library of Congress   88-38125
                                                                                       CIP

Printed in The Netherlands

Contents

SECTION II – BASIC CONCEPTS

Chapter 2
Basic mechanisms of adaptive immune system function
N. Bloksma and H.-J. Schuurman

Chapter 3
Theories of self tolerance and autoimmunity
A.C. Allison 67

Chapter 8
Halothane hepatitis – an example of possibly immune-mediated hepatotoxicity
J. Neuberger

Chapter 9
Metabolism of procainamide, hydralazine, and isoniazid in relation to autoimmune(-like) reactions
D.W. Hein and W.W. Weber

Chapter 13
Autoimmune reactions induced by dietary antigens with an emphasis on amino acids
E.J. Bardana, Jr., A. Montanaro and M.R. Malinow

Chapter 14
Autoimmune reactions induced by metals
P. Druet, L. Pelletier, J. Rossert, E. Druet, F. Hirsch and C. Sapin

III.	Experimental strategies	446
	1. Animal-related approaches	446
	(a) Short-term assays	446
	(b) Long-term experiments	447
	2. Chemical-related approaches	449
	(a) Chemical reactivity of parent compounds	450
	(b) Metabolism	451
	(c) Immunotoxicologically relevant targets	452
IV.	Conclusions	453
	References	453

Subject index   459

List of Contributors

M. Alarcón-Riquelme, Departamento de Immunología y Reumatología, Instituto Nacional de la Nutrición Salvador Zubirán, Calle Vasco de Quiroga 15, Delegación Tlalpan, 14000 Mexico D.F., Mexico

D. Alarcón-Segovia, Departamento de Immunología y Reumatología, Instituto Nacional de la Nutrición Salvador Zubirán, Calle Vasco de Quiroga 15, Delegación Tlalpan, 14000 Mexico D.F., Mexico

A.C. Allison, Department of Immunology, Syntex Research, 3401 Hillview Avenue, P.O. Box 10850, Palo Alto, CA 94304, USA

S. Ansar Ahmed, Clinical Immunology Section, Department of Medicine, The University of Texas Health Science Center at San Antonio, 7730 Floyd Curl Drive, San Antonio, TX 78284, USA

D.P. Aucoin, North Carolina State University, College of Veterinary Medicine, 4700 Hillsborough Street, Raleigh, NC 27606, USA

E.J. Bardana, Jr., Department of Medicine, Division of Allergy and Clinical Immunology, The Oregon Health Sciences University, 3181 SW Sam Jackson Park Road, L329, Portland, OR 97201, USA

N. Bloksma, Department of Basic Veterinary Sciences, Section of Immunotoxicology, Faculty of Veterinary Sciences, University of Utrecht, Postbox 80176, NL-3508 TD Utrecht, The Netherlands

J.H. Dean, Sterling-Winthrop Research Institute, Department of Toxicology, 81 Columbia Turnpike, Rensselaer, NY 12144, USA

E. Druet, Pathologie Rénale et Vasculaire (INSERM U 28), Hôpital Broussais, 96, rue Didot, F-75674 Paris Cedex 14, France

P. Druet, Pathologie Rénale et Vasculaire (INSERM U 28) Hôpital Broussais, 96, rue Didot, F-75674 Paris Cedex, France

P. Emery, Rheumatology Research Wing, The Medical School, University of Birmingham, Birmingham B15 2TJ, UK

E. Gleichmann, Division of Immunology, Medical Institute of Environmental Hygiene, University of Düsseldorf, Auf'm Hennekamp 50, D-4000 Düsseldorf 1, FRG

H. Gleichmann, Diabetes Research Institute, University of Düsseldorf, Auf'm Hennekamp 65, D-4000 Düsseldorf 1, FRG

D.W. Hein, Department of Pharmacology, The Morehouse School of Medicine, 720 Westview Drive, Atlanta, GA 30310-1495, USA

L.A. Th. Hilgers, Duphar B.V., Animal Health Division, Department of Veterinary Vaccines, P.O. Box 2, NL-1380 AA Weesp, The Netherlands

F. Hirsch, Pathologie Rénale et Vasculaire (INSERM U 28), Hôpital Broussais, 96, rue Didot, F-75674 Paris Cedex 14, France

M.E. Kammüller, Drug Safety Assessment − Toxicology, Sandoz Ltd., CH-4002 Basle, Switzerland

A. Kristofferson, Research Laboratories, Astra Alab AB, S-15185 Södertälje, Sweden

G.R.F. Krueger, Pathologisches Institut, Universität zu Köln, Joseph-Stelzmann-strasse 9, D-5000 Köln 41, FRG

M.R. Malinow, Oregon Regional Primate Research Center, Beaverton, OR 97006, USA

A. Montanaro, Department of Medicine, Division of Allergy and Clinical Immunology, The Oregon Health Sciences University, 3181 SW, Sam Jackson Park Road, L329, Portland, OR 97201, USA

J. Neuberger, The Liver Unit, The Queen Elizabeth Hospital, Edgbaston, Birmingham B15 2TH, UK

B.S. Nilsson, Medical Department, Astra Läkemedel AB, S-15185 Södertälje, Sweden

J. Nuyens, Central Laboratory of the Netherlands Red Cross Blood Transfusion Service, Plesmanlaan 125, NL-1066 CX Amsterdam, The Netherlands

G.S. Panayi, Rheumatology Unit, Division of Medicine, Guy's Hospital, London SE1 9RT, UK

L. Pelletier, Pathologie Rénale et Vasculaire (INSERM U 28), Hôpital Broussais, 96, rue Didot, F-75674 Paris Cedex 14, France

J. Rossert, Pathologie Rénale et Vasculaire (INSERM U 28), Hôpital Broussais, 96 rue Didot, F-75674 Paris Cedex 14, France

R.L. Rubin, Department of Basic and Clinical Research, Research Institute of Scripps Clinic, 10666 North Torrey Pines Road, La Jolla, CA 92037, USA

G.J. Rijkers, Department of Immunology, University Hospital for Children and Youth 'Het Wilhelmina Kinderziekenhuis', P.O. Box 18009, NL-3501 CA Utrecht, The Netherlands

C. Sapin, Pathologie Rénale et Vasculaire (INSERM U 28), Hôpital Broussais, 96, rue Didot, F-75674 Paris Cedex 14, France

J.G.M. Scharenberg, Department of Immunology, University Hospital for Children and Youth 'Het Wilhelmina Kinderziekenhuis', P.O. Box 18009, NL-3501 Utrecht, The Netherlands

H.-J. Schuurman, Department of Pathology, Faculty of Medicine, University of Utrecht, Pasteurstraat 2, NL-3511 HX Utrecht, The Netherlands

W. Seinen, Department of Basic Veterinary Sciences, Section of Immunotoxicology, Faculty of Veterinary Sciences, University of Utrecht, Postbox 80176, NL-3508 TD Utrecht, The Netherlands

E. Sim, Department of Pharmacology, University of Oxford, South Parks Road, Oxford OX1, 3QT, UK

H. Snippe, Laboratory for Microbiology, University of Utrecht, Catharijnesingel 59, NL-3511 GG Utrecht, The Netherlands

C. Stringer, Division of Immunology, Medical Institute of Environmental Hygiene, University of Düsseldorf, Auf'm Hennekamp 50, D-4000 Düsseldorf 1, FRG

N. Talal, Clinical Immunology Section, Audie L. Murphy Memorial Veterans Hospital, The University of Texas Health Science Center at San Antonio, 7730 Floyd Curl Drive, San Antonio, TX 78284, USA

H.-W. Vohr, Division of Immunology, Medical Institute of Environmental Hygiene, University of Düsseldorf, Auf'm Hennekamp 50, D-4000 Düsseldorf 1, FRG

J.G. Vos, National Institute of Public Health and Environmental Protection, Antonie van Leeuwenhoeklaan 9, NL-3720 BA Bilthoven, The Netherlands

W.W. Weber, Department of Pharmacology, University of Michigan, Ann Arbor, MI 48109, USA

B.J.M. Zegers, Department of Immunology, University Hospital for Children and Youth 'Het Wilhelmina Kinderziekenhuis', P.O. Box 18009, NL-3501 CA Utrecht, The Netherlands

G.J.W.J. Zigterman, Intervet International B.V., P.O. Box 31, NL-5830 AA Boxmeer, The Netherlands

Foreword

The main task of the immune system is to recognize and destroy foreign antigens (e.g. infectious agents and foreign material). To perform this task, the immune system must distinguish self from non-self. This capacity to distinguish between self and non-self is a unique feature of the immune system, and its regulation is crucial for the maintenance of health. In healthy individuals, autoreactive lymphocytes can occur, but their appearance is limited by normal regulatory mechanisms. However, under certain conditions autoreactive lymphocytes may become activated and produce autoimmune diseases in which the immune system attacks healthy tissue. Such an autoimmune pathogenesis has been established for many organ-specific and systemic diseases. In several of these autoimmune disorders a causal relationship with drugs and chemicals has been established. The list of drugs or chemicals that can induce autoimmune diseases continues to grow. In general, agents were identified as causing autoimmune diseases on the basis of clinical investigations in man only after the introduction of the drug in the market, and not during routine safety assessment in laboratory animals. Interest of scientists, including the editors of this book, in environmental chemical-provoked autoimmune disorders was triggered by an epidemic that broke out in Spain in 1981 following the consumption of chemically altered rapeseed oil. Many individuals suffering from this so-called 'toxic oil syndrome' showed numerous characteristics of autoimmune disease.

The main theme of this book, edited by Drs. M.E. Kammüller, N. Bloksma and W. Seinen, concerns experimental approaches to identify at a preclinical phase the potential of drugs and chemicals to induce autoimmune diseases, and reviews the literature surrounding this area. The first two sections contain an introduction to drug- or chemical-induced autoimmunity and its toxicological significances and chapters on the basic mechanisms of immunity, and theories on the induction of autoimmune diseases. In the next section, comprehensive reviews are given of different drugs that have been shown to induce autoimmune reactions in man. The fourth section discusses chemical characteristics and immunological properties of such drugs which provoke autoimmunity. The final section describes various experimental approaches and animal models for the detection of chemicals that induce autoimmunity. The concluding chapter, authored by the editors, provides a critical assessment of the limitations of routine toxicity tests, and a discussion of possible improvements as well as new experimental strategies which might assist in routine safety assessment. In this regard, a promising model is the popliteal lymph node assay, in which lymph node enlargement is measured following the local injection of a chemical or drug candidate. This assay appears to correlate fairly well with the potential of drugs and chemicals to induce autoimmune-like diseases in man. The future success of this area of investigative immunotoxicity depends on refinement and validation of predictive assays in experimental animals and rigorous clinical investigation when drug- or chemical-induced autoimmunity is suspected in man.

The editors as well as the authors of the individual chapters are to be complimented. This book represents a milestone volume on chemical-induced autoimmunity and should be of interest to toxicologists, immunologists, cell biologists, and clinicians who deal with drug- or chemical-induced autoimmunity. It is also highly recommended to scientists involved in the safety assessment of drugs and chemicals.

J.G. Vos
Director of Immunology
National Institute of Public Health and Environmental Protection
Bilthoven, The Netherlands

J.H. Dean
Director, Toxicology
Sterling-Winthrop Research
Rensselaer, NY, USA

Preface

Immunotoxicology is a relatively young branch of research which enjoys increasing interest from both disciplines, immunology and toxicology. From a historical perspective, important triggers for immunotoxicological research in immunology have been provided by the untoward immunosuppressive side effect of chemotherapy in cancer patients and by the toxicity of therapeutic application of immunosuppressive and immunostimulating agents. In toxicology, the majority of research has been directed to the immunosuppressive action of environmental agents, and various animal models for its detection have been developed. In experimental immunology and especially toxicology, however, hardly any attention has been focussed on autoimmune diseases as side effect of medication with or of exposure to low molecular weight compounds. This in spite of the large amount of literature documenting the potential of drugs and chemicals to induce or exacerbate autoimmune phenomenons, especially in man. The available data in combination with the fact that the compounds are chemically well-defined, in contrast to for instance the pathogens that have been associated with induction of autoimmune disease, provide a solid base for studying the etiopathology of autoimmune disorders by immunologists and toxicologists. However, attempts to develop animal models for the study of chemical-induced autoimmune disorders have been frustrating, and only recently several interesting and reproducible models have become available. Moreover, relevant data are widely dispersed throughout the literature, making access to the field difficult.

Therefore, the aim of this volume was to present the field in a cohesive manner by reviewing the subject from a basic immunological, clinical, chemical and toxicological perspective. It is primarily intended for toxicologists and immunologists in order to improve the understanding and accessibility of the area of chemical-induced autoimmune diseases. It was not intended to give a comprehensive listing and review of every single compound with the potential to induce or exacerbate autoimmune reactions. Only a selected number of compounds with such a potential has been reviewed, and attempts have been undertaken to dissect the conditions under which these compounds induce autoimmune disorders.

The editors would like to emphasize the invaluable contributions of all authors, enabling the realization of a multifaceted overview of the rather new and fascinating immunotoxicological research field: drug- and chemical-induced autoimmunity. It is expected to find its way to many scientists in this multidisciplinary field and to further stimulate research on the mechanisms leading to autoimmune disorders and on the structural requirements that endow chemicals with the ability to induce or exacerbate immune disregulation.

Utrecht

Michael Kammüller
Nanne Bloksma
Willem Seinen

List of abbreviations

ABTS	2,2′-azino-di-(3-ethylbenzthiazoline-6-sulfonic acid)
AchR	acetylcholine receptor
AD	autoimmune disease
ADA	adenosine deaminase
ADCC	antibody-dependent cell-mediated cytotoxicity
AF	2-aminofluorene
AMP	adenosine monophosphate
ANA	antinuclear antibodies
anti-nDNA	anti-native (double-stranded) DNA antibodies
anti-Sm	anti-Sm antibodies
APC	antigen-presenting cell
A-PE	3-(p-azobenzenearsonate)-N-acetyl derivative coupled to phosphatidylethanolamine
ATP	adenosine triphosphate
BGG	bovine gamma-globulin
BN (rat)	Brown-Norway (rat)
BP	basic protein
BSA	bovine serum albumin
cAMP	cyclic AMP
CD	cluster of differentiation. CD numbers refer to groups of antibodies that react with epitopes of the same human leukocyte differentiation antigens
C-gene segment	gene segment encoding the constant region of immunoglobulin L and H chains
CMV	cytomegalovirus
ConA	concanavalin A
CR	receptor for complement components
CTL	cytotoxic T lymphocyte
(d) Ado	(deoxy) adenosine
(d)ADP	(deoxy)adenosine di-phosphate
(d)AMP	(deoxy)adenosine mono-phosphate
DAT	direct antiglobulin test
(d)ATP	(deoxy)adenosine tri-phosphate
(d)CDP	(deoxy)cytidine di-phosphate
dCF	deoxycoformycin

(d)CTP	(deoxy)cytidine tri-phosphate
dCyd	deoxycytidine
DDA	dimethyldioctadecylammonium bromide
dDNA	denatured (single-stranded) DNA
D-gene segment	gene segment encoding the diversity region of immunoglobulin H chains
(d)GDP	(deoxy)guanosine di-phosphate
(d)GMP	(deoxy)guanosine mono-phosphate
(d)GTP	(deoxy)guanosine tri-phosphate
dGuo	deoxyguanosine
DHEA	dihydroepiandrosterone
DNP	dinitrophenol
DNP-BSA	dinitrophenol coupled to BSA
D-pen	D-penicillamine
DPH	phenytoin, diphenylhydantoin, dilantin
dsDNA	double-stranded (native) DNA
DTH	delayed-type hypersensitivity
EAE	experimental allergic encephalitis
EBV	Epstein-Barr virus
ELISA	enzyme-linked immunosorbent assay
ER	estrogen receptor
Fc	C-terminal region formed by the two H chains of an immunoglobulin
FDC	follicular dendritic cells
GBM	glomerular basement cell membrane
gld	(generalized lymphoproliferative disease) accelerator gene in mice
GM-CSF	granulocyte/macrophage colony stimulating factor
GST	glutathione-S-transferase
Guo	guanosine
GVH	graft versus host
H-2	histocompatibility-2 complex (the MHC of mice)
HAL	halothane
H chain	heavy polypeptide chain of immunoglobulins
HEV	high endothelial venules
HGG	human gamma globulin
HGPRT	hypoxanthine guanine phosphoribosyl transferase
HH	hydralazine hydrazone
HLA	human leukocyte antigen (the MHC of man)
HLB	hydrophilic-lipophilic balance
HPZ	4-hydrazinophthalazine-1-one
HSA	human serum albumin

HS-BSA	hexasaccharide fragment of the capsular polysaccharide of *Streptococcus pneumoniae* type 3 coupled to BSA
5-HT	serotonin
HTLV	human T cell leukemia virus
HZ	hydrazine
Ia	I region associated antigen(s), the MHC class II molecules of the mouse
ICAM	intercellular adhesion molecule
IDDM	insulin-dependent diabetes mellitus
IFN-γ	interferon-γ
Ig	immunoglobulin
IL	interleukin(s)
IL-1	interleukin 1
IL-2	interleukin 2
IL-2R	receptor for IL-2
IMDS	immune-mediated disease syndrome
IMP	inosine monophosphate
INH	isoniazid
J	dinitrophenyl-alanyl-alanyl-glycine
J-BSA	dinitrophenyl-alanyl-alanyl-glycine (J) coupled to BSA
J-gene segment	gene segment encoding the joining region of immunoglobulin L and H chains
J-PE	J coupled to phosphatidylethanolamine
kbp	kilobase pairs
L chain	light polypeptide chain of immunoglobulins
LE	lupus erythematosus
LEW	Lewis (rats)
LFA	leukocyte function associated antigen(s)
LMW	low molecular weight
lpr	(lymphoproliferation) accelerator gene in mice
LPS	lipopolysaccharide
LTT	lymphocyte transformation test
MAH	(mono)acetylhydrazine
MALT	mucosa-associated lymphoid tissue
MHC	major histocompatibility complex
MHCI	major histocompatibility complex class I
MHCII	major histocompatibility complex class II
MMI	methimazole
MTP	methyltriazolophthalazine
NAcHPZ	*N*-acetylhydrazinophthalazinone
NAPA	*N*-acetylprocainamide
NAT	*N*-acetyltransferase

NBP	non-ionic block polymer
$8NH_2Guo$	$8NH_2$-guanosine
NK	natural killer
NOD	non-obese diabetic
N-OH-AF	*N*-hydroxy-2-aminofluorene
Norzim-BGG	norzimeldine succinic acid amide BGG
5'-NT	5'-nucleotidase
OAT	*O*-acetyltransferase
ODC	ornithine decarboxylase
OH.MTP	3-hydroxymethyltriazolophthalazine
OS	obese strain
PA	procainamide
PAB	*p*-aminobenzoic acid
PAGE	polyacrylamide gel electrophoresis
PAHA	procainamide-hydroxylamine (4-hydroxylamino-*N*-(diethyl-aminoethyl) benzamide
PALS	periarteriolar lymphocyte sheath
PCA	passive cutaneous anaphylaxis
PH	phthalazine
PHA	phytohemagglutinin
PHZ	phenelzine
PLN (A)	popliteal lymph node (assay)
PNP	purine nucleoside phosphorylase
PO-BGG	penicilloylated bovine gammaglobulin
POE	polyoxyethylene
POP	polyoxypropylene
PPD	purified protein derivative
PRPP	phosphoribosyl pyrophosphate
PBS	phosphate-buffered saline
PTU	propylthiouracil
PU	propyluracil
PZ	phthalazinone
R-5-P	ribose-5-phosphate
RA	rheumatoid arthritis
RBC	red blood cells
RCM	radiographic contrast media
RF	rheumatoid factor
rr	homozygous slow acetylator
Rr	heterozygous acetylator
RR	homozygous rapid acetylator
RSA	rabbit serum albumin
RT1	MHC of the rat

RTE	rabbit thymus extract
SAC	protein of staphylococcus
SCID	severe combined immunodeficiency disease
SLE	systemic lupus erythematosus
SLP	sulfolipopolysaccharide
Sm antigen	Smith antigen
SMZ	sulfamethazine
SPD	semi-purified diet
SRBC	sheep red blood cell
ssDNA	single-stranded (denatured) DNA
STZ	streptozotocin
T4	thyroxine
T_h	T helper
T_k	T killer
T_s	T suppressor
TCR	T cell receptor
TFA	trifluoroacetyl
TLA	gene complex encoding class I molecules in mice and rats, named after one of the molecules, the thymus-leukemia antigen
TMAg	thyroid microsomal/microvillar antigen
TNBSA	trinitrobenzene sulfonic acid
TNF-α	tumor necrosis factor
TNF-β	lymphotoxin
TNP	trinitrophenol
TOS	Spanish toxic oil syndrome
TP	triazolophthalazine
V-gene segment	gene segment encoding the variable N-terminal polymorphic region of immunoglobulin L and H chains
V region	variable region of the N-terminal portion of L and H chains or complete antibodies
xid	X chromosome linked recessive immune deficiency gene

SECTION I

Introduction

M.E. Kammüller, N. Bloksma and W. Seinen (Eds.)
Autoimmunity and Toxicology
© 1989 Elsevier Science Publishers B.V. (Biomedical Division)

Autoimmunity and toxicology. Immune disregulation induced by drugs and chemicals

1

M.E. KAMMÜLLER*, N. BLOKSMA and W. SEINEN

Department of Basic Veterinary Sciences, Section of Immunotoxicology, Faculty of Veterinary Sciences, University of Utrecht, Yalelaan 2, NL-3508 TD Utrecht, The Netherlands

* Present address: Drug Safety Assessment-Toxicology, Sandoz Ltd., CH-4002 Basle, Switzerland

I. Scope

The purpose of this introduction is to give a bird's-eye view of some characteristics of idiopathic systemic autoimmune diseases (AD), notably systemic lupus erythematosus (SLE), and drug- and chemical-induced forms of this complex systemic disorder as they are observed in humans. Since there are several excellent recent reviews covering the clinical characteristics and possible pathogenic mechanisms of these disorders (reviewed in [1 – 4], see Chapter 3 by Allison), this chapter will attempt to emphasize some toxicological aspects of the subject. In order to enable dissection of host and environmental factors possibly involved in the etiology and pathogenesis of AD, different areas of research in immunology and toxicology are speculatively pulled together.

Research and discussion concerning the etiology and mechanisms of drug-induced AD have centered around a number of questions, which are still relevant: (1) Is SLE a single clinical entity or are there fundamentally different mechanisms leading to the same clinical syndrome? Is drug-induced SLE identical to idiopathic SLE? (2) Do drugs actually induce SLE de novo or do they activate a pre-existing lupus diathesis? What is the relative contribution of drugs to the etiopathogenesis of SLE? What makes some individuals more susceptible to the development of drug-induced AD than others? (3) Which particular chemical or pharmacological characteristics endow some low molecular weight (LMW) compounds (mol.wt. < 10 000) with the potential to provoke SLE? (4) Are there environmental or dietary chemicals contributing to the development and/or persistence of genetically determined AD? (5) Can drug-induced SLE be reproduced in animals? The following discussion attempts to address some of these questions.

II. Autoimmunity and autoimmune diseases

Until recently, autoimmunity, defined as immunity to self-components, has been considered abnormal. The current concept in immunology is that autoantibody-producing B lymphocytes and autoreactive T lymphocytes contribute to the complex mechanisms needed to maintain immunological homeostasis [5 – 7]. In this respect AD may be defined as diseases in which abnormal autoimmune responses are a primary cause or a secondary contributor. According to this definition organ-specific and systemic diseases with an enormous diversity of clinical and pathological manifestations are considered to be AD [7, 8]. A number of experimental animal models support the autoimmune pathogenesis of various diseases observed in man [3, 4, 9, 10]. Because clinical assessment of an AD is not easily achieved, unambiguous evidence for an autoimmune pathogenesis in several disorders is still lacking. However, the list of disorders with a proposed autoimmune pathogenesis is still growing. As pointed out by Nossal [8], one should not be too eager to promote every obscure chronic disease as an autoimmune condition, without direct or circumstantial evidence. 'In the future as in the past, each disease will have to be studied as an entity in its own right, with the autoimmune component seen as only one in a web of causative factors' [8].

The present discussion will be limited to systemic forms of AD. Syndromes considered to have an autoimmune pathogenesis include SLE, rheumatoid arthritis, scleroderma, Sjögren's syndrome, dermatomyositis and polymyositis, mixed connective tissue disease, glomerulonephritis, and certain forms of vasculitis, hepatitis, neuropathies and blood dyscrasias [7]. SLE is one of the best studied AD both clinically [2] and experimentally [3, 4]. Appearance, course and severity of the syndrome are highly variable, and overlap with other AD is not unusual [11]. Currently, any dogmatic categorization is not yet possible [11]. However, differential diagnosis and discrimination of subsets is aided by a still increasing list of serological parameters, particularly concerning the specificity of the autoantibodies [7, 12].

1. ANTIBODY- AND CELL-MEDIATED AUTOREACTIVITY

Autoantibodies found in the above-mentioned AD are principally directed towards integral components of all cell types, i.e. nucleus, nucleolus, cytoplasmic organelles and membrane components [12, 13], and hence are not tissue-specific. Common epitopes of the autoantibodies are found on native DNA (double-stranded; dsDNA) and denatured DNA (single-stranded; ssDNA), RNA, histone and non-histone proteins, as well as on phospholipids in cell membranes [14]. Presence and frequency of the autoantibodies appear to vary among different AD, and it is becoming established that each AD is associated with a characteristic pattern of autoantibodies ('diagnostic fingerprints') [12]. It, therefore, has been suggested that the autoantibody responses are antigen-driven or antigen-directed [12], rather than a random event or an epiphenomenon, although this is still subject for debate. Another point of discussion relates to the pathogenic significance of the autoantibodies in various AD. In SLE, it is generally agreed that certain autoantibodies are implicated in the pathogenesis [3, 7], and some investigators consider autoantibodies as primary cause of the immune complex-mediated disease. Others, however, emphasize that complement deficiencies and other defects leading to inadequate immune complex clearance would be the fundamental abnormality in SLE rather than abnormal and/or enhanced autoantibody formation [15].

The primary pathogenic significance of autoantibodies in other disorders, like scleroderma, is even less clear-cut. A relation between commonly determined autoantibodies and duration and clinical severity of the disease in man could not be found [7, 16], but recently a close association with autoantibodies directed to particular nucleolar antigens such as to Scl-70, a 70 kilodalton degradation product of native DNA topoisomerase I, centromere/kinetochore, and RNA polymerase I has been reported [12]. Because dermal cellular infiltrates correlated better with disease activity than autoantibody levels, it has also been suggested that scleroderma is primarily the result of cell-mediated autoreactivity [16, 17].

2. AUTOIMMUNE AND ALLERGIC DISEASES

Systemic disorders like erythema exsudativum multiforme, Stevens-Johnson syndrome and toxic epidermal necrolysis (Lyell syndrome) have an uncertain pathogenesis. According to some authors these diseases may represent different grades of severity of the same illness [18 – 21]. An allergic origin has been assumed on the basis of firm associations between exposure to various drugs and development of the syndromes [18, 22, 23]. The implicated drugs, however, are also known to induce a variety of AD and AD-like phenomena in man (see Section III.2. of this chapter), suggesting that an autoimmune component could be involved in the pathogenesis of the abovementioned disorders. This possibility is supported by observations that graft-versus-host (GVH) disease can evolve into toxic epidermal necrolysis in man [24] and hamsters [25], and into AD such as SLE, scleroderma and lichen planus in man [26, 27] and mice [9, 10].

Kawasaki's disease (mucocutaneous lymph node syndrome) is characterized by cutaneous, vascular and lymphoid lesions, especially in children, and bears several similarities with 'allergic' disorders such as erythema multiforme [28] and 'autoimmune' disorders like periarteritis nodosa [28, 29]. Some data indicate that excessive

T helper cell activity may be involved in the pathogenesis of Kawasaki's disease, similar to that observed in early GVH disease [30 – 32]. Although autoantibodies commonly detected in GVH disease and AD have not been found [33], circulating complement-fixing antibodies directed to monokine-inducible endothelial cell antigens have been detected in sera from patients with acute Kawasaki's disease [34]. Interestingly, the anticonvulsant drug diphenylhydantoin may induce lymphoproliferative disorders resembling Kawasaki's disease [28, 35, 36].

Data indicate that the border between systemic AD and systemic allergic manifestations is apparently diffuse. Furthermore, observations that clinical signs such as fever and various types of, exanthemas, usually associated with allergic diseases, precede or accompany several systemic AD, underline the similarities. Before the current concepts of autoimmunity were put forward, (auto)allergic reactions or hypersensitivities were considered as primary cause of syndromes like SLE [37]. A major argument for this view was the observation that forms of vasculitis are a basic pathologic feature of several systemic 'allergic' diseases (see above) as well as SLE, rheumatoid arthritis and scleroderma [1, 2, 29]. In fact, it is conceivable that some drug-induced allergic and autoimmune disorders are based on similar primary immunologic reactions, but that the clinical outcome is defined by secondary host and environmental factors (see Section II.4. of this chapter).

3. EPIDEMIOLOGY

Epidemiological data on AD are not easily obtained, because appropriate and unequivocal diagnostic criteria for the complex systemic diseases are frequently absent. Available figures, therefore, may be biased, but generally AD are relatively rare chronic disorders [11, 38, 39]. Prevalence and incidence rates of SLE and rheumatoid arthritis are given in Table 1. The average annual incidence rates of scleroderma, polymyositis and mixed connective tissue disease were found to be less than for SLE [40 – 42]. Most AD including SLE occur much more often in women than in man [11]. The age distribution differs between the various AD. Incidence rates of scleroderma and rheumatoid arthritis increase with age, whereas SLE ap-

TABLE 1

Epidemiological data of SLE and rheumatoid arthritis

Disease	Prevalence[a]	Incidence[b]	References
SLE	3 – 400	2 – 67	[11, 39]
Rheumatoid arthritis	400 – 1 400	28 – 97	[38]

[a] Cases/100 000 (proportion of cases found in a defined population at a given point or period of time).
[b] Cases/year/100 000 (rate of occurrence of new cases per year in a defined population).

pears to have its highest incidence in females at childbearing age [11, 38 – 42]. Reports documenting increases in incidence and prevalence among certain racial, religious, or geographic groupings are conflicting [11, 38, 39].

4. ETIOLOGIC AND PATHOGENIC FACTORS

The chance to develop AD appears to be highly influenced by individual as well as environmental factors [3, 4, 7, 43]. Implicated individual factors comprise the (patho)physiologic state and/or the genetic make-up of immune, metabolic and (neuro)endocrine systems. Environmental factors that have been related to the etiology of AD, notably SLE, are infectious agents, drugs, chemicals, some food constituents, radiation, and physical and emotional trauma [3, 7, 43, 44]. In general, more than one factor is considered to contribute to development of disease. For instance, SLE has been proposed to result from an interplay between genetic predisposition, sometimes referred to as 'lupus diathesis', and environmental influences [45, 46]. In individuals with a strong genetic predisposition, only minor environmental influences would suffice to cause development of full-blown SLE. On the other hand, powerful and often prolonged environmental triggers would be required to cause overt disease in genetically resistant individuals, if any at all. In such individuals without clinically manifest disease, however, circulating antinuclear and lymphocytotoxic antibodies may be detected, showing that besides induction of autoantibodies other individual and/or environmental factors define progression to, and, probably, severity of AD. Elegant experimental evidence showing the firm interaction between genetic factors and environmental agents in the development of murine AD has been provided by Hang et al. [47] using normal C57BL/6 and SLE-prone MRL/n mice. Transfer of the lpr (= lymphoproliferation) mutation, a single autosomal recessive gene, to SLE-prone MRL/n mice resulted in considerably faster progression of the disease and animals died much earlier of glomerulonephritis [47]. Similarly, chronic immunostimulation of MRL/n mice by the polyclonal B cell activator and adjuvant lipid-A accelerated the manifestations of autoimmunity and glomerulonephritis [47]. In normal C57BL/6 mice, either the lpr gene or endotoxin alone, caused autoantibody production with delayed minimal immunopathologic lesions, but simultaneous action of both immunostimulators caused early-onset, fatal glomerulonephritis [47]. Whether different combinations of factors may be active in different individuals, thus explaining the existence of subsets of SLE in humans [46], needs to be demonstrated. In murine lupus models, however, diverging manifestations reflecting different basic mechanisms have actually been demonstrated ([3, 4]; see Section IV.1. of this chapter).

Various defined host and environmental factors are known to be occasionally implicated in the etiology of AD in man or animals and will be briefly addressed.

The capacity of sex hormones to influence immune system function and development of AD has been firmly established (see Chapter 17 by Ansar Ahmed and

Talal). In general, estrogens were found to stimulate immunity and exacerbate AD in SLE-prone mice, while testosterones were found to have the opposite effect. The diverging actions of the sex hormones, therefore, are considered to largely explain the observed predominance of AD in female organisms. Besides an association between sex-related hormone production and SLE in man, abnormal oxidative metabolism of sex hormones has been observed in human SLE patients [48]. An impaired oxidative metabolism occurs relatively frequently in SLE patients, as examined with the antihypertensive drug debrisoquine, a commonly used probe to analyze patterns of xenobiotic oxidation [49] and may be involved in the pathogenesis of SLE (see Section III.3. of this chapter).

Deficiencies of the early complement components (C1q, C1r/s, C4, C2), leading to decreased solubilisation and removal of immune complexes, have been closely associated with SLE [15]. Individuals with homozygous complement deficiencies are rare, but are at high risk to develop SLE. Partial, heterozygous complement deficiencies are much more common and are well known for C4. The relative C4 deficiency, making the handling of antigen-antibody complexes inefficient, but not impossible, might be further enhanced by drugs such as hydralazine, procainamide and D-penicillamine, which have been shown to inactivate C4 in vitro (see Chapter 10 by Sim). It has been proposed that this mechanism may be involved in the induction of SLE by these drugs.

Ample data have shown that genes of the major histocompatibility complex (MHC) play a crucial role in immunoregulation, and interestingly several associations between the genetic make-up of MHC molecules and AD are known [43]. There is an increasing body of evidence suggesting that upregulation of MHC class II expression in organ-specific tissue is related to the induction of autoimmune reactions (see Chapter 3 by Allison; [50]). Some LMW compounds may enhance MHC expression by their ability to stimulate interferon production [51, 52]. Several drug- and chemical-induced AD also have been associated with particular MHC haplotypes [43]. HLA-DR4 and slow acetylation were found to be significantly associated with the tendency in females to develop hydralazine-induced SLE [53]. Further, HLA-DR3 was shown to be associated with D-penicillamine-induced renal, hematologic and cutaneous adverse reactions [54]. In patients with vinyl chloride induced scleroderma, severe symptoms were associated with the HLA-B8,DR3,DR5 haplotype, whereas DR5$^+$ individuals lacking the HLA-B8,DR3 haplotype only showed mild symptomatology [55]. Although associations are strong in some conditions, specific immunogenetic determinants are most likely not a direct cause of AD, but contribute to the predisposition of an individual to develop AD.

IgA fulfills a central function in the mucosal immune system. It is estimated that about 1 in 700 people in the general population has a selective IgA deficiency [56, 57]. Selective IgA-deficiency has been associated with AD such as SLE [58]. Further, increased frequencies of the HLA-A1,B8,DR3 haplotype, which is often associated with AD, have been found in IgA-deficient individuals [57]. Moreover,

drugs with a documented potential to induce AD, such as diphenylhydantoin and
D-penicillamine, have been shown to reduce secretory and/or serum IgA [59 – 61].
The mechanisms by which IgA deficiencies may contribute to the development of
AD are uncertain.

It should be noted that drugs with the potential to induce AD are given to patients
with a particular disease, implicating that the condition which is being treated may
predispose to the development of or is part of an AD. For instance grand mal and
petit mal epileptic seizures may be an initial symptom of SLE in some patients,
which may precede other features of the syndrome by years (see Chapter 5 by
Alarcón-Segovia and Alarcón-Riquelme; [2]). Therefore, antiepileptic drugs given
to treat the convulsions, may be mistakingly considered causative agents of the AD.
On the other hand, the relatively high frequency of epileptic seizures among the
general population [62] suggests that other host and environmental factors are likely
to be more important in provoking SLE. Another example of a possibly biased implication of drugs in the etiology of AD may be the relatively high incidence of immunological side effects observed during anti-infectious therapy with penicillins,

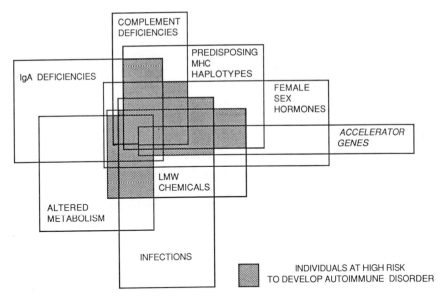

Fig. 1. Speculative representation of individual and environmental factors contributing to the development of AD. The listing of factors indicated is not exhaustive, but refers to those known to be occasionally implicated in the etiology of AD in humans and/or animals (for details see text). Each rectangle (arbitrary size) represents the population with a particular characteristic, which may be in itself not sufficient to produce AD. Although combinations of individual and environmental factors may increase the
risk of development and the progression of AD, it should be noted that not all factors indicated in Fig.
1 have to be present simultaneously in the same individual. The shaded area represents those individuals
at high risk to develop AD. (Modified after an idea of Dr. E. Sim, Chapter 10.)

sulfonamides and nitrofurantoin. A relation between the simultaneous presence of a particular drug and immune-modulating infectious organisms is likely, but not proven. Viruses have frequently been implicated in the etiology of human and murine SLE, but a clear causal relationship remains to be established [4, 7]. Data pointing at such a relationship come from observations with regard to development and clinical course of GVH reactions in humans, which are thought to be codetermined by infections [63].

The above listing of host and environmental factors possibly involved in the etiology and pathogenesis of AD, although most certainly not complete, clearly depicts the multifactorial nature of AD. This, at least partly, may explain the relatively low incidence of AD, as well as their complexity and variable severity among individuals with the same disease. The multiplicity of factors involved may also explain the unpredictability of drug- and chemical-induced AD in humans, and the difficulty to reproduce these syndromes in experimental animals (see Section IV.3. of this chapter). The chance to develop (chemical-induced) AD seems to be increased by certain combinations of individual factors either or not in interaction with one or more environmental factors. This is speculatively illustrated in Fig. 1.

III. Drug- and chemical-induced autoimmune diseases in humans

1. DRUG-INDUCED AND IDIOPATHIC SLE

Drug-induced lupus differs from idiopathic SLE in that it usually remits when drug therapy is discontinued. In most cases drug-induced SLE presents as a milder disease. Clinically manifest renal involvement, often a serious and sometimes fatal feature of progressive idiopathic SLE [2], is rarely observed in drug-induced SLE, although relatively frequent in the case of hydralazine and D-penicillamine [54, 64]. The milder course of drug-induced AD may be partially due to withdrawal of the drug upon diagnosis of AD, which may be far in advance to renal involvement.

Drug-induced and idiopathic lupus could also be distinguished as to the specificity of autoantibodies. Autoantibodies in idiopathic lupus appeared to be primarily directed against dsDNA, RNA, histone and other cellular autoantigens, while in drug-induced SLE autoantibody specificities seemed to be limited to ssDNA and particular histone proteins ([12]; see Chapter 4 by Rubin). In some cases, the autoantibodies may persist for months or years after withdrawal of the provoking drug. In idiopathic and vinyl chloride induced scleroderma, a remarkable similarity in clinical symptoms and in immunogenetic markers has been observed. However, in the chemically induced syndrome autoantibodies typical of idiopathic scleroderma appeared absent [55]. Currently, the reason for these similarities and differences is unclear.

The phenomenon of drug- and chemical-induced AD has frequently been reviewed since the first sulfadiazine-induced case of SLE was recognized by Hoffman in 1945 [64 – 74]. At first, the reports were sporadic, but gradually specific (groups of) drugs with the potential to induce SLE emerged (Fig. 2) [64, 74]. The potential to induce AD may reflect a particular chemical characteristic of the drugs, but may also be biased by the frequency of application. SLE is the most frequently observed drug-induced AD. Approximately 1 – 12% of all diagnosed cases of SLE have been attributed to drugs [42, 64, 74, 75].

As mentioned before, acute symptoms such as fever and exanthemas do not discern drug-induced allergic and autoimmune disorders, but detection of drug-specific antibodies may be of diagnostic value [76]. Whereas in drug-induced allergic diseases drug-specific antibodies, such as in allergic reactions to penicilline derivatives [66, 76], are frequently found, these are usually not detectable in drug-induced AD.

2. CLASSES OF DRUGS AND CHEMICALS

Drugs and chemicals known to incidentally induce or exacerbate AD-like side effects in susceptible individuals are LMW compounds (mol.wt. 100 – 500), which are generally considered to be not immunogenic themselves. Usually molecules having a mol.wt. above 10 000 have immunogenic potential. The LMW drugs belong to different chemical classes (Fig. 2) and include among others derivatives of aromatic amines (procainamide, practolol); hydrazines (hydralazine) (see Chapter 4 by Rubin, and Chapter 9 by Hein and Weber); hydantoins (phenytoin, mephenytoin, ethotoin, nitrofurantoin) (see Chapter 5 by Alarcón-Segovia and Alarcón-Riquelme); thioureylenes (methimazole, propylthiouracil) (see Chapter 12 by Aucoin); oxazolidinediones (trimethadione, paramethadione); succinimides (ethosuximide, methsuximide, phensuximide); dibenzazepines (carbamazepine); phenothiazines (chlorpromazine); sulfonamides (sulfasalazine, sulfadiazine); pyrazolones (phenylbutazone); amino acids (D-penicillamine (see Chapter 6 by Emery and Panayi), captopril, methyldopa); allyl amines such as zimeldine (see Chapter 7 by Kristofferson and Nilsson), furthermore halothane (see Chapter 8 by Neuberger); mercuric chloride (see Chapter 14 by Druet et al.); and gold preparations [64, 74]. From a pharmacological perspective, the majority of AD-inducing drugs can be ranked among anti-infectious agents, β-adrenergic receptor blocking compounds, and drugs acting at the central nervous system. With some exceptions compounds are heterocyclic and/or contain at least one aromatic group (Fig. 2).

Occupational exposure to chemicals may incidentally lead to AD-like syndromes. A SLE-like syndrome has been described after exposure to hydrazine [77]. Occupational exposure to monomeric vinyl chloride [55, 78, 79], trichloroethylene [80, 81], perchloroethylene [82], and epoxy resins [83] may induce scleroderma-like syndromes. Trichloroethylene has also been associated with Stevens-Johnson syndrome and jaundice [84]. Exposure to toluene di-isocyanate has been associated with the

12

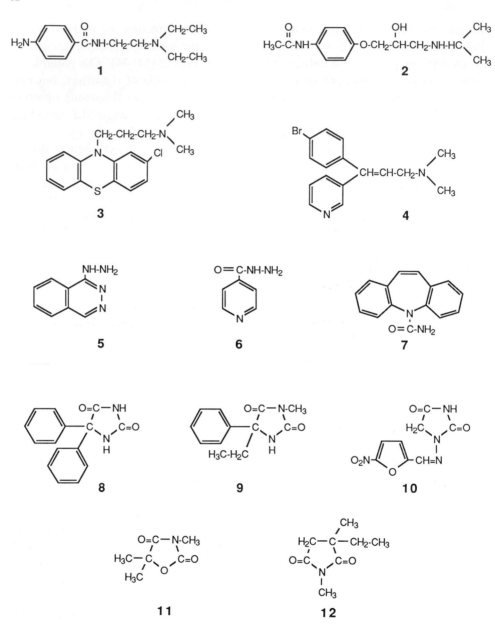

Fig. 2. Structures of several drugs and chemicals with documented potential to induce or exacerbate autoimmune-like disorders in humans, notably SLE [64, 66, 74]. Zimeldine has been reported to induce a Guillain-Barré-like neuropathy, halothane to induce hepatitis, vinyl chloride and trichloroethylene to induce scleroderma-like syndromes. 1, Procainamide (cardiac depressant); 2, practolol (β-adrenergic receptor blocker); 3, chlorpromazine (antipsychotic); 4, zimeldine (antidepressant); 5, hydralazine (antihypertensive); 6, isoniazid (antibacterial); 7, carbamazepine (anticonvulsant); 8, diphenylhydantoin (anticonvulsant); 9, mephenytoin (anticonvulsant); 10, nitrofurantoin (antibacterial); 11, trimethadione

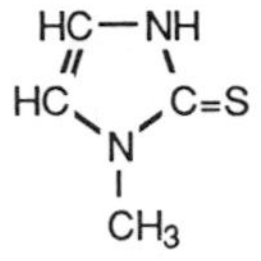

13

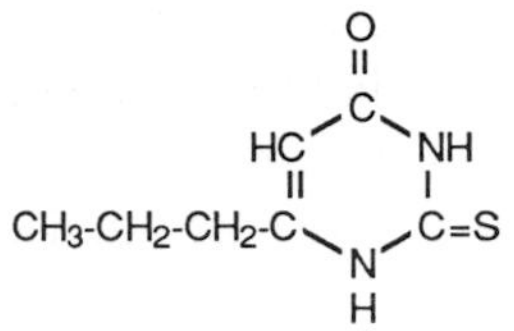

14

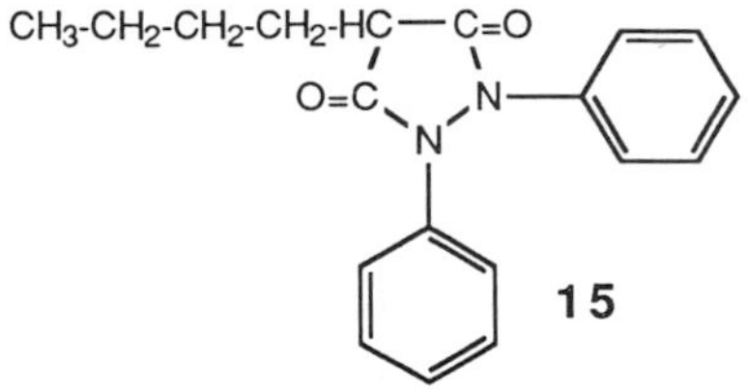

15

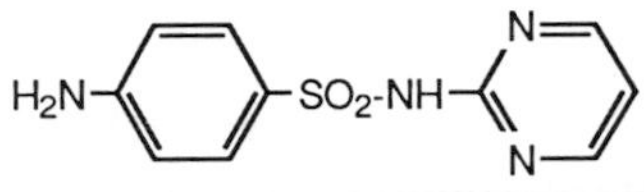

16

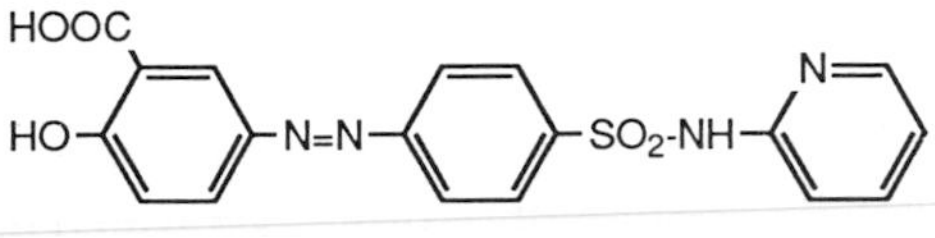

17

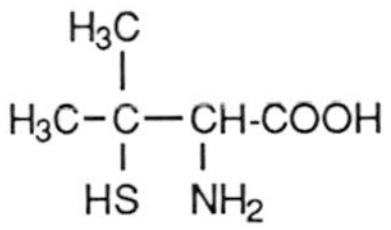

18

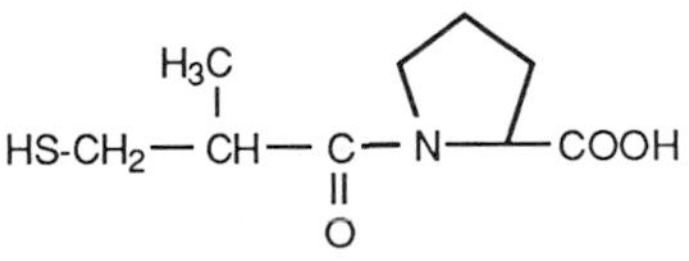

19

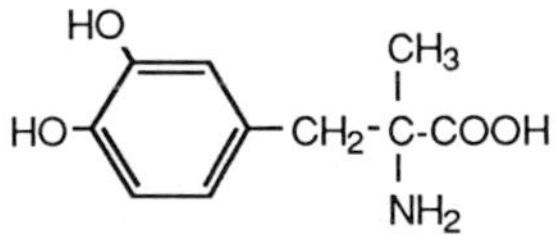

20

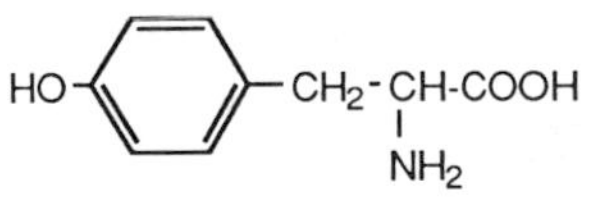

21

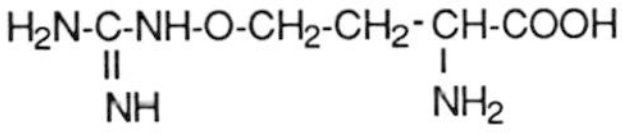

22

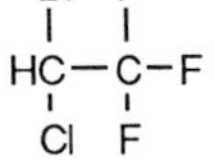

23

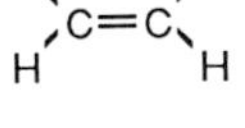

24

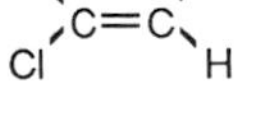

25

(anticonvulsant); 12, ethosuximide (anticonvulsant); 13, methimazole (antithyroidal); 14, propylthiouracil (antithyroidal); 15, phenylbutazone (anti-inflammatory); 16, sulfadiazine (antibacterial);
17, sulfasalazine (antibacterial); 18, D-penicillamine (chelating agent); 19, captopril (antihypertensive);
20, methyldopa (antihypertensive); 21, L-tyrosine; 22, L-canavanine; 23, halothane (anesthetic); 24, vinyl
chloride; 25, trichloroethylene.

induction of thrombocytopenic purpura [85]. The development of lichen planus has been reported after occupational exposure to photographic developers [27].

Data on food as a source of LMW AD-inducing compounds are scarce, although effects of lipid composition and caloric intake have been studied rather extensively in this context [44, 86]. Complexity of food matrices as well as variability of consumption behaviour hampers assessment of LMW food constituents as possible contributors to the course and severity of certain AD. However, a naturally occurring non-protein amino acid, L-canavanine (Fig. 2), has been demonstrated to induce or exacerbate pancytopenia and SLE in humans and monkeys ([87, 88]; see Chapter 13 by Bardana et al.). Furthermore, low phenylalanine and tyrosine diet has been observed to ameliorate clinical signs and to improve laboratory parameters of patients suffering from SLE, rheumatoid arthritis, scleroderma and dermatomyositis [89]. Administration of tyrosine aggravated disease symptoms in patients with these AD [90]. Studies with regard to other LMW food constituents with a similar potential have, as far as we know, not been performed, but it is likely that such compounds are present in the diet, either naturally occurring or formed upon processing or digestion. For example, a large variety of heterocyclic compounds among which 1,3-dimethylhydantoin, 3-ethyl-1-methylhydantoin, and 3,5-dimethyl-2,4-oxazolidinedione have been identified in boiled or roasted meat [91]. Further, it has been proposed that thiourea and possibly 2-thiohydantoin derivatives may be formed in the human diet due to reactions of naturally occurring isothiocyanates with amino acids and proteins [92, 93]. In this context it is interesting to note that albutoin (3-allyl-5-isobutyl-2-thiohydantoin), which can be formed by a reaction between allyl isothiocyanate and leucine, has been reported to induce exanthema in a clinical trial [94]. Since the above-mentioned compounds are closely related to AD-inducing drugs (see Fig. 2) and could be ingested chronically, it may be worthwhile to investigate their potential to induce or exacerbate AD and thereby their ability to contribute to the chronicity of AD in predisposed individuals.

The importance of research on immune disregulating agents in food is stressed by the observation that food-born allergic and AD-like syndromes can occur on an epidemic scale. In 1960, of an estimated 600 000 consumers of a new margarine brand in The Netherlands, 50 000 people developed an erythema-multiforme-like syndrome [95]. The disease was attributed to a novel emulsifier used in the margarine, but due to lack of animal models no unequivocal evidence for its etiological significance could be presented [95].

In 1981, a dramatic epidemic with many allergic and autoimmune characteristics broke out in Spain [96, 97]. The acute phase affected approximately 20 000 people and was characterized by a non-necrotizing vasculitis presenting with different combinations of symptoms [98 – 105]. After about 3 months a small portion of the patients, particularly women, developed a severe, invalidating neuromuscular and scleroderma-like syndrome [98]. The manifestations and biphasic evolution of the syndrome showed resemblances to acute and chronic GVH disease [105 – 107].

Overall, the syndrome has caused over 350 deaths to date. Some 6 weeks after the outbreak of the disease a link to the consumption of denatured rapeseed oil was suggested [104], and later on supported by several epidemiological studies [102, 108, 109] and case reports [110]. Hence, the disease has become known as toxic oil syndrome (TOS). Analysis of supposedly toxic oil samples has shown that most of the oils contained mainly low erucic acid rapeseed oil, severely contaminated with reaction products of aniline, especially fatty acid anilides [96, 97]. Toxicological research with fatty acid anilides and case-associated oil samples has not been able to reproduce (part of) the spectrum of symptoms observed in TOS [96, 97, 111]. On the basis of structural resemblances to AD-inducing drugs, it has been hypothesized that (cyclic) phenylthiourea derivatives, that may have been formed in adulterated rapeseed oil, might represent the etiologic factors of TOS [106, 107, 112]. Due to analytical difficulties relating to oil samples, and the lack of suitable animal models, convincing evidence could not be presented so far [113]. Taken together, the nature of the causative agent of TOS is still elusive.

3. ASPECTS OF METABOLISM AND DISPOSITION IN RELATION TO DRUG-INDUCED AUTOIMMUNE DISEASES

As mentioned above, polymorphisms of metabolism of endogenous or xenobiotic compounds may be involved in the pathogenesis of SLE [49]. Slow acetylators on medication with procainamide or hydralazine (Fig. 2) were found to have an increased chance to develop SLE-like symptoms (see Chapter 4 by Rubin, and Chapter 9 by Hein and Weber). Furthermore, slow acetylation was also associated with the development of systemic immunologically mediated disease during treatment with a triple sulfonamide preparation [114]. Impaired sulfoxidation of D-penicillamine (Fig.2) appeared to increase the chance to develop adverse renal effects, thrombocytopenia and cutaneous lesions (see Chapter 6 by Emery and Panayi).

For other drugs, such as diphenylhydantoin (Fig. 2), it is still a matter of debate whether the immunomodulating potential has to be attributed to the unmetabolized agent, its metabolites or both [115, 116]. It has been suggested that the covalent binding of arene oxide metabolites of diphenylhydantoin to macromolecules may give rise to SLE-like syndromes and other immunotoxic effects [115]. Wilson et al. [117], however, proposed that the unmetabolized drug might be the immunotoxic agent, because children developing generalised exanthemas during diphenylhydantoin medication had significantly higher plasma concentrations of the drug and a lower plasma 5 (p-hydroxyphenyl)-5-phenylhydantoin to diphenylhydantoin ratio. High plasma levels of diphenylhydantoin have been attributed to an impaired metabolism [118, 119], and this is possibly genetically determined, since interethnic differences in the rate of diphenylhydantoin metabolism have been reported [120, 121]. For the hydantoin drug mephenytoin (Fig. 2) very striking interethnic differences have been found. Oxidative metabolism of the drug appeared defective in

2 – 5% Caucasians and up to 23% Japanese [122 – 124], but an association with the potential immunotoxic effects of mephenytoin [125] has not been sought. The drug mephobarbital, however, whose metabolism cosegregates with the mephenytoin metabolism, induced approximately a six-fold higher incidence of, unfortunately unspecified, adverse effects in Japanese than in white Australians (cited in [124]).

Polymorphisms of drug metabolism may not only result in a slower elimination of the parent hydantoin compound and/or its metabolites, but also in formation of particular metabolites [126, 127]. Notably, the extent of formation of 5-ethyl-5-phenylhydantoin (Nirvanol®) from mephenytoin was found to be determined by a stereoselective metabolism of the R- and S-enantiomers [126]. As Nirvanol®, used at the beginning of this century for the treatment of chorea, was shown to cause a high incidence of mild to severe immunological disorders in children and adults [128], this particular metabolite may be implicated in the immunotoxic effects of mephenytoin.

Another noteworthy point in this context may be modulation of metabolism by immunologically active agents. Recently, the effect of influenza vaccine on serum anticonvulsant concentrations was investigated, and diphenylhydantoin levels were found to be significantly elevated 7 days after vaccination and back to prevaccination levels on day 28. However, no adverse effects were observed [129]. The increased serum levels have been attributed to a temporal depression of P-450 monooxygenase activity induced by the vaccine, as is well known for other interferon-inducing agents [130].

Thus, measurement of individual variation in metabolic pathways offers a potential way for investigating individual variations in susceptibility of subjects who have equal exposure to drugs or environmental chemicals, but diverging responses [127, 131 – 133]. To which extent inherited metabolic polymorphisms relate to the low incidence of hydantoin derivative induced AD is not known, but certainly merits further investigations.

IV. Mechanisms and animal models of idiopathic and chemical-induced autoimmune reactions

1. MECHANISMS OF SLE

Various subsets of SLE have been recognized in man [46] and mice [4], and the diverging manifestations of SLE, are thought to reflect different basic mechanisms [4, 32]. On the basis of experimental findings in lupus-prone mice, Theofilopoulos et al. [32] proposed two main categories of murine SLE: type 1 denotes primary B cell abnormalities which result in excessive and poorly regulated B cell activation, proliferation and differentiation notably in NZB, (NZB × NZW)F_1 and BXSB mice (see Section IV.2. of this chapter), and type 2 comprises primary defects of T cells, which produce excessive T helper cell factors notably in MRL mice, in this way leading to increased B cell activation. The importance of hyperactive B cells producing a spectrum of autoantibodies in murine lupus is evident. A convincing argument for the importance of B cells in the pathogenesis of murine SLE is provided by the beneficial effects of the *xid* gene, an X-chromosome-linked recessive immune deficiency gene, when introduced into lupus strains. In several SLE-prone murine strains, as well as in AD induced by GVH reactions in mice [134], the *xid* gene prevented maturation of B lymphocytes, and animals did not develop clinically manifest AD [135, 136]. The *xid* gene did not influence the abnormal T cell proliferation in MRL/Mp-*lpr/lpr* and C3H-*gld/gld* (*gld* = generalized lymphoproliferative disease) mice, but reduced autoantibody levels [135, 136].

Similarly, many cases of human SLE are considered to result from abnormal B cell regulation [2, 7]. Some syndromes showing resemblances to AD, such as mucocutaneous lymph node syndrome (Kawasaki's disease), are believed to result primarily from excessive T helper cell activity [30 – 32]. AD induced by GVH reactions have been demonstrated to be T cell-triggered as well [9, 10, 30, 32].

Thus, immunologic abnormalities in SLE relate to intrinsic B cell defects and/or altered T cell activity. Endocrine and biochemical abnormalities can also be involved in immune disregulation leading to AD. These include primary immunodeficiencies ([56]; see Chapter 18 by Zegers et al.), complement deficiencies ([15]; see Chapter 10 by Sim), perturbed production of and responsiveness to cytokines ([137]; see Chapter 3 by Allison), abnormal hormone metabolism ([48]; see Chapter 17 by Ansar Ahmed and Talal), and altered oxidative metabolism ([49]; see Chapter 9 by Hein and Weber, and Chapter 4 by Rubin).

2. ANIMAL MODELS OF SPONTANEOUS SLE

Mechanistic diversity has of course important implications for the development and application of animal models for investigation of idiopathic and drug-induced forms of SLE. Currently, several murine models of SLE exist, which may shed some light on the various etiologic mechanisms leading to syndromes diagnosed as SLE [3, 4, 138, 139]. New Zealand Black (NZB) and F_1 hybrids produced by mating with New Zealand White (NZW) mice ((NZB × NZW)F_1) were the first described murine models of spontaneous SLE. More recently other murine strains, including MRL/Mp-*lpr/lpr*, C3H/He-*gld/gld*, BXSB, C57BL/6-*me/me* (*me* = motheaten) and others have become known to spontaneously develop SLE-like syndromes (reviewed in [3, 4, 139, 140]).

(a) NZB and (NZB × NZW)F₁ mice

The major autoimmune characteristic in NZB mice (H-2^d) is hemolytic anemia, with IgG anti-erythrocyte antibodies, and antinuclear and anti-ssDNA antibodies of the IgM class [3]. Glomerulonephritis is also observed. (NZB × NZW)F$_1$ mice (H-2$^{d/z}$) develop anti-dsDNA and anti-ssDNA IgG autoantibodies and eventually die of severe glomerulonephritis. Both strains develop Sjögren's syndrome and only mild lymphoproliferation, as judged by spleen and lymph node weight increase. Primary B cell abnormalities are considered to contribute to the pathogenesis of AD in these strains. NZB mice show little sex predilection with regard to AD, but in (NZB × NZW)F$_1$ mice females are much more prone to develop AD than males. The autoimmune phenomena in these strains were found to be controlled by at least six autosomal genes, which makes it very difficult to dissect the relative contribution of various genetic factors to the development of the disease.

(b) BXSB mice

Male BXSB mice (H-2^b) show moderate lymphoproliferation, anti-ssDNA and anti-dsDNA IgG antibodies as well as other autoantibodies and early fatal glomerulonephritis, characteristics which appear much later in females. Although autoimmune phenomena are under control of multiple autosomal genes, a single accelerator gene on the Y-chromosome promotes the development of AD in males [3, 4].

(c) MRL/Mp-lpr/lpr and C3H/He-gld/gld mice

The *lpr* and *gld* genes are distinct mutations with markedly similar manifestations [135, 138, 139, 141]. MRL/Mp-*lpr/lpr* (H-2^k) and C3H/He-*gld/gld* (H-2^k) mice show massive early lymphoproliferation and subsequently autoantibody formation. High levels of anti-ssDNA, anti-dsDNA and other autoantibodies are detected. The anti-Sm antibody, which is highly restricted to human SLE and rarely found in other human AD [12], has also been found in MRL/Mp mice but not in other murine lupus models [139]. Expansion of an abnormal T lymphocyte population accounts for the early lymphoproliferation in these mice. MRL/Mp-*lpr/lpr* mice also show arteritis, Sjögren's syndrome, polyarthritis and severe glomerulonephritis [138, 139, 142], whereas C3H/He-*gld/gld* mice are susceptible to development of interestitial pneumonitis without major perivascular lymphoid infiltrations [141]. Both female and male MRL/Mp-*lpr/lpr* and C3H/He-*gld/gld* mice show early-onset of symptoms, but females die at an earlier age [139, 141].

The cause of the abnormal T cell proliferation has been related to defective regulation of the phosphorylation of tyrosine residues in particular subunits of the T cell antigen receptor [143]. The phosphorylation is an important step in the activation of T cells and was found to occur in normal T lymphocytes only upon activation by antigens or mitogenic lectins, but in T cells carrying the *lpr* or *gld* gene also in the absence of exogenous stimuli [143]. Whether this relates to the beneficial effect of tyrosine restriction in murine [144] and human AD (see Section III.2. of this chapter) is not known.

(d) Contribution of accelerator genes to development of AD

Transfer of the *lpr* gene to other inbred strains of mice, including AKR, BALB/c, C3H/He, C57BL/6, C57BL/10, and SJL appeared to result in lymphoproliferation and formation of autoantibodies as well, but pathologic manifestations of SLE were delayed and much less evident than in the MRL/Mp-*lpr/lpr* strain [4, 47, 139, 145]. This suggests that the *lpr* gene is able to induce autoantibody formation in normal mice, but that the full development of SLE requires additional genetic factors provided by the MRL background. The influence of the *lpr* gene on B cell activation and autoantibody production was limited to females only in C57BL/6-*lpr/lpr* mice, suggesting a strong sex influence, which was not manifested as clearly in the MRL/Mp-*lpr/lpr* and some other *lpr* congenic mouse strains [146]. As has been mentioned in Section II.4. of this chapter also exogenous factors were capable to interact with the *lpr* gene to stimulate development of AD [47].

Currently, no clear answer can be given why non-autoimmune mice carrying the *lpr* gene, despite autoantibody production, fail to develop early-onset lethal glomerulonephritis [47, 145]. The different effects of the *lpr* gene in lupus-prone and normal mice has been attributed to the class, affinity and epitope specificity of the autoantibodies formed [4, 47, 145]. Particularly the switch from IgM to IgG autoantibody class is thought to coincide with onset of clinically manifest AD in lupus-prone mice [32, 47]. Further, the decreased immune complex clearance and earlier development of renal lesions in MRL-*lpr/lpr* mice compared to MRL/n and other *lpr* congenic strains, may relate to impaired mononuclear phagocyte system function as superimposing factor in this strain [147].

The possibility to transfer accelerator genes such as *lpr* or *gld* into strains of mice with different backgrounds, allows a better dissection of the relative contribution of the genetic background in interaction with environmental agents to the etiology of AD. It is likely that these models will also have an important spin-off for immunotoxicology, i.e. the development of highly defined animal models that can predict the potential of (groups of) compounds to induce AD. This may allow risk-assessment studies in this field.

(e) GVH reactions

Diverging AD are a well-recognized consequence of GVH disease in man [26, 148]. GVH reactions in mice have shown that a similar spectrum of symptoms can be induced, and that the kind of developing symptoms are primarily defined by MHC haplotype differences between donor and recipient and/or the phenotype of donor T cells transferred ([10]; see Chapter 15 by Gleichmann et al.). The development of SLE has been attributed to a chronic activation of donor T helper cells by the allogeneic MHC class II molecules of the F_1 recipient, leading to a chronic production of helper factors. These in turn would enable autoantigen-recognizing B cells to proliferate and to differentiate into autoantibody-secreting plasma cells. GVH reactions may, therefore, provide valuable models of induced AD [9, 10].

An analogous mechanism has been proposed to underly induction of SLE syndromes by the drugs diphenylhydantoin and D-penicillamine ([10]; see Chapter 15 by Gleichmann et al.). It has been suggested that autologous T cells may be activated by drug-modified membrane determinants on B cells or macrophages in association with autologous MHC class II molecules, and so, upon chronic administration, evoke similar events.

3. ANIMAL MODELS OF DRUG-INDUCED AUTOIMMUNE REACTIONS

In view of the unpredictable nature and potentially fatal outcome of some drug- and chemical-induced AD in humans, it is essential to develop methods for (a) identification of drugs and chemicals which have the potential to provoke AD by virtue of their chemical or pharmacological properties, and (b) to identify and define endogenous and exogenous factors which make individuals susceptible. Generally, however, attempts to reproduce systemic autoimmune diseases in experimental animals during exposure to LMW drugs known to have this potential in humans, have been unsuccessful or have yielded contradictory results for some compounds [3, 64].

(a) Mouse models

Procainamide and hydralazine. Procainamide and hydralazine have been administered orally to groups of 250 A/J (H-2^a), BALB/cJ (H-2^d) and C57BL/6J (H-2^b) mice of both sexes during 10 months [149]. Both drugs significantly increased the frequency of antinuclear antibodies as compared to age-matched controls that showed a spontaneous increase with age [149]. The most marked increases were found in female A/J and BALB/cJ mice after 8 months of treatment. Induction of antinuclear antibodies in female BALB/c mice after 6 months of treatment with hydralazine has also been reported in another study [150]. In the moderately responding C57BL/6J strain, male mice were better responders than females [149]. Of all strains tested A/J mice were the first to show significantly elevated chemical-induced antinuclear antibody levels and C57BL/6J mice the slowest [149]. Further studies with the same mice revealed that hydralazine induced smooth muscle antibodies in A/J mice, but not in C57BL/6 and BALB/c mice [151] and splenomegaly in BALB/cJ and A/J mice [152]. Splenomegaly in response to procainamide was only seen in BALB/cJ. Signs of immune complex glomerulonephritis were observed more often in drug-treated mice than in age-matched controls, especially A/J mice [152].

In contrast to the findings of Ten Veen and coworkers, however, Tannen and Weber [153] found that procainamide given at a similar dosage during more than 9 months suppressed spontaneous antinuclear antibody formation in C57BL/6J mice. As found in the above-mentioned experiments procainamide was able to induce antinuclear antibodies in A/J mice [153]. The authors also paid attention to the role of acetylation polymorphisms, because in humans slow acetylation of procainamide was found to predispose to the development of antinuclear antibodies (reviewed in [133]). Backcross studies between phenotypically slow acetylator A/J and rapid acetylator C57BL/6J mice showed that slow acetylators in the F_2 generation, like A/J mice, had high spontaneous titers of antinuclear antibodies, but like C57BL/6 mice decreased antinuclear antibodies titers in response to procainamide [153]. The authors concluded that besides slow acetylation of procainamide, other predisposing factors define the ability of this drug to induce antinuclear antibodies.

Long-term treatment of (NZB × NZW)F_1 with procainamide did not show aggravation of the spontaneously developing lupus syndrome [154]. Experiments with inbred female and male lupus-prone NZB mice and outbred 'normal' HI mice showed that subcutaneous injection of procainamide three times a week for 30 weeks did not induce antinuclear antibodies, nor influence the age-related spontaneous increase of antinuclear antibodies [155].

5,5-Diphenylhydantoin.   Chronic oral exposure of C57BL/6 (H-2^b), C3Hf (H-2^k) and SJL (H-2^s) was shown to induce a dose-dependent transient lymphoid hyperplasia, but no signs of AD ([156]; see Chapter 16 by Krueger). As Atlas et al. [157] have demonstrated that C57BL/6 and C3H mice are fast metabolizers of diphenylhydantoin and SJL mice slow metabolizers, there is as yet no apparent relation between induction of hyperplasia and pharmacokinetics. SJL mice with a high spontaneous incidence of lymphomas, however, developed lymphomas earlier than age-matched controls ([156]; see Chapter 16 by Krueger). Functionally, non-specific immune suppression as judged by suppressed antibody production, is a frequently observed effect of diphenylhydantoin administration to mice [158, 159].

Besides the afore-mentioned experiments using systemic exposure to diphenylhydantoin, it has been demonstrated that a single subcutaneous injection of this compound into the hind footpad of mice, elicited a lymphoproliferative popliteal lymph node (PLN) reaction ([160]; see Chapter 15 by Gleichmann et al.). The kinetics and morphology of the diphenylhydantoin-induced PLN reactions beared resemblances to locally induced GVH reactions [161, 161a]. The degree of the PLN response appeared to be strain dependent [160 – 162], which could be attributed to certain MHC as well as undefined non-MHC haplotypes [161a, 162]. Furthermore, structure-activity studies with hydantoin, 3-methyl- and 3-phenyl-2-thiohydantoin derivatives indicated that combinations of aromatic as well as aliphatic lipophilic substituents at the 3- and 5-position of the molecule determined the capacity of this class of compounds to elicit a PLN response [163]. Results obtained so far indicate that the PLN assay may allow studies with regard to the type of lymphoproliferation as well as to the genetic dependence of the response, and investigations of structure-activity relationships. This approach may therefore be of value in immunotoxicological research (see Chapter 15 by Gleichmann et al., and last chapter of volume).

HgCl$_2$, gold sodium thiomalate, and D-penicillamine. An 8-month study using various inbred strains of mice revealed that HgCl$_2$ readily induced antinuclear antibodies in mice with the H-2^s haplotype, and to a lesser extent or not at all in H-2^b and H-2^f mice, depending on interaction with background genes [164]. Mice with H-2^a were resistant to induction of antinuclear antibodies by the chemicals, regardless of the genetic background. Similarly, gold sodium thiomalate and D-penicillamine induced antinuclear antibodies only in A.SW(H-2^s) mice, while other strains tested were resistant to this treatment [164].

Other studies have demonstrated the development of immune complex glomerulonephritis in female BALB/c (H-2^d) and SJL (H-2^s), but not in C57BL/6 (H-2^b) mice exposed to HgCl$_2$ by oral or parenteral administration up to 6 months [165, 166]. This again may reflect the resistance of the C57BL/6 (H-2^b) background to develop antinuclear antibodies and immune complex glomerulonephritis (see above). The immunoglobulin isotypes differed in the two responder strains [165, 166]. Oral administration of HgCl$_2$ to (C57BL/6 × C3H)F$_1$ (H-2$^{b/k}$) mice for 7 weeks resulted in suppressed T cell mitogen and mixed leukocyte responses [167].

(b) Rat models

Procainamide. Subcutaneous injection of procainamide three times a week for 30 weeks did not induce antinuclear antibodies in male and female Wistar rats [155].

5,5-Diphenylhydantoin. A 2-year study with Fischer 344 rats orally exposed to diphenylhydantoin did not reveal a higher incidence of lymphomas or signs of AD compared to controls [168].

HgCl$_2$. Transient, immunologically mediated glomerulonephritis induced by repeated injections of HgCl$_2$ in Brown Norway rats has been shown to be highly reproducible and several aspects have been studied in detail (see Chapter 14 by Druet et al.). In Brown Norway rats an initial HgCl$_2$-induced immunostimulation leading to renal lesions is followed by immunosuppression. HgCl$_2$ did not induce glomerulonephritis in Lewis rats, which has been attributed to an immediate induction of suppressor cells. The diverging immunologic reactions towards $HgCl_2$ have been demonstrated to depend on the MHC haplotype as similarly observed in mice [see Section IV.3.a.].

D-*Penicillamine and captopril.*   Brown Norway rats treated orally with D-penicillamine during 5 to 10 months developed antinuclear antibodies, circulating immune complexes, IgG deposits along the glomerular basement membrane and dermatitis [169]. No adverse effects were noted in Lewis and Sprague-Dawley rats treated with D-penicillamine, nor in Brown Norway and Lewis rats treated with captopril [169].

2-Amino-5-bromo-6-(3-fluorophenyl)-4-pyrimidinone.   This potent interferon inducer [51] has been shown to induce elevated serum IgG levels, lymphoid hyperplasia and adjuvant-like arthritis in Sprague-Dawley rats within 14 days of daily oral administration [52].

(c) Cat models

6-Propylthiouracil.   The antithyroidal drug 6-propylthiouracil has been shown to induce features of human SLE, such as antinuclear antibodies including the characteristic autoantibodies directed to dsDNA and Sm antigen (see [12]), lymphadenopathy and hemolytic anemia in cats after 2 – 10 weeks of treatment (see Chapter 12 by Aucoin). After cessation of the treatment the clinical signs resolved. Replacement of 6-propylthiouracil by the non-sulfur analog 6-propyluracil led to resolution of the syndrome, which indicates that the sulfur atom in 6-propylthiouracil appears to be an important structural requirement for induction of the disease (see Chapter 12 by Aucoin). Interestingly, in this model delayed clearance of the drug could be correlated with an increased chance to develop AD. Normal cats with longer elimination half-lives of 6-propylthiouracil than hyperthyroid cats developed the SLE-like syndrome considerably more frequently.

Mephenytoin.   Repeated oral administration of mephenytoin to cats has been shown to induce transient systemic lymphoid hyperplasia within several days [170].

(d) Dog models

Procainamide.   Oral administration of procainamide during 11 – 14 months has been shown to induce antinuclear antibodies in 3 – 6-year old, but not in 1-year-old, beagle dogs [171]. Similarly, Dubois and Strain [154] could not detect antinuclear antibodies in 2 – 12-month old dogs treated with procainamide up to 34 weeks. This suggests that age-related factors are contributory to the development of this autoimmune response in the dog. No overt signs of AD were observed.

Hydralazine. Findings of hydralazine-induced symptoms of lupus in dogs [172] could not be reproduced in another study [173].

(e) Monkey models

L-Canavanine. Alfalfa seeds containing the non-protein amino acid L-canavanine, as well as the pure compound itself, have been shown to induce SLE-like disease in monkeys within several weeks to months of oral treatment (see Chapter 13 by Bardana et al.). Withdrawal of alfalfa seeds from the diet resulted in improvement of the condition and return to normal hematologic parameters, although antinuclear and anti-dsDNA antibodies remained detectable for a considerable period.

(f) Toxicological considerations

Taken together, besides some promising recent models in inbred rats and outbred cats and monkeys, many attempts to reproduce drug-induced overt SLE in animals have yielded conflicting results. The afore-mentioned studies indicate that autoimmune phenomena such as antinuclear antibodies can indeed be produced in experimental animals, but that the genetic background, including both MHC and non-MHC genes, plays a crucial role. As pointed out by Festing [174], genetic background of animals in toxicological research and screening should acquire a much more important role. Usage of genetically highly defined strains may contribute to a more balanced evaluation of factors involved in the etiology and pathogenesis of systemic AD as observed in man. Moreover, this approach could allow risk assessment of the potential of chemicals to induce adverse systemic immunological reactions, which are at present recognized for the first time in humans. Some considerations which might be of value for immunotoxicological research with regard to drug- and chemical-induced AD will be dealt with in the last chapter of this volume.

V. Conclusions

There is no doubt that LMW drugs and chemicals have the potential to induce AD in man. However, the mechanisms by which LMW compounds induce immune disregulation leading to AD remain largely obscure. One obvious reason for this relates to the multifactorial etiology of AD, which probably involves interactions of host and environmental factors. Further, experimental toxicology and immunology do not yet dispose of enough knowledge and tools to recognize or demonstrate chemically induced diseases with an autoimmune pathogenesis.

Therefore, design and validation of experimental models is urgently needed. Drugs with an established capacity to induce immune derangements in man may be a suitable point of departure. Validated models will enable thorough mechanistic and structure-activity studies and so allow a risk assessment of the potential of environmental agents, including food components, to induce AD in genetically predisposed individuals.

Although infectious agents are often implicated in the etiology and pathogenesis of AD, available circumstantial data point at the likelihood that (yet unidentified) environmental chemicals may well provide another set of important etiologic factors of these complex disorders. Therefore, toxicology may contribute to a further understanding of AD.

References

1. Cruickshank, B. (1987) The basic pattern of tissue damage and pathology of systemic lupus erythematosus. In: D. J. Wallace and E. L. Dubois (Eds.), Dubois' Lupus Erythematosus, 3rd edn., Lea and Febiger, Philadelphia, pp. 53 – 104.

2. Dubois, E. L. and Wallace, D. J. (1987) Clinical and laboratory manifestations of systemic lupus erythematosus. In: D. J. Wallace and E. L. Dubois (Eds.), Dubois' Lupus Erythematosus, 3rd edn., Lea and Febiger, Philadelphia, pp. 317 – 449.

3. Hahn, B. H. (1987) Animal models of systemic lupus erythematosus. In: D. J. Wallace and E. L. Dubois (Eds.), Dubois' Lupus Erythematosus, 3rd edn., Lea and Febiger, Philadelphia, pp. 130 – 157.

4. Theofilopoulos, A. N. and Dixon, F. J. (1985) Murine models of systemic lupus erythematosus. Adv. Immunol. 37, 269 – 390.

5. Cohen, I. R. and Cooke, A. (1986) Natural autoantibodies might prevent autoimmune disease. Immunol. Today 7, 363 – 364.

6. Holmberg, D. and Coutinho, A. (1985) Natural antibodies and autoimmunity. Immunol. Today 6, 356 – 357.

7. Mackay, I. R. (1987) Autoimmunity in relation to lupus erythematosus. In: D. J. Wallace and E. L. Dubois (Eds.), Dubois' Lupus Erythematosus, 3rd edn., Lea and Febiger, Philadelphia, pp. 44 – 52.

8. Nossal, G. J. V. (1985) Autoimmunity of the future. In: N. R. Rose and I. R. Mackay (Eds.), The Autoimmune Diseases, Academic Press, Orlando, pp. 695 – 706.

9. Jaffee, B. D. and Claman, H. N. (1983) Chronic graft-versus-host disease (GVHD) as a model for scleroderma. I. Description of model systems. Cell. Immunol. 77, 1 – 12.

10. Gleichmann, E., Pals, S. T., Rolink, A. G., Radaszkiewicz, T. and Gleichmann, H. (1984) Graft-versus-host reactions: clues to the etiopathology of a spectrum of immunological diseases. Immunol. Today 5, 324 – 332.

11. Wallace, D. J. and Dubois, E. L. (1987) Definition, classification, and epidemiology of systemic lupus erythematosus. In: D. J. Wallace and E. L. Dubois (Eds.), Dubois' Lupus Erythematosus, 3rd edn., Lea and Febiger, Philadelphia, pp. 15 – 32.

12. Tan, E. M., Chan, E. K. L., Sullivan, K. F. and Rubin, R. L. (1988) Antinuclear antibodies (ANAs): diagnostically specific immune markers and clues toward the understanding of systemic autoimmunity. Clin. Immunol. Immunopathol. 47, 121 – 141.

13. Hardin, J. A. (1986) The lupus autoantigens and the pathogenesis of systemic lupus

erythematosus. Arthritis Rheum. 29, 457–460.

14. Janoff, A. S. and Rauch, J. (1986) The structural specificity of anti-phospholipid antibodies in autoimmune disease. Chem. Phys. Lipids 40, 315–332.

15. Lachmann, P. J. and Walport, M. J. (1987) Deficiency of the effector mechanisms of the immune response and autoimmunity. In: Autoimmunity and Autoimmune Disease (Ciba Foundation Symposium 129), John Wiley and Sons, Chichester, pp. 149–171.

16. Fleischmajer, R., Perlish, J. S. and Reeves, J. R. T. (1977) Cellular infiltrates in scleroderma skin. Arthritis Rheum. 20, 975–984.

17. Fleischmajer, R., Perlish, J. S. and Duncan, M. (1983) Scleroderma. A model for fibrosis (editorial). Arch. Dermatol. 119, 957–962.

18. Huff, J. C., Weston, W. L. and Tonneson, M. G. (1983) Erythema multiforme: a critical review of characteristics, diagnostic criteria and causes. J. Am. Acad. Dermatol. 8, 763–775.

19. Lyell, A. (1979) Toxic epidermal necrolysis (the scalded skin syndrome): a reappraisal. Br. J. Dermatol. 100, 69–86.

20. Rallison, M. L., Carlisle, J. W., Lee, R. E., Vernier, R. L. and Good, R. A. (1961) Lupus erythematosus and Stevens-Johnson syndrome. Occurrence as reactions to anticonvulsant medication. Am. J. Dis. Child. 101, 81–94.

21. Sontheimer, R. D. and Gilliam, J. N. (1981) Immunologically mediated epidermal cell injury. Springer Semin. Immunopathol. 4, 1–5.

22. Bianchine, J. R., Macaraeg, P. V. J., Lasagna, L., Azarnoff, D. L., Brunk, S. F., Hvidberg, E. F. and Owen, J. A. (1968) Drugs as etiologic factors in the Stevens-Johnson syndrome. Am. J. Med. 44, 390–405.

23. Kauppinnen, K. (1972) Cutaneous reactions to drugs with special reference to severe bullous mucocutaneous eruptions and sulphonamides. Acta Dermatol. Venereol. Suppl. 68, 1–89.

24. Peck, G. L., Herzig, G. P. and Elias, P. M. (1972) Toxic epidermal necrolysis in a patient with graft-versus-host reaction. Arch. Dermatol. 105, 561–569.

25. Streilein, J. W. and Billingham, R. E. (1970) An analysis of graft-versus-host disease in syrian hamsters. I. The epidermolytic syndrome: description and studies on its procurement. J. Exp. Med. 132, 163–180.

26. Graze, P. R. and Gale, R. P. (1979) Chronic graft versus host disease: a syndrome of disordered immunity. Am. J. Med. 66, 611–620.

27. Scully, C. and El-Kom, M. (1985) Lichen planus: review and update on pathogenesis. J. Oral Pathol. 14, 431–458.

28. Weston, W. L. and Huff, J. C. (1981) The mucocutaneous lymph node syndrome: a critical re-examination. Clin. Exp. Dermatol. 6, 167–178.

29. Fauci, A. S., Haynes, B. F. and Katz, P. (1978) The spectrum of vasculitis. Clinical, pathologic, immunologic, and therapeutic considerations. Ann. Intern. Med. 89 (part 1), 660–676.

30. Geha, R. S. and Rosen, F. S. (1983) Immunoregulatory T-cell defects. Immunol. Today 4, 233–236.

31. Leung, D. Y. M., Chu, E. D., Wood, N., Grady, S., Meade, R. and Geha, R. S. (1983) Immunoregulatory T cell abnormalities in mucocutaneous lymph node syndrome. J. Immunol. 130, 2002–2004.

32. Theofilopoulos, A. N., Prud'homme, G. J. and Dixon, F. J. (1985) Autoimmune aspects of systemic lupus erythematosus. Concepts Immunopathol. 1, 190–218.

33. Lee, L. A., Burns, M., Glode, C., Harmon, C. and Weston, W. (1983) No autoantibodies to nuclear antigens in Kawasaki syndrome. N. Engl. J. Med. 308, 1034.

34. Leung, D. Y. M., Geha, R. S., Newburger, J. W., Burns, J. C., Fiers, W., Lapierre, L. A. and Pober, J. S. (1986) Two monokines, interleukin 1 and tumor necrosis factor, render cultured vascular endothelial cells susceptible to lysis by antibodies circulating during Kawasaki syndrome. J. Exp. Med. 164, 1958–1972.

35. Anderson, V. M., Bauer, H. M. and Kelly, A. P. (1979) Mucocutaneous lymph node syndrome in adult receiving diphenylhydantoin. Cutis 23, 493 – 498.

36. Gams, R. A., Neal, J. A. and Conrad, F. G. (1968) Hydantoin-induced pseudopseudolymphoma. Ann. Intern. Med. 69, 557 – 568.

37. Rich, A. R. (1947) Hypersensitivity in disease with especial reference to periarteritis nodosa, rheumatic fever, disseminated lupus erythematosus and rheumatoid arthritis. Harvey Lect. 42, 106 – 147.

38. Gran, J. T. (1987) The epidemiology of rheumatoid arthritis. Monogr. Allergy 21, 162 – 196.

39. Nived, O. and Sturfelt, G. (1987) Epidemiology of systemic lupus erythematosus. Monogr. Allergy. 21, 197 – 214.

40. Medsger, T. A., Dawson, W. N. and Masi, A. T. (1970) The epidemiology of polymyositis. Am. J. Med. 48, 715 – 723.

41. Medsger, T. A. and Masi, A. T. (1971) Epidemiology of systemic sclerosis (scleroderma). Ann. Intern. Med. 74, 714 – 721.

42. Michet, C. L., McKenna, C. H., Elveback, L. R., Kaslow, R. A. and Kurland, L. T. (1985) Epidemiology of systemic lupus erythematosus and other connective tissue diseases in Rochester, Minnesota, 1950 through 1979. Mayo Clin. Proc. 60, 105 – 113.

43. Welsh, K. I. and Black, C. M. (1985) Genetic aspects of the acquired connective tissue diseases. Semin. Dermatol. 4, 152 – 163.

44. Homsy, J., Morrow, W. J. W. and Levy, J. A. (1986) Nutrition and autoimmunity: a review. Clin. Exp. Immunol. 65, 473 – 488.

45. Alarcón-Segovia, D. (1969) Drug-induced lupus syndromes. Mayo Clin. Proc. 44, 664 – 681.

46. Alarcón-Segovia, D. and Díaz-Jouanen, E. (1980) Lupus subsets: relationships to genetic and environmental factors. Semin. Arthritis Rheum. 10, 18 – 24.

47. Hang, L., Aguado, M. T., Dixon, F. J. and Theofilopoulos, A. N. (1985) Induction of severe autoimmune disease in normal mice by simultaneous action of multiple immunostimulators. J. Exp. Med. 161, 423 – 428.

48. Lahita, R. G., Bradlow, H. L., Fishman, J. and Kunkel, H. G. (1982) Abnormal estrogen and androgen metabolism in the human with systemic lupus erythematosus. Am. J. Kidney Dis. 2, 206 – 211.

49. Baer, A. N., McAllister, C. B., Wilkinson, G. R., Woosley, R. L. and Pincus, T. (1986) Altered distribution of debrisoquine oxidation phenotypes in patients with systemic lupus erythematosus. Arthritis Rheum. 29, 843 – 850.

50. Feldmann, M. (1987) Regulation of HLA class II expression and its role in autoimmune disease. In: Autoimmunity and Autoimmune Disease (Ciba Foundation Symposium 129), John Wiley and Sons, Chichester, pp. 88 – 108.

51. Fast, P. E., Hatfield, C. A., Sun, E. L. and Stringfellow, D. A. (1982) Polyclonal B-cell activation and stimulation of specific antibody responses by 5-halo-pyrimidinones with antiviral and antineoplastic activity. J. Biol. Response Mod., 1, 199 – 215.

52. Gray, J. E., Larsen, E. R., Fast, P. E. and Hamilton, R. D. (1985) Orally induced adjuvant-like arthritis in the rat. Toxicol. Pathol. 13, 266 – 275.

53. Batchelor, J. R., Welsh, K. I., Mansilla Tinoco, R., Dollery, C. T., Hughes, G. R. V., Bernstein, R., Ryan, P., Naish, P. F., Aber, G. M., Bing, R. F. and Russell, G. I. (1980) Hydralazine-induced systemic lupus erythematosus: influence of HLA-DR and sex on susceptibility. Lancet i, 1107 – 1109.

54. Emery, P., Panayi, G.S., Huston, G., Welsh, K. I., Mitchell, S.C., Shah, R. R., Idle, J. R., Smith, R. L. and Waring, R. H. (1984) D-Penicillamine induced toxicity in rheumatoid arthritis: the role of sulphoxidation status and HLA-DR3. J. Rheumatol. 11, 626 – 632.

55. Black, C. M., Welsh, K. I., Walker, A. E., Bernstein, R. M., Catoggio, L. J., McGregor, A. R. and Lloyd Jones, J. K. (1983) Genetic susceptibility to scleroderma-like syndrome induced by

vinyl chloride. Lancet i, 53 – 55.

56. Rosen, F. S. (1987) Autoimmunity and immunodeficiency disease. In: Autoimmunity and Autoimmune Disease (Ciba Foundation Symposium 129), John Wiley and Sons, Chichester, pp. 135 – 148.

57. Wilton, A. N., Cobain, T. J. and Dawkins, R. L. (1985) Family studies of IgA deficiency. Immunogenetics 21, 333 – 342.

58. Cleland, L. G. and Bell, D. A. (1978) The occurrence of systemic lupus erythematosus in two kindreds in association with selective IgA deficiency. J. Rheumatol. 5, 288 – 293.

59. Hjalmarson, O., Hanson, L. Å. and Nilsson, L. Å. (1977) IgA deficiency during D-penicillamine treatment. Br. Med. J. 1, 549.

60. Schmidt, D. and Seldon, L. (1982) Adverse effects of antiepileptic drugs. Raven Press, New York, pp. 42 – 48.

61. Seager, J., Jamison, D. L., Wilson, J., Hayward, A. R. and Soothill, J. F. (1975) IgA deficiency, epilepsy, and phenytoin treatment. Lancet ii, 632 – 635.

62. Janz, D. (1985) Epilepsy: seizures and syndromes. In: H.-H. Frey and D. Janz, Antiepileptic Drugs, Springer-Verlag, Berlin, pp. 3 – 34.

63. De Gast, G. C., Gratama, J. W., Ringden, O. and Gluckman, E. (1987) The multifactorial etiology of graft-versus-host disease. Immunol. Today 8, 209 – 212.

64. Dubois, E. L. and Wallace, D. J. (1987) Drugs that exacerbate and induce systemic lupus erythematosus. In: D. J. Wallace and E. L. Dubois (Eds.), Dubois' Lupus Erythematosus, 3rd edn., Lea and Febiger, Philadelphia, pp. 450 – 469.

65. Denman, A. M. and Pugh, S. (1982) Drug induced systemic lupus erythematosus. In: P. Dukor, P. Kallos, H. D. Schlumberger and G. B. West (Eds.), PAR, Pseudo Allergic Reactions, Vol. 3, Karger, Basel, pp. 18 – 47.

66. De Weck, A. L. (1983) Immunopathological mechanisms and clinical aspects of allergic reactions to drugs. In: A. L. De Weck and H. Bundgaard (Eds.), Allergic Reactions to Drugs, Springer Verlag, Berlin, pp. 75 – 133.

67. Bigazzi, P. E. (1985) Mechanisms of chemical-induced autoimmunity. In: J. H. Dean, M. I. Luster, A. E. Munson and H. Amos (Eds.), Immunotoxicology and Immunopharmacology, Raven Press, New York, pp. 277 – 290.

67a. Bigazzi, P. E. (1988) Autoimmunity induced by chemicals. Clin. Toxicol. 26, 125 – 156.

68. Duggan, M. A. K. and Court, J. B. (1981) A proposed mechanism of production of the autoimmune and lymphoproliferative side-effects of β-adrenergic-site-blocking drugs and hydantoin anticonvulsants. Ann. Clin. Res. 13, 406 – 418.

69. Harmon, C. E. and Portanova, J. P. (1982) Drug-induced lupus: clinical and serological studies. Clin. Rheum. Dis. 8, 121 – 135.

70. Hess, E. V. and Litwin, A. (1985) Drug-related rheumatic diseases. Basic mechanisms. In: S. Gupta and N. Talal (Eds.), Immunology of Rheumatic Diseases, Plenum, New York, pp. 651 – 668.

71. Russell, A. S. (1981) Drug-induced autoimmune disease. Clin. Immunol. Allergy 1, 57 – 76.

72. Schoen, R. T. and Trentham, D. E. (1981) Drug-induced lupus: an adjuvant disease? Am. J. Med. 71, 5 – 8.

73. Weinstein, A. (1980) Drug-induced systemic lupus erythematosus. Prog. Clin. Immunol. 4, 1 – 21.

74. Zürcher, K. and Krebs, A. (1980) Cutaneous Side Effects of Systemic Drugs. A Commentated Synopsis of Today's Drugs, Karger, Basel, pp. 165 – 191.

75. Siegel, M., Lee, S. L. and Peress, N. S. (1967) The epidemiology of drug-induced systemic lupus erythematosus. Arthritis Rheum. 10, 407 – 415.

76. Park, B. K., Coleman, J. W. and Kitteringham, N. R. (1987) Drug disposition and drug hypersensitivity. Biochem. Pharmacol. 36, 581 – 590.

77. Reidenberg, M. M., Durant, P. J., Harris, R. A., De Boccardo, G., Lahita, R. and Stenzel, K. H. (1983) Lupus erythematosus-like disease due to hydrazine. Am. J. Med. 75, 365 – 370.

78. Lange, C. E., Jühe, S., Stein, G. and Veltman, G. (1974) Die sogenannte Vinylchlorid-Krankheit – eine berufsbedingte Systemsklerose? Int. Arch. Arbeitsmed. 32, 1 – 32.

79. Ward, A. M., Udnoon, S., Watkins, J., Walker, A. E. and Darke, C. S. (1976) Immunological mechanisms in the pathogenesis of vinyl chloride disease. Br. Med. J. 1, 936 – 938.

80. Saihan, E. M., Burton, J. L. and Heaton, K. W. (1978) A new syndrome with pigmentation, scleroderma, gynaecomastia, Raynaud's phenomenon and peripheral neuropathy. Br. J. Dermatol. 99, 437 – 440.

81. Flindt-Hansen, H. and Isager, H. (1987) Scleroderma after occupational exposure to trichlorethylene and trichlorethane. Acta Dermatol. Venereol. 67, 263 – 264.

82. Sparrow, G. P. (1977) A connective tissue disorder similar to vinyl chloride disease in a patient exposed to perchlorethylene. Clin. Exp. Dermatol. 2, 17 – 22.

83. Yamakage, A., Ishikawa, H., Saito, Y. and Hattori, A. (1980) Occupational scleroderma-like disorder occurring in men engaged in the polymerization of epoxy resins. Dermatologica 161, 33 – 44.

84. Phoon, W. H., Chan, M. O. Y., Rajan, V. S., Tan, K. J., Thirumoorthy, T. and Goh, C. L. (1984) Stevens-Johnson syndrome associated with occupational exposure to trichloroethylene. Contact Dermatitis 10, 270 – 276.

85. Jennings, G. H. and Gower, N. D. (1963) Thrombocytopenic purpura in toluene di-isocyanate workers. Lancet i, 406 – 408.

86. Corman, L. C. (1985) The role of the diet in animal models of systemic lupus erythematosus: possible implications for human lupus. Semin. Arthritis Rheum. 15, 61 – 69.

87. Malinow, M. R., Bardana, E. J., Pirofsky, B., Craig, S. and McLaughlin, P. (1982) Systemic lupus erythematosus-like syndrome in monkeys fed alfalfa sprouts: role of non-protein amino acid. Science 216, 415 – 417.

88. Roberts, J. L. and Hayashi, J. A. (1983) Exacerbation of SLE associated with alfalfa ingestion. N. Engl. J. Med. 380, 1361.

89. Nishimura, N., Okamoto, H., Yasui, M., Maeda, K. and Ogura, K. (1959) Intermediary metabolism of phenylalanine and tyrosine in diffuse collagen diseases. II. Influences of the low phenylalanine and tyrosine diet upon patients with collagen disease. Arch. Dermatol. 80, 124 – 135.

90. Nishimura, N., Yasui, M., Okamoto, H., Kanazawa, M., Kotake, Y. and Shibata, Y. (1958) Intermediary metabolism of phenylalanine and tyrosine in diffuse collagen diseases. I. The presence of 2,5-dihydroxyphenylpyruvic acid in the urine of patients with collagen disease. Arch. Dermatol. 77, 255 – 262.

91. MacLeod, G. and Seyyedain-Ardebili, M. (1981) Natural and simulated meat flavors (with particular references to beef). CRC. Crit. Rev. Food. Sci. Nutr. 14, 309 – 437.

92. Langer, P. and Greer, M. A. (1977) Antithyroid Substances and Naturally Occurring Goitrogens, Karger, Basel, pp. 126 – 128.

93. Kammüller, M. E. and Seinen, W. (1988) Toxicology of naturally occurring isothiocyanates in the human diet – a short review. Hum. Toxicol. 7, 43 – 45.

94. Davis, J. P. and Schwade, E. D. (1959) Anticonvulsant effects 3-allyl-5-isobutyl-2-thiohydantoin (BAX 422). Fed. Proc. 18, 380.

95. Mali, J. W. H. and Malten, K. E. (1966) The epidemic of polymorph toxic erythema in The Netherlands in 1960. The so-called Margarine Disease. Acta Dermatol. Venereol. 46, 123 – 135.

96. Aldridge, W. N. (1985) Toxic oil syndrome. Hum. Toxicol. 4, 231 – 235.

97. Grandjean, P. and Tarkowski, S. (1984) Review of investigations and findings. In: P. Grandjean and S. Tarkowski (Eds.), Toxic Oil Syndrome: Mass Food Poisoning in Spain, WHO Regional Office for Europe, Copenhagen, pp. 3 – 30.

98. Alonso-Ruiz, A., Zea-Mendoza, A. C., Salazar-Vallinas, J. M., Rocamora-Ripoll, A. and Beltran-

Gutierrez, J. (1986) Toxic oil syndrome: a syndrome with features overlapping those of various forms of scleroderma. Semin. Arthritis Rheum. 15, 200–212.

99. Fernandez-Segoviano, P., Esteban, A. and Martinez-Cabruja, R. (1983) Pulmonary vascular lesions in the toxic oil syndrome in Spain. Thorax 38, 724–729.

100. Gomez-Reino, J. J. (1987) Immune system disorders associated with adulterated cooking oil. In: A. Berlin, J. Dean, M. H. Draper, E. M. B. Smith, F. Spreafico (Eds.), Immunotoxicology, Martinus Nijhoff Publ., Dordrecht, pp. 376–388.

101. Gutierrez, C., Gaspar, L., Muro, R., Kreisler, M. and Ferriz, P. (1983) Autoimmunity in patients with Spanish toxic oil syndrome. Lancet i, 644.

102. Kilbourne, E. M., Rigau-Perez, J. G., Heath, C. W., Zack, M. M., Falk, H., Martin-Marcos, M. and de Carlos, A. (1983) Clinical epidemiology of toxic oil syndrome. Manifestations of a new illness. N. Engl. J. Med. 309, 1408–1414.

103. Martinez-Tello, F. J., Navas-Palacios, J. J., Ricoy, J. R., Gil-Martin, R., Conde-Zurita, J. M., Colina-Ruiz, F., Teller, I., Cabello, A. and Madero-Garcia, S. (1982) Pathology of a new toxic syndrome caused by ingestion of adulterated oil in Spain. Virchows Arch. Abt. A, Pathol. Anat. 397, 261–285.

104. Tabuenca, J. M. (1981) Toxic-allergic syndrome caused by ingestion of rapeseed oil denatured with aniline. Lancet ii, 567–568.

105. Toxic Epidemic Syndrome Study Group (1982) Toxic epidemic syndrome, Spain, 1981. Lancet ii, 697–702.

106. Kammüller, M. E., Penninks, A. H. and Seinen, W. (1984) Spanish toxic oil syndrome is a chemically induced GVHD-like epidemic. Lancet i, 1174–1175.

107. Kammüller, M. E., Penninks, A. H., De Bakker, J. M., Thomas, C., Bloksma, N. and Seinen, W. (1987) An experimental approach to chemically induced systemic (auto)immune alterations: Spanish toxic oil syndrome as an example. In: B. A. Fowler (Ed.), Mechanisms of Cell Injury: Implications for Human Health. Dahlem Konferenzen, John Wiley and Sons, Chichester, pp. 175–192.

108. Kilbourne, E. M., Bernert, J. T., Posada de la Paz, M., Hill, R. H., Abaitua Borda, I., Kilbourne, B. W., Zack, M. M. and the Toxic-Epidemiologic Study Group (1988) Chemical correlates of pathogenicity of oils related to the toxic-oil syndrome epidemic in Spain. Am. J. Epidemiol. 127, 1210–1227.

109. Rigau-Perez, J. G., Perez-Alvarez, L., Duenas-Castro, S., Choi, K., Thacker, S. B., German, J. C., Gonzalez-de-Andres, G., Canada-Royo, L. and Perez-Gallardo, F. (1984) Epidemiological investigation of an oil associated pneumonic paralytic eosinophilic syndrome in Spain. Am. J. Epidemiol. 119, 250–260.

110. Posada, M., Castro, M., Kilbourne, E. M., Diaz de Rojas, F., Abaitua, I., Tabuenca, J. M. and Vioque, A. (1987) Toxic oil syndrome: case reports associated with the ITH oil refinery in Sevilla. Food Chem. Toxicol. 25, 87–90.

111. Tucker, S. P. and Cunningham, V. J. (1986) The incorporation of palmitic acid into lipids in the rat after treatment with oleylanilide. Biochem. Pharmacol. 35, 1764–1766.

112. Kammüller, M. E., Bloksma, N. and Seinen, W. (1988) Chemical-induced autoimmune reactions and Spanish toxic oil syndrome. Focus on hydantoins and related compounds. Clin. Toxicol. 26, 157–174.

113. Kammüller, M.E., Verhaar, H. J. M., Versluis, C., Terlouw, J. K., Brandsma, L., Penninks, A. H. and Seinen, W. (1988) 1-Phenyl-5-vinyl-2-imidazolidinethione, a proposed causative agent of Spanish toxic oil syndrome: synthesis, and identification in one of a group of case-associated oil samples. Food Chem. Toxicol. 26, 119–127.

114. Shear, N. H., Spielberg, S. P., Grant, D. M., Tang, B. K. and Kalow, W. (1986) Differences in metabolism of sulfonamides predisposing to idiosyncratic toxicity. Ann. Intern. Med. 105, 179–184.

115. Spielberg, S. P., Gordon, G. B., Blake, D. A., Goldstein, D. A. and Herlong, H. F. (1981) Predisposition to phenytoin hepatotoxicity assessed in vitro. N. Engl. J. Med. 305, 722 – 727.
116. Mullen, P. W. and Queiroz, M. L. S. (1983) Phenytoin and humoral immunity: background and a pharmacokinetic interpretation of recent findings. In: J. W. Hadden, L. Chedid, P. Dukor, F. Spreafico and D. Willoughby (Eds.), Advances in Immunopharmacology, 2, Pergamon Press, Oxford, pp. 3 – 9.
117. Wilson, J. T., Höjer, B., Tomson, G., Rane, A. and Sjöquist, F. (1978) High incidence of a concentration-dependent skin reaction in children treated with phenytoin. Br. Med. J. 1, 1583 – 1586.
118. Kutt, H., Wolk, M., Scherman, R. and McDowell, F. (1964) Insufficient parahydroxylation as a cause of diphenylhydantoin toxicity. Neurology, 14, 542 – 548.
119. De Wolff, F. A., Vermeij, P., Ferrari, M. D., Buruma, O. J. S. and Breimer, D. D. (1983) Impairment of phenytoin parahydroxylation as a cause of severe intoxication. Ther. Drug Monit. 5, 213 – 215.
120. Andoh, B., Idle, J. R., Sloan, T. P., Smith, R. L. and Woolhouse, N. (1980) Inter-ethnic and inter-phenotype differences among Ghanaians and Caucasians in the metabolic hydroxylation of phenytoin. Br. J. Clin. Pharmacol. 9, 282 – 283.
121. Kromann, N., Christiansen, J., Flachs, H., Dam, M. and Hvidberg, E. F. (1981) Differences in single dose phenytoin kinetics between Greenland Eskimos and Danes. Ther. Drug Monit. 3, 239 – 246.
122. Inaba, T., Jurima, M., Nakano, M. and Kalow, W. (1984) Mephenytoin and sparteine pharmacogenetics in Canadian caucasians. Clin. Pharmacol. Ther. 36, 670 – 676.
123. Jurima, M., Inaba, T., Kadar, D. and Kalow, W. (1985) Genetic polymorphism of mephenytoin p-(4')-hydroxylation: differences between Orientals and Caucasians. Br. J. Clin. Pharmacol. 19, 483 – 487.
124. Nakamura, K., Goto, W., Ray, W. A., McAllister, C.B., Jacqz, E., Wilkinson, G. R. and Branch, R. A. (1985) Interethnic differences in genetic polymorphism of debrisoquin and mephenytoin hydroxylation between Japanese and Caucasian populations. Clin. Pharmacol. Ther. 38, 402 – 408.
125. Lindquist, T. (1957) Lupus erythematosus disseminatus after administration of mesantoin. Acta Med. Scand. 158, 131 – 138.
126. Wedlund, P. J., Aslanian, W. S., Jacqz, E., McAllister, C. B., Branch, R. A. and Wilkinson, G. R. (1985) Phenotype differences in mephenytoin pharmacokinetics in normal subjects. J. Pharmacol. Exp. Ther. 234, 662 – 669.
127. Jacqz, E., Hall, S. D. and Branch, R. A. (1986) Genetically determined polymorphisms in drug oxidation. Hepatology 6, 1020 – 1032.
128. Pilcher, J. D. and Gerstenberger, H. J. (1930) Treatment of chorea with phenylethyl-hydantoin. Am. J. Dis. Child. 40, 1239 – 1249.
129. Jann, M. W. and Fidone, G. S. (1986) Effect of influenza vaccine on serum anticonvulsant concentrations. Clin. Pharmacol. 5, 817 – 820.
130. Mannering, G. J., Renton, K. W., Azhary, R. and Deloria, L. B. (1980) Effects of interferon-inducing agents on the hepatic cytochrome P-450 drug metabolizing systems. NY Acad. Sci. 350, 314 – 331.
131. Caldwell, J., Winter, S. M. and Hutt, A. J. (1988) The pharmacological and toxicological significance of the stereochemistry of drug disposition. Xenobiotica, 18, Suppl. 1, 59 – 70.
132. Smith, R. L. (1988) The role of metabolism and disposition studies in the safety assessment of pharmaceuticals. Xenobiotica 18, Suppl. 1, 89 – 96.
133. Weber, W. W. and Hein, D. W. (1985) N-Acetylation pharmacogenetics. Pharmacol. Rev. 37, 25 – 79.
134. Reeves, J. P. and Steinberg, A. D. (1985) Effect of the xid gene on graft-versus-host-induced

autoantibody production in nonautoimmune mice. Clin. Immunol. Immunopathol. 36, 320–329.

135. Seldin, M. F., Reeves, J. P., Scribner, C. L., Roths, J. B., Davidson, W. F., Morse, H. C. and Steinberg, A. D. (1987) Effect of *xid* on autoimmune C3H-*gld/gld* mice. Cell. Immunol. 107, 249–255.

136. Steinberg, E. B., Santoro, T. J., Chused, T. M., Smathers, P. A. and Steinberg, A. D. (1983) Studies of congenic MRL-*lpr/lpr.xid* mice. J. Immunol. 131, 2789–2795.

137. Revel, M. and Schattner, A. (1987) Interferons: cytokines in autoimmunity. In: Autoimmunity and Autoimmune Disease (Ciba Foundation Symposium 129), John Wiley and Sons, Chichester, pp. 223–233.

138. Andrews, B. S., Eisenberg, R. A., Theofilopoulos, A. N., Izui, S., Wilson, C. B., McConahey, P. J., Murphy, E. D., Roths, J. B. and Dixon, F. J. (1978) Spontaneous murine lupus-like syndrome. Clinical and immunopathological manifestations in several strains. J. Exp. Med. 148, 1198–1215.

139. Murphy, E.D. (1981) Lymphoproliferation (*lpr*) and other single-locus models for murine lupus. In: M. E. Gershwin and B. Merchant (Eds.), Immunologic Defects in Laboratory Animals, Plenum, New York, pp. 143–173.

140. Shultz, L. D. and Sidman, C. L. (1987) Genetically determined murine models of immunodeficiency. Ann. Rev. Immunol. 5, 367–403.

141. Roths, J. B., Murphy, E. D. and Eicher, E. M. (1984) A new mutation, *gld*, that produces lymphoproliferation and autoimmunity in C3H/HeJ mice. J. Exp. Med. 159, 1–20.

142. Alexander, E. L., Moyer, C., Travlos, G. S., Roths, J. B. and Murphy, E. D. (1985) Two histopathologic types of inflammatory vascular disease in MRL/Mp autoimmune mice. Model for human vasculitis in connective tissue disease. Arthritis Rheum. 28, 1146–1155.

143. Samelson, L. E., Davidson, W. F., Morse, H. C. and Klausner, R. D. (1986) Abnormal tyrosine phosphorylation on T-cell receptor in lymphoproliferative disorders. Nature 324, 674–676.

144. Dubois, E. L. and Strain, L. (1973) Effect of diet on survival and nephropathy on NZB/NZW hybrid mice. Biochem. Med. 7, 336–340.

145. Izui, S., Kelley, V. E., Masuda, K., Yoshida, H., Roths, J. B. and Murphy, E. D. (1984) Induction of various autoantibodies by mutant gene *lpr* in several strains of mice. J. Immunol. 133, 227–233.

146. Warren, R. W., Caster, S. A., Roths, J. B., Murphy, E. D. and Pisetsky, D. S. (1984) The influence of the *lpr* gene on B cell activation: differential antibody expression in *lpr* congenic mouse strains. Clin. Immunol. Immunopathol. 31, 65–77.

147. Jones, F.S., Pisetsky, D.S. and Kurlander, R. J. (1985) Defects in mononuclear phagocytic system (MPS) function in autoimmune MRL-*lpr/lpr* mice. Clin. Immunol. Immunopathol. 36, 30–39.

148. Santos, G. W., Hess, A. D. and Vogelsang, G. B. (1985) Graft-versus-host-reactions and disease. Immunol. Rev. 88, 169–192.

149. Ten Veen, J. H. and Feltkamp, T. E. W. (1972) Studies on drug induced lupus erythematosus in mice. I. Drug induced antinuclear antibodies (ANA). Clin. Exp. Immunol. 11, 265–276.

150. Cannat, A. and Seligmann, M. (1968) Induction by isoniazid and hydralazine of antinuclear factors in mice. Clin. Exp. Immunol. 3, 99–105.

151. Ten Veen, J. H. (1973) Studies on drug induced lupus erythematosus in mice. II. Drug-induced smooth muscle and skeletal muscle antibodies. Clin. Exp. Immunol. 15, 375–384.

152. Ten Veen, J. H. and Feltkamp-Vroom, T. M. (1973) Studies on drug induced lupus erythematosus in mice. III. Renal lesions and splenomegaly in drug-induced lupus erythematosus. Clin. Exp. Immunol. 15, 591–600.

153. Tannen, R. H. and Weber, W. W. (1980) Antinuclear antibodies related to acetylator phenotype in mice. J. Pharmacol. Exp. Ther. 213, 485–490.

154. Dubois, E. L. and Strain, L. (1972) Failure of procainamide to induce systemic lupus

erythematosus-like disease in animals. Toxicol. Appl. Pharmacol. 21, 253–259.

155. Whittingham, S., Mackay, I. R., Whitworth, J. A. and Sloman, G. (1972) Antinuclear antibody response to procainamide in man and laboratory animals. Am. Heart J. 84, 228–234.

156. Krüger, G. R. F. and Bedoya, V. A. (1978) Hydantoin-induced lymphadenopathies and lymphomas: experimental studies in mice. Recent Res. Cancer Res. 64, 265–270.

157. Atlas, S. A., Zweier, J. L. and Nebert, D. W. (1980) Genetic differences in phenytoin pharmacokinetics. In vivo clearance and in vitro metabolism among inbred strains of mice. Dev. Pharmacol. Ther. 1, 281–304.

158. Margaretten, N. C. and Warren, R. P. (1987) Effect of phenytoin on antibody production: use of a murine model. Epilepsia 28, 77–80.

159. Tucker, A. N., Hong, L., Boorman, G. A., Pung, O. and Luster, M. I. (1985) Alteration of bone marrow cell cycle kinetics by diphenylhydantoin: relationship to folate utilization and immune function. J. Pharmacol. Exp. Ther. 234, 57–62.

160. Gleichmann, H. (1981) Studies on the mechanism of drug sensitization: T-cell-dependent popliteal lymph node reaction to diphenylhydantoin. Clin. Immunol. Immunopathol. 18, 203–211.

161. Gleichmann, H., Pals, S. T. and Radaszkiewicz, T. (1983) T-cell-dependent B-cell proliferation and activation by administration of the drug diphenylhydantoin to mice. Hematol. Oncol. 1, 165–176.

161a. Kammüller, M. E. (1988) A toxicological approach to chemical-induced autoimmunity. PhD Thesis, University of Utrecht, Utrecht, The Netherlands.

162. Hurtenbach, U., Gleichmann, H., Nagata, N. and Gleichmann, E. (1987) Immunity to D-penicillamine: genetic, cellular and chemical requirements for induction of popliteal lymph node enlargement in the mouse. J. Immunol. 139, 411–416.

163. Kammüller, M. E. and Seinen, W. Structural requirements for hydantoins and 2-thiohydantoins to induce lymphoproliferative popliteal lymph node reactions in the mouse. Int. J. Immunopharmacol., in press.

164. Robinson, C. H. G., Balazs, T. and Egorov, I. K. (1986) Mercuric chloride-, gold sodium thiomalate-, and D-penicillamine-induced antinuclear antibodies in mice. Toxicol. Appl. Pharmacol. 86, 159–169.

165. Hultman, P. and Eneström, S. (1987) The induction of immune complex deposits in mice by peroral and parenteral administration of mercuric chloride: strain dependent susceptibility. Clin. Exp. Immunol. 67, 283–292.

166. Hultman, P. and Eneström, S. (1988) Mercury induced antinuclear antibodies in mice: characterization and correlation with renal immune complex deposits. Clin. Exp. Immunol. 71, 269–274.

167. Dieter, M. P., Luster, M. I., Boorman, G. A., Jameson, C. W., Dean, J. H. and Cox, J. W. (1983) Immunological and biochemical responses in mice treated with mercuric chloride. Toxicol. Appl. Pharmacol. 68, 218–228.

168. Jang, J. J., Takahashi, M., Furukawa, F., Toyoda, K., Hasegawa, R., Sato, H. and Hayashi, Y. (1987) Long-term in vivo carcinogenicity study of phenytoin (5,5-diphenylhydantoin) in F344 rats. Food Chem. Toxicol. 25, 697–702.

169. Donker, A. J., Venuto, R. C., Vladutiu, A. O., Brentjens, J. R. and Andres, G. A. (1984) Effects of prolonged administration of D-penicillamine or captopril in various strains of rats. Brown Norway rats treated with D-penicillamine develop autoantibodies, circulating immune complexes, and disseminated intravascular coagulation. Clin. Immunol. Immunopathol. 30, 142–155.

170. Kaslaris, E. (1953) Experimentelle Erzeugung von Lymphknotenschwellung durch Mesantoin. Wien. Klin. Wschr. 65, 1007–1008.

171. Balazs, T. and Robinson, C. (1983) Procainamide-induced antinuclear antibodies in beagle dogs. Toxicol. Appl. Pharmacol. 71, 299 – 302.
172. Comens, P. (1956) Experimental hydralazine disease and its similarity to disseminated lupus erythematosus. J. Lab. Clin. Med. 47, 444 – 454.
173. Dubois, E. L., Katz, Y. J., Freeman, V. and Garbak, F. (1957) Chronic toxicity studies of hydralazine (Apresoline) in dogs with particular reference to the production of the 'hydralazine syndrome'. J. Lab. Clin. Med. 50, 119 – 126.
174. Festing, M. F. W. (1987) Genetic factors in toxicology: implications for toxicological screening. CRC Crit. Rev. Toxicol. 18, 1 – 26.

SECTION II

Basic concepts

M.E. Kammüller, N. Bloksma and W. Seinen (Eds.)
Autoimmunity and Toxicology
© 1989 Elsevier Science Publishers B.V. (Biomedical Division)

Basic mechanisms of adaptive immune system function 2

NANNE BLOKSMA[a] and HENK-JAN SCHUURMAN[b]

[a] Section of Immunotoxicology, Department of Basic Veterinary Sciences, and [b] Division of Immunopathology, Departments of Internal Medicine and Pathology, University of Utrecht, The Netherlands

I. Introduction

The immune system serves to combat infectious agents and native cells that have undergone neoplastic transformation, in order to maintain homeostasis and health in the body. The components towards which the reactions of the immune system are directed, are called antigens. The immune system can be divided in two functional divisions, namely the innate immune system and the adaptive immune system. Both consist of a variety of molecules and cells distributed throughout the body in blood, lymph, lymphoid organs and other tissues. In the innate immune system the components do not have an intrinsic capacity of specific recognition of antigens, but some components have a restricted, primitive antigen-recognition repertoire. The components comprise among others complement, acute-phase proteins, mononuclear and polymorphonuclear phagocytic leukocytes, cells with natural killer activity and their soluble effector molecules. In the adaptive immune system specific antigen recognition by lymphocytes is the inciting stimulus. The antigen-specific effector components are the antibodies or other lymphocyte-derived soluble products and various subpopulations of the lymphocytes themselves. Part of the mediator and effector molecules secreted by the lymphocytes, however, are not antigen-specific.

There is considerable interaction and cooperation between the innate and adaptive immune system, and their functions are tightly controlled by the intricate communications network of the immune system itself. Further, homeostatic systems outside the immune system, namely the endocrine system and the nervous system, exercise control of the immune system, and vice versa. By virtue of the regulatory mechanisms a particular immune response in a normally functioning immune system can be strongly amplified or diminished, depending on the momentary needs of the organism. Defects in the function of the immune system, either being congenital or induced, can result in disease. The kind of disease varies with the nature and extent of the defect.

This book deals with disregulation of the immune system induced by low molecular weight compounds, which may result in specific immune reactions to self-components. Whereas the ability of drugs to cause autoimmune diseases in man is well documented, the mechanisms of these immunotoxic effects are poorly understood. Elucidation requires a thorough understanding of immune system function. Due to space limitation the overview of the immune system in this chapter does not aim at completeness. It will try to emphasize those aspects of the immune system that are in the authors' opinion most relevant to the subject.

II. Components of the immune system

1. CELLS AND TISSUES

All cells involved in immune reactions, except for some types of antigen-presenting cells and cells constituting the framework of lymphoid organs, originate from one progenitor stem cell in the bone marrow. In this lymphoid organ a process of differentiation, maturation and proliferation generates cells of the granulocyte, monocyte and lymphocyte lineages, which enter the circulation and lodge in other (lymphoid) tissues. The process is considered to be antigen-independent, and the bone marrow is therefore called a primary lymphoid organ. Soluble mediators generated during specific and non-specific immune responses, however, can influence leukopoiesis.

(a) Granulocytes

The major population of cells of the granulocyte lineage are the neutrophils. They are short-lived (2 – 3 days) upon release from the bone marrow, and represent about 55 – 65% of the total normal blood leukocytes in man. In mice and rats this figure is about 5 – 15%. Neutrophils are usually not very numerous at extravascular sites, but have an exquisite capability to accumulate at sites of acute inflammation induced by immunological as well as non-immunological mechanisms. Combined with their efficient ability of ingesting and destroying most invading micro-organisms, especially in cooperation with specific antibodies and complement components, neutrophils constitute a major effector defence against infection. Granulocyte effector reactions, however, can be accompanied by harmful tissue destruction and vascular damage. Whereas this can be considered acceptable in the defence against pathogens, tissue destruction by granulocytes in response to non-infectious agents rather is a nuisance.

(b) Monocytes and macrophages

Cells of the monocyte lineage leave the bone marrow as monocytes, and circulate in the blood with a half-life of about 1 day before emigration to extravascular sites. There they mature to tissue macrophages, such as Kupffer cells in the liver, histiocytes in the connective tissues, alveolar macrophages in the lung, Langerhans cells in the epidermis and interdigitating cells in the lymph nodes. Tissue macrophages show functional heterogeneity, i.e. different capacities to perform a particular function. For instance, Langerhans cells and interdigitating cells are highly specialized as antigen-presenting cells. The functional heterogeneity of the cells is thought to parallel different sublineages of differentiation. Among the numerous functions of macrophages in the organism, a wide variety of functions in the immune system has been recognized (Table 1).

(c) Lymphocytes

Two major subpopulations of lymphocytes are generated from the bone marrow, the so-called T and B cells. Other lymphocytes coming from the bone marrow cannot be classified into the lineages of T or B lymphocytes and their precursor cells. Based on the absence of typical T and B cell markers, the cells have been originally termed null cells. The cells are very heterogenous and some of them bear markers

TABLE 1

Role of monocytes/macrophages in the immune response

Uptake, processing, transportation and presentation of antigens to lymphocytes

Elimination of antigens without presentation

Non-specific phagocytosis and killing of micro-organisms

Non-specific cytostatic or cytocidal activity against extracellular micro-organisms and tumour cells

Production of complement components

Production of endogenous pyrogens (IL-1 and tumour necrosis factor)

Antibody-mediated phagocytosis and/or killing of micro-organisms and tumour cells

Effector cell of delayed type hypersensitivity reactions

Regulation of monocytopoiesis and granulocytopoiesis

Regulation of T cell, B cell, and NK cell functions

---

normally found on cells of the monocyte lineage. A large portion of the null cells exert natural killer activity, i.e. they can kill target cells without prior immunization. These so-called natural killer cells show an extensive overlap with a morphologically defined lymphocyte subset, the large granular lymphocytes, being cells with distinct azurophilic granules in their plasma. As the designation and classification of the cells is far from being resolved, we will refer to the population on the basis of their function, i.e. natural killer (NK) cells. The lymphoid cells represent about 20% of the leukocytes in human blood, and about 90% of the leukocytes in blood of mice and rats.

(d) B lymphocytes

In man, B cells account for about 10 – 15% of the circulating lymphoid pool, and in mice and rats for about 25%. Their 'trademark' is the expression of immunoglobulins, inserted into the surface membrane or present in the cytoplasm. Immunoglobulins are composed of two identical glycosylated heavy (H) polypeptide chains, and two identical light (L) chains, linked together by disulphide bonds. Based on differences in the H chains, different classes (isotypes) of immunoglobulins are distinguished. Immunoglobulins can specifically recognize and bind antigen. The antigen-combining site resides in the variable (V) region of the N-terminal portion of both the H and the L chain. These regions are encoded by a large set of V-gene segments, located at different chromosomes for the H and L chain. The selection of a V-gene segment for a particular V region is the result of a rearrangement of the V-gene segments in which the other segments are deleted. Similar processes underlie the selection of the remaining segments of the immunoglobulin chains, namely the joining (J) and constant (C) gene segments for the light chains and an additional diversity (D) segment for the heavy chain. After recombination of the gene segments, translation and transcription of the complete gene results in the production of immunoglobulin chains that combine to complete immunoglobulin molecules in the endoplasmic reticulum. The rearrangement process is the basis of the extensive repertoire of antigen recognition by B cells (about 10^7 in man) that can be elaborated from a relatively small set of V-gene segments (about 200 in man).

The process yielding mature B cells able to recognize antigen by surface immunoglobulin is thought to occur in the bone marrow and to be independent of antigen.

The surface immunoglobulins of B cells have a receptor-like function with regard to antigens, i.e. specific binding of a multivalent ligand, the antigen, results in cross-linking of the immunoglobulins and the generation of second messenger molecules. In concert with other signals, usually delivered by activated T helper cells, the antigen-activated B cells undergo clonal proliferation. A portion of these cells mature to plasma cells and secrete immunoglobulins of the same antigen specificity as the initially activated B cell. Thus, the antigen-combining site is still encoded by the same rearranged V-D-J-gene segments. The class of the secreted im-munoglobulin, however, may be different as a consequence of a new rearrangement of the C genes, a process termed H chain isotype switch or class switch, for instance, a switch from IgM to IgG_1. Secreted immunoglobulins are usually called antibodies when their function to bind antigen is denoted. The remainder of the antigen-activated B cells does not mature to effector cells and becomes memory cell after immunoglobulin class switch. The memory cells are long-lived recirculating cells. The majority of B cells in the circulation express immunoglobulins of the IgM as well as the IgD class. A minority of the cells express either IgG, IgA or IgE.

Besides immunoglobulins, B cells express many other membrane-bound func-

TABLE 2

Major surface markers of B cells

Surface molecule	Man	Mouse	Rat	CD[a]	Specificity
Immunoglobulin	+	+	+		All cells, plasma cells
MHC class II molecules	HLA-DR, DP, DQ	I-A, I-E (Ia)	RT1. B, D		Most cells
Differentiation marker[b]	T1/Leu-1[c]	Ly-1		5	Subset
Fcγ receptors[d]	+	+	+		All cells
Fcϵ receptors[e]	+			23	Activated cells
Complement receptor for C3b	CR1	CR1		35	Peripheral cells
Complement receptor for C3d	CR2	CR2		21	Mature cells
IL-2 receptor α chain	Tac	+	+	25	Activated cells
Transferrin receptor	+	+	+		Proliferating cells
Terminal deoxynucleo-tidyl transferase (TdT)[f]	+	+	+		Immature cells

[a] CD denotes cluster of differentiation. CD numbers refer to groups of antibodies that react with the same human leukocyte differentiation antigens. Antibodies have been assigned to the various clusters during international workshops (Paris, 1982; Boston, 1984; Oxford, 1986). Although developed for the human system, analogous molecules in other species are commonly designated in CD nomenclature as well.
[b] Marker for most T cells with unknown function.
[c] Marker detected by monoclonal antibodies T1(OKT1) and Leu-1.
[d] Receptor for the Fc part of IgG antibodies, if bound to antigen.
[e] Low affinity receptor for the Fc part of IgE.
[f] TdT is a nuclear marker, and is not expressed on the cell surface.

tional molecules (Table 2). An interesting small subset of B cells are those expressing a typical T cell marker (CD5), in man Leu-1 and in mice Ly-1. The CD5$^+$ B cells can constitutively produce antibodies, predominantly of the IgM class, which generally have low affinity for self antigens, like single- and double-stranded DNA, IgG and phospholipids. CD5$^+$ B cells are virtually absent in peripheral blood and lymph nodes of healthy adult organisms, but relatively high numbers are found in foetuses and neonates. In man with autoimmune diseases such as rheumatoid arthritis, and especially in some mouse strains with genetically determined autoimmune disease, the CD5$^+$ B cell population can be significantly increased. Whether the cells are a source of pathogenic autoantibodies in these instances is not yet known.

(e) T lymphocytes

About 70% of the blood lymphocyte pool of man, mice and rats are T cells. T cells leave the bone marrow as immature precursor cells. They undergo a step-wise process of maturation and differentiation in the microenvironment of the thymus. The process is thought to be independent of antigen; therefore, the thymus is considered a primary lymphoid organ. The maturation and differentiation process can be characterized by sequential changes in the expression of membrane surface molecules and the acquisition of specific antigen receptors leading to immunocompetence. The antigen receptor on T cells consists of two disulphide-linked polypeptide chains, α and β, which are physically linked at the cell surface with the CD3 protein. In this complex the α,β-heterodimer acts as the antigen recognition unit, while the CD3 molecule plays a role in transmembrane signal transduction. Like the immunoglobulin chains, the α and β chains of the T cell receptor contain a variable and a constant domain. A major difference with immunoglobulin-type of antigen receptor of B cells is the way of antigen recognition. Immunoglobulin molecules can interact with soluble antigen as such, while the α,β-heterodimer molecules interact with cell-bound antigen in the context of molecules of the major histocompatibility complex (see sections below).

More or less different functional subsets of T cells can be distinguished, namely helper, suppressor, cytotoxic, and delayed hypersensitivity T cells. The functional differences are rather well paralleled by the presence of distinct glycoproteins (markers) in the membrane of the cells (Table 3).

Blood lymphocytes represent only a minor portion of the total lymphocyte pool of an organism. In the human adult this figure is about 1% of a total of 10^{12} lymphocytes (about 1 kg). The cells exert a mobile surveillance function by their capacity to recirculate in the body. During this process of recirculation they leave the blood, usually in the lymphoid organs. At these sites the lymphocytes can be sequestered and undergo activation and differentiation following antigen recognition; such in close contact with the appropriate extravascular micro-environment. If antigen is not encountered, the lymphocytes return to the blood via the lymph.

TABLE 3

Major surface markers of T lymphocytes

Surface molecule	Man	Mouse	Rat	CD	Specificity
Differentiation marker		Thy-1 (θ)			All cells
Differentiation marker of T cell receptor	T3/Leu-4	+	+	3	Mature cells
Adhesion and regulatory molecule (LFA-2)	T11/Leu-5	+	+	2	All T cells with sheep erythrocyte receptors
Differentiation marker	T1/Leu-1	Ly-1	MRC Ox 19	5	Most cells
Cell interaction molecule	T4/Leu-3	L3T4	W3/25	4	Most helper T cells, most T_{DTH} cells
Cell interaction molecule	T8/Leu-2	Ly-2,3	MRC OX8	8	Most cytotoxic and suppressor T cells
IL-2 receptor α chain	Tac	+	+	25	Activated cells
Transferrin receptor	+	+	+		Proliferating cells
Terminal deoxynucleotidyl transferase (TdT)[a]	+	+	+		Immature cells
TLA complex class I molecule		Qa1	RT1C		Helper T cells, T_{DTH} cells
MHC class II molecule	HLA-DR	I-A, I-E (Ia)	RT1B, D		Activated cells

[a] Nuclear marker.

(f) Lymphoid organs

The mature cells of the non-recirculating lymphoid pool are primarily lodged in the secondary (peripheral) lymphoid organs, including spleen, lymph nodes and lymphoid tissues along the respiratory, gastrointestinal and urogenital tract. Secondary lymphoid organs are, unlike primary (central) lymphoid organs, not involved in the ontogeny and development of lymphocytes, but are the sites of cellular and humoral immune response initiated by immunogens. Bone marrow serves both functions, so it can be considered as primary and as secondary lymphoid organ. The architecture of secondary lymphoid organs diverges, but common characteristics can be recognized. All consist of a reticular network with areas containing predominantly T or B cells. The physiologic basis of the T and B cell compartmentalization resides in the specialized structure of the stromal reticulum. The stromal cells facilitate the residence and the generation of defined reactions of one of the two cell types. In the white pulp of the spleen, the periarteriolar lymphocyte sheath (PALS) lodges T cells and therefore is termed thymus-dependent area. The follicles inside the PALS and the marginal zone around the PALS harbour B cells. In the lymph nodes the follicles in the cortex constitute the B areas, and the interfollicular areas or the paracortex the T cell areas. The medulla is a third distinct region in the lymph node. Normally it contains moderate numbers of small lymphocytes, plasma cells and macrophages, but upon antigenic stimulation numerous lymphoblasts, plasma cells, macrophages and granulocytes can be seen.

Along the mucosal surface of the gastrointestinal and respiratory tract specialized lymphoid tissues, like Peyer's patches, appendix and tonsils can be found. Their organization is analogous to that of lymph nodes, but unlike lymph nodes these organs are not encapsulated and in close proximity of the external milieu. Peyer's patches, appendix and tonsils belong to the so-called mucosa-associated lymphoid tissue (MALT), being the microenvironment of the secretory immune system ('external' immune system). The designation MALT is based on common functions, like predominant production of antibodies of the IgA class and preferential migration of their lymphocytes from and to other members of the MALT. These include also lymphoid tissues along all other secretory epithelial sites (urogenital tract, gingiva, mammary gland) and draining, e.g. mesenteric, lymph nodes. In addition, the numerous segregate plasma cells and lymphocytes scattered throughout and underneath the epithelial layer (lamina propria) belong to the MALT. Since mucosal surfaces are constantly exposed to pathogens and foreign antigens, the MALT constitutes an important component of the local immunologic defence. This is reflected by the number of lymphocytes belonging to the MALT, being about half of the total number of lymphocytes in the body.

(g) Lymphocyte recirculation

As already indicated above, the migration of mature lymphocytes throughout the body from one lymphoid organ to another via blood and lymph is not an at random process. The extravasation of blood-born lymphocytes into the parenchyma of lymphoid organs, the spleen excepted, occurs in the venules of the T cell areas, which are lined by high cuboidal endothelium and designated high endothelial venules (HEV). A rapid increase of HEV is seen upon antigenic stimulation, so facilitating a local recruitment of lymphocytes. Their extravasation is among others mediated by distinct adhesion structures on the HEV endothelium and specific counter structures (homing receptors) on T and B cells. Their nature is an important basis of directed lymphocyte recirculation patterns in the body. The adhesion structures of HEV in Peyer's patches, which are also found on endothelium in the lamina propria and mammary gland, are different from those in peripheral lymph nodes, while HEV from mesenteric lymph nodes express both types of adhesion structures. As counterpart, there are two distinct types of homing receptors on lymphocytes, which recognize the respective adhesion structures. Lymphocytes can express either one type or both. The in this way controlled lymphocyte traffic segregates effector cells derived from stimulation in different tissues and increases the efficiency of organ-specific immune responses. It should be noted that the expression of homing receptors on lymphocytes is an exclusive property of the recirculating pool. Sessile cells, immature lymphocytes, and lymphocytes undergoing antigen-driven differentiation and proliferation within the lymphoid tissues do not recirculate and as a cause or consequence do not express homing receptors.

Lymphocyte traffic into the spleen is via the arterial circulation. Arterioles end in the marginal sinus at the periphery of the white pulp. From there the lymphocytes enter the marginal zone and compartments of the white pulp. Besides a supply of blood-born lymphocytes, all secondary lymphoid organs, the spleen and Peyer's patches excepted, are supplied of lymphocytes via the lymph. Lymph enters lymph nodes via the afferent lymphatic vessels that end in the subcapsular sinuses lying just under the lymph node capsule. The sinuses are drained by sinusoids in the paracortex and medulla, and terminate in the hilum where they form the efferent lymphatics.

2. MOLECULES

Numerous circulating, cell-bound and intracellular molecules contribute to normal immune system function. Classification of the molecules by their function is not useful, since generally most molecules exert various functions. Tables 2 and 3 give a compilation of some of the molecules or molecular complexes expressed on the surface of lymphocytes and, if known, their major roles in the immune response. Almost all these structures on the cell surface are nowadays routinely demonstrated with monoclonal antibodies coupled to a suitable signal molecule (fluorochrome, enzyme, gold label) or with antibodies and complement in a cytotoxicity assay. The reagents have become powerful tools for phenotyping and recognizing cells of the immune system for their class, subclass and state of maturation and/or activation. In terms of function, the surface expression of different molecules during maturation and their up or down regulation during antigen-induced cell activation provides the immune system of regulatory mechanisms by which particular subsets of cells can be selectively influenced or influence other cells.

In this paragraph we will focus on a few types of pivotal molecules in immune reactions, viz. proteins encoded by genes of the major histocompatibility complex, cell-bound leukocyte function-associated antigens, interleukins, antibodies and complement.

(a) Major histocompatibility complex (MHC) molecules

MHC molecules have initially been identified by serology and as target molecules in transplant rejection reactions. They, therefore, are often denoted transplantation antigens. Two major types of MHC-encoded molecules can be distinguished by their structure and function, class I and class II molecules. In mice and rats particular class I molecules are also encoded by the TLA (thymus-leukemia antigen) gene complex near the MHC. In man there is evidence for a similar gene complex. The tissue distribution of the MHC class I and II molecules is different. MHC class I molecules are expressed on all nucleated cells and platelets of humans, mice and rats. In the latter two species they are also found on erythrocytes. Class II expression is normally restricted to B cells, activated T cells, cells of the monocyte/macrophage series, endothelial cells, and epithelial cells. Class I molecules consist of two polypeptide chains. The larger polypeptide is encoded by the MHC. It is non-covalently linked to β_2-microglobulin, a small polypeptide encoded by a gene located at an other chromosome. Class II molecules consist of two non-covalently linked polypeptide chains encoded by the MHC. The MHC and its molecular products perform similar functions in different species, but the gene arrangements and the designation of the components are different. Table 4 shows the nomenclature of the MHC and the

TABLE 4

Gene complexes and the encoded class I and II molecules

	Man	Mouse		Rat	
MHC	HLA	H-2		RT1^a	
TLA complex			TLA		TLA
Chromosome	6	17	17		
Class I gene regions	B, C, A	K, D	Qa, Tla	F, H, A, E^b G, C	
Loci	B, C, A	K, D, L, R	Qa$_2$, Qa$_3$, Tla, Qa$_1$	A$_\alpha$, E$_\alpha$^{b} C$_\alpha$	
Class II gene regions	D	I		B, D	
Loci	SB$_\alpha$, DC$_\alpha$, DR$_\alpha$^{b} SB$_\beta$, DC$_\beta$, DR$_\beta$	A$_\alpha$, A$_\beta$, E$_\beta$, E$_\alpha$		B$_\alpha$, B$_\beta$, D$_\alpha$, D$_\beta$^{b}	
Specificities (serologic)	DP, DQ, DR	I-A, I-E			

The order of the gene regions in man is D, B, C, A; in mice K, I, D, Qa, Tla. Gene regions of the MHC encoding for complement components, sometimes referred to as class III molecules, have not been included.
^{a} Previously called Ag-B and H-1.
^{b} Precise order of regions or loci is not known.

TLA complex and their main products in the species man, mouse and rat. The nomenclature is rather confusing. For instance, the class II molecules of the mouse MHC, termed H-2 (histocompatibility-2), are encoded by genes of the I (capital i) region. Subregions of H-2I are frequently referred to as I-A and I-E, while their protein products are usually designated as Ia (I region-associated) antigens. Further, the genes of the MHC class II region of man (human leukocyte antigen-D; HLA-D), mice (H-2I) and rats (RT1.B and RT1.D) are very commonly called Ir (Immune response) genes.

In a random population the protein encoded by a gene at a particular MHC locus, for instance H-2K, is usually different between two individuals because of variant fine structure in some parts of the molecule. This polymorphism is seen for all class I and II molecules and is the result of multiple different alleles at each known locus. Differences in fine structures are demonstrated with a panel of allo-antisera and are distinguished in public and private specificities. Public specificities are found on some but not all K proteins, while private specificities are unique to a particular K protein. The whole set of public and private specificities of all the class I and class II molecules expressed by an individual makes up its MHC haplotype. In mice and rats the haplotype is indicated by a superscript, for example $H-2^d$ or $RT1^a$. The same is done with the polypeptide chains and the complete molecules. For instance the recombinant inbred mouse strain B10.A(2R) has the $H-2^{h4}$ haplotype, which is characterized by K^k, $I-A^k$ ($I-A_\alpha^k$, $I-A_\beta^k$), $I-E^d$ ($I-E_\alpha^d$, $I-E_\beta^d$), D^b. In man the average chance to find two individuals with the same MHC haplotype for the major HLA loci, A, B, C, and D, is estimated to be 1 : 20 000, but it varies with the haplotype. Haplotypes in man, therefore, are indicated by the specificities of the HLA molecules, for instance HLA-A1, A13, B3, B7, C2, C2, DR3, DR4.

Polymorphic differences between MHC haplotypes are usually based on a single or a few amino acid substitutions. Nevertheless, MHC molecules act as potent immunogens, i.e. transplantation antigens, in haplotype non-identical recipients. Strong immunogenicity in allograft situations, however, cannot be considered as the normal physiological function of the MHC molecules. Their main function is the regulation of several aspects of the immune response, particularly at the level of the T cell, because activation of any T cell is dependent on an interaction of its antigen receptor with a specific combination of foreign antigen and a self-MHC molecule. The formation of the MHC/antigen complex seems to be determined by the kind of antigen fragments created by the antigen-presenting cells, and the antigen fragment 'selected' by an MHC molecule to be presented to the T cell. The latter is influenced by polymorphic determinants in MHC molecules, which are involved in the binding of the antigen fragments. T cell activation, therefore, frequently differs between individuals with a different haplotype, both with regard to the antigenic fragment to which a T cell response is directed and the degree of activation. These processes also underlie the association of diseases with particular MHC haplotypes in animals and man.

(b) Leukocyte function-associated antigens

A second group of cell-bound molecules consists of the so-called leukocyte function-associated antigens (LFA). The molecules are required for mutual cell-cell contact between leukocytes, and between leukocytes and other cells. Three different types of LFA have been recognized, LFA-1, LFA-2, and LFA-3. LFA-1 belongs with the receptors for the complement components iC3b (CR3) and iC3b, C3d and C3dg (CR4) to a family of dimeric glycoproteins with identical β chains (CD18) and different α chains, designated CD11a, CD11b and CD11c, respectively. LFA-1 is found on all leukocytes and is involved in antigen- and lectin-induced T and B cell proliferation and in cytotoxicity mediated by cytotoxic T lymphocytes, NK cells and macrophages. Further, a role of LFA-1 in the extravasation of lymphocytes in the HEV has been claimed. The indispensibility of LFA-1 and congeners in normal immune system function is underscored by the recurrent life-threatening bacterial and fungal infections observed in cases of deficiency. Further, progressive periodontitis, lack of pus formation and leukocytosis are seen in such patients. A ligand recognized by LFA-1 is the so-called intercellular-adhesion molecule-1 (ICAM-1). Under normal conditions only endothelium exhibits strong ICAM-1 expression, but inflammation and cytokines like interleukin-1, tumour necrosis factor and interferon γ, induce a markedly increased expression of ICAM-1 on a large variety of other cells.

The LFA-2 molecule is better known as the sheep red blood cell receptor, T11 or CD2. It is expressed on virtually all T cells and a subset of NK cells, and serves as an interaction molecule in T cell proliferation against allogeneic class II molecules and in target cell killing by cytotoxic T lymphocytes and the NK cell subset. The counterstructure recognized by LFA-2 has been identified as LFA-3. This molecule is not only expressed on all blood leukocytes, but also on endothelium, fibroblasts, and smooth muscle cells, and in some species also on erythrocytes. Members of the LFA family probably function not merely as cellular adhesion molecules. There is evidence that LFA-1 and LFA-2 also function as signal transduction molecules for lymphocyte proliferation and differentiation.

(c) Interleukins

An important group of immunoregulating molecules is represented by the interleukins (IL). The term was introduced to indicate their production by leukocytes and their function of signalling between these cells. Also the terms lymphokines and monokines are still frequently used to denote production by lymphocytes and monocytes/macrophages, respectively. IL production, however, is generally not restricted to a single cell type, or to cells belonging to the immune system. Further, IL exert effects on various organs and cell types outside the immune system. This implies that a great number of cells all over the body express receptors for IL. A

TABLE 5

Interleukins and some of their regulatory functions in specific immunity

Factor(s)	Other names	Source	Effects
IL-1[a]	Lymphocyte activating factor, endogenous pyrogen, serum amyloid A inducer, and others	Monocytes/macrophages, and many other cell types	Promotes multiplication and activation of T and B cells; activates macrophages and NK cells; induces prostaglandin synthesis in many cell types; induces IL-6 production
IL-2	T cell derived growth factor	Helper T cells	(Co)stimulates T cell multiplication and effector functions; co-stimulates B cel multiplication and differentiation
IL-3	Mast cell growth factor, multiple colony stimulating factor, and others	Helper T cells	Stimulates mast cell multiplication; stimulates proliferation and differentiation of hemopoietic stem cells
IL-4	B cell stimulatory factor-1 B cell growth factor II, T cell growth factor II, macrophage activating factor, and others	Helper T cells, B cells[b]	Co-stimulates B cell multiplication and IgE and IgG_1 secretion; reduces IgG_{2a}, IgG_{2b}, IgG_3 and IgM secretion; enhances MHC class II expression on B cells and macrophages; T cell growth factor; activates macrophages
IL-5	T cell replacing factor, B cell growth factor II, Eosinophil differentiation factor, and others	Helper T cells	Co-stimulates B cell multiplication and antibody secretion; stimulates eosinophil differentiation
IL-6	Hybridoma growth factor, B cell differentiation factor, interferon-β_2, B cell stimulatory factor-2, and others	T cells, monocytes, fibroblasts	Co-stimulates growth and differentiation of B cells; co-promotes IL-2 production by mature T cells
Interferon-α[a]		Leukocytes	Differentiation of B cells; increases IgM and IgG production; enhances MHC class I expression lymphoid cells; potentiates IL-1 production by macrophages
Interferon-β_1		Fibroblasts, epithelial cells	Potentiates IL-1 production and decreases prostaglandin E production by macrophages

TABLE 5 (*continued*)

Factor(s)	Other names	Source	Effects
Interferon-γ	Macrophage activating factor	Helper T cells, cytotoxic T cells	Enhances MHC class II expression on macrophages; activates macrophages; induces MHC class II expression on epithelial and endothelial cells; antagonizes IL-4 effects on B cells; stimulates B cell multiplication and differentiation
Lymphotoxin[a]	Tumour necrosis factor β	Lymphocytes, NK cells	Effector molecule of T cell mediated cytostasis and cytolysis
Tumour necrosis factor	Tumour necrosis factor α, cachectin	Monocytes/macrophages, and other cell types	Enhances IL-2 receptor expression of T cells; inhibits antibody secretion; activates macrophages; (Co)promotes MHC class I and or II expression on various cells; induces IL-6

[a] Various subclasses have been found.
[b] The B cell product is very similar, if not identical, to the T cell product.

brief compilation of some major IL and their main effects on specific immune reactions has been given in Table 5. Actions of some molecules will be discussed in more detail below. The knowledge of IL and their function has explosively increased by the recent availability of highly purified molecules, produced by recombinant DNA techniques. It has become obvious that most, if not all, IL have multiple target cells in the immune system and that many of their effects are either dependent on or influenced by the concomitant action of other IL. The same is true for the control of the production of these molecules. This insight gives an indication of how the immune system with relatively few different cells and signalling molecules can efficiently perform a large variety of well-controlled reactions. Besides inter-interleukin control of immune reactions, IL also trigger feedback reactions by other systems. For example, IL-1 induces prostaglandin E production in a variety of cells, and glucocorticoid synthesis by stimulation of the pituitary-adrenal axis. These molecules, in their turn, can inhibit the immune response by various mechanisms, among others by down-regulation of IL synthesis at both the pretranslational and posttranslational level.

(d) Antibodies

In the strict sense, antibodies can be designated as IL. The molecules not only serve to eliminate foreign antigens, but also have, just like IL, a variety of immunoregulatory functions. Some of these are mediated by the Fc portion of the molecules, constituted by the C-terminal constant region of the H chains, upon binding to Fc receptors of a cell. Fc-mediated binding of antigen-complexed antibodies to macrophages, granulocytes and NK cells usually stimulates the cells to cytotoxicity or enhanced phagocytic capacity. If antigen-presenting cells are involved, this can lead to enhanced antibody formation by a more efficient antigen presentation to helper T cells. Most Fc-mediated signals, however, suppress antibody responses, especially those delivered by IgG molecules. After binding of IgG to B cells with the same antigen specificity, antigen causes direct down-regulation of B cell activation by cross-linking of antigen receptors and Fc receptors. The negative signal can be overcome by helper T cell factors, like IL-4 and IL-5. This kind of suppression, therefore, is only seen in the relative absence of T cell help. This is not the case with B cell suppression caused by T suppressor cells triggered by Fc-mediated binding of IgG. A mechanism that is supposed to counteract Fc-mediated suppression, is the formation of IgM antibodies directed towards the Fc portion of various subclasses of IgG. Production of these antibodies, known as rheuma factors, is a physiological concomitant of normal, notably secondary, immune responses to antigens and comes to an end when antigens disappear. If its production is less well controlled, however, disease may result.

Besides control of antibody formation by Fc-mediated interactions, control by interactions via antigen-combining sites occurs. This has been called idiotypic regulation, since the variable and hypervariable regions of the antigen-combining site constitute the idiotype of an antibody. The idiotypes can act as antigenic determinants, and can evoke the production of anti-idiotype antibodies. Thus, an antigen stimulates both the production of specific antibodies with particular idiotypes and anti-idiotype antibodies. These, in their turn, can induce anti-anti-idiotype antibodies and so on. In this way an idiotypic network is formed, which maintains a persistent state of activity via idiotypic-anti-idiotypic interactions. Its function is far from understood, but the network may contribute to homeostatic control of the antibody response, and direct the idiotypic repertoire of the antibody response. Idiotypic regulation, however, is complex and not well understood. This is illustrated by the ability of anti-idiotype antibodies to stimulate or suppress antibody responses towards an antigen. Stimulation of B cells may be caused by cross-linking idiotype-expressing surface immunoglobulins. In fact, the idiotype of anti-idiotype antibodies frequently mimicks the original antigen, being their 'internal image', and as such the antibodies can substitute for the antigen. The antibodies, however, contain Fc portions that can switch on feedback inhibitory signals, as mentioned above.

Idiotypic regulation appears not to be restricted to antibodies. There is ample evidence that helper and suppressor T cells function in part by idiotype specific interactions with antibodies, B cells and other T cells.

(e) Complement

A group of non-antigen-specific molecules with important defensive and regulatory functions is represented by the components of the complement system. Complement consists of a series of proteinase precursors that can be sequentially activated, i.e. a precursor enzyme is activated by the previously activated component through splitting off a small molecular weight peptide. An exception is formed by the third complement factor, C3, which shows a slow 'tick-over' in the steady state. The activation events are well-controlled by many inhibitory and regulatory proteins. Classical pathway activation of complement cascade is initiated by triggering of the first component (C1). The activation signal is usually delivered by the Fc portion of antibodies bound to antigen, for example a foreign cell or pathogen. Some tumour cells and virus-infected cells and many pathogens can also directly enhance activation of the third component in the absence of antibodies, in the so-called alternative pathway activation. The major complement components generated during activation bind as complex to the cell membrane. This can finally lead to lysis of the cell by formation of a transmembrane tube, in which the terminal complement components C5b till C9 are involved. Many pathogens, however, are resistant to complement-mediated lysis and can only be killed inside phagocytic cells. This process is facilitated by complement and termed opsonization. Binding of the activated third and fourth complement components, C3b and C4b, to the membrane of cells promotes their adherence to and ingestion by phagocytic cells through the C3b (CR1; CD35) and C4b (CR2) receptor. The process is independent of adherence and ingestion mediated by the Fc portion of antibodies, although antibody can mediate the deposition of the opsonizing complement components by classical pathway activation. Complement components also facilitate the removal of circulating immune complexes by phagocytic cells.

The released small molecular split products of the third and fifth complement factor, C3a and C5a, are known as anaphylatoxins. They promote inflammation by causing mast cell degranulation, lysosomal enzyme release, smooth muscle contraction and enhanced vascular permeability. C5a is 10 – 20 times more active than C3a in these respects. In addition, C5a is chemotactic for neutrophils, causes their margination to the endothelial lining of blood vessels, and triggers the bactericidal oxidative burst in these cells.

The beneficial role of complement in the elimination of pathogens and immune complexes is beyond doubt, but complement can be harmful to the organism by promoting inflammatory reactions. Tissue destruction can be the result. The pathological processes are known as antibody-dependent cytotoxic hypersensitivity and immune complex-mediated hypersensitivity, and underly the symptomatology of immune complex diseases and several autoimmune diseases, irrespective of the etiology.

Some complement components, particularly split products of C3 and C5, were shown to regulate specific immune responses. Generally, C3 split products inhibit lymphocyte blastogenesis and induction of antibody responses, while C5 split products are stimulatory. Further, complement components, especially C3, mediate adequate retention of antigen in the form of antigen-antibody complexes in the lymph node follicles. Such a retention is needed for IgG antibody formation upon primary immunization, and for induction of B cell memory. Finally, complement split products interfere with other activation systems of the body, like the coagulation system and the kallikrein system. Mediators generated from these systems can, in their turn, influence the immune system, but to a limited extent.

III. Antigens

1. DEFINITIONS

Immunogenicity is a property of a substance making it capable to provoke a detectable immune response when introduced into an organism. Such a substance is called an immunogen. The term antigen is frequently used instead, although the term has a broader meaning. It can also indicate that the substance can combine with an antibody of appropriate specificity, without implicitly pointing to immunogenicity.

Most natural antigens, like infective organisms, are composed of a set of many different molecules. Only a limited number of molecules appear to be involved in immune reactions to such infective agents and generally the response is directed only to some portions of these molecules. These constitute the antigenic determinants. If they are responsible for the induction of the immune response, the term immunogenic determinant is to be preferred. Immunogenic determinants for T cells have two distinct binding sites, called epitope and agretope. The epitope is specifically recognized by the T cell receptor, while the agretope is responsible for the interaction with the MHC class II molecule.

2. REQUISITES FOR IMMUNOGENICITY

Immunogenicity of a substance is dependent on intrinsic physical and chemical properties of the substance itself as well as other factors, like mode of encounter and various properties of the organism encountering the substance. Despite the wide variety of conditions that define immunogenicity of substances, some broad generalities can be made. These will be dealt with briefly.

(a) Foreignness

The ability of a normally functioning immune system to somehow discriminate between self and non-self components as to initiating an immune response implicates that only foreign antigens are immunogenic under normal conditions. In this respect it is probably correct to distinguish circulating self-antigens and tissue-specific self-antigens. Only the latter antigens, for example testis and brain antigens, can readily induce autoimmune reactions after immunization in conjunction with appropriate adjuvants.

(b) Molecular size

As a general rule substances with a molecular weight below 10 000 are poor immunogens, if immunogenic at all. The immunogenicity appears to increase with increasing molecular weight. Chemically reactive small molecular weight compounds, however, may induce specific immune reactions after binding to larger self-components. A classical example are penicillins and their metabolites. They bind to plasma proteins and can induce specific antibodies. Such small molecular weight compounds are called haptens. In the given example the haptens constitute immunogenic determinants for B cells, but binding of haptens can create immunogenic determinants for T cells as well. There is evidence that such events may underly induction of autoimmune reactions by small molecular weight compounds, as will be addressed by Allison in Chapter 3 in this book.

(c) Chemical complexity

Immunogens are rarely monotonous molecules like homopolymers, regardless of size. More heterogenously constituted molecules, especially those containing aromatic residues, generally have increased immunogenic potential. This may, in part, be related to the observations that aromatic groups are frequently included in the immunogenic determinants.

(d) Presence and accessibility of epitopes

Most natural antigens have to be recognized by different subsets of T cells, or both by T cells and B cells, to initiate an immune reaction. Thus, an antigen must contain accessible epitopes for these cells. The epitopes for B and T cells on protein antigens are almost without exception distinct. B cells preferentially recognize tertiairy structures on native proteins that are lost on denaturation. On the other hand, T cells do not distinguish between native and denatured proteins as antigen. Immunogenic T cell determinants from proteins investigated so far, appear to be peptide sequences of about 10 amino acids that assume an α-helix conformation. In the conformation the hydrophobic and hydrophilic side chains appear to line up on opposite sides, thereby forming the agretope and epitope, respectively.

It has been found that distinct T cell epitopes can contribute to antibody formation against one B cell epitope. Also, one T cell epitope can contribute to antibody formation against different B cell epitopes, provided that the T and B cell epitopes are not too close together.

Protein antigens can also contain suppressor determinants. These are much less defined, but the determinants appear capable to reduce or prevent immune responses to the whole molecule.

(e) Physico-chemical properties

Properties of antigens that are not perceived as immunologically specific signals can influence immunogenicity. Bacterial pathogens, for example, contain a lot of compounds that can non-specifically enhance or modify specific immune reactions to antigens exposed by the pathogens. Such compounds are referred to as adjuvants and will be addressed by Hilgers et al., in Chapter 11. Antigens consisting of a single molecule can also have intrinsic adjuvanticity. Properties like resistance to degradation, lipophilicity and ionic charge are known to influence antigen processing and localization, but it is beyond the scope of this chapter to go into further detail.

(f) Dose and mode of administration

Immunogenicity is highly defined by the dose and route of antigen and the frequency of administration. Generally, bell-shaped curves are seen on systemic administration of a range of doses of antigen. Too low or too high doses of antigen may induce specific unresponsiveness (tolerance), attributed to a temporal or more persistent functional elimination of antigen-specific T and B cells, respectively.

Systemic administration of antigen tends to favour antibody production, while the dermal route facilitates induction of T cell mediated immunity. Oral antigen encounter frequently leads to tolerance. By use of suitable adjuvants, however, the mode of immune response and its intensity can be modified. Adjuvants are also capable of preventing induction of tolerance and can even abolish established tolerance.

(g) Host factors

The genetic make-up of an organism plays a crucial role in its ability to mount an immune response to antigens. Not only the MHC haplotype is important in this respect, but non-MHC 'immune response' genes can have considerable influence as well. As a matter of fact, the immune response is under polygenic control. With so-called Biozzi mice the importance of genes controlling antigen processing by macrophages has been demonstrated. Biozzi mice are genetically stable lines of mice with high or low antigen-specific immune responsiveness to a panel of antigens. Such mouse lines are obtained from an outbred population by selective mating of brothers and sisters with either a high or low immune response to a particular antigen for 20 generations. The in this way obtained low responder line shows a high degree of antigen uptake and degradation by macrophages, and a short persistence of surface antigen expression, while the high responder line shows quite the opposite macrophage functions. Interestingly, the low responders demonstrate an increased non-specific resistance to intracellular pathogens as compared to the high responders.

Immune responsiveness is also influenced by the condition of the organism. Many factors including diet, medication, environmental agents, infections and other diseases are known to change the immune response in various ways. Studies on immune response modifiers have shown that their effects are highly dependent on the kind of modifier, route, dose and time of administration, all in relation to the particular antigen, host species, genetic make-up and other factors. Thus, effects of undeliberately encountered immune response modifiers are usually hard to predict and to evaluate.

IV. The immune response

1. HELPER T CELL ACTIVATION

The vast majority of antigens encountering the immune system are T cell dependent antigens, i.e. helper T cells have to be activated by the antigen to induce an immune response of whatever type. The few natural compounds that are T cell independent antigens comprise, usually mitogenic, polysaccharides with repeating antigenic determinants, for instance the lipopolysaccharides of gram-negative bacteria.

The induction of a specific immune response against foreign T cell dependent antigens manifests some main features: (a) encounter of the antigen and recognition as foreign substance; (b) amplification and diversification of the specific reaction; (c) effector reactions leading to elimination of the antigen; (d) memory induction, leading to accelerated and enhanced responses upon renewed antigen encounter. Normally, antigens enter the body via the skin or mucous surfaces of the respiratory, gastrointestinal or urogenital tracts. At these locations antigen encounters antigen-presenting cells. Most antigen-presenting cells belong to the monocyte/macrophage series. In skin epidermis they are represented by the Langerhans cells. After ingestion by the Langerhans cells, antigen is partially degraded or denatured. Then portions of the antigen, containing the immunogenic determinants, are associated with MHC class II molecules, and presented at the surface membrane. These events are known as antigen processing. The mechanisms underlying the processing are still not well understood, but are obviously influenced by the nature of the antigen. Some antigens probably do not require any intracellular processing at all. Subsequently, the Langerhans cells migrate via the lymph to the draining lymph node. During transport the cells can be recognized morphologically as so-called veiled macrophages. Upon arrival in the subcapsular sinus the veiled macrophages migrate to the paracortex and change their morphology to become interdigitating cells. The cells and their numerous protrusions have an intimate contact with many surrounding T cells with the helper phenotype, and so facilitate the presentation of processed antigen to helper T cells.

Antigens not always need to be transported by antigen-presenting cells to the draining lymph nodes. Antigens and antigenic fragments secreted after degradation in macrophages and granulocytes also may be carried free in solution to the lymph node and trapped by local antigen-presenting cells in the B or T cell areas. Lymphoid tissues along mucosal surfaces, e.g. the Peyers patches, are almost directly accessible to notably particulate antigens. Only passage of the flattened epithelium overlying the Peyer's patches is needed to enter the follicular or interfollicular areas. The epithelium is specialized for this purpose by the presence of so-called M (microfold) cells. After entrance antigen is ingested by macrophages and presented locally or, after transport, in the draining mesenteric lymph nodes. Soluble protein antigens in the gut lumen hardly enter Peyer's patches, but are ingested by enterocytes of the villi and end up in antigen-processing cells of the lamina propria. Antigens entering the body via the blood are mainly trapped by liver and spleen. In the liver the antigens are usually completely degraded, notably by Kupffer cells, and not presented to the immune system. Processing and presentation of T cell dependent antigens in the spleen are essentially similar as in lymph nodes. In addition, the spleen is essential for induction of primary immune responses to non-mitogenic T cell independent antigens, such as dextran and polyvinylpyrrolidone. These antigens are presented to B cells by specialized antigen-presenting cells, the marginal zone macrophages.

The helper T cell to which antigen is presented by the antigen-presenting interdigitating cells in a primary response expresses receptors which bind the foreign antigen in association with polymorphic determinants of a self-MHC class II molecule. The binding is intensified by an interaction of the CD4 molecules with a non-polymorphic determinant of the class II molecules, and probably also by binding of LFA-1 to its counterstructure. The final result is cross-linking of the antigen receptors and the generation of transmembrane signals by the CD3 molecules of the T cell receptor. Subsequently, the second messenger molecules diacylglycerol and inositol-1,4,5-triphosphate are formed, and the activation proceeds with DNA, RNA, and protein synthesis. The process of T cell activation is supported by IL-1 produced by the antigen-presenting cells. It induces in association with antigen stimulation the expression of high-affinity IL-2 receptors (IL-2R) on the T cell membrane and stimulates the T cells to release the growth-promoting IL-2. In this way, a rather selective expansion of the antigen-activated T cells is induced in an autocrine or paracrine manner. Resting lymphocytes, however, can be activated in the absence of antigen by rather high concentrations of IL-2. This effect is mediated through the low-affinity receptor for IL-2, IL-2R$_\beta$, a peptide chain that is constitutively expressed on the T cell membrane in moderate amounts. Antigens trigger enhanced IL-2R$_\beta$ expression and induce the surface expression of IL-2R$_\alpha$ chains, known as the Tac antigen. The associated α and β chain constitute the high-affinity IL-2 receptor, that confers responsiveness to low concentrations of IL-2.

Following activation of helper T cells, the antigen-specific immune response starts its diversification. Three main types of immune reactions can be generated: antibody responses, cytolytic T cell responses and delayed-type hypersensitivity responses.

2. ANTIBODY RESPONSES

For antibody or humoral responses, surface immunoglobulins of B cells have to recognize the same antigenic fragment as the helper T cells, but the immunogenic determinants recognized by the respective cells on the antigenic fragment are essentially different. Antigen-specific activation of resting B cells is known to be restricted by MHC class II molecules on the B cell membrane. Whether the activation involves an interaction between the B cells and helper T cells or B cells and antigen-presenting cells is not known. Direct T-B cell interaction is thought to be mediated by mutual antigen recognition and binding of MHC class II molecules by the T cells. Antigen-presenting cells may interact with the B cells by collecting antigen-specific helper T cell factors on their membrane, which bind both the antigen and MHC class II molecules. The cell-cell interaction finally leads to cross-linking of the immunoglobulin receptors and the generation of the same intracellular second messengers as in antigen-activated T cells. Full clonal expansion, heavy chain class switch and further differentiation to antibody-secreting plasma cells, however, is dependent on helper factors synthesized by T cells (Table 5). In the mouse not all antigen-specific CD4$^+$ helper T cells appear to have the same capacity to do so. Therefore, two different types of T cells have been distinguished, T$_H$1 and T$_H$2. The T$_H$1 type cells produce IL-2 and interferon γ, and provide moderate B cell help, while the T$_H$2 type cells produce IL-4 and IL-5, and provide strong B cell help.

The exact location of B cell stimulation short after antigen stimulation in a primary immune response to T cell dependent antigens is not known. A few days after antigen stimulation germinal centres arise in the follicles of the stimulated lymph nodes. These can be identified histologically by a central light area in the follicles containing large-sized proliferating B cells, starry sky macrophages and follicular dendritic cells. The latter cells are specialized reticulum cells of uncertain origin (bone marrow or mesenchyme) with antigen-presenting function. They do not process antigen, but retain it in the form of antigen-antibody complexes on their dendritic processes by a complement-dependent mechanism. Antigens bound in this form can persist for very long times and cause a continuous activation of the B cells, so contributing to the persistence of B cell memory. In the absence of persistent antigen, B cell memory is short-lived and negligible. A role of helper T cells and their products in the ongoing B cell stimulation is presupposed by the presence of helper T cells in the germinal centres, but not exactly defined.

Whereas the germinal centres are the sites of B cell proliferation, memory B cell formation and probably heavy chain class switch, the plasma cells generated in a primary response are found at the periphery of the germinal centres and more prominently in the medullary cords. The antibodies produced by the plasma cells in the lymph nodes are mainly IgM and IgG and are drained via the lymph to the blood. In the lymphoid tissues belonging to the MALT the major class of antibody produced is IgA. Most of the synthesized IgA is dimeric and appears in the mucosal fluids with a polypeptide chain, called secretory component, attached to it. The polypeptide is synthesized by epithelial cells. It is required for the transport of IgA across the epithelium into the lumen and renders the molecule more resistant to the nonphysiologic conditions in the alimentary and respiratory tract. Part of the dimeric IgA synthesized at external sites can enter the blood circulation and so contribute to the internal host defence. In rodents the dimeric IgA in the blood is efficiently removed by the liver. Their hepatocytes express secretory component, that acts as receptor for the dimeric IgA and facilitates the transport into the bile and from there into the gut lumen. In other species, like dog, rabbit, and man this transport way does not exist, as the hepatocytes do not express secretory component.

Serum IgA in rodents is predominantly dimeric, but in man only 10% is dimeric and polymeric. The origin of serum IgA in man is not fully elucidated, but circumstantial evidence indicates that part of it is derived from the MALT. In rodents a large portion of serum dimeric IgA is derived from the MALT. Also IgA formation by spleen and peripheral lymph nodes upon oral or parenteral immunization with certain antigens contributes to the serum IgA pool.

On second encounter of antigen the antibody response is quantitatively and qualitatively different from the primary antibody response. Secondary antibody responses have accelerated kinetics and the amount of antibody produced is much higher. Further, the affinity of the antibodies is usually much greater. This is attributed to a more selective expansion of clones with higher affinity to the antigen, but somatic mutation during clonal expansion is thought to be involved as well. The contribution of IgM to the response has been markedly decreased, in favour of IgG production. The site of antibody production changes as well. Whereas the antibody production in primary responses is mainly restricted to plasma cells in the stimulated lymphoid organs, the antibody production in secondary and subsequent responses is usually more systemic, since memory B cells have become distributed all over the body as a consequence of recirculation. A considerable portion of antibody forma-

60

tion in secondary-type responses occurs in the bone marrow, especially after systemic immunization.

The main function of antibodies in the organism is elimination of antigens from circulation and tissues, and prevention of the entrance of antigens into the body via the mucosal surfaces. Elimination can occur by lysis of antibody-coated cells in cooperation with complement (see above) or by Fc-mediated phagocytosis of antigen-antibody complexes. Monocytes, macrophages and natural killer cells can also kill antibody-coated extracellular pathogens or cells after binding through the Fc-receptors. This process is known as antibody-dependent cell-mediated cytotoxicity (ADCC).

3. CYTOTOXIC T LYMPHOCYTE RESPONSES

As mentioned above, helper T cell involvement in immune system function is not restricted to humoral immunity. T cell help is also required for the formation of cytotoxic T lymphocytes (CTL) from precursor cells in a primary response. CTL have initially been studied for their cytotoxic action against cells with allogeneic MHC molecules, leading to transplant rejections. Later, it has been recognized that tumour cells, viruses, intracellular bacteria and several other antigens, including synthetic small molecular weight compounds (haptens), can elicit CTL. In these instances, only those virus-infected or antigen-bearing target cells are lysed which display MHC molecules of the same haplotype as the precursor CTL. CTL and their precursors differ in some respects from helper T cells. They express CD8 molecules instead of CD4 molecules and display MHC class I restriction instead of class II restriction. It should be realized, however, that this is not a general rule. Among others, class II restricted CD4$^+$ or CD8$^+$ CTL and class I restricted CD8$^+$ helper T cells have been found. The antigen receptor of class I restricted precursor CTL is similar to that of helper T cells, i.e. a CD3 molecule linked to an antigen recognition unit consisting of a polymorphic, α,β-heterodimer.

Activation of MHC class I restricted precursor CTL by foreign antigens, like viruses, as well as allogeneic cells requires accessory antigen-presenting cells and helper T cells. CD4$^+$ helper T cells recognize either viral antigens or allogeneic class I molecules in the context of self class II molecules on the antigen-presenting cells. The helper cells then aid the development of CTL from CD8$^+$ precursor CTL. The latter cells acquire sensitivity to T cell help after binding the viral antigens in association with self-MHC class I molecules or the allogeneic class I molecules. In an allogeneic response help can also be generated by CD4$^+$ or CD8$^+$ helper T cells after recognition of allogeneic class II and class I molecules, respectively, on the allogeneic accessory cells. Thus, allogeneic MHC molecules apparently resemble self-MHC molecules associated with foreign antigen fragments. This is also indicated by observations that many allospecific T cells cross-reactively recognize self-MHC in the context of conventional foreign antigens.

The need for helper T cells in the generation of CTL can probably be reduced to the need for IL-2. Precursor CTL react with an upregulation of their IL-2 receptors after antigen recognition, but not with the production of IL-2. In the presence of IL-2, proliferation and acquisition of cytolytic activity ensues. The cytolytic process can be divided in various stages and is cyclic, i.e. after lysis of a target cell the CTL can interact with additional targets. The conjugation between CTL and target starts with the recognition of allogeneic or antigen-altered class I molecules. The cell-cell interaction is intensified on the one hand by interactions of the CD8 molecule with non-polymorphic determinants of class I molecules, and on the other hand by binding of the adhesion molecules LFA-1 (CD11a) and LFA-2 (CD2) to their ligands. The conjugation does not require protein, RNA and DNA synthesis, but it is an energy- and Mg^{2+}-dependent process. Subsequent events are energy-independent, but are inhibited by increased cAMP levels in the effector cell. The lysis of the target cells is the result of the formation of a hydrophobic pore through the membrane of the target cell, which is very similar to the complement lesion. The pores are formed by polymerization of pore-forming proteins (polyperforins, cytolysins) stored in the granula of the CTL and released into the gap between effector and target cell. Killing by the CTL can continue until the granula are exhausted and can be regenerated by IL-2. Pore-forming proteins are not the only cytotoxic effector molecules of CTL. Non-pore-forming cytotoxic molecules, like lymphotoxins, tumour necrosis factor, interferons and neutral proteases may be induced concomitantly. Most of these molecules are known to bind to target cells via specific receptors and have a more restricted array of target cells than the pore-forming proteins. Generally, their mode of action is not yet well understood. Also their contribution to CTL-mediated killing is not clear.

During a primary CTL response memory cells with specificity for the antigen are generated. The duration of memory is among others dependent on the kind of antigen. In general, memory cells induced by allogeneic cells seem more persistent than those induced by small molecular weight compounds. Further, the duration of memory differs as to the species, being much shorter in mice than in man. The need for helper T cells in secondary CTL responses has not been studied very extensively. There is evidence that secondary responses are largely, if not completely, independent of helper T cells, unless the dose of antigen in the challenge is very low.

Apart from the 'true', MHC-restricted CTL that recognize antigen through the α,β-heterodimer, other T cells with cytotoxic capacity exist. In mice and humans a small subset of $CD2^+$, $CD3^+$, $CD4^-$, $CD8^-$ cytotoxic T cells has been recognized. The cells are able to kill allogeneic and syngeneic tumour cells without prior antigenic stimulation or apparent MHC restriction. The cells do not utilize the CD3-linked α,β-heterodimer of classical CTL for antigen recognition. Instead they express a γ,γ- or γ,δ-dimer in association with CD3. The dimers possess variable domains, indicative of reactions with a polymorphic ligand. The variability of the γ chain, however, is limited in comparison with α and β chains. Thus the cells, frequently referred to as Tγ cells, probably have a restricted antigen recognition repertoire. Other lymphoid cells with MHC non-restricted killer activity and the ability to mediate antibody-dependent cell-mediated cytotoxicity have the phenotype: $CD2^+$, $CD3^-$, $CD4^-$, $CD8^{+/-}$, Fc receptor$^+$. Such NK cells are probably important in the immune system for their ability to kill virus-infected cells, especially when virus-specific CTL have not yet been generated. Further, they play a role in the prevention of tumour metastasis and in artificial models of bone marrow graft rejection. NK cell function is stimulated by interferons that are produced by virus-infected cells, lymphocytes and, upon activation by the target cell, by NK cells themselves. The interferons act by transforming non-cytolytic precursor cells into a lytic state, by enhancing the lytic capacity and the array of target cells of already activated NK cells. Further, interferons induce IL-2 receptors on NK progenitors and so promote their proliferation in response to IL-2. In these ways helper T cells can stimulate NK cell function. On the other hand, interferons can induce T cells to inhibit NK cell activity. The cytotoxic effector mechanisms of NK cells are probably very similar to those of CTL.

4. DELAYED TYPE HYPERSENSITIVITY

The third major type of immunity in which helper T cells are required is delayed-type hypersensitivity (DTH). DTH is a generic term for T cell induced inflammatory reactions that become manifest about 24 – 96 h after application of antigen to sensitized individuals. In a locally challenged skin the reaction can be characterized by erythema and induration, as seen in the classical example of the Mantoux reaction in individuals sensitized to *Mycobacterium tuberculosis*. The macroscopic and microscopic aspects of DTH reactions, however, can vary considerably between different antigens in the same species and among different species.

DTH reactions are initiated by antigen-specific and MHC-restricted activation of T cells. The activated T cells release, besides interferon-γ and IL-2, numerous other mediators that cause, among others, enhanced vasopermeability, chemotaxis of granulocytes and monocytes, and retention and activation of monocytes/macrophages. The macrophages, in their turn, release IL-1 and probably tumour necrosis factor, both capable to activate granulocytes, and to co-stimulate T cell proliferation. The whole reaction results in an enhanced capacity of the phagocytes to eliminate microorganisms, virus-infected cells, and neoplastic cells either intracellularly or extracellularly by release of oxygen radicals, proteolytic enzymes and other factors. DTH reactions are not only induced against particulate antigens, but also against proteins, polysaccharides and small molecular weight compounds. In the latter instance it is usually called contact sensitivity. Further, DTH is considered to play an important role in transplant rejection.

The T cells that provide help for the triggering of DTH reactions can have the $CD4^+$ or $CD8^+$ phenotype and recognize the antigen in the context of MHC class

II or I molecules, depending on the antigen involved. They are frequently called T_{DTH} cells, but it is doubtful whether they represent a separate functional subset of T cells. For instance, it has been shown that cloned CD8$^+$ CTL against influenza-infected cells and cloned CD4$^+$ helper T cells for antibody formation against sheep erythrocytes could transfer DTH reactions to the respective antigens upon transfer in mice. That T cells are not strictly committed to a certain type of immune response is further supported by observations that induction of contact sensitivity frequently elicits a concomitant antigen-specific CTL response and that DTH reactions to various antigens are often transient and replaced by IgG antibody formation to the antigens. Also, antibody and CTL responses to the same antigen, for instance viruses, can be observed at the same time. The ability of pathogens to switch on more than one type of immune reaction does not imply that their elimination is enhanced by all the pathways. Rather, it can occur that e.g. antibody formation interferes with the elimination of pathogens by CTL or DTH.

V. Regulation of the immune response

1. FEEDBACK REGULATION

Immune responses are a necessary evil to maintain health in a non-sterile environment. They are based on a rapid amplification and activation of certain types of cells and thus inherent to a disturbance of internal homeostasis and integrity. Therefore, it is not surprising that many negative feedback signals from inside and outside the immune system are generated during an immune response. Various inhibitory control mechanisms have already been mentioned. Suppressor T cells have been mentioned only casually. Because their mode of action is subject of much controversy, and apparently very complex, suppressor T cells will be addressed only briefly. There is ample evidence that T cells can down-regulate afferent and/or efferent limbs of immune responses. Generally, it concerns CD8$^+$ cells, and their suppressive action can be directed at helper T cells, other T cells or B cells. The down-regulation can be antigen-specific, idiotype-specific or nonspecific. Some data indicate that development of suppressor activity would be the result of complex interactions of three subsets of T suppressor cells and their respective soluble suppressor factors. Evidence for the existence of T cell subsets with contrasuppressive activity suggests that the regulation is even more complex. Others, however, question whether there are distinct and specialized subsets of T cells with suppressor activity.

2. TOLERANCE

Down-regulation of immune responses not only serves to temper and to terminate

64

antigen-driven reactions, but also to prevent the onset of responses in the presence of antigen. The latter, known as tolerance, is due to antigen-specific activation of suppressor cells, and can be transferred with T cells to virgin recipients. Induction of tolerance is frequently seen after oral administration of antigens and after intravenous injection of a high dose of antigen. Unresponsiveness to antigens is not always the result of induced tolerance, but can also be due to the absence of T cells that can recognize the antigen. Whether this 'hole' in the T cell repertoire is caused by a specific deletion of the T cells during ontogeny of the immune system or is defined by the genetic make-up is not clear at present.

The tolerance phenomenon is obviously very important in the prevention of unwanted immune reactions to self-antigens. Healthy normal organisms possess autoreactive B and T cells, but activation of the cells is probably very well-controlled by regulatory mechanisms to prevent development of autoimmune disease.

Bibliography

GENERAL TEXTBOOKS

Advanced Immunology (1987) D. Male, B. Champion and A. Cooke (Eds.), J. B. Lippincott Company, Philadelphia.
Fundamental Immunology (1984) W. E. Paul (Ed.), Raven Press, New York.
General Immunology (1982) E. L. Cooper (Ed.), Pergamon Press, Oxford.
Basic and Clinical Immunology, 6 edn. (1987) D. P. Stites, J. D. Stobo and J. V. Wells (Eds.), Appleton and Lange, Norwalk, Connecticut.
Essential Immunology, 6th edn. (1988) I. M. Roitt (Ed.), Blackwell Scientific Publ., Oxford.
Immunology (1985) I. M. Roitt, J. Brostoff and D. K. Male (Eds.), Churchill Livingstone, Edinburgh.
Immunology, Immunopathology, and Immunity, 4th edn. (1987) S. Sell (Ed.), Elsevier Publ., Barking.

REVIEW JOURNALS/BOOKS

Annual Review of Immunology
Advances in Immunology
Immunological Reviews
Immunology Today
Progress in Allergy
Progress in Immunology

SELECTED REVIEWS

Nossal, G. J. V. (1987) Immunology. The basic components of the immune system. N. Engl. J. Med. 316, 1320 – 1325.

Frank, M. M. (1987) Complement in the pathology of human disease. N. Engl. J. Med. 316, 1525 – 1530.

Burdette, S. and Schwartz, R. S. (1987) Idiotypes and idiotypic networks. N. Engl. J. Med. 317, 219 – 224.

Malech, H. L. and Gallin, J. I. (1987) Neutrophils in human diseases. N. Engl. J. Med. 317, 687 – 694.

Dinarello, C. A. and Meir, J. W. (1987) Lymphokines. N. Engl. J. Med. 317, 940 – 945.

Royer, H. D. and Reinherz, E. L. (1987) T lymphocytes: ontogeny, function, and relevance to clinical disorders. N. Engl. J. Med. 317, 1136 – 1141.

Back, F. H. and Sachs, D. H. (1987) Transplantation immunology. N. Engl. J. Med. 317, 489 – 492.

Serafin, W. E. and Austen, K. F. (1987) Mediators of immediate hypersensitivity reactions. N. Engl. J. Med. 317, 30 – 34.

Cooper, M. D. (1987) B lymphocytes: normal development and function. N. Engl. J. Med. 317, 1452 – 1456.

M.E. Kammüller, N. Bloksma and W. Seinen (Eds.)
Autoimmunity and Toxicology
© *1989 Elsevier Science Publishers B.V. (Biomedical Division)*

Theories of self tolerance and autoimmunity

3

ANTHONY C. ALLISON

Department of Immunology, Syntex Research, Palo Alto, CA 94304, USA

I. Introduction

One of the fundamental concepts on which the science of immunology was founded about the beginning of the twentieth century was the recognition that animals do not as a rule make antibodies against their own body constituents. In 1900, Ehrlich and Morgenroth [1] injected goats with blood of other goats and observed the formation of antibodies able to lyse blood cells of donor goats but not those of the recipients. Ehrlich recognized that 'the organism has contrivances by means of which the immunity reaction, so easily produced by all kinds of cells, is prevented from reacting against the organism's own elements and so give rise to autotoxins . . . Only when the internal regulating contrivances are no longer intact can great dangers arise'. Thus arose the term 'horror autotoxus' [1].

The distinction between self and non-self became blurred when Traub [2] observed in 1938 that mice infected *in utero* with lymphocytic choriomeningitis virus carried the virus for the rest of their lives without detectable immune responses, whereas mice infected as adults produced a typical antibody response. In 1945, Owen [3] found that in binovular twin cattle sharing a common placenta 'erythrocyte precursors from each twin fetus had become established in the other and had conferred on their new host a tolerance towards foreign cells that lasted throughout life'. On the basis of these two observations Burnet and Fenner [4], in 1949, predicted that an antigen introduced into the body during embryonic life, before the immune system had matured, would not elicit an immune response at that time or if reintroduced later in life. They adopted Owen's designation 'tolerance' for the phenomenon. In 1953, Billingham et al. [5] reported that mice of some strains inoculated at birth with spleen cells from another strain later accept skin grafts from the donor strain, another example of acquired tolerance.

The nature of the internal regulating contrivances preventing autoimmunity postulated by Ehrlich remained without explanation until 1957 when Burnet [6], developing the clonal selection theory, proposed that the contact of antibody-forming cells with self antigens during fetal or early postnatal life leads to destruction or inactivation, with consequent elimination of the corresponding clones. In this way self-reactive clones are avoided unless they arise later in life by somatic mutation of lymphocytes. Burnet suggested that the proliferation of such mutant cells, termed forbidden clones, gives rise to self-reacting antibodies.

Burnet's classical clonal deletion hypothesis was modified in 1970 by Bretscher and Cohn [7] in their 'two signal' hypothesis, according to which contact of an antigen-reactive cell with antigen alone (signal one) in the absence of a second triggering signal from a collaborating cell (signal two) leads to irreversible inactivation of that cell.

By that time it was known that the formation of autoantibodies can easily be elicited: for example, immunization with thyroglobulin produces autoantibodies against thyroglobulin and thyroiditis, whereas immunization with testicular antigens produces antibodies against acrosomes and orchitis. It seemed inconceivable to me that the first procedure would produce somatic mutations leading to antibodies against thyroglobulin and the latter to mutations resulting in the formation of autoantibodies against acrosomes. Selection of pre-existing clones of B lymphocytes able to produce autoantibodies seemed more probable. For this reason in 1971 we challenged the interpretations of Burnet, Bretscher and Cohn, and proposed that B lymphocytes able to bind autoantigens and respond by producing autoantibodies, are not deleted or inactivated [8, 9]. We suggested that tolerance of self antigens occurs for two reasons: first, because T lymphocytes are more readily rendered unresponsive to self antigens than are B lymphocytes, and, second, because a subset of T lymphocytes can suppress the formation of autoantibodies. According to the first hypothesis, any situation that can by-pass the requirement for helper T lymphocytes reactive with self antigens can give rise to autoimmunity. Examples of such situations are infections, the use of adjuvants and graft-versus-host (GVH) reactions. For these reasons tolerance is precarious and is backed up by active suppression. Weigle [10] independently proposed a theory of selective tolerance of T cells, but made no mention of suppressor T cells which for a long time he regarded as unimportant for maintenance of immunological unresponsiveness [11].

The first prediction of our hypothesis was that B lymphocytes binding self antigens, and responding to them by production of autoantibodies, will be present in normal humans and experimental animals. We confirmed this by demonstrating in normal humans lymphocytes binding human thyroglobulin with high affinity [12]. Such autoantigen-binding cells have since been found by many other investigators and have been shown to be increased in autoimmune diseases. An extension of this prediction is that elimination of B lymphocytes binding self antigens will prevent the formation of autoantibodies and autoimmune disease. We [13] and Clagett and Weigle [14] showed that if B lymphocytes binding highly radioactive thyroglobulin are inactivated, mice do not develop autoantibodies to thyroglobulin and thyroiditis, although responses to other antigens are unimpaired. Our demonstration of autoantigen binding by B lymphocytes assumes added significance in the light of recent evidence that these cells can present antigens to T lymphocytes.

The second prediction was that if self antigens form complexes with immunogens of exogenous origin, e.g. virus antigens, which activate T lymphocytes (helper determinants), autoantibodies can be produced. An analogous situation is when exogenous antigens share determinants with self antigens; in that case exogenous T determinants can act as helpers for the formation of autoantibodies binding the shared determinants. Modification of autoantigens so as to reveal helper determinants not normally available for presentation to the immune system could have the same effect. These predictions were soon validated, as discussed below.

The third prediction was that any procedure non-specifically activating lymphocytes, such as the use of an adjuvant or a GVH reaction, should stimulate the formation of autoantibodies. Since self antigens, such as thyroglobulin administered in Freund's complete adjuvant, were known to elicit the formation of autoantibodies, the first point was already established. We used immunoglobulin (Ig) allotype markers to show that when parental lymphocytes are injected into F_1 mice and produce a GVH reaction the recipients form autoantibodies against nuclear antigens resembling those in systemic lupus erythematosus (SLE) [15]. Subsequently, there have been many investigations of autoimmunity associated with GVH reactions.

The fourth prediction was that T lymphocytes should be able to suppress manifestations of autoimmunity. In our original paper [8], evidence was presented that when spleen cells are transferred from old to young NZB mice there is transient production in some recipients of autoantibodies against erythrocytes; if the recipients are deprived of T lymphocytes, the proportion producing autoantibodies is increased and the phenomenon persists. This was the first experimental evidence that T lymphocytes can suppress autoantibody formation, although Gershon and Kondo [16], independently and at the same time, concluded that T lymphocytes can suppress the formation of antibodies against foreign erythrocytes.

The principal paper embodying our concepts of self-tolerance and autoimmunity [8] became a Citation Classic [17] and influenced a generation of investigators. Only a few examples of the ensuing studies can be mentioned in this introduction: others will be discussed below. Different manifestations of autoimmunity associated with GVH reactions have been documented particularly by Gleichmann et al. [18] and Pollard et al. [19]. The formation of autoantibodies in mice injected with rat red blood cells (RBC) was analysed in terms of our theoretical framework by Cox and his colleagues [20, 21]. Our observations [8, 13] that T lymphocytes from young

NZB mice can suppress autoimmunity was confirmed and extended in the laboratory of Steinberg [22], and the role of suppressor T cells in preventing thyroiditis in rats was documented by Penhale et al. [23].

Five years after the original publication I was able to report that our concepts had survived the risky perinatal period, when many theories succumb, and showed signs of healthy growth and development [24]. I am now glad to have the opportunity to update and extend the concepts after 17 years and point out that they fit in well with contemporary immunological thinking and experimentation. Demonstration of the roles of major histocompatibility (MHC) glycoproteins in cellular interactions, and definition of cytokines, their activities and factors controlling their formation, have extended the earlier theoretical framework. In this chapter the argument will be presented that self tolerance is a quantitative phenomenon, depending on the concentrations of antigens, MHC glycoproteins and cytokines. Triggering an immune response is a threshold phenomenon rather than a graded response. The threshold level is set in the course of ontogenic development in a way that normally limits autoimmune manifestations. This is likely to be due to the generation of an 'off' signal rather than merely engagement of receptors for antigen in the absence of a second signal. If the ontogenetic threshold is exceeded because of disordered regulation of cytokine production and/or MHC expression (in genetically predisposed humans or experimental animals), or if there is non-specific stimulation of the immune system as a result of infection, GVH reactions or another process, autoimmunity can occur. The possible extension of these concepts to autoimmune responses associated with drugs or other chemicals will be discussed. In the space available data supporting the many theories of self tolerance and autoimmunity cannot be comprehensively reviewed. A few examples are given in support of each concept, followed by a brief personal assessment of their relative importance. Other authorities may, of course, rank their relative importance in a different way.

II. Qualitative and quantitative requirements for activation of T lymphocytes

B lymphocytes bind free antigen whereas T lymphocytes recognize antigens associated with MHC glycoproteins, a phenomenon termed MHC restriction. Class I MHC glycoproteins (MHCI) consist of a varying α chain of relative molecular mass 45 000 (M_r = 45 kDa) each complexed with an invariant β_2-microglobulin chain (12 kDa). MHCI are expressed on most cells of the body. Class II MHC glycoproteins (MHCII) are heterodimers consisting of α and β chains (32 kDa and 28 kDa respectively) termed I-A and I-E in mice and HLA-DP, HLA-DQ and HLA-DR in humans [25]. MHCII are expressed only in certain cell types: epithelial cells and dendritic cells in the thymus (discussed below in the context of clonal deletion), B lymphocytes, monocytes and macrophages, specialized antigen-presenting cells (APC) such as Langerhans cells and follicular dendritic cells (FDC) [25], and also chondrocytes (discussed in the context of APC).

APC are thought to degrade protein antigens to relatively short peptides which can selectively bind MHCII [26, 27]. Genetic restriction of responses to antigens is attributed to the efficiency of such binding, which depends on the complementarity of antigens and MHC glycoproteins.

Antigen associated with MHCII binds the T lymphocyte receptor for antigen (TCR, i.e. α-β heterodimer and the T3 (CD3) complex) and triggers a first set of cellular activation signals. The extent of activation of T lymphocyte populations by antigen depends on the concentration of antigen on APC, reflecting a requirement for multivalent interaction between TCR and epitopes on antigen [28]. Only a sufficient number of epitopes, binding to TCR with sufficiently high affinity, will trigger responses. In addition CD4 molecules on the surface of a subset of T lymphocytes bind MHCII glycoproteins [29, 30]; this binding may supplement the binding of T lymphocytes to APC and/or amplify activation signals.

The second signal for activation is the binding of a co-stimulator, e.g. interleukin-1 (IL-1) produced by APC or other accessory cells such as macrophages, to its specific receptor on the T lymphocyte. When the T lymphocyte receives the first and second signals at nearly the same time, it is activated to proliferate, produce IL-2 and other lymphokines and express receptors for IL-2.

CD4-bearing T cells should be regarded as MHCII selective rather than being of the helper phenotype. In mice $CD4^+$ T cells show functional differences at both the clonal and population levels [30]. One functional subset co-ordinately produces a group of lymphokines including IL-4 [31], which helps B lymphocytes to produce antibodies of the IgG_1 and IgE classes [32]. A second subset of $CD4^+$ T cells in mice produces interferon-γ (IFN-γ) [31], which, among other effects, increases the production of antibodies of the IgG_{2a} class [33]. Lymphokines produced by $CD4^+$ cells can also have effects on other cell types: for example both IFN-γ and IL-4 can increase MHCII expression in cells of the monocyte-macrophage lineage and activate these cells for various functions [34, 35]. Cytotoxicity of T cells for target cells infected with Epstein-Barr virus and cytomegalovirus is MHCII restricted [36, 37]. Replication of the viruses in B cells and monocytes allows association of viral antigens with MHCII for presentation to $CD4^+$ cells.

Nevertheless cytotoxic T cells are usually MHCI restricted and of the $CD8^+$ phenotype. Again binding of CD8 to MHCI amplifies signals following binding of TCR to MHCI-associated antigen [28, 29]. Often the antigen, e.g. a virus surface or internal component, is produced within the target cell [38], but influenza virus peptides added to target cells can be recognized in the content of MHCI and trigger cytotoxic reactions [39]. A soluble protein, ovalbumin, can elicit in mice cytotoxic T lymphocytes specific for ovalbumin peptides and MHCI restricted [40]. In general, from a qualitative point of view, antigen presentation to T cells exhibits symmetry: some antigens bind preferentially to MHCI and stimulate $CD8^+$ cells while others, often following partial degradation in APC, bind preferentially to

MHCII and stimulate CD4$^+$ cells.

Considering the quantitative aspects of autoimmune responses, the first point to be made is that the concentrations of autoantigens to which lymphocytes are exposed vary greatly. Some autoantigens such as myelin basic protein are normally secluded from lymphocytes altogether, others such as thyroglobulin circulate in low concentrations (of the order of 10^{-9} M), while still others such as serum albumin circulate in high concentrations (of the order of 10^{-6} M). This is relevant to the concentrations of self antigens required to activate autoreactive T and B lymphocytes; perhaps it is less relevant to the concentrations required for induction of tolerance than was formerly thought.

The second point is that there is no all-or-none distinction between autoantigens and foreign antigens. A receptor on a human T or B lymphocyte for a self-determinant may bind the corresponding determinant from a subhuman primate with the same or somewhat lower affinity (depending upon the extent of amino acid conservation or substitution in the epitope). The same antigen receptor will probably bind the corresponding determinant in a molecule from a non-primate with still lower affinity. Some epitopes in micro-organisms cross-react with self antigens. In other words, given a large population of receptors, there will be a continuum of affinities for autoantigens and foreign antigens. The only clones of lymphocytes relevant to the discussion in this chapter are those with receptors binding autoantigens in the concentrations seen by the lymphocytes in the body with sufficiently high affinity to trigger immune responses.

Quantitative requirements for T cell activation and self-tolerance have recently been discussed by Blanden et al. [28]. They review evidence that activation of lymphocyte populations by antigens is not a graded response but an all-or-none response occurring when the concentrations of antigen, MHC glycoproteins and co-stimulators exceed a threshold level. Some cloned T lymphocytes require contact with a single target cell for triggering lymphokine production [41], whereas others require contact with two target cells [42]. Nevertheless, in both cases the dose-response curves are consistent with a model of stimulation based on all-or-none triggering [42].

The above considerations apply not only to the concentrations of antigens but also to those of MHC glycoproteins. This is nicely shown with L cells (transformed fibroblasts) which do not express Ia (MHCII), even in response to regulatory signals such as IFN-γ, and by transfection obtain L cells displaying the same Ia molecules but varying more than 15-fold in membrane expression [43]. Using these cells in dose-response titrations, a dependent relationship between the antigen (Ag) concentration and Ia concentration required to elicit a T cell response has been obtained such that: Response = k[(Ia) × (Ag)] over the range studied. Tumors often have low MHCI expression, and increasing this by transfection allows tumors to be rejected [44].

Several immunological paradoxes are explained by taking into account levels of

MHC expression, including some types of one-way graft rejection and T cell reactivity observed in chimeras [28]. An example is the observation that in some strains of mice females reject male skin grafts but not vice versa. An antigen designated H-Y reacts with a monoclonal antibody; absorption tests show the antigen to be present in both male and female cells but in higher concentration in the males [45]. Thus, the higher concentration of the H-Y antigen on the surface of male cells may exceed the threshold for unresponsiveness set by the lower concentration of H-Y antigen on the surface of female cells.

III. T cell clonal elimination in the thymus

Classical observations [2, 3, 5] established that tolerance to self antigens is acquired during development of the immune system. Nevertheless, under suitable experimental conditions the formation of autoantibodies can be elicited. It follows that antigen receptors of T and B cells can be encoded in the germ line but not normally expressed in peripheral lymphoid tissues (the spleen, lymph nodes and circulation). Evidence is accumulating that autoreactive T cells are deleted in the thymus. Kappler and colleagues [46] have used a monoclonal antibody against a specific T cell receptor reacting with I-E to show that T cells expressing this receptor are present in large numbers in the immature thymocyte population of I-E-expressing animals but are eliminated from their mature thymocyte pool and peripheral T cells. In an analogous way T cells expressing TCR $V_{\beta 8.1}$ reacting with MHC products encoded or modified by the M/S locus are deleted in the thymus [47, 48]. These results support the interpretation that in normal animals tolerance to self-MHC is due to clonal elimination rather than suppression. Moreover, they suggest that tolerance induction occurs in the thymus at the time that thymocytes are selected to move into the mature thymocyte pool. The cell types in the thymus and mechanisms involved in the induction of MHC restriction and MHC tolerance are not yet understood. Epithelial cells and macrophages (dendritic cells of bone marrow origin) both express MHCII [28]. Binding of thymocytes to these cells may impose negative selection of thymocytes with a high affinity for self-MHC. Evidence has been presented that epithelial cells impose MHC restriction on differentiating lymphocytes [49], while cells of the macrophage lineage prevent T cells from reacting against self-MHC and autoantigens associated with self-MHC [50]. This process of T cell tolerance induction, like T cell responsiveness, is MHC restricted [51].

Blanden et al. [28] reviewed evidence that the level of MHCII expression on thymic epithelial cells and macrophages sets the level at which T cell tolerance is induced. If in extra-thymic sites sufficient antigen is presented in association with concentrations of MHC exceeding those expressed by thymic cells, in the presence of co-stimulating factors, T cell will respond to the antigen. This may also be true for self antigens, so that the relative levels of MHC expression and of cytokine production in the thymus and periphery are key factors in the pathogenesis of autoimmunity.

Observations consistent with the interpretation that failure of T cell clonal elimination can lead to the autoimmunity comes from studies of non-obese diabetic (NOD) mice [52]. These mice spontaneously develop insulin-dependent diabetes mellitus (IDDM) with infiltration of pancreatic islets by CD4-bearing T cells and loss of insulin-secreting β cells. The disease can be transferred by autoreactive CD4$^+$ cells. This situation is analogous to findings in human IDDM. Genetic analyses in mice show that two recessive genes on independent chromosomes contribute to the development of insulitis. One of these is linked to the MHC, and the pattern of MHCII expression in these mice is unique. No messenger RNA for the α chain of I-E is detectable. Transgenic mice expressing I-E on the same genetic background are protected from autoimmune insulitis [52], suggesting that MHCII molecules are involved in the deletion, inactivation or functional suppression of autoreactive T cells. Whether this is due to clonal elimination of autoreactive T cells or active suppression remains to be determined. In several models I-E constitution influences the generation of suppressor T cells (reviewed in [52]).

I-A and HLA-DQ constitution is also relevant in NOD mice and human IDDM: a single amino acid substitution (specifically, the absence of aspartic acid at residue 57) in mouse I-Aβ or its human correlate HLA-DQβ chain is highly correlated with the propensity to develop IDDM [53, 54].

IV. Antigen-presenting cells (APC)

Although many cell types bearing the appropriate MHC glycoproteins can function as APC, most attention has been focused on macrophages [55]. While these are useful model cells, and may function as APC when activated by infection, evidence is accumulating that other cell types more efficiently present antigens under normal circumstances. These include Langerhans cells as antigen presenters to T lymphocytes and follicular dendritic cells (FDC) as APC for B lymphocytes. Furthermore, B lymphocytes can present antigens to T lymphocytes.

1. THE LANGERHANS CELL LINEAGE

Labeling with tritiated thymidine or uridine has shown that cells of this lineage originate in the bone marrow, reside in the skin (and presumably other tissues) for a relatively short period (a few days to 1 week), and migrate through afferent lymphatics to the paracortical thymus-dependent areas of lymph nodes of the drainage chain [56]. These cells are termed veiled cells in afferent lymph and interdigitating cells in the lymph nodes because they have finger-like cytoplasmic extensions among T lymphocytes.

Langerhans cells in the skin, and malignant cells of the same lineage (histocytosis X cells), express MHCII and CD4 [57]. Confined to cells of this lineage are CD6 and strong membrane ATPase reactions. Langerhans cells can be isolated from human skin by rosetting procedures and be maintained in culture. They efficiently present antigens, including herpesvirus antigens, to elicit immune responses by histocompatible T lymphocytes [58]. Dendritic cells isolated from lymphoid tissues [59] have similar properties and may be of the same lineage. Because of possible confusion with FDC, which have a different location and properties, the term Langerhans cells is used in this chapter. These cells efficiently present antigens associated with their surfaces, for example contact-sensitizing chemicals and myelin basic protein, to elicit T lymphocyte dependent immune responses [59, 60].

2. FOLLICULAR DENDRITIC CELLS (FDC)

As their name implies, these cells are found in lymphoid follicles, where their branching cytoplasmic extensions are closely related to B lymphocytes. FDC express CD4, MHCII and complement receptors CR1, CR2 and CR3 [62]. The origin of FDC and their relationship to other cell types is unknown, but mouse reconstitution experiments suggest that they are not derived from precursors in bone marrow [63]. Isolation of FDC without damaging them has been difficult and has impaired analysis of their immune functions. Immune complexes activating complement injected into mice become localized on FDC, and this process appears to be required for the generation of B lymphocyte memory, in other words, proliferation of clones of B lymphocytes responding to the antigen [64]. The high-affinity C3b receptor (CR1) expressed on FDC is presumably involved in the localization of the complexes. Immune complexes binding FDC become associated with beaded cell membrane extensions which are readily taken up by follicular MHCII$^+$ B lymphocytes [65].

3. B LYMPHOCYTES

During the past few years evidence has accumulated that B lymphocytes efficiently present antigens to T lymphocytes [66]. In fact, depletion of B cells by treatment of neonatal mice with antibody against the μ chain of Ig markedly decreases the capacity of T cells in lymph nodes to respond to later antigenic stimulation [67]. A major role of surface membrane Ig receptors for antigen on B cells may be to bind antigen at limiting concentrations for its subsequent presentation to helper T cells. There is no fundamental difference between MHCII-restricted or cognate help and unrestricted or factor-mediated T cell help. The observed differences are largely due to differences in antigen concentration, which cells present antigens and the concentrations of cytokines (helper factors) that accumulate in the local microenvironment [66].

Because the concentrations of autoantigens (e.g. thyroglobulin, DNA and microsomal antigens) are usually low, the antigen-focusing effect of B cells with specific receptors for autoantigens and their presentation to T cells is highly relevant. Since B cells binding autoantigens with high-affinity circulate in normal humans and experimental animals [12], the cells required for autoantigen presentation to T cells are not limiting, whereas responses of helper T cells to autoantigens are deficient, as we originally postulated [9, 10]. The limiting factor may be the production of adequate concentrations of appropriate cytokines in the microenvironment in which autoantigens are presented.

4. MHCII EXPRESSION ON OTHER CELL TYPES

Bottazzo et al. [68] have emphasized the role of aberrant MHCII expression in the pathogenesis of autoimmunity. They propose that since only cells expressing MHCII can function as antigen-presenting cells for T cells, persistent MHCII expression in sites where they are not normally present could result in autoimmunity. DR antigens have been demonstrated on thyroid epithelial cells of patients with Graves' disease and Hashimoto's thyroiditis [68]. Transcripts of DRα chain are observed in Graves' thyroid tissue and thyroid cells in culture [69]. The induction of MHCII expression in thyroid epithelial cells by IFN-γ and other mediators is discussed below. Cultured thyroid epithelial cells expressing MHCII can act as antigen-presenting cells for T cells [70], and, in autoimmune thyroiditis, infiltrating T cells specifically recognize thyroid epithelial cells expressing MHCII [71]. DR antigens are expressed on the β cells of pancreatic islets in type I IDDM [72].

These observations are interesting, and are discussed below in the context of viral infections. However, in view of the efficiency with which B cells present antigens to T cells [66] it is not clear whether aberrant MHCII expression on thyroid and pancreatic cells is required for the development of autoimmunity or is a manifestation of autoimmunity following local production of cytokines that can increase MHC expression. Conceivably supranormal concentrations of MHCII on B cells in these sites, because of the presence of cytokines increasing MHC expression, facilitates the development of autoimmunity. In MRL-*lpr/lpr* mice genetically predisposed to autoimmunity, the concentration of MHCII on B lymphocytes is increased [73]. In patients with recent onset Graves' hyperthyroidism, but not in hyperthyroid patients with subacute thyroiditis, there is a marked increase in presumably activated T cells expressing MHCII [74]. In the majority of IDDM patients, T lymphocytes expressing MHCII are also present [74]. A high level of expression of MHCII on thyroid and pancreatic β cells could certainly focus the effector functions of CD4$^+$ T lymphocytes on those sites, with production of mediators affecting function or viability and even MHCII-restricted cytotoxicity (analogous to that in the Epstein-Barr virus and cytomegalovirus systems).

The expression of MHCII on chrondrocytes in articular cartilage in normal and arthritic joints is also of interest. Tiku and colleagues [75] found that 29 – 46% of normal rabbit chrondrocytes displayed Ia compared with 49 – 60% of spleen cells. The chondrocytes were as efficient as spleen cells in the presentation of an antigen (ovalbumin) to T lymphocytes from immunized animals. Human articular chondrocytes from patients with rheumatoid arthritis and osteoarthritis express MHCII (HLA-DR), which was considered to be a marker of activation [76]. However, MHCII expression may be constitutive in articular chrondrocytes, and increased by cytokines (e.g. IFN-γ, tumor necrosis factor (TNF-α), and granulo-cyte/macrophage-colony stimulating factor (GM-CSF)). Normal cartilage is thought to be immunologically privileged because of the absence of a blood and lymphatic supply. However, some chrondrocytes may be accessible on the periphery of articular cartilage, and degradation of matrix in arthritis would allow further contact of chondrocytes and lymphocytes. Introduction of ovalbumin into the joints of immunized rabbits produces a chronic arthritis with pathology analogous to rheumatoid arthritis [77]; chondrocyte presentation of antigen to sensitized T cells may be involved in the pathogenesis. Among all joint components cartilage plays a special role, as suggested by the finding that the only type of collagen able to induce autoimmune arthritis is type II, which is present in cartilage but not other cell types [78]. An antigen in mycobacteria cross-reacting with an antigen in cartilage plays a pathogenetic role in adjuvant arthritis in the rat [79]. Some of the cells in rheumatoid arthritis synovial tissue expressing MHCII may be chondrocytes derived from eroded cartilage.

V. Regulation of MHC expression

For reasons just discussed the regulation of MHC expression is relevant to theories of autoimmunity. The first cytokines shown to change MHC expression were IFN-α and IFN-β, which were found to increase MHCI expression on several cell types [80]. Later, IFN-γ was found to increase expression of MHCII on macrophages [81] and on several other cell types, an effect correlated with increased transcription of MHCII genes [82]. The effects of IFN-γ on cultured cells are parallelled by regulatory effects on MHC expression in vivo. Skoskiewicz et al. [83] administered recombinant murine IFN-γ intraperitoneally to mice for 6 days or longer and found substantial increases in MHCI and MHCII expression. This effect was selective, for example occurring in proximal but not distal convoluted tubules in the kidney and on basal but not apical aspects of their cell membranes. In the pancreas and small intestine the expression of MHCI was increased 13- to 17-fold, whereas in the heart, kidney and adrenals the increase was 4- to 8-fold. Increases of MHCII expression were greatest in the hart, kidney, pancreas, lung, liver, adrenal and small intestine, with lesser increases in the thymus and spleen and they were undetectable in lymph nodes. It is remarkable that the tissues in which IFN-γ increases MHC expression and the number of MHCII-bearing dendritic cells (potential APC) are those in which disorders are known or believed to have an autoimmune basis.

IL-4 augments MHCII expression in B cells [84] as well as monocytes and macrophages [34, 35]. TNF-α also increases MHCII expression and acts synergistically with IFN-γ. In cultured human pancreatic β cells IFN-γ or TNF-α induce expression of HLA-A, B, C but not HLA-DR; however, IFN-γ and TNF-α together induce MHCII expression in β cells [85]. In inducing expression of MHCII on thyroid epithelial cells in culture, IFN-γ and thyrotropin have synergistic effects [86]. In Hashimoto's disease thyrotropin levels are increased and in Graves' disease thyroid-stimulating autoantibodies may play a similar role.

Colony-stimulating factors can also regulate MHC expression. In mouse macrophages GM-CSF increases MHCII gene transcription whereas M-CSF (= CSF-1) decreases it (C. Willman and C. Stewart, personal communication). IL-6 increases MHCI expression in human fibroblasts [87]. Glucocorticoids and prostaglandin E_1 inhibit murine macrophage Ia expression [87, 88].

VI. Increased MHCII expression in autoimmune mice

Increased macrophage Ia expression in mice genetically predisposed to develop autoimmunity has been reported by several groups of investigators [73, 88, 89]. Peritoneal macrophage Ia expression has been found to increase coincidentally with the development of lymphoid hyperplasia and lupus nephritis in MRL-*lpr/lpr* mice [88, 89]. The number of Ia-positive peritoneal cells also increases in NZB mice coincidentally with the appearance of autoimmune disease [88]. Although lymphadenopathy and B cell activation are also observed in *lpr/lpr*-bearing C3H, B6 and AKR strains, only those that are genetically predisposed to develop autoimmunity (MRL-*lpr/lpr* and NZB-*lpr/lpr*) also show increased Ia expression [73]. This may be secondary to unregulated production of cytokines (e.g. IFN-γ or GM-CSF) increasing MHCII expression. Ageing MRL-*lpr/lpr* mice spontaneously produce IFN-γ in spleen and lymph nodes (C.L. Martens, personal communication).

It is of interest that repeated administration of agents decreasing MHCII expression, such as glucocorticoids [87, 87a], and PGE$_1$ [88] reduce manifestations of autoimmunity [88]. Repeated administration of TNF-α to mice, which elevates serum PGE$_2$ levels [90], delays the onset of lupus-like disease in (NZB $\times$ NZW)F$_1$ mice [91]. In contrast, administration of IFN-γ, which increases MHCII expression, accelerates and exacerbates manifestations of autoimmunity while monoclonal antibody to IFN-γ delays the disease in (NZB $\times$ NZW)F$_1$ mice [92]. Although these agents have other effects, the observations are consistent with the hypothesis that expression of MHC above a threshold level is part of the setting in which autoimmunity develops. Additional evidence for that interpretation is the finding that administration of monoclonal antibodies against I-A can prevent autoimmune diseases such as diabetes mellitus and thyroiditis in genetically predisposed BB rats and *db/db* mice [93, 94], and allergic encephalomyelitis in mice immunized with myelin basic protein [95]. Administration of monoclonal antibodies (anti-L3T4) against the CD4$^+$ subset of T lymphocytes which interacts preferentially with MHCII prevents autoimmunity in NZB mice [96] and experimental allergic encephalomyelitis in mice [97].

VII. Control of expression of genes for MHC glycoproteins and cytokines

For reasons discussed above the genetic control of expression of genes for MHC glycoproteins and cytokines is important in autoimmunity. The regulation of gene expression in mammalian cells is an area of intense current research. Nuclear proteins, present in a variety of cell types, have been shown to regulate RNA polymerase II mediated transcription units. Several of these proteins have been purified, and the genes encoding them have been cloned. An emerging rule concerning regulatory elements controlling several widely expressed genes is that multiple DNA regions are required for the expression of each gene [98]. The functionally defined DNA elements are recognized by different proteins found in particular cell types, and this interaction is required for active transcription. In addition to promoters and repressors, *cis*-acting DNA sequences that increase the levels of transcription when placed in either orientation at large distances from the promoter, have been identified in mammalian cells; they are termed enhancers. Some genes are transcribed in many cell types, e.g., most histones, RNA polymerase II and thymidine kinase, whereas other genes are expressed in only one or a few cell types. Evidence is accumulating that the proteins regulating such transcription are confined to the cell types in question and can regulate several genes in a co-ordinate fashion. In the liver, four different regulatory sites are required for transcriptional stimulation by the enhancers of two unrelated genes, encoding the acute-phase proteins α_1-antitrypsin and transthyretin. These bind the same nuclear protein, which is found mainly in the liver [98]. Such proteins may provide a basis for co-ordinate, hepatocyte-specific control of gene transcription, which can be increased by IL-6 [99].

The expression of MHCI in both human and murine cells can be induced by α-, β- and γ-IFN. This is controlled, at least in part, at the level of transcription. A common sequence has been found in the promotor region of several human genes responsive to IFN-α [100]. The promoters of H-2K^b and several other mouse class I genes contain a similar IFN-response sequence. The H-2K^b promoter can be induced by all three types of IFN, and the IFN-response sequence is necessary for induction to occur [100]. However, the response sequence is active only when associated with a functional enhancer sequence in the promoter region of other class I genes. The combination of these two sequences can make a heterologous promoter responsive to IFN, irrespective of its orientation relative to the cap site.

The regulated and co-ordinate expression of MHCII genes to give non-covalently linked $\alpha\beta$ heterodimers on the surface of APC is critical for the initiation of immune responses. Human patients with a hereditary immunodeficiency (class II bare lymphocyte syndrome) have intact MHCII genes but they are not transcribed even in the presence of IFN-γ; the locus in question is not on chromosome 6 which encodes the human MHCII genes [101]. The expression of the entire family of MHCII genes is normally controlled by a *trans*-acting regulatory gene which controls the formation of a product necessary for the action of IFN-γ on MHCII gene expression [101]. Recent genetic and biochemical studies [102] show that the constitutive high expression of MHCII in B lymphocytes is the result of tissue-specific enhancer elements, transcriptionally active promoters and the absence of negative regulatory factors. One of the regulatory sequences is an octamer (ATTTGCAT) which is found in the promoters of Ig light- and heavy-chain genes, as well as in the transcriptional enhancer of the Ig heavy-chain gene; the octamer can function as a B cell specific transcriptional activator [102]. Another regulator of MHCII expression is the sequence CCAAT to which a ubiquitous cellular CCAAT transcription factor can bind, and two more have been identified [102]. Infection of B lymphocytes with Epstein-Barr virus further increases MHCII expression [103], which may contribute to the autoimmune responses observed following infectious mononucleosis (see below). In IFN-γ-inducible cells the tissue-specific enhancer elements do not function; repressors acting at the promoter can be modified through the action of IFN-γ-inducible factors [102]. In activated T cells MHCII can also be expressed. Glucocorticoids decrease levels of MHCII messenger RNA in murine B lymphocytes and expression of Ia on the surface of the cells [87a].

Less is known about the control of cytokine expression. We have recently shown that glucocorticoids selectively inhibit transcription of the IL-1β gene in cells of the monocyte lineage and decrease stability of the corresponding messenger RNA [104]. The inference is that the glucocorticoid receptor, a nuclear protein, binds to a regulatory element of the IL-1β gene. Murine helper T lymphocytes are of two types, Th1 and Th2 [31]. Th1 clones produce messenger RNAs for IL-2, IFN-γ and lymphotoxin (TNF-β) whereas Th2 clones produce messenger RNAs for IL-4 and IL-5 [31]. These findings suggest that the expression of the IL-2 and IFN-γ genes may be co-ordinately regulated by one set of promoters, enhancers and repressors while the formation of IL-4 and IL-5 genes is co-ordinately controlled by another set of regulatory elements.

VIII. Graft-versus-host (GVH) reactions

The primary event in GVH reactions is the response of donor CD4$^+$ (L3T4$^+$) T lymphocytes to MHCII glycoproteins of the recipient, with consequent production of cytokines which help the proliferation of, and antibody formation by, B lymphocytes of host origin. The latter can produce autoantibodies. In non-irradiated F_1 recipient mice undergoing systemic GVH reactions, lymphoid stimulation is induced by donor T cells, including CD4$^+$ cells reacting against host MHCII [18] and involves recruitment and proliferation of B cells of host origin [105]. There is consequent lymphoreticular hyperplasia with germinal center enlargement and plasmacytosis. According to the T lymphocyte by-pass concept, in a normal animal autoantibody formation does not occur because T lymphocytes are unable to respond self antigens. However, when T lymphocytes are non-specifically stimulated, as in GVH reactions, there is an 'allogeneic effect' leading to production of antibodies which normally require T lymphocyte help [106]. In this way the need for carrier-specific T lymphocytes in the immune response can be by-passed. Hence we postulated that in GVH reactions the formation of autoantibodies would be expected [9], and we were soon able to show the production of antibodies against nuclear antigens in such reactions [15]. Ig allotypic markers were used to demonstrate that the autoantibodies were of host and not donor origin, a procedure that has been used in subsequent investigations.

The autoantibodies produced in GVH reactions have been analysed systematically by Gleichmann et al. [18]. Non-irradiated (C57BL/10 × DBA/2) F_1 mice can be induced to develop a variety of pathological syndromes following the injection of parental T cells. The injection of C57BL/10 T cells leads to acute GVH reactions, with runting and severe lymphadenopathy, whereas injection of DBA/2 T cells leads to chronic GVH disease with the production of autoantibodies and a syndrome like SLE. Among the autoantibodies produced in chronic GVH reactions are those against erythrocytes, thymocytes and nuclear antigens, including antibodies against double-stranded DNA (dsDNA). Pollard et al. [19] used spleen cells from such animals to generate hybridomas producing antibodies with the specificities described above, including some reacting with dsDNA. Such antibodies, which are characteristic of SLE, are difficult to raise by conventional immunization, confirming the usefulness of the model.

The mechanisms by which GVH reactions produce autoimmunity have not yet been analysed in detail, although a speculative interpretation of the sequence of events can be offered. One effect of GVH reactions is the induction of MHCII expression in host epidermal cells, gut epithelium, renal tubular cells and presumably in other cell types. This induction was analysed in rats by Barclay and Mason [107]. The Ia expression in epidermal and gut epithelial cells was found to be of host origin but not acquired from bone marrow derived cells. Donor lymphocytes infiltrating the skin and intestine presumably produce cytokines increasing Ia expression in host cells; IFN-γ is known to do this for keratinocytes [108]. Increased Ia expression in various host cells and in B lymphocytes may facilitate host antigen presentation to T cells. GVH reactions in mice are also associated with migration of lymphocytes into the gut mucosa and increased intestinal epithelial Ia expression [109]. The principal mechanism of epithelial damage does not appear to be direct cytotoxicity and may be due to the release of TNF-β or other cytokines. GVH reactions also induce transcription of MHCII genes in mouse renal tubular cells [110].

Possibly expression of MHCII genes in host B cells is also increased, thereby augmenting their capacity to present autoantigens to donor T cells. Donor class II restricted L3T4$^+$ (CD4$^+$) T cells provide allogeneic help for autoantibody formation by recipient B cells in 'class II' GVH reactions; host L3T4$^+$ T cells are depleted [18, 111]. One of the cytokines mediating allogeneic help for antibody formation is IL-6, and W. Fiers and A.L. Goldberg (personal communication) find high levels of IL-6 production by macrophages of mice undergoing GVH reactions. When autoantigens such as DNA, other nuclear factors, erythrocyte antigens and renal tubular antigens are presented to T and B lymphocytes in the presence of these helper factors, and possibly others not yet defined, and in the absence of T cell mediated suppression, autoantibody formation is elicited. This is the mechanism underlying the 'allogeneic effect'.

IX. Factors increasing B cell proliferation and/or differentiation

Overproduction of cytokines increasing the proliferation of B lymphocytes and/or their differentiation into antibody-forming cells, or increased responsiveness of B cells to such stimuli, could be factors leading to autoimmunity. Two common features of autoimmune disease are polyclonal B cell activation and Ig (including autoantibody) production.

Factors produced by helper T lymphocytes and other accessory cells which increase proliferation and/or differentiation of B lymphocytes are currently being defined. Already the information is too extensive to review comprehensively in this chapter; a convenient summary and list of references has recently been published [112]. IL-1, IL-2 and IFN-γ can all act as co-factors increasing proliferation of and/or antibody production by B cells under some circumstances. Three more recently cloned and expressed cytokines, IL-4, IL-5 and IL-6, have major effects on B lymphocytes in addition to effects on other cell types.

IL-4 (M_r = 15 – 20 kDa), previously known as B cell stimulatory factor 1 (BSF-1), is produced by activated T cells, mast-cells and a B cell line (CH12) in the mouse [32] and by activated human T cells [113]. IL-4 acts on resting B cells to increase MHCII expression, proliferation and production of IgE; in the mouse it also increases formation of IgG$_1$ [32]. IL-4 is also a growth factor for T cells, and it increases MHCII expression and cytocidal capacity of human monocytes and mouse macrophages [34, 35].

IL-5 (M_r = 45 – 60 kDa) is produced by activated murine and human T cells [112]. It increases proliferation of B cells stimulated with lipopolysaccharide (LPS) (mouse) or protein A of *Staphylococcus* (SAC) (human) and augments IgA secretion. It also induces differentiation of eosinophils in both species.

IL-6 was previously known as IFN-β_2 and BSF-2. The M_r varies from $20-30$ kDa depending on the extent of glycosylation. One cell type producing IL-6 in the human is the activated peripheral blood monocyte [114], and it is also produced by the mouse macrophage cell line P388D1 [112]. Human T cell leukemia virus (HTLVI) transformed human T cells and activated murine T cells produce IL-6 [115], as do activated human fibroblasts and cells of a murine bone marrow stromal cell line [112]. Several human tumors, or cell lines derived from them, including human cardiac myxomas, cervical carcinoma cells and osteosarcoma cells, produce IL-6 [115]. A major effect of murine and human IL-6 is induction of the formation of acute-phase proteins, including fibrinogen and proteinase inhibitors, by hepatocytes and hepatoma cells [99].

Observations have accumulated suggesting that the production of, or response to, B lymphocyte growth and differentiation factors is abnormal in mice genetically predisposed to develop autoimmunity. Although the information is still incomplete, it is highly suggestive and opens the way for a detailed analysis of the disordered regulation of cytokine production in relation to autoimmunity.

Mice homozygous for the allelic, recessive single-gene mutations termed motheaten and viable motheaten (gene symbols *me* and *me*^{v}, respectively) show the most severe genetically determined autoimmune syndromes known, including rapidly progressive glomerulonephritis. Sidman et al. [116] reported that sera and tissue culture supernatants of cells from lymphoid tissues of *me*^{v}/*me*^{v} mice contain a factor that directly drives the maturation of normal or malignant B cells to a state of active Ig secretion. The factors produced in these mice have not yet been identified. McCoy et al. [117] reported that splenic macrophages of motheaten mice spontaneously produce colony stimulating activity, and N. Windsor and J. Claggett (personal communication) have found that such cells spontaneously produce GM-CSF and IL-6 messenger RNAs. Hence overproduction of GM-CSF and IL-6 could be a basic disorder in motheaten mice, although this remains to be fully documented.

MRL-*lpr*/*lpr* mice spontaneously develop an autoimmune disease manifested clinically by arthritis, vasculitis and immune complex glomerulonephritis, which is regarded as a murine model for SLE. Lu and Unanue [89] described spontaneous T cell lymphokine production in *lpr*/*lpr* mice. Prud'homme et al. [118] reported that MRL-*lpr*/*lpr* mice develop a T cell lymphoproliferative syndrome with hypersecretion of factors that increase proliferation of B cells and their differentiation into Ig-secreting cells. Rosenberg and her colleagues [73] established T cell lines from MRL-*lpr*/*lpr* mice and found that they spontaneously produce IL-2, express IL-2 receptors and proliferate in the absence of added antigen, mitogen or growth factor. They also spontaneously produce colony-stimulating factor, IFN (presumably IFN-γ) and factors increasing B cell proliferation and differentiation into Ig-secreting cells. The latter have properties suggestive of IL-4 and IL-6. Unregulated production of these factors, including IFN-γ, could account for the greatly increased numbers of cells secreting Ig, particularly IgG, in *lpr/lpr* mouse strains [119].

A rare syndrome has suggested that overproduction of IL-6, irrespective of the site at which this occurs, may be associated with autoimmunity in humans [115]. Patients with cardiac myxoma show fever, arthralgia, hypergammaglobulinemia, elevated erythrocyte sedimentation rate and Raynaud's phenomenon. Among the autoantibodies produced are those against nuclear antigens and DNA as well as rheumatoid factor. Six cardiac myxomas were found to produce substantial amounts of IL-6. The same was true of a cervical carcinoma in a woman with autoantibodies against nuclear antigens, anti-sicca syndrome A antibody and Raynaud's phenomenon. The latter may be related to increased fibrinogen levels, blood viscosity and sedimentation rate. The symptoms and signs associated with the myxomas, including autoantibodies, disappeared following surgical removal of the tumors, suggesting that products of the myxomas contributed to their pathogenesis. Rheumatoid arthritis synovial tissue produces IL-6, which may be one factor driving the high level of Ig production by B cells in that tissue (Y. Nawata, E.M. Eugui, S.W. Lee and A.C. Allison, unpublished).

An alternative explanation for polyclonal activation of B cells in animals genetically predisposed to autoimmunity is that they are hyper-responsive to proliferation signals. Prud'homme et al. [118] reported that this is true of B cells of young NZB/W and B × SB mice. In contrast, the B cells of MRL-*lpr/lpr* mice were found to respond normally to growth and differentiation factors, while the production of such factors is increased, as described above.

T lymphocytes of obese (OS) chickens, which develop autoimmune thyroiditis, produce more IL-2 and less of an inhibitory product than lymphocytes from other chickens [120]; in the lymphocytes of the OS chickens there was also higher expression of IL-2 receptors. This is consistent with a disorder of immunoregulation in OS chickens as compared with the Cornell C strain from which they were derived and other strains.

The situation in human autoimmune diseases is too complex to review comprehensively here. It has been claimed [121] that decreased IL-2 production plays a role in defective self recognition and autoimmunity. However, when T cells producing cytokines are separated from cells exerting suppressive effects, lymphokine production is not inhibited. Thus T cells expressing MHCII, a marker of activation, are observed in patients with SLE and they spontaneously produce factors increasing IgG synthesis by B lymphocytes [122]. The situation resembles that described above for T cells from MRL-*lpr/lpr* mice which spontaneously produce lymphokines but produce less IL-2 when artificially stimulated than normal T cells [73].

In general, substantial evidence has accumulated that there is disregulation of cytokine production in autoimmune diseases of experimental animals and of humans. An important task for future research is definition of the molecular biological basis for such disregulation, and analysis of the sequence of events by which this contributes to the pathogenesis of autoimmunity.

X. Use of transgenic mice for investigating autoimmunity

The processes which have been discussed above for inducing autoimmunity, e.g. GVH disease, act non-specifically to increase both MHCI and MHCII expression, as well as the production of cytokines, in several different tissues. A more refined experimental procedure is the selective induction of MHCI or MHCII expression, or cytokine production, in a particular cell type to ascertain whether autoimmunity develops under these conditions. Transgenic mice can be used for that purpose. Sarvetnick et al. [123] produced transgenic mouse strains with MHCII α and β chain genes linked to an insulin promoter. These mice express both MHCII chains in β cells of the islets of Langerhans in the pancreas. When these mice are aged about 2 months, the insulin-producing β cells disappear from the pancreas and IDDM develops.

Sarvetnick et al. [123] also produced transgenic mice with the IFN-γ gene linked to an insulin promoter. In these transgenic strains IFN-γ genes were expressed in pancreatic β cells, and destruction of islets was associated with an inflammatory reaction involving mainly lymphocytes and cells of the monocyte-macrophage lineage. Although the inflammatory reaction was focused on the islets, it also involved the exocrine pancreas to some extent.

Independently, Allison and her colleagues [124] have over-expressed MHCI in β cells of pancreatic islets, using a similar procedure in transgenic mice. Again IDDM developed and β cells were found to be markedly depleted. However, there was no infiltration of lymphocytes into the pancreatic islets. While all these findings are interesting, the explanation of the diabetes is not yet clear. There is no evidence of autoimmunity (antibodies against β cells or T cells specifically recognizing them in the context of overexpressed MHC). As the authors recognize, the possibility that MHC glycoproteins may influence cellular events by non-immune mechanisms has not been excluded, for example association with membrane receptors involved in metabolism [125].

Increased expression of MHCII in transgenic mice does not always increase predisposition to IDDM. In fact, increased expression of I-E, not confined to the pancreas, protects genetically predisposed mice from the disease [52]. This is discussed above in the context of clonal elimination of T cells in the thymus.

The general strategy of selectively inducing the expression of MHC glycoproteins and cytokines in different tissues, using transgenic mice or other experimental manipulations, for analysing mechanisms of tolerance and autoimmunity, is appealing and will doubtless be widely applied in the next decade.

XI. Lack of tolerance to self antigens in B lymphocytes

According to Burnet's clonal selection hypothesis [6], lymphocytes producing antibodies against self antigens are deleted or inactivated in the course of ontogeny; autoimmunity results from somatic mutation allowing the emergence of forbidden clones producing antibodies against self. In fact, it has proven easy to produce autoantibodies against a variety of antigens by experimental manipulations such as immunization with a foreign protein or cell having epitopes cross-reactive with self antigens. This was first shown for the thyroid [126] and extended to thyroglobulin; patients with Hashimoto's thyroiditis were also found to have autoantibodies against thyroglobulin [127].

Thyroglobulin has been studied as a model autoantigen for several reasons. It circulates in concentrations of about 10^{-9} M, and can be regarded as representative of autoantigens circulating in low concentrations but still able to bind to and saturate high-affinity lymphocyte receptors for antigen. Thyroglobulin can be heavily iodinated without denaturation, and, as just mentioned, the formation of autoantibodies against thyroglobulin is associated with thyroiditis.

Because of the ease with which autoantibody formation can be elicited, we postulated in 1971 that tolerance for self antigens is selective for T cells and is not true for B cells [9]. We predicted that B cells able to bind self antigens with high affinity should be present in normal persons and experimental animals, and that those B cells would be required to produce autoantibodies and most autoimmune diseases. In 1973, we showed that normal humans have in their peripheral blood B lymphocytes binding human thyroglobulin [12]. This has been confirmed in other laboratories, and the number of thyroglobulin-binding cells was found to be considerably increased in patients with Hashimoto's thyroiditis [128]. Mice were also found in our laboratory and that of Weigle to have B cells binding thyroglobulin with high affinity [13, 14]. If X-irradiated mice were reconstituted with spleen cells incubated with highly radioactive thyroglobulin such B cells were inactivated; the mice were then unable to produce autoantibodies against thyroglobulin and thyroiditis when suitably immunized, although they responded normally to other antigens. B lymphocytes binding many other self antigens have been described, including native dsDNA [129] and erythrocyte antigens [130]; patients with SLE show increased numbers of DNA-binding B lymphocytes and mice with autoimmunity increased numbers of B cells binding erythrocyte antigens. Thus, autoimmunity can result from expansion of pre-existing clones of B cells with receptors for self antigens.

The presence of autoantibodies to thyroglobulin, actin, tubulin, fetuin, myoglobin, albumin, transferrin, collagen and cytochrome c in normal humans and mice [131] is discussed further below. The frequencies of murine B cell precursors developing into clones secreting antibodies which bind to autologous (mouse) or heterologous (rabbit or human) forms of the same protein antigens (myosin and albumin), have been measured [132]. These antigens were taken as representative of intracellular and extracellular antigens present in high concentrations. The authors conclude that their findings exclude, on a quantitative basis, any form of inactivation or deletion of such cells.

B lymphocytes from healthy children and young adults who were seronegative for autoantibodies, and B lymphocytes from umbilical cord blood of newborns, were induced by Epstein-Barr virus infection to secrete a variety of autoantibodies [133]. These autoantibodies recognized normal cellular components including nuclear, cytoskeletal and other cytoplasmic antigens. Such autoantibody-secreting clones were obtained from tonsils as well as peripheral blood in frequencies of 1 in $10^6 - 10^7$ of mononuclear cells. The authors concluded that self-reactive clones were not eliminated during ontogeny [133]. The studies quoted in the last two paragraphs can be criticized because the affinities of the autoantibodies formed were not measured accurately; however, competition experiments did not show any differences between reactions with corresponding self and foreign proteins.

Despite all the evidence summarized above, Nossal [134] has fought a gallant rearguard action defending Burnet's hypothesis that 'functional silencing of particular elements in the immunological repertoire is an important mechanism in immunological tolerance for both B and T lymphocyte classes'. Nossal has adopted the Bretscher and Cohn [7] hypothesis that contact of a B lymphocyte with an antigen in the absence of a second signal from T cells or macrophages renders B cells anergic, and the Klinman hypothesis [135] that such anergy is more likely to occur in pre-B cells than in B cells. Hence exposure to antigens before the immune system is fully mature increases the probability of 'functional silencing'. Nossal and his colleagues have found such unresponsiveness induced by some multivalent antigens (review [134]), yet many self antigens are univalent.

The clonal abortion hypothesis as expounded by Nossal has recently been challenged by Diener and Waters [136] on the basis of their findings with antigens administered transplacentally. They conclude that many antigens capable of receptor cross-linking fail to induce tolerance in B cells regardless of the ontogenetic state of these cells. It is notable that even B cells reactive to autologous serum albumin, the self antigen circulating in highest concentration and present in the extravascular compartment, were not eliminated [131, 132], which is consistent with the finding that autoantibodies against albumin can be produced [137]. Thus, the balance of evidence supports our interpretation that there is qualitative difference between T cells and B cells such that the former are much more easily rendered tolerant to self antigens, perhaps because of the special process of maturation in the thymus.

Even the distinction between immune responses in fetal and postnatal life is not all-or-none. Fetal lambs and monkeys produce antibodies to a variety of antigens and can reject skin grafts [138, 139], and suitable regimes can render adult animals unresponsive to foreign serum proteins and other antigens [140 – 142]. At least some of these examples of unresponsiveness are due to suppressor T cells (see below).

XII. Selective tolerance in T lymphocytes

In 1969 Taylor [141] showed in mice injected with bovine serum albumin, and in 1970 Chiller et al. [142] in mice injected with human γ-globulin, that low doses of antigen induce unresponsiveness selectively in helper T lymphocytes, leaving responses of B lymphocytes to the antigens unimpaired. These results are relevant to self tolerance, as pointed out independently by Allison [9] and Weigle [10] in 1971. Many autoantigens, including thyroglobulin and polypeptide hormones, circulate in low concentrations ($10^{-8}-10^{-9}$ M). The affinities of receptors for these hormones are, in fact, of the same order as the affinities of receptors for antigens on lymphocytes. In these cases only T lymphocytes may be tolerant, leaving B lymphocytes able to respond to autoantigens suitably presented to them with T lymphocyte help. One mechanism allowing the requirement for T lymphocytes to be bypassed is association of an autoantigen with a carrier epitope able to activate T lymphocytes (e.g. a foreign protein or cell with xenogeneic and cross-reactive epitopes, a viral antigen or a chemical that can act as a carrier). Examples of each of these will be given. Other mechanisms by-passing the requirement for autoreactive T cells involve non-specific activation of T cells by a GVH reaction, infection or exposure to a stimulatory microbial product.

First, evidence for selective T cell tolerance will be reviewed. Gammon et al. [143] presented observations suggesting that neonatal T cell tolerance to minimal immunogenic peptides is produced by clonal inactivation. They analysed T cell responses to three cytochrome c peptides differing by only a single amino acid substitution in the epitope recognized. Following exposure of neonatal mice to the antigens, each peptide induced tolerance to itself, while the response to variants was unchanged. In this system T cell clonal deletion or inactivation rather than suppression appears to be the mechanism of neonatally induced tolerance.

The cytoplasmic protein F (M_r = 40 kDa) occurs in two forms in mice, F^1 and F^2. In some strains of mice alloimmunization can lead to an autoantibody response directed against determinants common to F^1 and F^2 [144]. Responses of T cells to F can be measured by recording the proliferation of F-primed T cells exposed to F-pulsed splenic adherent cells. Syngeneic F antigen does not elicit such responses whereas allogeneic F antigen elicits strong responses [144]. Thus, there is selective unresponsiveness of T cells, but not B cells, to F autoantigenic determinants. Attempts to demonstrate suppression in this system have failed.

It has long been known that animals immunized with thyroglobulin from other species develop autoantibodies to thyroglobulin and thyroiditis. The autoantibodies can be absorbed by the heterologous thyroglobulins, showing that they are all directed to cross-reactive determinants and are not produced as a result of non-specific polyclonal stimulation. The most economical explanation of the observations is that T lymphocytes responding to allogeneic determinants on thyroglobulin exert help for the formation of autoantibodies against shared determinants [10, 24].

An analogous situation is the formation of autoantibodies against erythrocytes by mice injected with rat erythrocytes [20, 21, 145]. The recipients develop autoantibodies against erythrocyte antigens, remove RBC from the circulation more rapidly than normal and show reticulocytosis. Thus they develop clinically typical autoimmune hemolytic anemia. The mouse autoantibodies are absorbed by rat erythrocytes but not erythrocytes of other species of animals, showing that they are directed against antigenic determinants shared by rat and mouse erythrocytes. T cell deprived mice do not produce autoantibodies when injected with rat erythrocytes [145]. These observations are consistent with the interpretation that T lymphocytes reacting with rat erythrocyte determinants are able to provide help for B lymphocytes producing antibodies against determinants shared by rat and mouse erythrocytes, in other words autoantibodies, supporting the T cell by-pass model. There is no evidence that normal mice have functional helper T lymphocytes responding to mouse erythrocytes in vivo, although T lymphocytes proliferating in response to mouse erythrocytes in culture can be observed [146]. This may be related to the presence in mice of T cells able to suppress autoantibody formation against erythrocytes, as discussed below.

Relevant to autoimmunity following exposure to drugs is the finding that small molecules can act in an analogous function as carriers. Potent stimulators of T cells are arsanilic acid and dinitrophenol (DNP), a contact sensitizer. Rabbit thyroglobulin coupled with arsanilic and sulfanilic acids elicits the formation of autoantibodies to thyroglobulin in the rabbit, even in the absence of adjuvant [147]. Coupling of DNP groups to myeloma proteins has been used to elicit the formation of anti-idiotypic antibodies in syngeneic mice sensitized to DNP [148]. Complexing of virus antigens with self antigens to elicit autoantibody formation is considered in the section on viruses.

XIII. T lymphocyte mediated suppression of autoimmunity

For several years it was thought that T lymphocytes have two functions: as effectors of cell-mediated immunity and as helpers in antibody formation. In 1971, evidence was independently obtained, in several laboratories using different models, that T lymphocytes can also suppress immune responses. Gershon and Kondo [16] showed this for responses of mice to sheep erythrocytes, following analogous experiments by McCullagh [149] in rats. Herzenberg and colleagues [150] found that allotype suppression in mice is mediated by T cells. Okumura and Tada [151] showed that T cells can suppress the formation of IgE antibodies. Allison et al. [8] presented evidence that T cells can suppress the formation of autoantibodies against erythrocytes in NZB mice. Since this finding is pertinent to the distinction between tolerance and autoimmunity, the evidence is discussed in more detail.

NZB mice develop a Coombs-positive autoimmune hemolytic anemia from about the age of 4 months. If spleen cells are transferred from old to young NZB mice, about one half of the recipients show positive Coombs tests, which usually disappear in a few weeks. If recipients are depleted of T lymphocytes, a higher proportion develop positive Coombs tests, and these usually remain positive until the death of the animals [8]. The simplest explanation of these observations is that T cells in the young animals exert an inhibitory influence on the B lymphocytes that are producing autoantibodies against erythrocytes. In keeping with this interpretation, repeated transfers of thymus cells from young NZB mice to ageing NZB mice were found in our laboratory [13] and that of Steinberg [22] to delay the onset of hemolytic anemia.

The evidence that has since accumulated supporting the interpretation that T lymphocytes can suppress autoimmune reactions, is too extensive to review comprehensively; only selected examples can be given. Two experimental manipulations have facilitated the distinction between helper T lymphocytes, which are required for autoimmunity, and suppressor T lymphocytes, which prevent it. First, the suppressor subset is more sensitive to ionizing radiation than the helper subset [152]. Second, the helper subset of T cells migrates from the thymus to peripheral tissues in the first few days after birth, whereas the suppressor subset remains in the thymus longer. Hence, by thymectomizing mice 2 – 4 days after birth it is possible to tip the balance towards help rather than suppression.

Wistar rats do not normally show thyroiditis, but if thymectomized at the age of 3 weeks and given sublethal radiation (4×200 R X-rays), the majority was found to have thyroiditis when examined 2 months later [23]. Irradiation of the thyroid alone had no such effect, and, when the rats were given 10^8 syngeneic lymphocytes after radiation, the development of thyroiditis was prevented; the active cells were eliminated by an antiserum reacting selectively with T cells.

Taguchi, Nishizuka and their colleagues have exploited the second strategy, thymectomizing mice during the critical period 2 – 4 days after birth when helper T cells but not suppressors have migrated from the thymus to peripheral lymphoid tissues (review [153]). This procedure, without any sensitization with exogenous antigens, resulted in the production of autoantibodies and the development of several organ-specific autoimmune diseases (thyroiditis, gastritis with macrocytic anaemia, oophoritis, orchitis and prostatitis). These diseases could be prevented by transfers of T cells from normal adult mice. Thymectomy 2 – 4 days after birth preferentially depletes the Ly-1$^+$ T cell subset, which includes the cells suppressing autoimmunity. Reconstitution of BALB/c nude mice with anti-Ly-1-treated spleen cells, without any other manipulation, produced organ-related autoimmune diseases like those observed in 2 – 4 day thymectomized mice [154]. Restoration of T cell functions in BALB/c nude mice by transplantation of rat thymic rudiments was likewise associated with production of autoantibodies and organ-specific autoimmune diseases [153]. Possibly T lymphocytes able to respond to autoantigens were not eliminated by interaction with MHCII on rat thymic epithelial cells (see discussion on genetic restriction of clonal elimination in the thymus). An alternative explanation is that suppressor T lymphocytes are not efficiently activated by interaction with rat cells because of genetic restriction. These alternatives can be tested by appropriate cell transfer experiments.

Chickens are convenient experimental animals, since it is possible to deplete selectively B lymphocytes by bursectomy or T lymphocytes by thymectomy. Hormonal bursectomy by injection of androgen into obese strain chick embryos or surgical bursectomy in ovo abolished or markedly reduced the autoimmune thyroiditis characteristic of this strain [155]. In contrast, thymectomy of newly hatched obese chickens accelerated and aggravated the lymphoid infiltration of the thyroid, and raised the incidence of birds with antibodies to thyroglobulin [155]: whole-body X-radiation after hatching also produced more severe disease [155].

As discussed above, tolerance to autologous erythrocytes can be terminated in mice by injections of rat erythrocytes [21]. This elicits the formation of both antibodies to rat erythrocytes and autoantibodies to determinants on mouse erythrocytes cross-reactive with rat erythrocytes. If mice are given lymphocytes from donors immunized in this way and then challenged with rat erythrocytes, their autoantibody response is suppressed while their response to rat erythrocytes is normal or increased [156]. The cells transferring suppression are Ly-1$^+$2$^-$ T cells, although B memory cells increase the efficiency of the transfer (possibly by functioning as APC). Nude mice receiving spleen cells from mice immunized with rat erythrocytes produce normal levels of autoantibodies and anti-rat erythrocyte antibodies, but are unable to generate suppressor cells [156]. This implies that T cells are required in the recipients and are stimulated to become effector suppressor cells.

The distinction between memory and effector T suppressor (Ts) cells has been shown in studies using foreign serum proteins. Loblay et al. [157] analysed the role of these cells in high-dose tolerance of mice to human gamma globulin (HGG). The T suppressor cells specific for HGG were found in two distinct functional states in the tolerant animals: effector cells and memory cells. The activity of the former was demonstrable in standard adoptive mixing experiments shortly after tolerance induction, but their presence was transient by comparison with the duration of the tolerant state. In contrast, memory T suppressor cells did not express effector functions in adoptive transfer studies unless they were first reactivated by secondary antigenic stimulation. Nevertheless, these latent T suppressor cells were long lived and able to respond rapidly to antigenic stimulation in adoptive tests for effector function. The properties of memory T suppressor cells (suppressor-inducer cells) make them good candidates for the long-term maintenance of tolerance to foreign antigens and, by implication, self antigens.

However, when tolerance is induced to exogenous antigens such as foreign serum proteins, there is always some concern whether the models are relevant to naturally induced tolerance. It is, therefore, comforting to know that similar mechanisms operate for proteins normally presented to the immune system. Harris et al. [158]

analysed mice that were identical genetically except for the ability to produce the fifth component of complement (C5). The mice lacking C5 could be immunized to form antibodies against C5 whereas those producing C5 were unresponsive. Nevertheless, the unresponsive mice had B cells that could be activated by C5, as shown in transfer experiments. Unresponsiveness required the continued presence of antigen and could be transferred by T lymphocytes.

Studies of cytotoxic and helper T cells have been greatly advanced by three developments: cloning the separate subsets of cells, characterizing their receptors for antigens and defining the lymphokines they produce when activated. Suppressor T cells have been known for 17 years, and it is to be hoped that in the next decade their properties, receptors for antigen and major products will become as well-characterized as those of other subsets of lymphocytes. That will facilitate understanding of their role in maintaining self tolerance and, thereby, preventing autoimmunity.

XIV. Idiotypic regulation of autoimmunity

Jerne's network theory of the immune system [159] has attracted a great deal of attention, and his concepts have been extended to autoimmunity by several investigators (reviews [160, 161]). In principle, antibodies against idiotypes could induce autoimmune disease or suppress it. If the latter is true, anti-idiotypic antibodies might be used for therapy of autoimmune diseases in a manner analogous to the prevention of hemolytic disease of the newborn by antibodies against Rh blood groups.

Idiotypy and autoimmunity is a large subject which cannot be reviewed comprehensively in this chapter. Only a few pertinent points will be discussed. Rats injected with anti-insulin antibodies produce anti-idiotypic antibodies which bind to insulin receptors of the rat [162]. Anti-insulin receptor antibodies in humans with IDDM may arise as auto-anti-idiotypic antibodies [163]. In an analogous manner, immunization with thyrotropin elicits antibodies reacting with and stimulating thyrotropin receptors on thyroid epithelial cells [164]. In each case, administration of an idiotype induced an autoimmune response dominated by clones expressing a particular auto-idiotype. Such phenomena may occur spontaneously in autoimmune diseases.

Klinman and Steinberg [161] postulate that auto-anti-idiotypic antibodies might facilitate the development of autoimmunity by interfering with the tolerization of autoreactive B cells. However, since the importance of such tolerization is questionable (see above) extension to anti-idiotypic responses is even more questionable. In fact, regulation of the formation of anti-idiotypic antibodies may be moderated by T helper and/or suppressor cells rather than by antibodies. Whether antibodies, and the idiotypes they present, are required for the generation of suppressor T cells is also uncertain. A model has been discussed above in which mice injected with rat erythrocytes produce autoantibodies against shared erythrocytic determinants. The mice also develop suppressor-inducer cells which, when transferred to naive recipients, regulate the production of autoantibodies but not anti-rat erythrocyte agglutinins. CBA/N mice (which express an X-linked genetic B lymphocyte defect) immunized with rat erythrocytes produced no autoantibodies but normal levels of antibodies against rat erythrocytes and suppressor-inducer cells [156]. The authors conclude that suppressor-inducer cells are carrier-specific and are not stimulated by idiotypes on either autoantibody or autoreactive B cells.

In summary, while anti-idiotypic responses regulate autoimmunity in some experimental and clinical situations, there is at present no evidence that idiotypic networks play a major role in the prevention of autoimmunity or in the pathogenesis of most autoimmune diseases.

XV. Seclusion of autoantigens from the immune system

Burnet [6] suggested that autoantigens are often secluded from the immune system. However, many antigens formerly thought to be secluded, such as thyroglobulin and protein hormones, are now known to circulate even in the sera of newborns (about 100 ng per ml, or 10^{-9} M, in the case of thyroglobulin [165]). The cytoplasmic protein F in liver and other tissues circulates in concentrations of between 10^{-8} M and 10^{-9} M. These concentrations are sufficient to bind to lymphocytes with high-affinity receptors for the antigens and induce T cell tolerance.

However, there may well be seclusion of some antigens from immunocompetent cells in normal hosts. For example, the lens is segregated from blood vessels and lymphatics, and its constituents do not normally elicit immune responses, as the acceptance of lens homografts shows. Cartilage is likewise segregated from blood vessels and lymphatics and constituents such as type II collagen may not have induced T cell tolerance, which would account for the ease with which immune responses to type II collagen, in contrast to other types, can be elicited [78]. The basic protein of myelin may be effectively secluded from the immune system, which could explain the reaction of T cells to this antigen in autoimmune encephalomyelitis. Some antigens are organ-specific and insoluble in aqueous solvents. These include organ-specific microsomal antigens of the thyroid, gastric parietal cells and other cell types. The microsomal/microvillar antigen (TMAg) of thyroid epithelial cells may provide an example of a secluded antigen. The surface expression of this molecule is normally restricted to the apical border facing the interior of thyroid follicles where it is not exposed to the immune system. However, in the autoimmune disease, Graves' thyrotoxicosis, follicles can express TMAg on their basal vascular border where it is exposed to cells of the immune system [86]. In this condition autoantibodies against TMAg are characteristically present.

XVI. Partial degradation of autoantigens

Most macromolecular antigens are thought to be partially broken down in APC to release peptides that bind to MHC glycoproteins [26, 27]. As we first showed [166], many drugs are taken up into and concentrated in endocytic compartments [167]; some selectively inhibit proteinases and could inhibit or modify such processing. An example of partial degradation modifying immunogenicity is the use of rabbit thyroglobulin digested with papain or leukocyte proteases to immunize rabbits without adjuvants [168, 169]. Many bacterial, viral and parasitic infections are associated with transient positive tests for antiglobulins of rheumatoid factor type. Enzyme-treated Ig is more immunogenic than native Ig [170], and the possibility that proteinases of microbial or host origin modify Ig to make it more im-munogenic, deserves consideration. Antigen-antibody complexes induce in ex-perimental animals the formation of antiglobulins [171] as well as anti-idiotypic an-tibodies [64]. Such complexes are efficiently localized on FDC [64], and in these or other APC the complexes may be processed differently from normal processing of host Ig.

Following coronary thrombosis autoantibodies against heart antigens are observ-ed [172]. These may be the result of modification of autoantigens by partial degradation or some other mechanism such as oxidation mediated by free oxygen radicals.

XVII. Cross-reactivity of exogenous and self antigens

The concept that autoimmunity can result from cross-reactivity of exogenous and self antigens has been discussed for a long time. A classical example is sharing of antigenic determinants by streptococci and heart muscle, which is believed to play a role in the pathogenesis of rheumatic fever [173]. The formation of antinuclear antibodies is characteristic of SLE and a group of related diseases. Many of the specificities of such antibodies, reacting with nuclear proteins, have now been defin-ed. Antibodies against native dsDNA, characteristically produced in SLE, have at-tracted special interest. Definition of antibodies against DNA has been facilitated by the development of human and murine hybridomas using cells from patients and mice with autoimmune disease [174]. Many anti-DNA monoclonal antibodies were found to be cross-reactive with various nucleic acids as well as cardiolipin and other phospholipids, presumably involving recognition of suitably spaced phosphodiester groups. Others stained cytoskeletal intermediate filaments because of reaction with vimentin. Monoclonal antibodies raised against measles virus phosphoprotein also cross-react with intermediate filaments [175].

Antigenic epitopes shared between mycobacteria and cartilage are believed to play a role in the pathogenesis of adjuvant arthritis in the rat. This is a chronic disease inducible in rats by inoculation of *Mycobacterium tuberculosis*. Clones of T cells able to produce arthritis in rats were obtained in the laboratory of Cohen [176] and shown to respond to an antigen shared by *M. tuberculosis* and joint cartilage. The epitope recognized by the T cells is formed by amino acids at positions 180 – 188 in the sequence of a 65 kDa antigen from *M. tuberculosis* cloned and expressed in *E. coli* [79]. Administration of this antigen to rats produced resistance to subsequent attempts to induce adjuvant arthritis. The fraction of cartilage proteoglycan recognized by the T lymphocyte may be the link protein which binds the core protein to hyaluronic acid [177]. T lymphocytes from patients with rheumatoid arthritis sometimes also respond to the mycobacterial antigen, but whether this reactivity plays any role in the pathogenesis of the disease is at present unknown; it might be a consequence of the arthritis. Sharing of bacterial and self epitopes might play a role in the pathogenesis of arthritis in Reiters' disease, which is associated with *Klebsiella, Yersinia* and other infections in genetically predisposed persons, often of the HLA-B27 haptotype [178].

In general, there is no doubt that cross-reactivity of microbial antigens and host antigens *can* produce autoimmune disease. This is a plausible model for the pathogenesis of rheumatic fever, but its role in the pathogenesis of autoimmune diseases currently prevalent remains to be established. Attempts to immunize humans against autoimmunity by eliciting anti-idiotypic or anti-TCR responses [177] require validation of the model.

XVIII. Virus infections

It has long been known that human infections with viruses, including influenza, measles, varicella and herpes simplex viruses, are sometimes followed by autoimmune manifestations, including antibody-mediated thrombocytopenia and positive Coombs tests [179]. Autoantibodies are more consistently observed following mononucleosis associated with Epstein-Barr virus (EBV) and cytomegalovirus (CMV) infections. Autoantibodies observed after EBV infections include those directed against nuclear antigens [180], lymphocytes and erythrocytes [181] and smooth muscle [182] and its constituent actin [183].

The initial event in EBV mononucleosis is proliferation of B lymphocytes, which show increased MHCII expression [103]; later reactive, proliferating T lymphocytes predominate [184]. The B cells with increased MHCII expression could present antigens, including autoantigens, to T cells; even cytotoxic T cells in this system are MHCII-restricted [36]. The reactive T cells presumably produce several lymphokines. Thus, the conditions required for induction of autoantibody formation, increased MHCII expression in the presence of autoantigens and cytokines, are all present. Possibly the polyclonal B cell proliferation stimulus provided by EBV itself could be an additional mechanism favoring the development of autoimmunity.

Viral antigens may also function as helper determinants for autoantigens. The abundant cytoskeletal protein actin is considered to be a weak antigen because of its highly conserved structure. Nevertheless, autoantibodies reacting with actin have been found in the sera of patients following several viral illnesses including acute hepatitis, infectious mononucleosis and measles virus infections [183]. Actin has been identified in many enveloped viruses and is believed to play a part in their assembly [185]. As a model, M protein purified from Newcastle disease virus has been found to bind to rabbit skeletal muscle actin non-covalently, but with high affinity, and to increase the antigenicity of actin in rabbits [186]. The same is true in mice; moreover, T lymphocytes from immunized mice respond to M protein but not to actin (W.T. Anomasiri and D.L.J. Tyrrell, personal communication). This supports the interpretation that the viral protein is acting as a helper determinant increasing autoantibody formation against actin. Rats infected with Friend leukemia virus develop Coombs-positive autoimmune hemolytic anemia [187]. The virus buds from the surface of erythroblasts and could presumably function as a helper in production of autoantibodies against an antigen or antigens on the surface of normal erythrocytes.

A third hypothesis associating virus infections and autoimmunity has been proposed by Bottazzo and his colleagues [68]. They postulate that virus infections, especially those of endocrine organs, result in the production of IFN-γ which increases local MHCII expression, presentation of autoantigens and subsequent induction of autoimmune T cells. The latter would, in turn, activate effector B and T cells. This mechanism of autoimmune induction would explain 'vague associations with virus infections and long latency periods before disease becomes manifest and gives a simple explanation for the well-documented association between HLA-DR and autoimmune disease'. This hypothesis may explain some associations between virus infections and subsequent autoimmunity. However, for reasons discussed in the section on antigen presentation, it is unknown whether expression of MHCII on thyroid epithelial cells and pancreatic islet β cells is a cause of the autoimmune disease or a manifestation of it. Moreover, virus infections can actually protect genetically predisposed BB rats and non-obese diabetic mice from later development of diabetes mellitus [188, 189]. Hence, the relationship between virus infections and later expression of autoimmunity is complicated.

XIX. Bacterial infections and products

Bacterial infections and products can stimulate the immune system in a variety of ways. Some bacteria and bacterial products are adjuvants, able to increase cell-mediated and humoral responses against unrelated antigens. Well-known examples are LPS of Gram-negative bacteria, *Bordetella pertussis* organisms, and mycobacterial cell walls and their muramyl dipeptide components [190]. Some bacterial products are polyclonal B cell mitogens, e.g. LPS in mice and protein A of *Staphylococcus* in humans.

Partly for these reasons and partly because of their immunogenicity, bacteria can strongly stimulate macrophages, B and T lymphocytes, with consequent production of cytokines. A classical system for production of IFN-γ is sensitization with mycobacteria and challenge with tuberculin [191], whereas that for production of TNF-α is similar sensitization and challenge with LPS [192]. LPS and other bacterial products induce production of GM-CSF [193]. These mediators are likely to increase MHCII expression, for example in the heart in rheumatic fever. LPS also induces the release of IL-6 [112] and presumably other mediators promoting proliferation of B cells and their differentiation into antibody-forming cells.

In addition, bacteria may share determinants with autoantigens, as discussed above. Thus, the conditions required for formation of autoantibodies are all present, and it has long been known that bacterial infections or repeated injections of bacteria are associated with the production of autoantibodies. Well-known examples include autoantibodies to myocardial antigens in rheumatic fever [173], antibodies to cardiolipin and cold autoantibodies to erythrocytes in syphilis, autoantibodies to lung antigens in tuberculosis, various autoantibodies in leprosy and antiglobulins in animals repeatedly injected with bacteria (review [24]).

Repeated injections of LPS in mice elicit the formation of many autoantibodies, with specificity for DNA [194] and other antigens. This has been attributed to polyclonal B cell activation [194], but the adjuvant activity of LPS [190] should also be considered.

XX. Autoimmunity following administration of drugs

Some autoimmune manifestations following drug administration are remarkably specific. In patients treated with α-methyldopa Coombs-positive autoimmune hemolytic anemias are not uncommon [195]. Often the autoantibody is IgG directed against the antigen of the Rh series. The production of antibodies against denatured DNA and histones and a syndrome-like SLE occurs in patients treated with procainamide or hydralazine [196]. Autoantibodies from patients with drug-induced or idiopathic SLE react with epitopes of the amino and carboxyl termini of histone [197].

The first explanation proposed for drug-induced autoimmunity was binding of the drug or a metabolite to an autoantigen; it was postulated that if host T lymphocytes can react against antigenic determinants of the drug, autoantibodies could be formed through a helper effect [8]. As discussed above, small molecules able to stimulate T lymphocytes, such as arsanilic acid or dinitrophenol, when coupled with autologous thyroglobulin or Ig, can elicit autoantibodies against thyroglobulin and anti-idiotypic antibodies [147, 148]. Mouse T lymphocytes were sensitized to *p*-

aminobenzoic acid (PAB) by immunization with a hapten-isologous protein conjugate, and then the animals were challenged with PAB-conjugated isologous mouse erythrocytes. They developed Coombs-positive autoimmune hemolytic anemias. Evidence was presented that reactive helper T cells were essential for the production of the autoantibodies [198]. A lupus-like syndrome with pulmonary reactions has also been described in patients treated with nitrofurantoin. Such patients show evidence of cell-mediated reactions to nitrofurantoin but no binding of the drug by antibodies [199]; this is consistent with the interpretation that the drug is functioning as a helper determinant. Binding of procainamide and hydralazine to DNA and nucleoproteins, which has been observed (review [197]), could likewise allow the drugs to function as helper determinants. In nitrofurantoin treatment a variety of autoantibodies, including some with specificity for human serum albumin, have been found [137]. Tailing of albumin on electrophoretic strips occurred because of the formation of complexes with polyclonal IgG autoantibodies. As discussed above, the production of autoantibodies against human serum albumin, together with other evidence [132], suggests that even in the case of self antigens circulating in high dose, B lymphocytes able to react to them are not deleted.

A second explanation for drug-induced autoimmunity is polyclonal activation of B lymphocytes. Mercuric chloride induces in Brown-Norway (BN) rats, but not in Lewis rats, the production of autoantibodies against basement membranes followed by an immune complex disease [200]. Mercuric chloride was found to be a polyclonal activator of rat spleen cells, but not of isolated B lymphocytes [201]. The authors conclude that polyclonal activation may play a role in the pathogenesis of $HgCl_2$-induced disease of BN rats.

A third explanation for drug-induced autoimmunity has been proposed by Gleichmann and Gleichmann [202]. They review evidence that, following administration of diphenylhydantoin to some human patients and experimental animals, there is widespread lymphoid hyperplasia and plasmacytosis, with the formation of autoantibodies reacting against nuclear antigens, erythrocytes and lymphocytes. They propose that hydantoin derivatives become attached to the surface of lymphoid cells and modify their MHC antigens in such a way that autologous T lymphocytes recognize them as 'foreign' and react to them. Thereafter, the sequence of events would be analogous to that in GVH reactions. Autoimmune manifestations in patients treated with D-penicillamine have been explained in a similar way [203]. In some persons, D-penicillamine treatment has produced myasthenia gravis with autoantibodies against the acetylcholine receptor, pemphigus with autoantibodies to the intercellular substance of dermal epithelial cells, and a syndrome like SLE with antibodies against nuclear antigens and immune complex glomerulonephritis. Nagata et al. [203] found that D-penicillamine, when presented on the surface of stimulator cells from mouse spleen, can stimulate specific Ly-1$^+$2$^-$ T cells. They postulate that if D-penicillamine were to generate stimulator cells in some humans, this could lead to T cell responses comparable to those in GVH reactions. As discussed above, such reactions could increase MHCII expression and production of cytokines required for activation of autoantibody-producing B cells. This explanation and the helper effect mentioned above are not mutually exclusive. In fact, drugs acting as helper determinants for autoantigens might focus GVH-type reactions. For example, suppose that D-penicillamine can bind to the surface of APC such as Langerhans cells and to the acetylcholine receptor. The former might elicit T cell clones reactive with D-penicillamine, and those T cells might then react with the drug bound to the acetylcholine receptor, thereby helping the formation of autoantibodies against the receptor.

A fourth explanation has been mentioned above in the context of degradation of autoantigens. As we first showed [166], many drugs are concentrated in lysosomal or other endocytic compartments [167]. Some such drugs are known to inhibit proteolytic and other degradative pathways which can modify presentation to the immune system and produce autoimmunity [168, 169]. Production of immunogenic peptides from large molecules, and their binding to MHC glycoproteins, is now being studied in detail [26, 27] so that it would therefore be possible to analyse effects of drugs on such processing of foreign antigens and self antigens more precisely.

A fifth explanation for drug-induced autoimmunity is that drugs might increase MHC expression or cytokine production. Glucocortocoids and E-type prostaglandins decrease MHCII expression in macrophages [87, 88] and responses of lymphocytes to mitogenic stimulation [204]. The latter has been attributed to activation of adenylate cyclase, the best-known mode of action of E-type prostaglandins [204]. However, activation of adenylate cyclase in other cell types might increase expression of MHCII or other markers. For example, thyrotropin activates adenylate cyclase in thyroid epithelial cells [205] and is a co-factor increasing MHCII expression in these cells [86]. Agents increasing cyclic AMP levels augment the expression of Thy-1 on murine T cells [206]. Remarkably little is known about intracellular mechanisms by which MHC expression and cytokine production are regulated. Many drugs exert their effects by perturbing such second messenger systems, and some could well act as co-factors increasing MHC expression and/or cytokine production. One consequence could be to tip the balance between help and suppression by T lymphocytes.

An example of a drug having a differential effect on a lymphocyte subset is the iodinated benzofuran derivative amiodarone, which has antianginal and antiarrhythmic activity. Known side effects include hyper- and hypothyroidism, with antibodies against thyroglobulin, thyroid microsomal antigens and thyrotropin receptor. Amiodarone therapy is associated in most patients with a marked increase in circulation of a recently discovered subset of T cells expressing a complex ganglioside antigen reacting with monoclonal antibody 3G5 [207]. One patient was hyperthyroid and had T cells expressing MCHII which disappeared 3 weeks after discontinuing the drug. The presence of T cells expressing MCHII in recent-onset Graves' disease [74] is discussed above in the context of APC.

In general, several mechanisms have already been postulated by which drugs could precipitate organ-specific autoimmunity, and doubtless other mechanisms not yet recognized exist. It will be necessary to examine carefully each combination of drug and host to ascertain which mechanism is operative.

XXI. Holes in the repertoire of receptors for antigen

One interpretation of tolerance to self is that there has been selection against V regions of T cell antigen receptors and immunoglobulins with specificity for self. This may be true in some cases, for example the observation in Klinman's laboratory that even pre-B cells of mice cannot respond to an amino-terminal peptide of cytochrome *c* well conserved in evolution [208]. The argument could be extended to postulate selection against MHCI and II glycoproteins able to bind autoantigens. However, this cannot be the explanation for acquired tolerance, e.g. chimerism, since adult animals can efficiently mount immune responses against the alloantigens in question. Integration of insulin-promoted T antigen of SV40 into the genome of mice has shown that tolerance to a foreign antigen can be induced [209].

XXII. Ly-1$^+$ B cells in mice and Leu-1$^+$ B cells in humans

In mice T lymphocytes express the Ly-1 glycoprotein and in humans T lymphocytes express the Leu-1 (CD5) glycoprotein. During the past few years it has been recognized that in mice there is a subset of B lymphocytes expressing Ly-1 at low density (Ly-1$^+$ B cells) and in humans a subset of B lymphocytes expressing Leu-1 at low density (Leu-1$^+$ B cells). In mice Ly-1$^+$ B cells are found predominantly in the peritoneal cavity and spleen [210]. In viable motheaten mice, which develop severe autoimmunity, all B cells express Ly-1 [211], and NZB mice have a high proportion of Ly-1$^+$ B cells [212], whereas the SJL strain has few cells of this subset. Ly-1$^+$ B cells produce nearly all IgM autoantibodies in mice [210] and in motheaten mice they also produce IgG$_3$ [211].

In humans, up to 30% of B cells in peripheral blood have been found to express Leu-1 [212, 213]. Casali et al. [212] stimulated Leu-1$^+$ B cells with Epstein-Barr virus and found production of IgM antibodies reacting with ssDNA and IgG(Fc), in other words rheumatoid factor. Hardy et al. [213], using Leu-1$^+$ B cells and the polyclonal stimulant *Staphylococcus aureus*, obtained similar results. Leu-1$^+$ B cells from immunized persons produced IgM antibodies against tetanus toxoid; Leu-1$^-$ B cells produced IgG antibodies. Plater-Zyberk [214] reported that the proportion of Leu-1$^+$ B cells is higher in patients with rheumatoid arthritis than in controls: however, there was no correlation in individual patients between the number of Leu-1$^+$ B cells and clinical disease activity.

The recognition of the existence of this subset of cells producing IgM autoantibodies, and in one strain of mice IgG_3 antibodies, is interesting. Little is known about cytokines regulating production of antibodies by these subsets of B cells in mice and in humans. It seems certain that autoantibodies produced by this subset play a role in the pathogenesis of disease in viable motheaten mice. Whether Leu-1^+ B cell products are important in the pathogenesis of autoimmune diseases in humans is still an open question.

XXIII. Autoantibodies in normal persons

It has been known for two decades that healthy persons can have autoantibodies against thyroglobulin, especially as they age. In such persons autoantibodies can be demonstrated against actin, tubulin, fetuin, albumin, transferrin, collagen and cytochrome c as well as thyroglobulin, and natural autoantibodies constitute a substantial part of normal circulating immunoglobulins [131]. Results of fusing lymphocytes from non-immunized young mice with a non-secreting myeloma line indicated the existence in mice of B cell clones reactive with self antigens, notably cytoskeletal proteins and DNA [131]. Nevertheless, levels of antibodies against cytoskeletal proteins such as actin can be considerably raised by virus infections or by appropriate immunization (see section on viruses). Monoclonal autoantibodies from 31 patients with gammopathies showed similar specificities to those naturally occurring; in none of these patients could clinical symptoms be related to the presence of the autoantibodies [131].

Why some autoantibodies produce pathology while others do not is an important and only partially resolved question. The properties of the autoantibodies, e.g. affinity and isotype, as well as the epitopes recognized, are important. Autoantibodies of the IgG_1 or IgG_3 isotypes in humans, reacting with erythrocyte antigens with reasonably high affinity, are likely to produce hemolytic anemia because they sensitize the cells to lysis by monocytes. Some autoantibodies to thyrotropin receptors stimulate the thyroid while others do not: in this case the epitopes on the receptor recognized are important. Most autoimmune diseases are antibody-mediated rather than cell-mediated [24]. However, it is possible to envisage a sequence of events in which an autoantibody interacting with a target tissue, e.g. the thyroid, produces immune complexes, stimulates mediator production and increases MHC expression to a level which allows T cells to react with autoantigens, thereby perpetuating the immunopathological process.

XXIV. Somatic mutation and forbidden clones

As stated in the introduction, the formation of autoantibodies can readily be elicited in young experimental animals. The autoantibodies formed depend on the antigen used – thyroglobulin, acetylcholine receptor, acrosomal, etc. No mechanism is known by which antigenic stimulation could selectively induce somatic mutations leading to production of autoantibodies reacting selectively with the antigen used. The frequent presence in humans and mice of autoantibodies, and the sharing of idiotypes with monoclonal autoantibodies naturally occurring and experimentally produced, has convinced most investigators [131], including some in institutes formerly directed by Burnet [215], that autoimmunity results from expansion of pre-existing clones of B cells. As Davidson et al. [216] point out, cross-reactive idiotypes on anti-DNA antibodies suggest that the same germline genes or gene families are used to encode anti-DNA antibodies in unrelated patients with SLE. They nevertheless suggest that anti-DNA antibodies may represent somatic mutants of antibodies made in response to a microbial antigen. This is an *ad hoc* hypothesis for which there is at present no evidence. Comparison of base sequences encoding the autoantibodies with germline V_H sequences should provide an unambiguous answer to the question of whether somatic mutation is a requirement for the formation of autoantibodies.

XXV. Old and new hypotheses for the development of autoimmunity

Many studies carried out during the past 17 years support our hypothesis made in 1971 [8, 9]:
(a) deletion or inactivation of clones of B lymphocytes reacting with self antigens is not a major mechanism of self tolerance;
(b) deletion of inactivation of T lymphocytes with receptors for self antigens occurs;
(c) by-passing the requirement for self-reactive T lymphocytes by the use of carrier epitopes stimulating T cells can give rise to the production of autoantibodies. Such carrier epitopes can occur on foreign proteins or cells with cross-reactive B cell epitopes, or on viral antigens or drugs binding to self antigens. Examples of all of these are listed above;
(d) T lymphocytes can suppress autoimmune responses;
(e) non-antigen specific stimulation of immune responses as a result of GVH reactions, infections or administration of adjuvants can give rise to the production of autoantibodies.

Major advances in immunology made during the past decade have allowed analysis of the mechanisms by which non-antigen-specific stimulation of immune responses increases the production of autoantibodies. Immune responses require (i) an adequate concentration of antigen; (ii) an adequate concentration of MHC glycoproteins in the presence of antigen to stimulate T lymphocytes efficiently; and (iii) adequate concentrations of stimulatory cytokines. Adequate concentrations of self antigens are usually present, although sometimes they have to be released from seclusion. Hence two major requirements for autoimmunity are (i) increasing MHC expression on host cells above a threshold level and (ii) augmenting cytokine production. Either of these two mechanisms increases the probability of developing autoimmunity, but they are likely to have synergistic effects.

Studies of experimental animals genetically predisposed to develop autoimmunity show (i) spontaneous production of cytokines by lymphocytes and by other cell types such as macrophages, and (ii) increased MHCII expression. It is difficult to escape the conclusion that a coincidence of these two abnormalities is required for early and consistent manifestation of autoimmune disease. Thus the *lpr* gene, irrespective of the genetic background of mice, gives rise to lymphoproliferation, which is presumably a consequence of spontaneous cytokine production. However, mice homozygous for *lpr* develop autoimmunity only when they also show increased MHCII expression in peritoneal macrophages (MRL-*lpr/lpr* and NZB *lpr/lpr*). It can, therefore, be postulated that the MRL or NZB genetic backgrounds allow increased MHCII expression in response to the cytokines produced by *lpr/lpr* mice. Other mutations predisposing to autoimmunity (e.g *me* and *me^v*) are likewise associated with spontaneous cytokine production and high MHCII expression.

The new hypothesis can be made that the *lpr* and *me^v* mutations each involve an element regulating cytokine production, e.g. defective production of a repressor, modification of a DNA sequence to which a repressor binds, excessive production of a promoter or enhancer or modification of a DNA sequence to which these elements bind, or absence of a ribonuclease degrading cytokine mRNA. An extension of the hypothesis is that MRL and NZB mice should have mutations in regions regulating expression of MHCII. Increased expression of MHCII in B lymphocytes and other APC may initiate systemic autoimmune responses while MHCII expression on parenchymal cells (thyroid epithelial cells, articular chondrocytes, etc.) may focus the effector phase of the immune response on a particular target. This, again, is a testable hypothesis. Augmenting MHC expression on thyroid epithelial cells by IFN-γ and thyrotropin should increase their susceptibility to damage by clones of T lymphocytes with appropriate specificity. Humans with SLE, thyroiditis and other autoimmune diseases should likewise have defects in the regulation of cytokine production and/or MHC expression in appropriate cell types, not necessarily peripheral blood monocytes. As DNA sequences and proteins regulating MHC expression and cytokine production become defined, these hypotheses are testable.

On this hypothesis a quantitative increase of MHC expression and cytokine production is sufficient to trigger autoimmunity. However, qualitative differences in MHC structure could also focus the manifestations of autoimmunity on a particular target, for example the relationship of I-A and DQ constitution to type I insulin-dependent diabetes mellitus [53, 54].

When more is known about suppressor T lymphocytes and the factors controlling

104

their activities, the hypothesis that lack of suppression is required for autoimmunity can be tested further. Of course that hypothesis is not mutually exclusive with those previously listed: for example, increased MHC expression or spontaneous cytokine production might be associated with decreased T lymphocyte mediated suppression.

These hypotheses have the advantage of being open to experimental verification or exclusion. Regulation of MHC expression and cytokine production, as well as definition of suppressor T cells, are high priority subjects for research in the next decade, and perhaps the findings will explain why the common types of autoimmunity occur.

References

1. Ehrlich, P. and Morgenroth, J. (1910) Collected Studies in Immunity, John Wiley, New York.
2. Traub, E. (1938) Factors influencing the persistence of lymphocytes choriomeningitis virus in the blood of mice following clinical recovery. J. Exp. Med. 68, 229–250.
3. Owen, R. D. (1945) Immunogenetic consequences of vascular anastomoses between bovine twins. Science 102, 400–401.
4. Burnet, F. M. and Fenner, F. (1949) The Production of Antibodies, 2nd edn., Macmillan, London.
5. Billingham, R. E., Brent, L. and Medawar, P. B. (1953) Actively acquired tolerance of foreign cells. Nature 172, 603–606.
6. Burnet, F. M. (1957) A modification of Jerne's theory of antibody production using the concept of clonal selection. Aust. J. Sci. 20, 67–69.
7. Bretscher, P. and Cohn, M. (1970) A theory of self-nonself discrimination: paralysis and induction involve the recognition of one and two determinants on an antigen, respectively. Science 169, 1042–1049.
8. Allison, A. C., Denman, A. M. and Barnes, R. D. (1971) Co-operating and controlling functions of thymus-derived lymphocytes in relation to autoimmunity. Lancet ii, 135–140.
9. Allison, A. C. (1971) Unresponsiveness to self antigens. Lancet ii, 1401–1403.
10. Weigle, W. O. (1971) Recent observations and concepts in immunological unresponsiveness and autoimmunity. Clin. Exp. Immunol. 92, 437–447.
11. Parks, D. E., Doyle, M. V. and Weigle, W. O. (1979) Induction and mode of action of suppressor cells generated against human gamma globulin: an immunologic unresponsive state devoid of demonstrable suppressor cells. J. Exp. Med. 148, 625–638.
12. Bankhurst, A. D., Torrigiani, G. and Allison, A. C. (1973) Lymphocytes binding human thyroglobulin in healthy people and its relevance to tolerance for autoantigens. Lancet i, 226–229.
13. Allison, A. C. (1974) Interactions of T and B lymphocytes in self tolerance and autoimmunity. In: D. H. Katz and B. Beracerraf (Eds.), Immunological Tolerance. Mechanisms and Potential Therapeutic Applications, Academic Press, New York, pp. 25–59.
14. Clagett, J. A. and Weigle, W. O. (1974) Roles of T and B lymphocytes in the termination of unresponsiveness to autologous thyroglobulin in mice. J. Exp. Med. 139, 643–660.
15. Fialkow, P., Gilchrist, C. and Allison, A. C. (1973) Autoimmunity in chronic graft-versus-host disease. Clin. Exp. Immunol. 13, 479–486.
16. Gershon, R. K. and Kondo, K. (1971) Infectious immunological tolerance. Immunology 21, 903–914.
17. Allison, A. C., Denman, A. M. and Barnes, R. D. (1980) Citation classic – co-operating and

controlling functions of thymus-derived lymphocytes in relation to autoimmunity. Current Contents/Clinical Practice N24, pp. 10–12.

18. Gleichmann, E., Pals, S. T., Rolink, T., Radaszkiewicz, T. and Gleichmann, H. (1984) Graft-versus-host reactions: clues to the etiopathology of a spectrum of immunological diseases. Immunol. Today 5, 324–328.

19. Pollard, K. M., Chan, E. K. L., Rubin, R. L. and Tan, E. M. (1987) Monoclonal autoantibodies to nuclear antigens from murine graft-versus-host disease. Clin. Immunol. Immunopathol. 44, 31–40.

20. Cox, K. O. and Keast, D. (1974) Autoimmune haemolytic anaemia induced in mice immunized with rat erythrocytes. Clin. Exp. Immunol. 17, 319–327.

21. Cox, K. O. (1987) Mouse models of autoantibody production against red blood cells in health and disease. In: Ballière's Clinical Immunology and Allergy, D. Doniach and G. F. Bottazzo (Eds.), Vol. 1, Ballière, London, pp. 1–23.

22. Gershwin, M. E. and Steinberg, A. D. (1975) Suppression of autoimmune hemolytic anemia in New Zealand (NZB) mice by syngeneic young thymocytes. Clin. Immunol. Immunopathol. 4, 38–45.

23. Penhale, W. J., Farmer, A. and Irvine, W. J. (1975) Thyroiditis in T-cell depleted rats. Influence of strain, radiation dose, adjuvants and antilymphocyte serum. Clin. Exp. Immunol. 21, 362–375.

24. Allison, A. C. (1977) Autoimmune diseases: concepts of pathogenesis and control. In: N. Talal (Ed.), Autoimmunity: Genetic, Immunologic, Virologic and Clinical Aspects, Academic Press, New York, pp. 91–139.

25. Germain, R. N. and Malissen, B. (1986) Analysis of the expression and function of class II major histocompatibility complex-encoded molecules mediated by gene transfer. Ann. Rev. Immunol. 4, 281–315.

26. Babbitt, B., Allen, P., Matsueda, G., Haber, E. and Unanue, E. (1985) Binding of immunogenic peptides to Ia histocompatibility molecules. Nature 317, 359–361.

27. Brus, S., Sette, A., Cohn, S., Miles, C. and Grey, H. (1987) The relation between major histocompatibility complex (MHC) restriction and capacity of Ia to bind immunogenic peptides. Science (Wash. D.C.) 235, 1353–1358.

28. Blanden, R. V., Hodgkin, P. D., Hill, A, Sinickas, V. G. and Müllbacher, A. (1987) Quantitative considerations of T-cell activation and self-tolerance. Immunol. Rev. 98, 75–93.

29. Swain, S. L. (1983) T-cell subsets and the recognition of MHC class. Immunol. Rev. 74, 129–142.

30. Janeway, C. A. Jr., Carding, S., Jones, B., Murray, J., Pontoles, P., Rasmussen, R., Rojo, J., Saizawa, K., West, J. and Bottomly, K. (1988) CD4$^+$ T-cells: specificity and function. Immunol. Rev. 101, 39–80.

31. Cherwinski, H. M., Schumacher, J. H., Brown, K. D. and Mossmann, T. R. (1987) Two types of mouse helper T-cell clone. III. Further differences in lymphokine synthesis between Th1 and Th2 clones revealed by RNA hybridization, functionally monospecific bioassays, and monoclonal antibodies. J. Exp. Med. 166, 1229–1244.

32. Paul, W. E. and Ohara, J. (1987) B-cell stimulatory factor/interleukin 4. Annu. Rev. Immunol. 5, 429–460.

33. Snapper, C. M. and Paul, W. E. (1987) Interferon-γ and B-cell stimulatory factor-1 reciprocally regulate Ig isotype production. Science (Wash. D.C.) 236, 944–947.

34. Crawford, R. M., Finbloom, D. S., Ohara, J., Paul, W. E. and Meltzer, M. S. (1987) B-cell stimulatory factor-1 (interleukin 4) activates macrophages for increased tumoricidal activity and expression of Ia antigens. Immunology 139, 135–141.

35. Te Velde, A. A., Klamp, J. P. G., Ward, B. A., De Vries, J. and Figdor, C. G. (1988) Modulation of phenotypic and functional properties of human peripheral blood

monocytes by IL-4. J. Immunol. 140, 1548 – 1554.

36. Misko, I. S., Pope, J. H., Hütler, R., Soszynski, T. J. and Kane, R. G. (1984) HLA-DR antigen associated restriction of EBV-specific cytotoxic T-cell colonies. Int. J. Cancer 33, 239 – 243.

37. Lindsley, M. D., Torpey, D. J. and Rinaldo, C. R. (1984) Restriction of lymphocyte-mediated cytotoxicity of cytomegalovirus-infected human monocytes by the HLA-DR locus. In: S. Plotkin (Ed.), Pathogenesis and Prevention of Human Cytomegalovirus Disease, Alan R. Liss, New York, pp. 429 – 433.

38. Morrison, L. A., Lukacher, A. E., Braciale, V. L., Fan, D. P. and Braciale, T. J. (1986) Differences in antigen presentation to MCH class I and MHC class II-restricted influenza virus-specific T lymphocyte clones. J. Exp. Med. 163, 903 – 921.

39. Townsend, A. R. M., Rothbard, J., Gotch, F. M., Bahadur, G., Wraith, D. and McMichael, A. J. (1986) The epitopes of influenza nucleoprotein recognized by cytotoxic T lymphocytes can be defined with short synthetic peptides. Cell 44, 959 – 968.

40. Staerz, U. D., Karasuyama, H. and Garner, A. M. (1987) Cytotoxic T lymphocytes against a soluble protein. Nature 329, 449 – 451.

41. Sinickas, V. G., Ashman, R. B. and Blanden, R. V. (1987) The cytotoxic response to murine cytomegalovirus. IV. Requirements for the generation of MCMV-specific target cells. Immunol. Cell Biol. (Australia) 65, 173 – 182.

42. Mc Kinnon, D. and Hodgkin, P. D. (1987) A model of T-cell-target cell interaction leading to lymphokine release. Immunol. Cell Biol. (Australia) 65, 431 – 443.

43. Lechler, R. I., Norcross, M. A. and Germain, R. N. (1955) Qualitative and quantitative studies of antigen presenting cell function using I-A expressing L cells. J. Immunol. 135, 2914 – 2922.

44. Tanaka, K., Gorelik, E., Watanabe, M., Hozumi, N. and Jay, G. (1988) Rejection of B16 melanoma induced by expression of a transfected major histocompatibility complex class I gene. Mol. Cell. Biol. 8, 1857 – 1861.

45. Brunner, M., Jaswaney, V. and Wachtel, S. (1987) Reaction of monoclonal H-Y antibody in the ELISA. J. Reprod. Immunol. 11, 181 – 191.

46. Kappler, J. W., Roehm, N. and Marrack, P. (1987) T-cell tolerance by clonal elimination in the thymus. Cell 49, 273 – 280.

47. Kappler, J. W., Staerz, V., White, J. and Marrack, P. C. (1986) Self tolerance eliminates T-cells specific for M/S-modified products of the major histocompatibility complex. Nature 323, 36 – 44.

48. MacDonald, H. R., Schneider, R., Lees, R. K., Howe, R. C., Acha-Orbea, H., Festenstein, H., Zinkernagel, R. M. and Hengartner, H. (1988) T-cell receptor $V\beta$ use predicts reactivity and tolerance to M/S^a encoded antigens. Nature 332, 40 – 45.

49. Lo, D. and Sprent, J. (1986) Identity of cells that imprint H-2-restricted T-cell specificity in the thymus. Nature 319, 672 – 675.

50. Ready, A. R. (1984) Successful transplantation across major histocompatibility barrier of deoxyguanosine-treated embryonic thymus expressing class II antigens. Nature 310, 231 – 233.

51. Matzinger, P., Zamoyska, R. and Waldmann, H. (1984) Self tolerance is H-2-restricted. Nature 308, 738 – 741.

52. Nishimoto, H., Kikutani, H., Yamamura, K.-I. and Kishimoto, T. (1987) Prevention of autoimmune insulitis by the expression of I-E molecules in NOD mice. Nature 328, 432 – 434.

53. Acha-Orbea, H. and Mc Devitt, H. O. (1987) The first external domain of the nonobese diabetic mouse class II I-A$_\beta$ chain is unique. Proc. Natl. Acad. Sci. USA 84, 2435 – 2439.

54. Todd, J. A., Bell, J. I. and Mc Devitt, H. O. (1987) HLA-DQ$_\beta$ gene contribute to susceptibility and resistance to insulin-dependent diabetes mellitus. Nature 329, 559 – 604.

55. Unanue, E. R. (1984) Antigen-presenting function of the macrophage. Annu. Rev. Immunol. 2, 395 – 428.

56. Balfour, B. M., Drexhage, H. A., Kamperdijk, E. W. A. and Hoefsmit, E. C. M. (1981) Antigen-presenting cells, including Langerhans cells, veiled cells and interdigitating cells. Ciba Found.

Symp. 84, 281 – 293.

57. Schmitt, D., Foure, M., Dambuyant-Dezutter, C. and Thivolet, J.   (1984)   The semi-quantitative distribution of T4 and T6 surface antigens on human Langerhans cells. Br. J. Dermatol. 111, 655 – 661.

58. Bjercke, S., Elg, J., Braathen, L. and Thorsby, E.   (1984)   Enriched epidermal Langerhans cells are potent antigen-presenting cells for T-cells. J. Invest. Dermatol. 83, 286 – 289.

59. Steinman, R. M. and Nussenzweig, M. C.   (1980)   Dendritic cells: features and functions. Immunol. Rev. 53, 127 – 147.

60. Knight, S. C., Krejci, J., Malkovsky, M., Colizzi, V., Gautam, A. and Asherson, G. L.   (1985)   The role of dendritic cells in the initiation of immune responses to contact sensitizers. Cell. Immunol. 94, 427 – 434.

61. Knight, S. C., Mertin, J., Stackpole, A. and Clarke, S.   (1983)   Induction of immune responses in vivo with small numbers of veiled (dendritic) cells. Proc. Natl. Acad. Sci. USA 80, 6032 – 6035.

62. Reynes, M., Aubert, J. P., Cohen, J. H., Audoin, J., Tricollet, V., Diebald, J. and Kazatchkine, M. D.   (1985)   Human follicular dendritic cells express CR1, CR2 and CR3 complement receptor antigens. J. Immunol. 135, 2687 – 2694.

63. Humphrey, J. H., Grennan, D. and Sundaram, V.   (1984)   The origin of follicular dendritic cells in the mouse and the mechanism of trapping of immune complexes on them. Eur. J. Immunol. 14, 859 – 863.

64. Klaus, G. G., Humphrey, J. H., Kunkl, A. and Dongworth, D. W.   (1980)   The follicular dendritic cell: its role in antigen presentation in the generation of immunological memory. Immunol. Rev. 53, 3 – 28.

65. Szakal, A. K., Kosco, M. H. and Tew, J. G.   (1988)   A novel in vivo follicular dendritic cell-dependent iccosome-mediated mechanism for delivery of antigen to antigen-processing cells. J. Immunol. 140, 341 – 353.

66. Abbas, A. K.   (1988)   A reassessment of the mechanisms of antigen-specific T-cell-dependent B-cell activation. Immunol. Today 9, 89 – 94.

67. Ron, Y. and Sprent, J.   (1987)   T-cell priming in vivo: a major role for B-cells in presenting antigen to T-cells in lymph nodes. J. Immunol. 138, 2848 – 2856.

68. Bottazzo, G. F., Pujol-Borrell, R., Hanafusa, T. and Feldmann, M.   (1983)   Role of aberrant HLA-DR expression and antigen presentation in induction of endocrine autoimmunity. Lancet ii, 1115 – 1119.

69. Piccinini, L. A., Schachter, B. S., Durgerian, S. and Davies, T. F.   (1988)   HLA-DR gene expression in human thyroid tissue and cultured human thyroid cells. Ann. NY Acad. Sci. 475, 391 – 394.

70. Londei, M., Lamb, J. R., Bottazzo, G. F. and Feldmann, M.   (1984)   Epithelial cells expressing aberrant MHC class II determinants can present antigen to cloned human T-cells. Nature 312, 639 – 641.

71. Londei, M., Bottazzo, G. F., Feldmann, M.   (1985)   Human T-cell clones from autoimmune thyroid glands: specific recognition of autologous thyroid cells. Science (Wash. D.C.) 228, 85 – 89.

72. Foulis, A. K., Farqhuarson, M. A. and Hardman, R.   (1987)   Aberrant expression of class II major histocompatibility complex molecules by insulin containing islets in type 1 (insulin-dependent) diabetes mellitus. Diabetologia 30, 333 – 343.

73. Rosenberg, Y. J., Goldsmith, P. K., Ohara, J., Steinberg, A. D. and Ohriner, W.   (1986)   Ia antigen expression and autoimmunity in MRL-*lpr/lpr* mice. Ann. NY Acad. Sci. 475, 251 – 266.

74. Jackson, R. A., Haynes, B. F., Burch, W. M., Shimuzu, K., Bowring, M. A. and Eisenbarth, G. S.   (1984)   Ia$^+$ T cells in new onset Graves' disease. J. Clin. Endocrinol. Metab. 59, 187 – 190.

75. Tiku, M. L., Liu, S., Weaver, C. W., Teodorescu, M. and Skosey, J. L.   (1985)   Class II histocompatibility antigen-mediated immunologic function of normal articular chondrocytes. J. Immunol. 135, 2923 – 2928.

76. Burmester, G. R., Menche, O., Merryman, P., Klein, M. and Winchester, R. O.   (1983)   Appli-

cation of monoclonal antibodies to the characterization of cells eluted from human articular cartilage. Arthritis Rheum. 26, 1187 – 1195.

77. Consden, R., Doble, A., Glynn, L. E. and Nind, A. P. (1971) Production of chronic arthritis with ovalbumin, its retention in rabbit knee joints. Ann. Rheum. Dis. 30, 307 – 315.

78. Stuart, J. M., Townes, A. S. and Kong, A. H. (1984) Collagen autoimmune arthritis. Annu. Rev. Immunol. 2, 199 – 218.

79. Van Eden, W., Thole, J. E. R., Van der Zee, R., Noordzij, A., Van Embden, J. D. A., Hensen, E. J. and Cohen, I. R. (1988) Cloning of the mycobacterial epitope recognized by T lymphocytes in adjuvant arthritis. Nature 331, 171 – 173.

80. Lindahl, P., Leary, P. and Gresser, I. (1973) Enhancement by interferon of the expression of surface antigens on murine leukemia L1210 cells. Proc. Natl. Acad. Sci. USA 70, 2785 – 2788.

81. Steeg, P. S., Moore, R. N., Johnson, H. M. and Oppenheim, J. J. (1982) Regulation of murine macrophage Ia expression by a lymphokine with immune interferon activity. J. Exp. Med. 156, 1780 – 1793.

82. Collins, T., Korman, A. J., Wake, C. T., Boss, J. M., Kappes, D. J., Fiers, W., Ault, K., Gimbrone, M. A., Strominger, J. L. and Pober, J. S. (1984) Immune interferon activates multiple class II major histocompatibility genes and the associated invariant chain gene in human endothelial cells and dermal fibroblasts. Proc. Natl. Acad. Sci. USA 81, 4917 – 4921.

83. Skoskiewicz, M. J., Colvin, R. B., Schneeberger, E. E. and Russell, P. S. (1985) Widespread and selective induction of major histocompatibility complex-determined antigens in vivo by γ-interferon. J. Exp. Med. 162, 1645 – 1664.

84. Noelle, R., Krammer, P. H., Ohara, J., Uhr, J. W. and Vitetta, E. S. (1984) Increased expression of Ia antigens in resting B-cells: an additional role for B-cell growth factor. Proc. Natl. Acad. Sci. USA 81, 6149 – 6153.

85. Pujol-Borrell, R., Todd, I., Doshi, M., Bottazzo, G. F., Sutton, R., Gray, D., Adolf, G. R. and Feldmann, M. (1987) HLA class II induction in human islet cells by interferon-γ plus tumour necrosis factor or lymphotoxin. Nature 326, 304 – 306.

86. Todd, I., Londei, M., Pujol-Borrell, R., Mirakian, R., Feldmann, M. and Bottazzo, G. F. (1986) HLA-D/DR expression on epithelial cells: the finger on the trigger? Ann. NY Acad. Sci. 475, 241 – 250.

87. May, L. T., Helfgott, D. C. and Seghal, P. B. (1986) Anti-β-interferon antibodies inhibit the increased expression of HLA-B7 in RNA in tumor necrosis factor treated human fibroblasts: structural studies of the β_2 interferon involved. Proc. Natl. Acad. Sci. USA 83, 8957 – 8961.

87. Synder, D. S. and Unanue, E. R. (1982) Corticosteroids inhibit murine macrophage Ia expression and interleukin-1 production. J. Immunol. 129, 1803 – 1805.

87a. McMillan, V. M., Dennis, G. J., Glimcher, L. H., Finkelman, F. D. and Mond, J. J. (1988) Corticosteroid induction of Ig$^+$Ia$^-$ B-cells in vitro is mediated via interaction with the glucocorticoid cytoplasmic receptor. J. Immunol. 140, 2549 – 2555.

88. Kelley, V. E. and Roths, J. B. (1982) Increase in macrophage Ia expression in autoimmune mice: role of the *lpr* gene. J. Immunol. 129, 923 – 925.

89. Lu, C. Y. and Unanue, E. R. (1982) Spontaneous T-cell lymphokine production and increased macrophage Ia expression in autoimmune mice: role of the *lpr* gene. J. Immunol. 125, 871 – 873.

90. Kettelhut, I. C., Fiers, W. and Goldberg, A. L. (1987) The toxic effects of tumor necrosis factor in vivo and their prevention by cyclooxygenase inhibitors. Proc. Natl. Acad. Sci. USA 84, 4273 – 4277.

91. Jacob, C. O. and Mc Devitt, H. O. (1988) Tumour necrosis factor-α in murine autoimmune 'lupus' nephritis. Nature 331, 356 – 358.

92. Jacob, C. O., Van der Meide, P. H. and Mc Devitt, H. O. (1987) In vivo treatment of (NZB $\times$ NZW)F$_1$ lupus-like nephritis with monoclonal antibodies to γ-interferon. J. Exp. Med. 166, 798 – 803.

93. Boitard, C., Michie, S., Serrurier, P., Butcher, G. W., Larkins, A. P. and Mc Devitt, H. O. (1985) In vivo prevention of thyroid and pancreatic autoimmunity in the BB rat by antibody to class II major histocompatibility gene products. Proc. Natl. Acad. Sci. USA 82, 6627–6631.

94. Singh, B. and Cliffe, W. J. (1986) Treatment of diabetic (db/db) mice with anti-class-II MHC monoclonal antibodies. Ann. NY Acad. Sci. 475, 353–355.

95. Siram, S. and Steinman, L. (1983) Anti-I-A antibody suppresses active encephalomyelitis. Treatment model for diseases linked to IR genes. J. Exp. Med. 158, 1362–1367.

96. Wofsy, D. and Seaman, W. E. (1985) Successful treatment of autoimmunity in NZB/NZW F1 mice with monoclonal antibody to a T cell subset marker (L3T4). J. Exp. Med. 161, 378–391.

97. Waldor, M., Siram, S., Hardy, R., Herzenberg, L. A., Herzenberg, L. A., Lanier, L., Lim, M. and Steinman, L. (1985) Reversal of experimental allergic encephalomyelitis with a monoclonal antibody to a T cell subset marker. Science 227, 415–417.

98. Grayson, D. R., Costa, R. H., Xanthopoulos, K. G. and Darnell, J. E. (1988) One factor recognizes liver-specific enhancers in α_1-antitrypsin and transthyretin genes. Science 239, 786–788.

99. Gauldie, J., Richards, C., Harnish, D., Landsdorf, P. and Baumann, H. (1987) Interferon β_2/B-cell stimulatory factor type 2 shares identity with monocyte-derived hepatocyte-stimulating factor and regulates the major acute-phase protein response in liver cells. Proc. Natl. Acad. Sci. USA 84, 7251–7255.

100. Israel, A., Kimura, A., Fournier, A., Fellous, M. and Kourilsky, P. (1986) Interferon response sequence protentiates activity of an enhancer in the promotor region of a mouse H-2 gene. Nature 322, 743–746.

101. De Préval, C., Lisowska-Grospierre, B., Loche, M., Griscelli, C. and Mach, B. (1985) A trans-acting class II regulatory gene unlinked to the MHC controls expression of HLA class II genes. Nature 318, 291–293.

102. Sullivan, K., Calman, A. F., Nakanishi, M., Tsang, S. Y., Wang, Y. and Peterlin, B. M. (1987) A model for the transcriptional regulation of MHC class II genes. Immunol. Today 8, 289–293.

103. McCune, J. M., Humphreys, R. E., Yocum, R. R. and Strominger, J. L. (1975) Enhanced representation of HL-A antigens on human lymphocytes after mitogenesis induced by phytohemag-glutinin or Epstein-Barr virus. Proc. Natl. Acad. Sci. USA 72, 3206–3209.

104. Lee, S. W., Tsou, A.-P., Chan, H., Thomas, J., Petrie, K., Eugui, E. M. and Allison, A. C. (1988) Glucocorticoids selectively inhibit the transcription of the interleukin 1β gene and decrease the stability of interleukin 1β mRNA. Proc. Natl. Acad. Sci. USA 85, 1204–1208.

105. Romano, T. J., Ponzio, N. M. and Thorbecke, G. J. (1976) Graft-versus-host reactions in F_1 mice induced by parental lymphoid cells: nature of the recruited F_1 cells. J. Immunol. 116, 1618–1623.

106. Katz, D. H. (1972) The allogeneic effect on immune responses: model for regulatory influences of T lymphocytes on the immune system. Transplant. Rev. 12, 141–179.

107. Barclay, A. N. and Mason, D. W. (1982) Induction of Ia antigen in rat epidermal cells and gut epithelium by immunological stimuli. J. Exp. Med. 156, 1665–1676.

108. Basham, T. Y., Nickoloff, B. J., Merigan, T. C. and Morhenn, V. B. (1984) Recombinant gamma interferon induces HLA-DR expression in cultured human keratinocytes. J. Invest. Dermatol. 83, 88–91.

109. Guy-Grand, D. and Vassalli, P. (1986) Gut injury in mouse graft-versus-host reaction. Study of tsi occurrence and mechanisms. J. Clin. Invest. 77, 1584–1595.

110. Sinclair, G. D., Wadgymar, A., Halloran, P. F. and Delovitch, T. L. (1984) Graft-vs.-host reactions induce H-2 class II gene transcription in host kidney cells. Immunogenetics 20, 503–511.

111. Moser, M., Mizuochi, T., Sharrow, S. O., Singer, A. and Shearer, G. M. (1987) Graft-versus-host reaction limited to a class II MHC difference results in a selective deficiency in L3T4$^+$ but

not in Lyt-2$^+$ helper function. J. Immunol. 138, 1355–1362.

112. O'Garra, A., Umland, S., De France, T. and Christiansen, J. (1988) 'B-cell factors' are pleiotropic. Immunol. Today 9, 45–54.

113. Yakota, T., Otsuka, T., Mosmann, T., Benckereau, J., De Frances, T., Blanchard, D., De Vries, J. E., Lee, F. and Arai, K.-I. (1986) Isolation and characterization of a human interleukin cDNA clone, homologous to mouse B-cell stimulatory factor 1, that expresses B-cell and T-cell stimulating activities. Proc. Natl. Acad. Sci. USA 83, 5894–5898.

114. Tosato, G., Seaman, K. B., Goldman, N. D., Sehgal, P. B., May, L. T., Washington, G. C., Jones, K. D. and Pike, S. E. (1988) Monocyte-derived human B-cell growth factor identified as interferon-β_2 (BSF-2, IL-6). Science 239, 502–504.

115. Hirano, T., Toga, T., Yasukawa, K., Nakajima, K., Nakano, N., Takatsuki, T., Shimizu, M., Murashima, A., Tsunasawa, S., Sakijama, F. and Kishimoto, T. (1987) Human B-cell differentiation factor defined by an anti-peptide antibody and its possible role in autoantibody production. Proc. Natl. Acad. Sci. USA 84, 228–231.

116. Sidman, C. L., Marshall, J. D., Masiello, N. C. and Roths, J. B. (1984) Novel B-cell maturation factor from spontaneously autoimmune viable motheaten mice. Proc. Natl. Acad. USA 81, 7199–7202.

117. Mc Coy, K. L., Nielson, K. and Clagett, J. (1984) Spontaneous production of colony-stimulating activity by splenic Mac-1 antigen-positive cells from autoimmune motheaten mice. J. Immunol. 132, 272–276.

118. Prud'homme, G. J., Fieser, T. M., Dixon, F. J. and Theofilopoulos, A. N. (1984) B-cell-tropic interleukins in murine systemic lupus erythematosus. Immunol. Rev. 78, 159–183.

119. Warren, R. W., Caster, S. A., Roths, J. B., Murphy, E. D. and Pisetsky, D. S. (1984) The influence of the *lpr* gene on B-cell activation: differential antibody expression in *lpr* congenic mouse strains. Clin. Immunol. Immunopathol. 31, 65–77.

120. Schauenstein, K., Krömer, G., Sundick, R. S. and Wick, G. (1985) Enhanced response to Con A and production of TCGF by lymphocytes of obese strain (OS) chickens with spontaneous autoimmune thyroiditis. J. Immunol. 134, 872–879.

121. Smith, J. B. and Talal, N. (1982) Significance of self-recognition and IL-2 for immunoregulation, autoimmunity and cancer. Scand. J. Immunol. 16, 269.

122. Koide, J. (1985) Functional property of Ia-positive T-cells in peripheral blood from patients with systemic lupus erythematosus. Scand. J. Immunol. 22, 577–584.

123. Sarvetnick, N., Liggitt, D., Pitts, S. L., Hansen, S. and Stewart, T. A. (1988) Insulin dependent diabetes mellitus induced in transgenic mice by ectopic expression of class II MHC and interferon-gamma. Cell 52, 773–782.

124. Allison, J., Campbell, IL., Morahan, G., Mandel, T. E., Harrison, L. and Miller, J. F. A. P. (1988) Diabetes in transgenic mice associated with over-expression of class I histocompatibility molecules in pancreatic islets. Nature 333, 529–533.

125. Schreiber, A. B., Schlessinger, J. and Edidin, M. (1984) Interactions between major histocompatibility antigens and epidermal growth factor receptors on human cells. J. Cell Biol. 98, 725–731.

126. Witebsky, E. and Rose, N. R. (1956) Studies on organ specificity; production of rabbit thyroid antibodies in rabbit. J. Immunol. 74, 408–416.

127. Roitt, I. M., Doniach, D., Campbell, N. and Hudson, R. V. (1956) Autoantibodies in Hashimoto's disease. Lancet ii, 820–821.

128. Roberts, I. M., Whittingham, S. and Mackay, I. R. (1973) Tolerance to an autoantigen-thyroglobulin. Antigen-binding lymphocytes in thymus and blood in health and autoimmune disease. Lancet ii, 936–940.

129. Bankhurst, A. D. and Williams, R. C. Jr. (1975) Identification of DNA-binding lymphocytes in patients with systemic lupus erythematosus. J. Clin. Invest. 56, 1378–1385.

130. De Heer, D. H. and Edgington, T. S. (1976) Specific antigen binding and autoantibody secreting lymphocytes associated with the erythrocyte autoantibody responses of NZB and genetically correlated mice. J. Immunol. 116, 1051 – 1058.

131. Dighiero, G., Lymberi, P., Guilbert, B., Terrynck, T. and Avrameas, S. (1986) Natural autoantibodies constitute a substantial part of normal circulating immunoglobulins. Ann. NY Acad. Sci. 475, 135 – 145.

132. Karray, S., Lymberi, P., Avrameas, S. and Coutinho, A. (1986) Quantitative evidence against inactivation of self-reactive B-cell clones. Scand. J. Immunol. 23, 475 – 480.

133. Uhlig, H., Rutter, G. and Derrick, R. (1985) Self-reactive B lymphocytes detected in young adults, children and newborns after in vitro infection with Epstein-Barr virus. Clin. Exp. Immunol. 62, 75 – 84.

134. Nossal, G. J. V. (1983) Cellular mechanisms of immunologic tolerance. Annu. Rev. Immunol. 1, 33 – 62.

135. Metcalf, E. S. and Klinman, N. R. (1977) In vitro tolerance of bone marrow cells: a marker for B-cell maturation. J. Immunol. 118, 2111 – 2116.

136. Diener, E. and Waters, C. A. (1986) Immunological quiescence towards self: rethinking the paradigm of clonal abortion. In Immunological Paradoxes, G. W. Hoffman, J. G. Levy and G. I. Nepom (Eds.). CRC Press, Boca Raton, FL, pp. 27 – 40.

137. Teppo, A. M., Haltia, K. and Wager, O. (1976) Immunoelectrophoretic 'tailing' of albumin line due to albumin-anti Ig antibody complexes: a side effect of nitrofurantoin treatment? Scand. J. Immunol. 5, 249 – 261.

138. Silverstein, A. M., Prendergast, R. A. and Kramer, K. L. (1964) Fetal response to an antigenic stimulus. IV. Rejection of skin homograft by the fetal lamb. J. Exp. Med. 119, 955 – 964.

139. Cotes, P. M., Hobbs, K. E. and Bangham, D. R. (1966) Development of the immune response in the foetal and newborn rhesus monkey. Immunology 11, 185 – 198.

140. Dresser, D. W. (1962) Specific inhibition of antibody production. I. Protein overloading paralysis. Immunology 5, 161 – 168.

141. Taylor, R. B. (1969) Cellular cooperation in the antibody response of mice to two serum albumins: specific function of thymus cells. Transplant. Rev. 1, 114 – 149.

142. Chiller, J. M., Habicht, G. S. and Weigle, W. O. (1970) Kinetic differences in unresponsiveness of thymus and bone marrow cells. Science (Wash. D. C.) 171, 813 – 815.

143. Gammon, G., Dunn, K., Shastri, N., Oki, A., Wilbur, J. and Sercarz, E. E. (1986) Neonatal T-cell tolerance to minimal immunogenic peptides. Nature 319, 413 – 415.

144. Iverson, G. M. and Lindenmann, J. (1972) The role of a carrier determinant and T-cells in the induction of liver-specific autoantibodies in the mouse. Eur. J. Immunol. 2, 195 – 197.

145. Keast, D. and Calagero, C. (1977) Erythrocyte autoantibodies induced in mice immunized with rat antigen. Aust. J. Exp. Biol. Med. Sci. 55, 359 – 362.

146. Hooper, D. C. (1987) Self tolerance for erythrocytes is not maintained by clonal deletion of T helper cells. Immunol. Today 8, 327 – 330.

147. Weigle, W. O. (1965) The production of thyroiditis and antibody following injection of unaltered thyroglobulin without adjuvant into rabbits previously stimulated with altered thyroglobulin. J. Exp. Med. 122, 1049 – 1062.

148. Iverson, G. M. (1970) Ability of CBA mice to produce anti-idiotypic sera to 5563 myeloma protein. Nature 227, 273 – 274.

149. McCullagh, P. J. (1970) The immunological capacity of lymphocytes from normal donors after their transfer to rats tolerant of sheep erythrocytes. Aust. J. Exp. Biol. Med. Sci. 48, 369 – 379.

150. Herzenberg, L. A., Jacobsen, E. B., Herzenberg, L. A. (1971) Chronic allotype suppression in mice: an active regulatory process. Ann. NY Acad. Sci. 190, 212 – 220.

151. Okumura, K. and Tada, T. (1971) Regulation of homocytotropic antibody formation in the rat. VI. Inhibiting effect of thymocytes on the homocytotropic antibody response. J. Immunol. 107, 1682 – 1689.

152. Moticka, E. (1983) Regulation of naturally occurring autoantibody secretion by a radiosensitive lymphocyte: initial characterization and ontogeny. Cell. Immunol. 81, 36 – 44.

153. Taguchi, O., Takahashi, T., Seto, M., Namikawa, R., Matsuyama, M. and Nishizuka, Y. (1986) Development of multiple organ-localized autoimmune diseases in nude mice after reconstitution of T-cell function by rat fetal thymus graft. J. Exp. Med. 164, 60 – 71.

154. Sakaguchi, S., Fukuma, K., Kuribayashi, K. and Matsuda, T. (1985) Organ-specific autoimmune diseases induced in mice by elimination of a T-cell subset. I. Evidence for the active participation of T-cells in natural self-tolerance; deficit of a T-cell subset as a possible cause of autoimmune disease. J. Exp. Med. 161, 72 – 87.

155. Wick, G., Kite, J. H. Jr. and Witebsky, E. (1970) Spontaneous thyroiditis in the obese strain of chickens. J. Immunol. 104, 43 – 53.

156. Watt, G. J., Russell, J. and Elson, C. J. (1986) Carrier-specific induction of suppressor cells controlling anti-erythrocyte autoantibody production in mice. Scand. J. Immunol. 24, 39 – 43.

157. Loblay, R.H., Fazekas de St. Groth, B., Pritchard-Briscoe, H. and Basten, A. (1983) Suppressor T-cell memory. II. The role of memory suppressor T-cells in tolerance to human gamma globulin. J. Exp. Med. 157, 957 – 973.

158. Harris, D. E., Cairns, L., Rosen, F. J. and Borel, Y. (1983) A natural model of immunological tolerance: tolerance to murine C5 is mediated by T-cells and antigen is required to maintain unresponsiveness. J. Exp. Med. 156, 567 – 584.

159. Jerne, N. K. (1974) Towards a network theory of the immune system. Ann. Immunol. (Paris) 125C, 373 – 389.

160. Roitt, I. M., Male, D. K., Cooke, A. and Lydyard, P. M. (1983) Idiotypes and autoimmunity. Springer Semin. Immunopathol. 6, 51 – 66.

161. Klinman, D. M. and Steinberg, A. D. (1986) Idiotypy and autoimmunity. Arthritis Rheum. 29, 697 – 705.

162. Sege, K. and Peterson, P. A. (1978) Use of anti-idiotypic antibodies as cell surface receptor probes. Proc. Natl. Acad. Sci. USA 75, 2443 – 2447.

163. Shoelson, S. E., Marshall, S., Horikoshi, H., Kolteman, O. G., Rubenstein, A. H. and Olefsky, J. M. (1986) Anti-insulin receptor antibodies in an insulin-dependent diabetic may arise as autoanti-idiotypes. J. Clin. Endocrinol. Metab. 63, 56 – 61.

164. Islam, M. N., Pepper, B. M., Brione-Urbina, R. and Farid, N. R. (1983) Biological activity of anti-thyrotropin anti-idiotypic antibodies. Eur. J. Immunol. 13, 57 – 66.

165. Torrigiani, G., Danich, D. and Roitt, I. M. (1969) Serum thyroglobulin levels in healthy subjects and in patients with thyroid disease. J. Clin. Endocrinol. Metab. 29, 305 – 314.

166. Allison, A. C. and Young, M. R. (1964) Uptake of dyes and drugs into lysosomes. Life Sci. 3, 1407 – 1412.

167. De Duve, C., De Barsy, T., Poole, B., Trouet, A., Tulkens, P. and Van Hoof, F. (1974) Lysosomotropic agents. Biochem. Pharmacol. 23, 2495 – 2531.

168. Anderson, C. L. and Rose, N. R. (1971) Induction of thyroiditis by intravenous injection of papain-treated rabbit thyroglobulin. J. Immunol. 107, 1341 – 1348.

169. Weigle, W. O., High, G. J. and Nakamura, R. M. (1969) Role of mycobacteria and the effect of proteolytic degradation of thyroglobulin on the production of autoimmune thyroiditis. J. Exp. Med. 130, 243 – 260.

170. Williams, R. C. and Kunkel, H. H. (1963) Antibodies to rabbit-γ-globulin after immunizing with various preparations of autologous γ-globulin. Proc. Soc. Exp. Biol. Med. 112, 554 – 561.

171. Aho, K. and Wager, P. (1961) The production of rheumatoid factor by immunization with bacteria. Acta Med. Exp. Biol. Fenn. 39, 79 – 89.

172. De Scheerder, I., Vanderckhove, J., Rolrecht, J., Algold, L., De Buyzere, M., De Langhe, J., De Schreijver, G. and Clement, D. (1985) Post-cardiac injury syndrome and an increased humoral immune response against the major contractile proteins (actin and myosin). Am. J. Cardiol. 56, 631 – 633.

173. Kaplan, M. H. (1965) Autoantibodies to heart and rheumatic fever: the induction of autoimmunity to heart by streptococcal antigen cross reactive with heart. Ann. NY Acad. Sci. 124, 904 – 915.
174. Stollar, B. D. and Schwartz, R. S. (1986) Monoclonal anti-DNA antibodies: the targets and origins of SLE autoantibodies. Ann. NY Acad. Sci. 475, 192 – 199.
175. Fujinami, R. S., Oldstone, M. B. A., Wroblewska, Z., Frankel, M. E. and Koprowski, H. (1983) Molecular mimicry in virus infection: cross reaction of measles virus phosphoprotein or of herpes simplex virus protein with human intermediate filaments. Proc. Natl. Acad. Sci. USA 80, 2346 – 2350.
176. Holoshitz, J., Matitiau, A. and Cohen, I. R. (1984) Arthritis in rats by cloned T lymphocytes responsive to mycobacteria but not to collagen type II. J. Clin. Invest. 73, 211 – 215.
177. Cohen, I. R. (1988) The self, the world and autoimmunity. Scientific American 258, 52 – 60.
178. Ebringer, A., Baines, M. and Ptaszynska, T. (1985) Spondyloarthritis, uveitis, HLA-B27 and Klebsiella. Immunol. Rev. 86, 101 – 116.
179. Dacie, J. V. (1963) The Haemolytic Anaemias, Congenital and Acquired. Churchill, London. Part II.
180. Kaplan, M. E. and Tan, E. M. (1968) Antinuclear antibodies in infectious mononucleosis. Lancet i, 561 – 563.
181. Stites, D. P. and Leikola, J. (1971) Infectious mononucleosis. Semin. Hematol. 8, 243 – 260.
182. Holborow, E. J., Hemsted, E. H. and Meads, S. V. (1973) Smooth muscle autoantibodies in infectious mononucleosis. Br. Med. J. 3, 323 – 325.
183. Fagraeus, A. and Norberg, R. (1978) Anti-actin antibodies Curr. Topics Microbiol. Immunol. 82, 1 – 13.
184. Svedmyr, E. and Jondal, M. (1975) Cytotoxic effector cells specific for B-cell lines transformed by Epstein-Barr virus are present in patients with infectious mononucleosis. Proc. Natl. Acad. Sci. USA 72, 1622 – 1626.
185. Guiffre, R. M., Tovell, D. R., Kay, C. M. and Tyrell, D. L. J. (1982) Evidence for an interaction between the membrane protein of a paramyxovirus and actin. J. Virol. 42, 963 – 968.
186. Tyrrell, D. L. J., Taechaudomitavorn, W., Lund, G. A. and Tovell, D. R. (1987) The mechanism by which paramyxoviruses break tolerance to actin. In: B. J. Mahy and J. Kolakofsky (Eds.), The Biology of the Negative Strand Viruses, Elsevier, Amsterdam, pp. 304 – 308.
187. Kuzumaki, N., Koama, T., Takeushi, N. and Kobayashi, H. (1974) Friend lymphatic leukemia virus-induced autoimmune hemolytic anemia with glomerulonephritis in the rat. Int. J. Cancer 14, 483 – 492.
188. Dyrberg, T., Schwimmbeck, P. L. and Oldstone, M. B. A. (1988) Inhibition of diabetes in BB rats by virus infection. J. Clin. Invest. 81, 928 – 931.
189. Oldstone, M. B. A. (1988) Prevention of type I diabetes in nonobese diabetic mice by virus infection. Science (Wash. D.C.) 239, 500 – 502.
190. Allison, A. C. (1979) Mode of action of immunological adjuvants. J. Reticuloendothelial Soc. 26 (Suppl.), 619 – 630.
191. Youngner, J. S. and Salvin, S. B. (1973) Production and properties of migration inhibitory factor and interferon in the circulation of mice with delayed hypersensitivity. J. Immunol. 111, 1914 – 1922.
192. Carswell, E. A., Old, L. J., Kassel, R. L., Green, S., Fiore, N. and Williamson, B. (1975) An endotoxin-induced serum factor that causes necrosis of tumors. Proc. Natl. Acad. Sci. USA 72, 3666 – 3670.
193. Metcalf, D. and Moore, M. A. J. (1971) Haemopoietic Cells. North-Holland Publ. Co., Amsterdam.
194. Izui, S. T., Kobayokawa, T., Zryd, M. J., Louis, J. and Lambert, P. H. (1977) Mechanisms for induction of anti-DNA antibodies by bacterial lipopolysaccharides in mice. II. Correlation be-

tween anti-DNA induction and polyclonal antibody formation by various polyclonal B-lymphocyte activators. J. Immunol. 119, 2157 – 2162.

195. Worrledge, S. M., Carstairs, K. C. and Dacie, J. V. (1966) Autoimmune haemolytic anaemia associated with α-methyldopa therapy. Lancet ii, 135 – 139.

196. Rubin, R. L., Reimer, G., McNally, E. M., Nusinow, S. R., Searles, R. P. and Tan, E. M. (1986) Procaineamide elicits a selective autoantibody immune response. Clin. Exp. Immunol. 63, 58 – 67.

197. Gohill, J., Cary, P. D., Couppez, M. and Fritzler, M. J. (1985) Antibodies from patients with drug-induced and idiopathic lupus erythematosus react with epitopes restricted to the amino and carboxyl termini of histone. J. Immunol. 135, 3116 – 3121.

198. Yamashita, U., Takami, T., Hamasaka, T. and Kitagawa, M. (1976) The role of hapten-reactive T-lymphocytes in the induction of autoimmunity in mice. II. Termination of self-tolerance to erythrocytes by immunization with hapten-isologous erythrocytes. Cell. Immunol. 25, 32 – 40.

199. Pearsall, H. R., Ewalt, J., Tsoi, M. S., Sumida, S., Packinos, D., Winterbauer, R., Webb, D. and Jones, H. (1974) Nitrofurantoin lung sensitivity: report of a case with prolonged nitrofurantoin lymphocyte sensitivity and interaction of nitrofurantoin-stimulated lymphocytes with alveolar cells. J. Lab. Clin. Med. 83, 728 – 737.

200. Hirsch, F., Kuhn, J., Ventura, M., Vial, M.-C., Fourné, G. and Druet, P. (1986) Autoimmunity induced by $HgCl_2$ in Brown-Norway rats. I. Production of monoclonal antibodies. J. Immunol. 136, 3272 – 3276.

201. Hirsch, F., Couderc, J., Sapin, C., Fourné, G. and Druet, P. (1982) Polyclonal effect of $HgCl_2$ in the rat, its possible role in an experimental autoimmune disease. Eur. J. Immunol. 12, 620 – 625.

202. Gleichmann, E. and Gleichmann, H. (1976) Graft-versus-host reaction: a pathogenetic principle for the development of drug allergy, autoimmunity, and malignant lymphoma in non-chimeric individuals. Z. Krebsforsch. 85, 91 – 109.

203. Nagata, N., Hurtenbach, U. and Gleichmann, E. (1986) Specific sensitization of $Lyt-1^+2^-$ T cells to spleen cells modified by the drug D-penicillamine or a stereoisomer. J. Immunol. 136, 136 – 142.

204. Goodwin, J. S. and Cueppens, J. (1983) Regulation of the immune response by prostaglandins. J. Clin. Immunol. 3, 295 – 315.

205. Lissitzky, S., Fayet, G. and Verrier, B. (1975) Thyrotropin-receptor interaction and cyclic AMP-mediated events on thyroid cells. In: G. I. Drummond, P. Greengard and G. A. Robison (Eds.), Advances in Cyclic Nucleotide Research, Vol. 5, Raven Press, New York, pp. 133 – 152.

206. Bach, M.-A., Fournier, C. and Bach, J.-F. (1975) Regulation of θ-antigen expression by agents altering cyclic AMP level and by thymic factor. Ann. NY Acad. Sci. 249, 316 – 320.

207. Rabinowe, S. L., Larsen, P. R., Artman, E. M., George, K. L., Friedman, P. L., Jackson, R. A. and Eisenbarth, G. S. (1986) Amiodarone therapy and autoimmune thyroid disease. Increase in a new monoclonal antibody-defined T-cell subset. Am. J. Med. 81, 53 – 57.

208. Jemmerson, R., Morrow, P. and Klinman, N. (1982) Antibody responses to synthetic peptides corresponding to antigenic determinants on mouse cytochrome c. Fed. Proc. 41 (3), 420.

209. Adams, T. E., Alpert, S. and Hanahan, D. (1987) Non-tolerance and autoantibodies to a transgenic self antigen expressed in pancreatic B-cells. Nature 325, 223 – 228.

210. Hayakawa, K., Hardy, R. R. and Herzenberg, L. A. (1986) Peritoneal Ly-1 B-cells: genetic control, autoantibody production, increased light chain expression. Eur. J. Immunol. 16, 450 – 506.

211. Sidman, C. L., Shultz, L. D., Hardy, R. R., Hayakawa, K. and Herzenberg, L. A. (1986) Production of immunoglobulin isotypes by $Ly-1^+$ cells in viable motheaten and normal mice. Science (Wash. D.C.) 232, 1423 – 1425.

212. Casali, P., Burastero, S. E., Nakamura, M., Inghirama, G. and Notkins, A. L. (1987) Human lymphocytes making rheumatoid factor and antibody to ssDNA belong to $Leu-1^+$ B-cell subset.

Science (Wash. D.C.) 236, 47 – 80.

213. Hardy, R. R., Hayakawa, K., Shimizu, M., Yamasaki, K. and Kishimoto, T.   (1987)   Rheuma-toid factor secretion from human Leu-1[+] B-cells. Science (Wash. D.C.) 236, 81 – 83.

214. Plater-Zyberk, C., Maini, R. N., Lam, K., Kennedy, T. D. and Janossy, G.   (1985)   A rheumatoid arthritis B-cell subset expresses a phenotype similar to that in chronic lymphocytic leukemia. Arthritis Rheum. 28, 971 – 976.

215. Mackay, I. R.   (1983)   Natural autoantibodies to the fore-forbidden clones to the rear? Immunol. Today 4, 340 – 342.

216. Davidson, A., Halpern, R. and Diamond, B.   (1986)   Speculation on the role of somatic muta-tion in the generation of anti-DNA antibodies. Ann. NY Acad. Sci. 475, 174 – 180.

SECTION III

Autoimmune(-like) reactions in humans induced by drugs and chemicals

M.E. Kammüller, N. Bloksma and W. Seinen (Eds.)
Autoimmunity and Toxicology
© *1989 Elsevier Science Publishers B.V. (Biomedical Division)*

Autoimmune reactions induced by procainamide and hydralazine

4

ROBERT L. RUBIN

Department of Basic and Clinical Research, Research Institute of Scripps Clinic, 10666 North Torrey Pines Road, La Jolla, CA 92037, USA

I. Introduction

1. DEFINITION OF AUTOIMMUNE-LIKE REACTIONS INDUCED BY PROCAINAMIDE AND HYDRALAZINE

A side effect of therapy with a wide variety of drugs is a syndrome resembling the autoimmune disease systemic lupus erythematosus (SLE). Procainamide and hydralazine are the most common offenders and have been demonstrated by prospective studies to induce in a minority of treated patients some of the symptoms commonly associated with SLE or rheumatoid arthritis [1]. Drug-induced lupus usually occurs after several months or years of therapy and should be distinguished from the short-term toxic side effects termed 'early toxicity' by Perry [2]. Soon after the initiation of treatment for hypertension with hydralazine many patients develop headache, palpitation, anorexia, nausea, tachycardia and less commonly conjunctivitis, nasal congestion, edema, fever and other symptoms [2]. These acute complications usually resolve within a few weeks. Procainamide has a substantially lower incidence of causing such problems, which is why procainamide would be the preferred therapy for treating cardiac arrhythmias if the 'late toxicity' of drug-induced lupus did not occur.

As discussed in greater detail in Sections II and III of this chapter, many patients treated with hydralazine and most patients treated with procainamide develop circulating antibodies reactive with cell nuclei. These anti-nuclear antibodies (ANA) are clearly drug-induced and, as with the lupus-like symptoms, gradually subside

120

after discontinuation of therapy. However, only a small percentage of patients who develop ANA will progress to symptomatic disease, and, consequently, the term drug-induced autoimmunity better describes the phenomenon of ANA induction. The mechanism of ANA induction is of considerable interest even in individuals who remain asymptomatic, and ANA provides the best objective marker for drug-induced autoimmune-like phenomena in humans and experimental systems.

2. HISTORICAL PERSPECTIVE

The first report of a hydralazine-induced lupus-like disease was that of Morrow et al. [3], in which 14 of 253 treated patients developed rheumatologic symptoms after 4 – 23 months of therapy. Subsequently Dustan et al. [4], and a flurry of reports during the next few years verified the syndrome of hydralazine-induced lupus in 5 – 20% of patients undergoing long-term therapy. Although procainamide was introduced at about the same time for treatment of cardiac arrhythmias, it was not until 1962 that the single case report of Ladd et al. [5] appeared, describing a patient who developed joint pain, muscle soreness and bilateral pleuritic chest pain after 6 months of procainamide therapy. Numerous subsequent studies showed that the incidence of symptomatic procainamide-induced lupus is approximately 10 – 20% after 1 year of therapy [6], although some reports were as high as 30% [7, 8]. These studies also demonstrated that almost all patients treated with procainamide for 1 year or more developed ANA [6], although many of these patients remained asymptomatic throughout subsequent years of therapy [9].

Application of an immunofluorescence assay in which nuclei are reconstituted with histones revealed the near universal presence of anti-histone antibodies in sera from patients with procainamide-induced lupus [10]. Similarly, application of solid-phase immunoassays to sera from patients with hydralazine-induced lupus showed that these patients also had anti-histone antibodies [11]. Antibodies to denatured (d) DNA (single-stranded, ssDNA) are also common in patients treated with these drugs [9, 12, 13]. The mechanism of autoantibody induction and the role of autoantibodies in disease pathogenesis continue to be the subject of intensive study.

II. Features of procainamide-induced autoimmunity

1. TIME COURSE AND DOSE DEPENDENCY

Because of therapeutic necessity to maintain uniform blood levels, procainamide is usually taken in equally divided doses at 3-h intervals for the standard procainamide HCl and at 6-h intervals for the slow-release form (Procan SR). Plasma drug concentrations necessary to abolish ventricular arrhythmia are generally 4 – 10 μg/ml (15 – 37 μM) [14], although Greenspan et al. [15] required plasma concentrations up

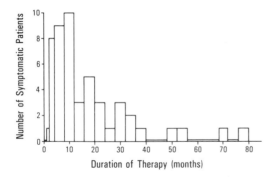

Fig. 1. Incidence of procainamide-induced lupus. The ordinate is the number of patients developing symptoms during the indicated time interval. Data was compiled from Sonnhag et al. [8], Woosley et al. [6] and Totoritis et al. [18].

to 32 μg/ml to maintain therapeutic control in some patients. Because of this variation in therapeutic response as well as differences in drug clearance and metabolism, daily intake of procainamide may vary from 0.25 – 6 g/day [7, 15, 16]. In light of this wide range in daily dose, it is not surprising that the time for manifestation of lupus-like symptoms varies greatly among the patient population as shown in Fig. 1. This cumulative tabulation of 50 patients who developed drug-induced lupus had a distribution of symptom onset with a median at approximately 10 months, but approximately one-fourth of the patients did not develop symptoms until 2 years or more of therapy. Even with patients showing the most rapid onset of symptoms, at least 2 months of therapy with a total dose of 140 g of procainamide was required.

ANA appearance follows a time course similar to that of symptom onset. All patients with symptoms have ANA [17], suggesting that ANA elicitation precedes or occurs coincident with clinical symptoms. After 12 months of treatment approximately 75% of patients are ANA positive [7, 16], and conversion to ANA positivity approached, but did not reach, 100% of patients treated for 2 years or more [6, 17]. In addition to the higher titer of ANA in symptomatic compared to asymptomatic patients [7, 8, 17], there are major differences in the immunoglobulin class and fine specificity of the autoantibodies which arise in these two groups of patients as described in Section II.3(a) in this chapter.

2. CLINICAL AND LABORATORY FEATURES

A compilation of the clinical symptoms and laboratory signs of procainamide-induced lupus is shown in Table 1. Although joint pain is the most common complaint, frank joint swelling is relatively unusual and deformities have not been reported. Lung involvement, particularly pleuritic chest pain and effusions, are notably present in approximately one-half of the patients. Constitutional symptoms of fever, weight loss and fatigue are also observed in approximately half the pa-

TABLE 1

Major clinical and laboratory abnormalities in procainamide-induced lupus

Clinical		Laboratory	
symptom	prevalence (%)	sign	prevalence (%)
Arthralgias	85	ANA	> 95
Lung involvement	50	LE cells	80
Fever/weight loss	45	Anti-dDNA	50
Myalgias	35	RF	30
Splenomegaly	25	Anemia (+ / − Coombs +)	20
Arthritis	20	Leukopenia	15
Pericarditis	15		

Data was compiled from Weinstein [109], Harmon and Portanova [41] and Russell [110], and each prevalence represents a consensus figure ± 5%. Abnormalities reported in < 10% of patients are not included.

tients. Similar symptoms are observed in idiopathic SLE but tend to be of a more severe nature, longer duration and more prevalent. In addition, SLE is commonly associated with skin rash, lymphadenopathy, renal involvement and to a lesser extent Raynaud's phenomenon and central nervous system disease, symptoms that have only rarely been reported for procainamide-induced lupus. Onset of symptoms is generally insidious, developing in intensity during 1 – 2 months before diagnosis can be made, although some individuals develop symptoms abruptly [7]. If symptom categories are grouped into pain (arthritis, arthralgias and/or myalgias), pleuro-pulmonary complaints or pericarditis, constitutional symptoms (fever, weight loss and/or malaise) and hematologic disorders (leukopenia, anemia and/or thrombocytopenia), 20% of patients have only one symptom (usually pain), 25% had two and 55% had three or more symptoms [18].

The major laboratory abnormality in procainamide-induced lupus is ANA. As described in detail below, these are anti-histone antibodies and are responsible for the positive lupus erythematosus (LE) test and deoxyribonucleoprotein binding [9, 19, 20], reactivities previously thought to be due to separate antibody populations. Antibodies to dDNA are present in approximately half the patients [9, 12, 21 – 23]. Rheumatoid factor (RF) was reported in earlier reports [9], but prospective studies indicated that RF is not drug-induced but merely reflects the increased incidence of this antibody in the elderly population commonly treated with procainamide [13]. Antibodies to lymphocytes [24], to ribonucleoprotein [25] and to procainamide [26] were reported, but these specificities were not observed in subsequent studies [20, 13, 22], although unidentified bands were detected by ^{35}S and ^{32}P immunoprecipitation in 4 of 29 sera from procainamide-treated patients [13].

ANA is also present in essentially all patients with SLE but is not restricted to anti-histone antibodies. SLE patients commonly have antibodies to native DNA, Smith (Sm) antigen, nuclear ribonucleoprotein and/or Sjögren's syndrome A antigen, reactivities generally not observed in drug-induced lupus [10, 13, 27] other than the earlier reports of Molina et al. [19] and Klajman et al. [22]. The greater heterogeneity of autoantibodies in SLE over procainamide-induced lupus may reflect the enhanced immunologic intensity and duration of the idiopathic disease, as also manifested by the higher incidence of leukopenia, anemia and hypocomplementemia in SLE. However, it should be noted that anti-histone antibodies and antibodies to dDNA are the most prevalent autoantibodies in both drug-induced and idiopathic SLE.

3. IMMUNOLOGICAL ABNORMALITIES

(a) Humoral autoimmune abnormalities

Autoantibodies in patients treated with procainamide are largely restricted to histones and dDNA, and the prevalence of these antibodies in symptomatic and

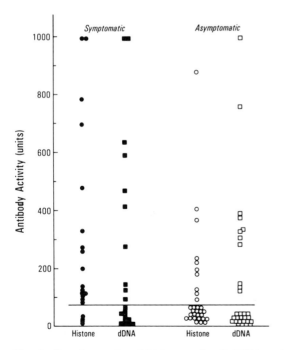

Fig. 2. Prevalence of anti-histone and anti-dDNA antibodies in symptomatic and asymptomatic procainamide-treated patients. Antibody activity was determined by ELISA using either total histones or dDNA in the solid phase.

asymptomatic patients is shown in Fig. 2. The close correlation between the ANA titer and the titer of histone-reactive ANA [10, 11], and the observation that absorption with nucleohistone efficiently removed both the ANA and the anti-histone activities [13], indicate that anti-histone antibodies largely account for the ANA activity. Antibodies to dDNA generally do not bind nucleohistone, although a recent report suggests that interaction may be possible with certain preparations of chromatin [28]. Antibodies to dDNA tend to be of higher titer in patients treated with procainamide who remain asymptomatic than in patients with procainamide-induced lupus [23], and a major subset of these antibodies reacts with the nucleoside guanosine [29]. Anti-dDNA idiotypes characteristic of patients with SLE were found in approximately one-third of the patients treated with procainamide [30].

Typical kinetics of autoantibody elicitation by procainamide are shown in Table 2. IgG and IgM anti-dDNA antibodies appear to develop concordantly, although it is possible that shorter time intervals would reveal an earlier IgM response. Anti-histone activity also often develops during the same period but tends to be confined to IgM response, especially in patients who remain asymptomatic. The de novo production of anti-histone and anti-dDNA antibody and their disappearance after withdrawal of procainamide is the sine qua non of the procainamide-induced autoimmunity phenomenon. However, the remarkably slow kinetics of this process and the apparent concordant appearance of IgG and IgM antibodies do not suggest

TABLE 2

Kinetics of autoantibody elicitation by procainamide (PA)

Patient	PA therapy duration (months)	Antibody activity (optical density units)			
		Anti-histone		Anti-dDNA	
		IgG	IgM	IgG	IgM
E.M.	1	0	0.13	0.27	0.47
	2	0	0.40	0.77	1.19
	9	0	1.69	2.82	2.91
J.F.	1	0.08	0.26	0.45	0.23
	2.5	0.04	0.96	0.99	1.50
	10	0.18	1.51	5.27	2.10
J.S.	0	0	0.07	0.13	0.19
	2	0.09	0.29	1.83	0.73
	13	2.56	1.62	0.95	0.75

Antibody activity was determined by ELISA using solid-phase histone or dDNA and immunoglobulin class specific detecting reagents. These patients remained asymptomatic.

a classical immunization phenomenon underlying the genesis of these autoantibodies. Furthermore, the simultaneous development of anti-histone and anti-dDNA antibodies is not readily explainable by immunization with native chromatin because this material lacks the epitope of denatured DNA.

Total histones consist of five major polypeptides separable by polyacrylamide gel electrophoresis (PAGE). Using Western blot formats, a unique pattern of reactivity with individual histones of sera from patients with procainamide-induced lupus has been claimed, but since there is little agreement in the predominant antigens (H1, H2A and H2B, in Gohill et al. [31]; H3, H2B and H2A, in Portanova et al. [32]; H2B, H1 and H3, in Craft et al. [33]), the significance of these observations is unclear. Discrepancies among these studies may be due to the small sample sizes, differences in detecting reagent (protein A from *Staphylococcus aureus* versus anti-immunoglobulins) and other methodology differences. Taken collectively, these studies suggest that there is considerable patient-to-patient variation in reactivity with individual histones. Furthermore, reliance on Western blot techniques may exclude epitopes determined by higher ordered structures in the protein and often requires interpretations which are subjective or arbitrary.

An alternative procedure for examining anti-histone fine specificity involves the use of purified histones or histone complexes in solid-phase immunoassays such as enzyme-linked-immunosorbent assays (ELISA). As shown in Fig. 3, histones occur in the nucleus in a highly organized structure called the nucleosome. The core of this structure consists of three subunits, two H2A-H2B dimers flanking an H3-H4 tetramer and surrounded by approximately two turns of DNA. A linear array of nucleosomes held together by a shorter piece of linker DNA along with bound H1 generates the 100-Å diameter primary polynucleosome fiber. Physiologic en-

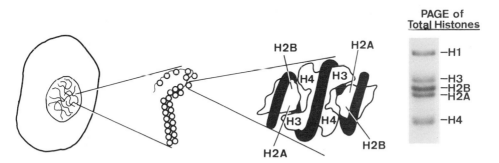

Fig. 3. Organization of histones in the nucleus. Chromatin fibers in the nucleus consist of nucleosomes interconnected by DNA. The core particle of the nucleosome is a tripartite structure held together by histone-histone interactions and stabilized by a cord of DNA 146 base pairs long. (The DNA diameter is shown at approximately 50% correct relative size for clarity.) The four core histones along with H1 can be extracted for chromatin and separated biochemically or by gel electrophoresis (PAGE). Core particle structure is derived from Burlingame et al. [112]. The exact position of H1 is unknown, but one molecule of H1 is presumably associated with the linker DNA between adjacent nucleosomes.

vironments tend to promote internucleosomal interactions, resulting in polynucleo-somal compaction and supercoiling. The resultant 300-Å diameter solenoid-like structure supercoils into even higher ordered structures, eventually visible in the light microscope as a chromosome.

Application of individual histones and histone-histone complexes to an ELISA format is shown in Fig. 4. Although considerable variation was displayed, a common denominator for patients with procainamide-induced lupus was a predominant IgG reactivity with a complex of histones H2A-H2B [23]. These sera also displayed weak reactivity with the monomers H2A and H2B, consistent with the Western blot studies previously discussed but demonstrating that this is only a minor component of the anti-histone response. In a larger multi-center study, all patients with well-defined symptomatic procainamide-induced lupus displayed enhanced reactivity with the H2A-H2B dimer compared to its denatured histone components [18]. Anti-(H2A-H2B) also binds well to native chromatin [11], trypsin digested chromatin and the H2A-H2B complex derived from it [32]. These studies indicate that the epitope for these antibodies does not involve the disordered regions of the amino terminus

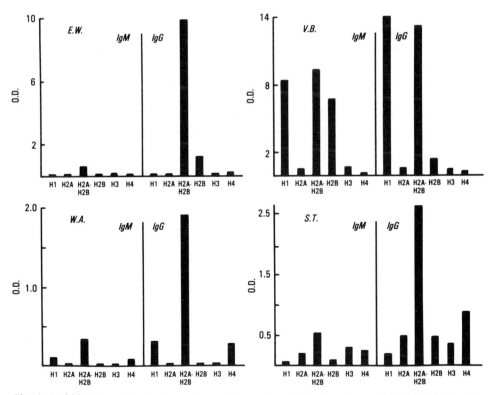

Fig. 4. Anti-histone activity in four patients with procainamide-induced lupus. Antibody binding to individual histones and to the H2A-H2B dimer was detected by ELISA using class-specific anti-immunoglobulin [23] and is expressed as optical density (O.D.) units.

of H2A and H2B and carboxyl terminus of H2A which are removed by trypsin digestion, but requires the highly structured regions of H2A and/or H2B necessary for dimer stability. This is in contrast to the apparent requirement for the trypsin-sensitive termini for antigenicity of the individual core histones in Western blot [31, 33]. Analysis of procainamide-induced lupus sera with fragments of H1 generated by protease digestion demonstrated predominant reactivity with the carboxyl terminal half of H1 [34], similar to the H1 domain reactivity observed for SLE sera [35, 36].

In contrast to symptomatic procainamide-induced lupus, the anti-histone specificity of patients who remain asymptomatic while taking procainamide tends to be restricted to an IgM response. IgM reactivity to all histones can often be quite elevated in these patients, whereas IgG reactivity is absent or limited often to only one or two individual histones [23]. Particularly noteworthy was the absence of IgG anti-(H2A-H2B) in 94% of 31 asymptomatic patients treated with an average dose of 2.5 g procainamide per day for an average of 31 months [18]. The maintenance for years of elevated IgM anti-histone antibodies as a result of procainamide treatment without switching to IgG isotypes is unlike classical (T cell dependent) antigen-driven immune responses. Since these individuals are without clinical symptoms, IgM anti-histone antibodies (and anti-dDNA antibodies which are also common in these patients) presumably are non-pathogenic. Nevertheless, these antibodies remain as objective markers for a procainamide-induced immune derangement with characteristics of an autoimmune phenomenon, since IgM anti-histone antibodies react readily with host nuclei.

As previously discussed and summarized in Table 1, anti-dDNA and anti-histone antibodies are the only humoral abnormalities shown by prospective studies to be regularly induced in the majority of procainamide-treated patients. Antibodies bound to red blood cells were detected in 21% of patients receiving procainamide for an average of 24 months (positive direct Coombs test), and 14% of these patients had hemolytic anemia [37], suggesting that anti-red blood cell antibodies may be an important although infrequent autoantibody induced by procainamide. Anemia, thrombocytopenia, leukopenia or neutropenia are generally detected in less than 20% of procainamide-treated patients [9, 37–39]; however, cytopenia is not necessarily the result of an antibody-mediated cytolytic process but may be an effect of procainamide on lympho- or hematopoiesis [40]. Slightly elevated gammaglobulins have been reported in procainamide-treated patients [7, 12, 16, 20, 38], but hypergammaglobulinemia is generally not observed in most patients. However, in a prospective study in which immunoglobulin levels were assayed during the course of therapy with procainamide, increased gammaglobulins of one or more class were commonly detected (Table 3). Although the levels of IgG, IgA and/or IgM that developed during therapy with procainamide were usually below the threshold for objective hypergammaglobulinemia because of the wide range of this laboratory parameter in the normal population, the temporal relationship between

TABLE 3

Immunoglobulin levels and antibodies to exogenous antigens during therapy with procainamide

Patient	Duration of therapy (months)	Ig level (mg/dl)			Antibody activity (optical density units)		
		IgG	IgA	IgM	tetanus	pneumococci	mumps
J.F.	1	976	7	64	0.1	0.2	0.5
	2.5	948	23	72	0.1	0.2	0.4
	10	1031	22	84	0.1	0.2	0.3
E.M.	1	1300	175	210	0.2	0.6	0.2
	2	1450	235	266	0.2	0.6	0.2
	9	1310	262	303	0.1	0.6	0.2
	13	1580	204	286	0.2	0.6	0.2
S.A.	0	1045	318	80	0.1	0.2	0
	3.5	1555	248	87	0.1	0.3	0
	12	1400	256	113	0.1	0.2	0

Immunoglobulin levels were determined by radial immunodiffusion, and specific antibodies were determined by ELISA using solid-phase antigens derived from vaccines and a polyvalent detecting reagent. These patients were asymptomatic.

immunoglobulin increase and drug therapy clearly indicates that this is a drug-induced process. After withdrawal of therapy, a 50 – 100% decrease in IgM and/or IgG immunoglobulins was commonly observed (unpublished data). This result is consistent with the splenomegaly that has occasionally been reported in procainamide-treated patients [41], and suggests that procainamide may cause a non-specific or polyclonal activation of immunoglobulin-secreting cells. However, as shown in Table 3, no increase in the levels of antibodies to exogenous agents such as tetanus toxoid, mumps virus of pneumococcus polysaccharide was detected during the period in which immunoglobulins were increasing, consistent with the high degree of specificity in the autoimmune response in these patients. It is unlikely that autoantibodies can account for the increased immunoglobulin levels, although these processes may be linked, as suggested by the observation that immune responses to T-dependent antigens result not only in specific antibodies but also in immunoglobulin of undetermined specificity secreted by lymphocytes in the spleen [42].

Although common in idiopathic SLE, hypocomplementemia is generally considered rare in drug-induced lupus. Hypocomplementemia has been reported in procainamide-induced lupus [43] but the vast majority of patients has a normal total hemolytic complement activity (CH_{50}), and C3 concentrations are usually within the normal range [9, 26, 44]. However, in vivo complement activation can be readily

TABLE 4

Complement activation in procainamide-treated patients

Symptomatic		Asymptomatic	
patient	C4d/C4	patient	C4d/C4
W.A.	1.2	J.F.	1.0
W.B.	1.5	R.H.	1.4
F.D.	1.0	F.H.	1.0
A.H.	1.4	W.J.	1.0
E.S.	2.6	H.K.	1.0
E.W.	1.8	R.P.	1.0
		M.S.	1.0
		J.S.	1.0

C4 and C4d were quantitated by rocket immunoelectrophoresis as described by Nitsche et al. [111]. C4d/C4 ratios > 1.1 are abnormal.

detected in patients with procainamide-induced lupus by the appearance of C4d, a fragment of C4 generated during classical pathway activation. As shown in Table 4, five out of six symptomatic patients had elevated C4d/C4 ratios whereas only one out of eight asymptomatic patients treated with procainamide displayed evidence of complement activation. Furthermore, in a prospective study of a patient who developed procainamide-induced lupus, C4 cleavage was detected 13.5 months after initiation of therapy, continued to increase during development of clinical drug-induced lupus, and returned to the normal range 2.5 months after discontinuation of procainamide therapy [45]. The correlation between complement activation and IgG anti-(H2A-H2B) in patients with procainamide-induced lupus supports the view that these antibodies are pathogenic and contribute to a immune complex mediated inflammatory process. Consistent with this notion is the observation that the anti-histone antibodies in procainamide-induced lupus are of the complement fixing isotypes, IgG_1 and IgG_3 [46].

(b) Cellular immune abnormalities

The effect of procainamide on cellular immune function has been examined in vivo and in vitro. Some reports showed procainamide-mediated enhancement of the in vitro activation of lymphocytes by phytohemagglutinin [24, 47] or pokeweed mitogen [48], or inhibition of immunoglobulin secretion by B cells [47]. However, these effects were small, or required relatively high concentrations of procainamide. Evaluation of the in vivo cellular immune status of procainamide-treated patients has led to conflicting results. Yu and Ziff [49] observed normal numbers and ratios of helper and suppressor T cells and normal concanavalin A induced suppressor cell activity. They also observed a 4-fold reduction in the number of pokeweed mitogen induced immunoglobulin-secreting cells, and mixing experiments indicated that both T helper cell and B cell activity were decreased in half the patients and B cell activity only was decreased in 25% of the patients. These results tend to contrast with the previous in vitro data of this group [48] in which the enhancing effect of procainamide on the number of immunoglobulin-secreting cells was attributed to inhibition of suppressor T cell activity, and the report by Miller and Salem [50], who observed an increased accumulation of immunoglobulin by pokeweed mitogen stimulated lymphocytes from patients treated with procainamide. Since these reports there has been little attempt to resolve these discrepancies. It is also possible that some of the observed effects may be due to the diethylaminoethylbenzamide moiety of procainamide rather than the autoimmunity-inducing para-amino group (see next section in this chapter). Procainamide may non-specifically suppress lymphocyte function through action of the hydrophobic portions of the molecule, analogous to the anesthetic action of procaine [51], by intercalation into the plasma membrane [52]. Furthermore, the necessity of restricting examination to only peripheral blood lymphocytes from procainamide-treated patients may exclude the hyper-responding, autoantibody-secreting cells which presumably reside mainly in the spleen.

4. GENETIC FACTORS

Acetylation of the amino group of procainamide and the hydrazine group of hydralazine is the predominant metabolic pathway of these drugs in humans. Acetyltransferase activity is found mainly in the liver, and its level is genetically controlled. Rapid acetylation is an autosomal dominant characteristic and occurs in approximately 50% of the North American Caucasian and Negroid races. Slow acetylators are homozygous for a recessive gene controlling hepatic acetyltransferase activity and will tend to have approximately 2-fold higher blood levels of the unacetylated drug at equivalent therapeutic doses. A strong association is observed between acetylator phenotype and the incidence of autoantibodies and drug-induced lupus as shown in Table 5. During the first 2 years of therapy with hydralazine, autoantibodies and clinical symptoms occur virtually exclusively in patients with the slow acetylator phenotype [53]. However, after extensive therapy rapid acetylators develop ANA, although out of a total of 25 patients with symptomatic hydralazine-induced lupus accumulated over a 16-year period, only one was a rapid acetylator [2]. With procainamide treatment ANA also appear more quickly in slow acetylators, and this phenotype predominates in the symptomatic patients during the first 6 months of therapy [6]. Although procainamide-induced lupus is not uncommon in rapid acetylators, exposure for an average of 48 ± 22 months was required, as opposed to a mean duration of 12 ± 5 months for symptom development in patients with the slow acetylator phenotype [6]. The importance of the unacetylated amino group on procainamide for induction of autoimmunity is further supported by the observation that N-acetyl-procainamide did not induce lupus symptoms, ANA or anti-dDNA [54, 55], and brought about the remission of procainamide-induced lupus and ANA during successful control of cardiac arrhythmias [56]. In fact, if the procainamide dose is adjusted so that the same steady-state plasma concentration was maintained in all patients by increasing the dose for rapid acetylators, there was no difference in the duration of therapy between slow and rapid acetylators for development of ANA or SLE-like symptoms [8].

Requirement for the primary amino or hydrazine group has been interpreted in two ways. A commonly held view is that these chemical moieties play a direct role in induction of autoimmunity, a concept which underlies all the in vitro studies in which direct effects of the parent molecule on lymphocyte function or binding to putative antigens or complement proteins are examined. An alternative explanation for the requirement of a free amino group is that in vivo metabolism of the drug at this chemical moiety generates an active compound, and that N-acetylation blocks these reactions. Reactive metabolites rather than the parent molecule would interact with a key immune target, leading to induction of autoimmunity. The failure of previous studies to demonstrate an immunologically specific effect of procainamide in vitro and its general immunosuppressive properties in vivo, in parallel with the recent identification of a reactive procainamide metabolite (Section V in this chapter) favors the view that metabolism of these drugs at the amino group is a prerequisite for their autoimmunity-inducing potential.

TABLE 5

Incidence of ANA and symptoms in fast and slow acetylators (Ac) treated with procainamide or hydralazine

Drug	Therapy period (months)	% Positive ANA		Number symptomatic	
		fast Ac	slow Ac	fast Ac	slow Ac
Hydralazine	13 – 26	0	60	0	3
	27 – 80	33	71	0	5
	81 – 200	86	75	0	4
Procainamide	1 – 2.5	0	20	0	0
	3 – 6	40	100	0	2
	7 – 77	80	0	7	12

Results are expressed as the percentage or number of patients with fast or slow acetylator phenotype undergoing therapy for the indicated period who developed abnormalities during that period. The hydralazine data is based on Perry et al. [53], assuming an average dose of 0.5 g hydralazine/day. Procainamide data is from Woosley et al. [6].

Other than acetyltransferase levels, no genetic factors predisposing procainamide-treated patients to autoimmunity have been identified. An early concept that some people have a 'lupus diathesis', a fertile genetic background for induction of disease by environmental factors such as drugs [57], has come under disfavor by the realization that almost all people treated with procainamide eventually develop some form of autoimmunity (i.e. ANA) and that procainamide-induced lupus almost always resolves within a few months after withdrawal of therapy. However, it is possible that genetic factors determine why only some patients develop anti-(H2A-H2B) and symptomatic drug-induced lupus. The human histocompatibility leukocyte antigens (HLA) are likely candidates for such a genetic predisposition, but we failed to detect an abnormal prevalence of any HLA antigen encoded at the A, B, C or D loci in six patients with procainamide-induced lupus [18], and no reports using a larger sample size have been published. The sex of the patient is generally considered unimportant, in contrast to idiopathic SLE in which there is a vast female predominance. However, most patients treated with procainamide are males, and there appears to be a disproportionate prevalence of procainamide-induced lupus in women. In the study of Henningsen et al. [7], procainamide-induced lupus was observed in 7 out of 12 female but only in 5 out of 30 male procainamide-treated patients, and Sonnhag et al. had similar results, with 4 out of 9 female compared to 5 out of 19 male patients with symptoms. Our experience is consistent with these older studies in that the male-to-female ratio was 1.9 in symptomatic but 5.2 in asymptomatic procainamide-treated patients [18]. Although these differences are not statistically significant, they do suggest that women are at greater risk for developing symptoms of procainamide-induced lupus, and that, as in the idiopathic form of SLE, sex hormones may be an accelerating factor in drug-induced lupus.

III. Features of hydralazine-induced autoimmunity

1. TIME COURSE AND DOSE DEPENDENCY

Control of hypertension by hydralazine requires a daily dose that can vary up to 20-fold, and some patients are maintained on hydralazine for over 10 years. Hydralazine plasma concentrations vary from $0.2-1.6$ μg/ml ($1.2-10$ μM) [58], and plasma half-life is 1.92 ± 0.11 h [58a]. In recent prospective studies in the United Kingdom, overall incidences of hydralazine lupus at 6.7% after 3 years' treatment [59] and 4.3% during 13 years [60] were observed. As with procainamide, there is a strong correlation between total cumulative dose of hydralazine and likelihood for development of lupus symptoms (Table 6), but precipitation of hydralazine-induced lupus tends to require a substantially longer period of therapy. A few patients develop lupus within 6 months of therapy, but the vast majority of patients require between 6 months and 2 years exposure [2]. However, it is not un-

133

TABLE 6

Incidence of lupus-like symptoms in patients treated with hydralazine

Hydralazine dose (mg/day)	Exposure duration (years)				
	0 – 0.5	0.5 – 1	1 – 2	2 – 4	4 – 8
100 – 200	0	0	3	0	0
200 – 400	2	1	5	2	0
400 – 800	1	6	8	2	1
800 – 1600	0	5	13	9	0

Values are the percentage of patients ingesting hydralazine at the indicated dose range who developed symptoms during the indicated time period. Data is from Perry [2], based on a population of 371 hydralazine-treated patients, 44 of whom developed lupus-like symptoms.

common for a patient to require > 1 kg of hydralazine during treatment for > 3 years before symptoms become manifested. Symptoms usually resolve within 1 month after discontinuation of therapy [60]. Readministration of hydralazine induced symptoms promptly in 3 out of 11 patients, and after weeks to months in another 5 out of 11, but 3 patients remained asymptomatic despite extensive retreatment [2].

Essentially, all patients with hydralazine-induced lupus are ANA positive [59, 60, 78] as well as approximately one-fourth of asymptomatic patients treated with hydralazine for 0.5 – 11 years [61]. Antinuclear antibodies induced by hydralazine tend to persist for as long as 10 years after discontinuation of therapy [2]. The incidence of ANA positivity in asymptomatic patients has been reported as low as 15% in patients treated with hydralazine for an average of 33 months [62], to a high of 44% in a group of 162 patients treated with hydralazine for 3 years [61].

2. CLINICAL AND LABORATORY FEATURES

Table 7 lists the major clinical symptoms and laboratory signs of hydralazine-induced lupus. Symptom onset is usually insidious and vague and often requires 3 months for diagnosis [59]. As with procainamide-induced lupus, joint involvement is the most common feature. However, objective arthritis is more remarkable in hydralazine lupus; this is non-deforming, polyarticular and tends to involve mainly the small joints. Fever, malaise and weight loss are commonly observed, and slightly enlarged spleens can sometimes be detected. Skin rash is more common in hydralazine-induced lupus than in procainamide-induced lupus and has been reported in the butterfly area of the face [2]. Unlike procainamide lupus, pericarditis has only rarely been reported [59] and, other than one report [63], myalgias are remarkably unusual. Renal involvement is generally considered uncommon,

134

TABLE 7

Major clinical and laboratory abnormalities in hydralazine-induced lupus

Clinical		Laboratory	
symptom	prevalence (%)	sign	prevalence (%)
Arthralgias	80	ANA	> 95
Arthritis	50 – 100	LE cells	50
Fever/weight loss	40 – 50	Anti-dDNA	50 – 90
Rash	25	Elevated ESR	60
Splenomegaly	15	Anemia	35
Lung involvement	10 – 30	RF	25
		Elevated γ-globulins	10 – 50

Data is based on Alarcon-Segovia et al. [72], Hahn et al. [68], Perry et al. [2], Cameron and Ramsay [59], and Russell et al. [60]. Abnormalities reported in < 10% of patients are not included.

although individual case reports of glomerulonephritis in patients taking hydralazine occasionally appear [64, 65]. However, it is not clear whether renal disease is a drug-induced phenomenon, related to the underlying hypertension or coincidentally due to other causes such as streptococcus infection.

As with procainamide-induced lupus, the major laboratory abnormality is ANA and the prevalences of other laboratory findings are similar in both hydralazine-and procainamide-induced lupus. The ANA are due to anti-histone antibodies but are of a different fine specificity than those in procainamide-induced lupus (see below). Antibodies to deoxyribonucleoprotein have been commonly reported [66, 67], but are probably the same as anti-histone antibodies. Other than in one report [68], antibodies to native DNA are not observed. Although anti-lymphocyte antibodies were detected in 4 out of 7 hydralazine-induced lupus patients, a similar prevalence was observed in asymptomatic hydralazine-treated patients [69] and in untreated controls [62], suggesting that if these antibodies are induced by hydralazine, they are not pathogenic.

3. IMMUNOLOGICAL ABNORMALITIES

(a) Humoral autoimmune abnormalities

The ANA isotype in asymptomatic hydralazine-treated patients was predominantly IgM as opposed to IgG ANA in symptomatic hydralazine-induced lupus [62]. Although hydralazine-induced ANA do not react after extraction of nuclei with 0.1 N HCl, a procedure which depletes nuclei of histones [70], histones do not reconstitute ANA in these sera. However, the sera showed good binding to histones in solid-phase assays [71]. The discrepancy between solid-phase and immunofluorescence assays was resolved by the observation that hydralazine-induced lupus sera are deficient in antibodies reactive with histones H2A, H2B and H1 and contain predominant reactivity with histones H3 and H4 [11], which apparently do not bind to histone-depleted nuclei. Unlike patients with procainamide-induced lupus, most patients with hydralazine-induced lupus do not react with the H2A-H2B complex, although they may contain antibodies to the monomers H2A and/or H2B [23]. By Western blot, H3 and H4 were the predominant targets for IgG antibodies in hydralazine-induced lupus [32], although another recent report showed predominant reactivity with H3, H2B, H2A and less commonly H1 and H4 [33]. Despite these discrepancies, there is general agreement that histone reactivity is preserved after trypsin digestion of chromatin [32, 33], indicating that the predominant epitope for these antibodies does not reside in the trypsin-sensitive tails of the antigenic histones. These antibodies do not bind well to native chromatin (unpublished observation), and give an ANA titer on intact nuclei which is on the average one log lower than that produced by procainamide-induced lupus sera [11]. These studies suggest that, in contrast to procainamide-induced anti-histone antibodies, antibodies in hydralazine-induced lupus sera show preferential reactivity with histone epitopes that are relatively inaccessible in native chromatin.

Antibodies to the drug itself were suggested to play an important role in the pathogenesis of hydralazine-induced lupus, since 4/4 patients with this syndrome had significantly elevated agglutination activity with hydralazine-coated red blood cells [68]. However, inhibition of this reaction required high hydralazine concentrations, and antibodies to hydralazine were not detected in 8 out of 8 asymptomatic patients treated with a similar dose of hydralazine for an average of 7 years or in eight patients with a prior history of hydralazine-induced lupus. Carpenter et al. [66] also reported antibodies to hydralazine, but 15 out of 16 of these patients were asymptomatic, and the one patient with mild hydralazine-induced lupus had a similar anti-hydralazine antibody titer prior to initiation of therapy with hydralazine. These discrepancies, along with the inability of Litwin et al. [62] to detect antibodies to hydralazine in 26 out of 27 asymptomatic patients treated with the drug for over 2 years and one patient with symptomatic hydralazine-induced lupus, raise some doubt about the immunologic relevance of this activity. Cross-reactions between anti-hydralazine and anti-DNA or anti-deoxyribonucleoprotein were not detected [66 – 68].

Antibodies to dDNA have been consistently observed in hydralazine-treated patients [23, 62, 68, 72]. Anti-dDNA were detected in over 60% of slow acetylators treated with hydralazine for over 2 years and in one-third of rapid acetylators, and even higher incidences of antibodies reacting with single- or double-stranded synthetic RNAs containing polyadenylic acid [62].

(b) Cellular immune abnormalities

Little in the way of abnormalities in the cellular immune system has been reported in hydralazine-treated patients. Skin tests for delayed-type hypersensitivity and responses of peripheral blood lymphocytes to a battery of standard mitogens were all within the normal range [62]. Evidence for hydralazine activation of peripheral blood lymphocytes was obtained by Hahn et al. [68], in which 4 out of 4 patients with active hydralazine-induced lupus but not asymptomatic patients showed a 50% stimulation index upon incubation with soluble hydralazine, and a study by Litwin et al. [62], in which 6 out of 12 asymptomatic hydralazine-treated patients displayed a 3- to 4-fold stimulation index, when incubated with hydralazine covalently bound to albumin. Whether these observations reflect a drug hypersensitivity reaction in vivo, a non-specific in vitro phenomenon or an important mechanism underlying autoimmunity, has not been explored. Peripheral blood lymphocytes from patients with hydralazine-induced lupus responded to dDNA in a proliferation assay [68], suggesting that antigen-specific T cells exist in the circulation.

4. GENETIC FACTORS

The importance of the slow acetylator phenotype as a predisposing element for development of hydralazine-induced autoimmunity was discussed in Section II.3(c) of this chapter. Although a subsequent study by Batchelor et al. [73] confirmed the original observations of Perry et al. [53] on this tight association, a rapid acetylator developing hydralazine-induced lupus was described [74], and 4 out of 20 hydralazine-induced lupus patients in a prospective study were rapid acetylators [60]. These exceptions reaffirm that the significance of the slow acetylator phenotype association with symptomatic drug-induced lupus is merely to decrease the duration of treatment (i.e. total cumulative dose of drug) required for development of autoimmunity. The lack of an association between acetylator phenotype and induction of ANA by isoniazid [75] or by captopril [76], as well as in idiopathic SLE [77], indicates that the slow acetylator phenotype is not a general predisposing element underlying autoimmunity nor is it genetically linked to a putative auto-immunity-inducing or -accelerating gene.

The association between sex and symptomatic drug-induced lupus may be stronger for hydralazine than procainamide. A $2-4/1$ preponderance of women over men for development of hydralazine-induced lupus has been reported [59, 60, 73]. In the longitudinal study of Cameron and Ramsay [59], the overall incidence of hydralazine-induced lupus during a 4-year observation period was 11.6% in women and 2.8% in men, and women treated with a daily dose of 200 mg hydralazine had a 3-year incidence of 19.4%. However, no significant difference in the incidence of ANA between men and women during 3 years of treatment with hydralazine were reported [63].

Racial differences have been consistently noted. Blacks develop hydralazine-induced lupus 4-fold [78] to 6-fold [2] less frequently than whites.

Considerable interest was generated by the study of Batchelor et al. [73] on the increased frequency of HLA-DR4 in patients with hydralazine-induced lupus. In a sample of 25 hydralazine-induced lupus patients, 19 (73%) were DR4 positive, compared to a frequency of 25% in asymptomatic hydralazine-treated patients, producing a relative risk for DR4 subjects of 8.1 [73]. However, HLA-phenotyping data on 15 hydralazine-induced lupus patients from the Melbourne (Australia) region failed to observe any increased frequency of HLA-DR4 or any other DR antigen, when compared to a control sample [79]. Another English study reported an HLA-DR4 frequency of 70% in hydralazine-induced lupus, but six patients were the same in both English studies [60]. A recalculated frequency after excluding these six patients was not reported, so whether a unique HLA phenotype occurs in hydralazine-induced lupus remains unresolved.

IV. Interactions of hydralazine and procainamide with macromolecules

1. BINDING TO DNA AND NUCLEOPROTEIN

Interaction of hydralazine with DNA or deoxyribonucleoprotein has been inferred from a variety of physical and chemical studies. Hydralazine increased the viscosity of soluble nucleoprotein and inhibited its sensitivity to trypsin digestion as assessed by antibody binding from a patient with hydralazine-induced lupus [80]. Hydralazine covalently bound to the pyrimidines, thymidine and deoxycytidine [81], although binding to DNA was not reported. At $> 50 \mu M$ hydralazine induced initiation of DNA repair in primary cultures of rat hepatocytes and was mutagenic in the Ames test at a concentration of 6 mM, suggesting an interaction with DNA [82].

Blomgren et al. [9] showed that a complex between procainamide and denatured DNA could be generated by a photo-oxidation reaction mediated by a variety of photodynamic agents. Direct interaction between procainamide and DNA was suggested by alteration in optical rotation and thermal stability when DNA was mixed with 50 mM procainamide [83]. Thomas and Messner [84] also observed a destabilizing effect of procainamide on double-stranded DNA and a facilitation of the B to Z transition of a synthetic polynucleotide having a propensity for Z conformations. Hydralazine showed similar effects [83, 84] and, importantly, N-acetyl procainamide was inactive [84]. However, by direct binding using radiolabelled procainamide no stable interaction between procainamide and DNA was observed [9, 85], and only $1/10^7$ molecules of radiolabeled procainamide remained bound to nuclei or nucleoprotein [85]. Furthermore, procainamide was only weakly mutagenic in the microsome-facilitated Ames test [86] and did not bind to microsomal proteins [87] or to DNA [88] unless it underwent biotransformation in vitro.

2. IMMUNOGENICITY STUDIES

The immunogenicity of covalent complexes of procainamide or hydralazine with DNA produced by a variety of chemical reactions has been examined. A photo-oxidized DNA-procainamide complex showed unique antigenicity, but was not a better immunogen for eliciting anti-dDNA antibodies than DNA alone and did not show enhanced reactivity with serum from patients with procainamide-induced lupus [9]. Complexes between procainamide and DNA or nucleoprotein formed by diazotization induced antibodies against procainamide and a small amount of transient reactivity with DNA [85]. Covalent complexes between hydralazine and albumin elicited anti-hydralazine antibodies in rabbits, and antibodies to denatured DNA were also detected if hydralazine was conjugated to human but not to rabbit albumin [89]. Reciprocal inhibition studies suggested that a component of the immune response in these animals was an antibody activity which cross-reacted with hydralazine and denatured DNA. However, although antibodies to denatured DNA are relatively common in drug-treated patients, cross-reacting anti-hydralazine antibodies have not been found (Section III.3(a) in this chapter), and antibodies reacting with procainamide have generally not been observed. These observations coupled with the need for an artificial covalent complex and complete Freund's adjuvant for elicitation of an anti-drug/dDNA response, indicate that the natural autoimmune response which arises in drug-treated patients has not been mimicked by direct immunization experiments.

3. BINDING TO COMPLEMENT

Studies by Sim et al. [90] demonstrated inhibition of complement component C4 binding to Cls by hydralazine, and that the C4A isotype was particularly susceptible [91]. It was suggested that hydralazine may interfere with immune complex clearance by disruption of complement pathways, especially in individuals with the C4B null allele. However, inhibition was only observed above 100 μM hydralazine and even higher concentrations of procainamide [90], concentrations 10 – 100-fold above the therapeutic plasma level of these drugs [58, 58a]. Therefore, if these in vitro phenomena are relevant to pathogenesis of drug-induced lupus, a drug-concentrating mechanism or involvement of a more reactive metabolite would have to be proposed.

4. SUMMARY

Little evidence exists for a stable interaction between procainamide or hydralazine and DNA, nucleoprotein or other macromolecules. Interactions were detected by physical studies or by biologic effects, but these required high drug concentrations or high ratios of drug to macromolecule. Such interactions may not reflect a specific, site-binding property of the drugs and, therefore, are of questionable relevance to the in vivo environment.

V. Oxidative metabolism of procainamide and hydralazine

Procainamide and hydralazine contain a nucleophilic nitrogen which has potential for undergoing oxidative reactions to reactive metabolites. Some of these products may be important for induction of autoimmunity because blocking oxidation by N-acetylation inactivates autoimmunity-inducing capacity [54–56]. Incubation of procainamide with rodent or human hepatic microsomes and an NADPH-generating system results in formation of an unstable product, the hydroxylamine derivative of procainamide (PAHA) [92, 93]. This metabolite readily forms covalent bonds with proteins (but not DNA) in an oxidizing environment [88] and is highly cytotoxic to a variety of cell types [94]. Cytotoxicity and covalent binding require further, non-enzymatic oxidation to a nitroso compound, a hypothetical intermediate with a relatively low redox potential. Rapidly dividing cells with high intrinsic biochemical reducing capacity are the most sensitive to PAHA, suggesting that redox cycling between hydroxylamine- and nitroso-procainamide within the cell may deplete cell-reducing potential, enhancing toxicity as shown in Fig. 5. This may explain why resting lymphocytes, which are only slowly killed by PAHA, contain massive single-stranded DNA breakage [94], since the deoxyribonucleotide substrates needed for DNA repair cannot be generated in an NADPH-depleted environment [95]. It appears, therefore, that PAHA has profound chemical, biochemical and biologic properties, implicating it as a key candidate for induction of autoimmunity.

Procainamide (PA)   Hydroxylamine-PA   Nitroso-PA

R: $CNH (CH_2)_2 N (CH_2CH_3)_2$, $\parallel$ O

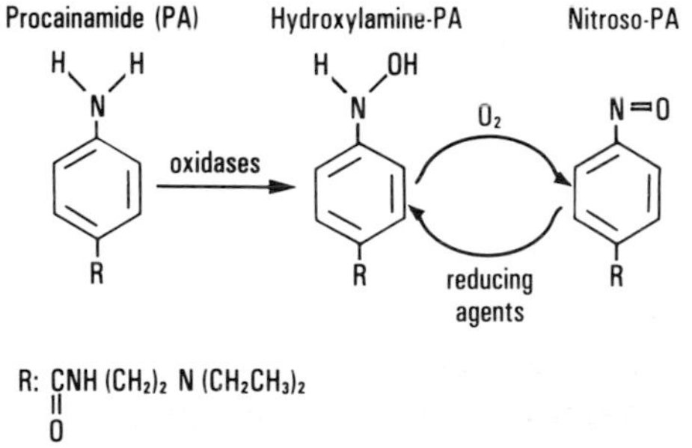

Fig. 5. Oxidative metabolism of procainamide. Procainamide can be oxidized to the hydroxylamine derivative (PAHA) by hepatic mixed-function oxidases and by neutrophils. Further oxidation by molecular oxygen generates the hypothetical nitroso intermediate. Nitroso-PA may be re-converted to PAHA by intracellular reduction reactions. Redox cycling between PAHA and nitroso-PA may deplete intracellular reducing potential, leading to DNA damage and cell death [88, 93, 94].

If PAHA formation is restricted to liver microsomal compartments, it is unlikely that substantial amounts could reach other tissues or organs, since microsomal proteins readily bind this metabolite [88] and serum proteins quench cytotoxicity [94]. However, peripheral blood neutrophils activated with opsonized zymosan can readily metabolize procainamide to the cytotoxic PAHA product (manuscript in preparation). These results raise the possibility of localized production of PAHA within a lymphoid tissue, lending credence to the importance of this reactive intermediate in the induction of autoimmunity and/or the pathogenesis of drug-induced lupus.

Hydralazine displays substantial chemical reactivity, and its metabolism is complex [96]. NADPH- and O_2-dependent biotransformation of hydralazine by microsomal enzymes produce a metabolite which covalently binds microsomal proteins, suggesting that mixed function oxidases metabolize hydralazine to a reactive electrophilic intermediate [97]. In vivo studies indicate that essentially all the introduced hydralazine is metabolized to a variety of products in the rat, some of which were detected covalently bound to the aorta, lungs and spleen [97].

VI. Animal models of procainamide- or hydralazine-induced autoimmunity

The inability to elicit ANA in rabbits, guinea pigs, rats, or mice injected with procainamide three times a week for 30 weeks [98] contrasts with other reports describing some success using oral administration of procainamide and/or hydralazine as summarized in Table 8. Cannat and Seligmann [99] obtained significant increases in the incidence of ANA in C57BL/6 mice continuously given oral hydralazine for 6 months, and female mice were particularly susceptible. Ten Veen and Feltkamp [100] obtained similar results and extended the study to procainamide and to two other mouse strains. A/J mice displayed the highest conversion to ANA positivity by hydralazine (80%) or procainamide (64%) compared to control mice (29%). Tannen and Weber [101] also were successful in eliciting ANA in A/J mice by procainamide, but contrary to the previous two reports observed suppression of spontaneous ANA induction by procainamide in C57BL/6 mice after 9 months of treatment. Although A/J mice were slow acetylators of procainamide using an in vitro assay involving blood hemolysates [101], analysis of urine levels showed no significant difference in acetylator phenotype among various mice strains [101]. More recent studies, using 24-h urinary collection in seven strains of mice, showed procainamide acetylation extents of 7 – 13% [102]. Although BALB/c and CD1 strains had a significantly lower acetylation rate, all strains of mice were remarkably slow acetylators compared to human standards and, therefore, would be expected to be a good species for drug-induced autoimmunity studies. In contrast six strains of rats were all rapid acetylators and showed no evidence for acetylation polymorphism [102].

The value of these murine models is compromised by their long duration, and

TABLE 8

Elicitation of ANA in mice by procainamide (PA) and hydralazine (HY)

Drug	Dose (mg/day)	Duration (months)	ANA incidence			Reference
			strain	group	% + ANA	
HY	0.5 – 1	6	C57BL/6	Ctl	12%	[99]
				HY	34%	
HY	1	8	C57BL/6	Ctl	16%	[100]
PA	20	8		HY	46%	
				PA	43%	
			A/J	Ctl	29%	
				HY	80%	
				PA	64%	
			BALB/c	Ctl	16%	
				HY	52%	
				PA	58%	
PA	24	9	C57BL/6	Ctl	33%	[101]
				PA	13%	
			A/J	Ctl	36%	
				PA	73%	

Hydralazine and procainamide were given continuously in the drinking water for the period shown. The incidence of positive ANA was significantly different in the drug-treated animals compared to untreated controls (Ctl) in all cases shown. Values from the study of Tannen and Weber [101] are estimates.

repetition of these results has not been reported. A major deficiency in these studies was the failure to measure procainamide blood levels. Drug clearance rates in mice are generally at least ten times the rate in humans [103], so at equivalent weight-adjusted doses mice would be expected to have much lower steady-state blood levels of procainamide and hydralazine than man. Because of the aversion of mice to higher oral doses, a different drug delivery system may need to be devised in order to increase blood levels and decrease exposure time to more practical periods.

VII. Possible mechanisms underlying drug-induced autoimmunity

1. IMMUNE RESPONSE TO DRUG OR TO DRUG-ALTERED ANTIGEN

This view is based on the precedents of allergic-like hypersensitivity reactions to drugs such as penicillin [104], in the context of the altered antigen concepts of Weigle [105] and Allison [106]. Drug bound to an endogenous structure may act as a hapten, rendering itself or an altered region on the conjugated macromolecule immunogenic, and antibodies raised against the hapten or the modified conjugate may cross-react with a native autoantigen. Alternatively, the drug-modified region may act as the carrier (T cell) epitope, activating drug-specific helper T cells which cooperate with B cells specific to epitopes on the macromolecule to elicit autoantibodies. Although the parent molecules, procainamide and hydralazine, are unlikely to act as haptens or carriers because of their inability to form covalent complexes with DNA or other macromolecules at therapeutically relevant concentrations, reactive metabolites may be produced in vivo. However, artificially prepared complexes of procainamide or hydralazine with macromolecules elicited antibodies which did not resemble the specificity of those which arise during drug-induced autoimmunity (Section IV.2 in this chapter). Furthermore, the slow kinetics of the drug-induced autoimmune response and its restriction to IgM antibodies in asymptomatic patients is not typical of a classical drug allergy. Allergic reactions are frequently localized to a single organ or tissue where hapten conjugation took place, and the patient is generally hypersensitive to challenge with drug. In contrast, procainamide- and hydralazine-induced lupus are systemic diseases and, although few studies have been done, rechallenge with low doses of either drug did not precipitate an immediate autoimmune reaction in most patients (this chapter, Section III.1.). Although the autoantibodies that arise in drug-induced autoimmunity are restricted to dDNA and histones, they are polyclonal and diverse in fine specificity in that many epitopes on nucleoprotein appear to be targeted. If the drug/carrier mechanism underlies this phenomenon, the drug must complex with either a macromolecule possessing many potential epitopes or with an array of its degradation products. Chromatin, polynucleosomes or subnucleosomal particles would be reasonable candidates for such macromolecules.

2. DRUGS ACT AS POLYCLONAL ACTIVATORS EITHER BY DIRECT STIMULATION OF B OR T CELLS OR THROUGH AN ADJUVANT EFFECT

This view is supported by in vitro studies demonstrating a stimulation of lymphocyte function by procainamide or hydralazine, and by the observation of frequently elevated immunoglobulins in drug-treated patients. However, the general hyporeactivity of lymphocytes isolated from procainamide-treated patients and the absence of diverse autoantibodies and of antibodies to exogenous agents are not consistent with this view. Although this concept also appears to be insufficient to explain the fine specificity of the autoantibodies which develop, some form of non-specific immune activation may be a component of the drug-induced autoimmune response. Such a phenomenon may reduce the threshold necessary to break tolerance to autoantigens.

3. DRUGS AFFECT ANTIGEN CATABOLISM OR PROCESSING

Rather than causing structural alterations in specific macromolecules rendering them immunogenic, procainamide or hydralazine may merely bring about an increase in the localized concentration of the target macromolecules. This could come about by an effect of the drugs on susceptibility of the macromolecules to enzymatic catabolism, clearance by the reticuloendothelial system, or by autoantigen release due to cytotoxic reactions of reactive drug metabolites. The specificity of the immune response to histones and dDNA can be accounted for by the predilection of antigens with rigid backbones containing repeating identical epitopes and/or extreme electrical charge to engage in multivalent high avidity binding directly to B-cell receptors. The repetitive, polynucleosome structure (Fig. 3), which contains the epitopes for anti-histone antibodies, fits in well with this concept, although it may be necessary to also invoke a drug-altered antigen model to explain elicitation of anti-dDNA antibodies.

4. PERTURBATION OF LYMPHOCYTE RECOGNITION MECHANISMS

The best model for this mechanism is the murine graft-versus-host reaction in which anti-histone and anti-DNA antibodies are induced in (C57BL/6 $\times$ DBA/2)F_1 mice by infusion of parental DBA/2 T cells [107]. H-2 mapping studies indicated that autoantibody induction required the interaction of DBA/2 alloreactive Ly-1$^+$ T cells with class II histocompatibility antigens on F_1 non-T cells [108]. Presumably endogenous autoantigen drives host B cells, and donor T helper cells contribute growth and differentiation factors to allow clonal expansion of antigen-activated B cells. In drug-induced autoimmunity procainamide, hydralazine or a metabolite of these drugs would bind Ia antigen on non-T cells, resulting in stimulation of pre-existing T helper cells recognizing allogeneic (drug-altered) Ia (major histocompatibility class II molecules). As with the previous mechanism, immune specificity could be provided by the unique polyvalent structure of deoxyribonucleoprotein, causing B cell stimulation.

VIII. Summary and future directions

The clinical and laboratory manifestations of drug-induced autoimmunity develop surprisingly slowly for an immunologic reaction, often taking months and sometimes years. For the subset of patients who develop clinical disease, the symptoms and signs induced by procainamide and hydralazine are remarkably similar. Nevertheless, subtle differences in symptoms induced by these two drugs have been detected, such as a higher incidence of pleuropulmonary symptoms and myalgias for procainamide and of arthritis and rash for hydralazine. Drug-related differences in the fine specificity of anti-histone antibodies can also be observed. Symptomatic lupus induced by procainamide is associated with anti-(H2A-H2B) dimer and lupus induced by hydralazine with antibodies to individual histones. Unlike the idiopathic form of lupus, autoantibodies in drug-induced lupus are largely restricted to histones and dDNA, with no enhanced immune reactivity to exogenous antigens. Nevertheless, evidence for generalized immune dysregulation is suggested by the overall reduction in peripheral T cell and B cell activities as well as the increase in circulating immunoglobulins. Genetic factors which accelerate drug-induced autoimmunity onset are the loose associations with females, Caucasians and possibly HLA phenotypes and especially with low level hepatic acetyltransferase activity. The latter association appears to relate to the importance of metabolism of these drugs at the primary amino or hydrazine group, transforming the parent molecule to a reactive intermediate which may be responsible for induction of autoimmunity.

The slow kinetics and dose dependency of the autoimmune phenomenon elicited by procainamide and hydralazine imply that a sequence of two or more events, or perhaps a coincidence of events needs to occur before autoimmunity can become manifested. Determining which mechanisms are involved demands a systematic study of the immunologic events leading up to autoimmunity. Currently, humans are the best 'animal model' for drug-induced lupus, and a prospective examination of the appropriate parameters as autoimmunity unfolds in these patients may yet be illuminating. However, practical considerations as well as decreasing availability of a sufficient patient sample size make development of an appropriate animal model even more urgent. Although drug-related autoimmunity is not a major medical problem, understanding the basis for this phenomenon promises to shed light on idiopathic autoimmune diseases and perhaps the normal functioning of the immune system.

Acknowledgements

This work was supported in part by Grants AR34358 from the National Institutes of Health and RR00833 from the U.S. Public Health Service. I thank Dr. Eng M. Tan for his years of encouragement and generous support and the staff of the BCR Wordprocessing Center for their valued help in the preparation of this manuscript. This is publication No. 5231BCR from the Research Institute of Scripps Clinic, La Jolla.

References

1. Lee, S. L. and Chase, P. H. (1975) Drug-induced systemic lupus erythematosus: a critical review. Semin. Arthritis Rheum. 5, 83 – 103.

2. Perry, H. M., Jr.   (1973)   Late toxicity of hydralazine resembling systemic lupus erythematosus or rheumatoid arthritis. Am. J. Med. 54, 58 – 72.

3. Morrow, J. D., Schroeder, H. A. and Perry, H. M., Jr.   (1953)   Studies on the control of hypertension by hyphex. II. Toxic reactions and side effects. Circulation 8, 829 – 839.

4. Dustan, H. P., Taylor, R. D., Corcoran, A. C. and Page, I. H.   (1954)   Rheumatic and febrile syndrome during prolonged hydralazine treatment. J. Am. Med. Assoc. 154, 23 – 29.

5. Ladd, A. T.   (1962)   Procainamide-induced lupus erythematosus. N. Engl. J. Med. 267, 1357 – 1358.

6. Woosley, R. L., Drayer, D. E., Reidenberg, M. M., Nies, A. S., Carr, K. and Oates, J. A.   (1978)   Effect of acetylator phenotype on the rate at which procainamide induces antinuclear antibodies and the lupus syndrome. N. Engl. J. Med. 298, 1157 – 1159.

7. Henningsen, N. C., Cederberg, A., Hanson, A. and Johansson, B. W.   (1975)   Effects of long-term treatment with procaine amide. Acta Med. Scand. 198, 475 – 482.

8. Sonnhag, C., Karlsson, E. and Hed, J.   (1979)   Procainamide-induced lupus erythematosus-like syndrome in relation to acetylator phenotype and plasma levels of procainamide. Acta Med. Scand. 206, 245 – 251.

9. Blomgren, S. E., Condemi, J. J. and Vaughan, J. H.   (1972)   Procainamide-induced lupus erythematosus. Am. J. Med. 52, 338 – 348.

10. Fritzler, M. J. and Tan, E. M.   (1978)   Antibodies to histones in drug-induced and idiopathic lupus erythematosus. J. Clin. Invest. 62, 560 – 567.

11. Portanova, J. P., Rubin, R. L., Joslin, F. G., Agnello, V. D. and Agnello, V. D.   (1982)   Reactivity of antihistone antibodies induced by procainamide and hydralazine. Clin. Immunol. Immunopathol. 25, 67 – 79.

12. Winfield, J. B. and Davis, J. S.   (1974)   Anti-DNA antibody in procainamide-induced lupus erythematosus. Arthritis Rheum. 17, 97 – 110.

13. Rubin, R. L., Reimer, G., McNally, E. M., Nusinow, S. R., Searles, R. P. and Tan, E. M.   (1986)   Procainamide elicits a selective autoantibody immune response. Clin. Exp. Immunol. 63, 58 – 67.

14. Giardina, E.-G. V., Heissenbuttel, R. H. and Bigger, J. T., Jr.   (1973)   Intermittent intravenous procaine amide to treat ventricular arrhythmias. Ann. Intern. Med. 78, 183 – 193.

15. Greenspan, A. M., Horowitz, L. N., Speilman, S. R. and Josephson, M. E.   (1980)   Large dose procainamide therapy for ventricular tachyarrhythmia. Am. J. Cardiol. 46, 453 – 462.

16. Blomgren, S. E., Condemi, J. J., Bignall, M. C. and Vaughan, J. H.   (1969)   Antinuclear antibody induced by procainamide: A prospective study. N. Engl. J. Med. 281, 64 – 66.

17. Kosowsky, B. D., Taylor, J., Lown, B. and Ritchie, R. F.   (1973)   Long-term use of procaine amide following acute myocardial infarction. Circulation 47, 1204 – 1210.

18. Totoritis, M. C., Tan, E. M., McNally, E. M. and Rubin, R. L.   (1988)   Association of anti-histone (H2A-H2B) complex antibody with symptomatic procainamide induced lupus. N. Engl. J. Med. 318, 1431 – 1436.

19. Molina, J., Dubois, E. L., Bilitch, M., Bland, S. L. and Friou, G. J.   (1969)   Procainamide-induced serologic changes in asymptomatic patients. Arthritis Rheum. 12, 608 – 614.

20. Klajman, A., Camin-Belsky, N., Kimchi, A. and Ben-Efraim, S.   (1970)   Occurrence, immunoglobulin pattern and specificity of antinuclear antibodies in sera of procaineamide treated patients. Clin. Exp. Immunol. 7, 641 – 649.

21. Koffler, D., Carr, R. I., Agnello, V., Thoburn, R. and Kunkel, H. G.   (1971)   Antibodies to polynucleotides in human sera: antigenic specificity and relation to disease. J. Exp. Med. 134, 294.

22. Klajman, A., Farkas, R., Gold, E. and Ben-Efraim, S.   (1975)   Procainamide-induced antibodies to nucleoprotein, denatured and native DNA in human subjects. Clin. Immunol. Immunopathol. 3, 525 – 530.

23. Rubin, R. L., McNally, E. M., Nusinow, S. R., Robinson, C. A. and Tan, E. M.   (1985)   IgG

antibodies to the histone complex H2A-H2B characterize procainamide-induced lupus. Clin. Immunol. Immunopathol. 36, 49 – 59.

24. Bluestein, H. G., Zvaifler, N. J., Weisman, M. H. and Shapiro, R. F. (1979) Lymphocyte alteration by procainamide: relation to drug-induced lupus erythematosus syndrome. Lancet ii, 816 – 819.

25. Winfield, J. B., Koffler, D. and Kunkel, H. G. (1975) Development of antibodies to ribonucleoprotein following short-term therapy with procainamide. Arthritis Rheum. 18, 531 – 534.

26. Russell, A. S. and Ziff, M. (1968) Natural antibodies to procaine amide. Clin. Exp. Immunol. 3, 901 – 909.

27. Tan, E. M. (1982) Autoantibodies to nuclear antigens. Their immunobiology and medicine. Adv. Immunol. 33, 167 – 240.

28. Faiferman, I. and Koffler, D. (1987) Reaction of antipolynucleotide antibody from systemic lupus erythematosus patient serum with double-stranded DNA complexed to protein. Arthritis Rheum. 30, 814 – 818.

29. Weisbart, R. H., Yee, W. S., Colburn, K. K., Whang, S. H., Heng, M. K. and Boucek, R. J. (1986) Antiguanosine antibodies: A new marker for procainamide-induced systemic lupus erythematosus. Ann. Intern. Med. 104, 310 – 313.

30. Shoenfeld, Y., Vilner, Y., Reshef, T., Klajman, A., Skibin, A., Kooperman, O. and Kennedy, R. C. (1987) Increased presence of common systemic lupus erythematosus (SLE) anti-DNA idiotypes (16/6 Id, 32/15 Id) is induced by procainamide. J. Clin. Immunol. 7, 410 – 419.

31. Gohill, J., Cary, P. D., Coupper, M. and Fritzler, M. J. (1985) Antibodies from patients with drug-induced and idiopathic lupus erythematosus react with epitopes restricted to the amino acid and carboxyl termini of histone. J. Immunol. 135, 3116 – 3121.

32. Portanova, J. P., Arndt, R. E., Tan, E. M. and Kotzin, B. L. (1987) Anti-histone antibodies in idiopathic and drug-induced lupus recognize distinct intrahistone regions. J. Immunol. 138, 446 – 451.

33. Craft, J. E., Radding, J. A., Harding, M. W., Bernstein, R. M. and Hardin, J. A. (1987) Autoantigenic histone epitopes: a comparison between procainamide- and hydralazine-induced lupus. Arthritis Rheum. 30, 689 – 694.

34. Gohill, J. and Fritzler, M. J. (1987) Antibodies in procainamide-induced and systemic lupus erythematosus bind the C-terminus of histone 1 (H1). Mol. Immunol. 24, 275 – 285.

35. Hardin, J. A. and Thomas, J. O. (1983) Antibodies to histones in systemic lupus erythematosus: localization of prominent autoantigens on histones H1 and H2B. Proc. Natl. Acad. Sci. USA 80, 7410 – 7414.

36. Costa, O., Tchouatcha-Tchouassom, J. C., Roux, B. and Monier, J. C. (1986) Anti-H1 histone antibodies in systemic lupus erythematosus: epitope localization after immunoblotting of chymotrypsin-digested H1. Clin. Exp. Immunol. 63, 608 – 613.

37. Kleinman, S., Nelson, R., Smith, L. and Goldfinger, D. (1984) Positive direct antiglobulin tests and immune hemolytic anemia in patients receiving procainamide. N. Engl. J. Med. 311, 809 – 812.

38. Dubois, E. L. (1969) Procainamide induction of a systemic lupus erythematosus-like syndrome. Presentation of six cases, review of the literature, and analysis and followup of reported cases. Medicine 48, 217 – 228.

39. Ellrodt, A. G., Murata, G. H., Riedinger, M. S., Stewart, M. E., Mochizuki, C. and Gray, R. (1984) Severe neutropenia associated with sustained-release procainamide. Ann. Intern. Med. 100, 197 – 201.

40. Pisciotta, A. V. (1973) Immune and toxic mechanisms in drug-induced agranulocytosis. Semin. Hematol. 10, 279 – 310.

41. Harmon, C. H. and Portanova, J. P. (1982) Drug-induced lupus: clinical and serological studies. Clin. Rheum. Dis. 8, 121 – 135.

42. Rosenberg, Y. J. and Chiller, J. M. (1979) Ability of antigen-specific helper cells to effect a class-restricted increase in total Ig-secreting cells in spleens after immunization with the antigen. J. Exp. Med. 150, 517 – 530.

43. Utsinger, P. D., Zvaifler, N. J. and Bluestein, H. G. (1976) Hypocomplementemia in procainamide-associated systemic lupus erythematosus. Ann. Intern. Med. 84, 293.

44. Klajman, A., Farkas, R. and Ben-Efraim, S. (1972) Reactions of procaine amide-induced antinuclear antibodies with fractions derived from calf thymus nuclei. Int. Arch. Allergy 43, 630 – 638.

45. Rubin, R. L., Nusinow, S. R., Johnson, A. D., Rubenson, D. S., Curd, J. G. and Tan, E. M. (1986) Serological changes during induction of lupus-like disease by procainamide. Am. J. Med. 80, 999 – 1002.

46. Rubin, R. L., Tang, F-L., Lucas, A. H., Spiegelberg, H. L. and Tan, E. M. (1986) IgG subclasses of anti-tetanus toxoid antibodies in adult and newborn normal subjects and in patients with systemic lupus erythematosus, Sjögren's syndrome, and drug-induced autoimmunity. J. Immunol. 137, 2522 – 2527.

47. De Boccardo, G., Drayer, D., Rubin, A. L., Novogrodsky, A., Reidenberg, M. M. and Stenzel, K. H. (1985) Inhibition of pokeweed mitogen-induced B cell differentiation by compounds containing primary amine or hydrazine groups. Clin. Exp. Immunol. 59, 69 – 76.

48. Ochi, T., Goldings, E. A., Lipsky, P. E. and Ziff, M. (1983) Immunomodulatory effect of procainamide in man. J. Clin. Invest. 71, 36 – 45.

49. Yu, C.-L. and Ziff, M. (1985) Effects of long-term procainamide therapy on immunoglobulin synthesis. Arthritis Rheum. 28, 276 – 284.

50. Miller, K. B. and Salem, D. (1982) Immune regulatory abnormalities produced by procainamide. Am. J. Med. 73, 487 – 492.

51. Seeman, P. (1972) The membrane actions of anesthetics and tranquilizers. Pharmacol. Rev. 24, 583 – 653.

52. Goldstein, D. B. (1984) The effects of drugs on membrane fluidity. Annu. Rev. Pharmacol. Toxicol. 24, 43 – 64.

53. Perry, H. M., Jr., Tan, E. M., Cormody, S. and Sakamato, A. (1970) Relationship of acetyltransferase activity to antinuclear antibodies and toxic symptoms in hypertensive patients treated with hydralazine. J. Lab. Clin. Med. 76, 114 – 125.

54. Lahita, R., Kluger, J., Drayer, D. E., Koffler, D. and Reidenberg, M. M. (1979) Antibodies to nuclear antigens in patients treated with procainamide or acetylprocainamide. N. Engl. J. Med. 301, 1382 – 1385.

55. Roden, D. M., Reele, S. B., Higgins, S. B., Wilkinson, G. R., Smith, R. F., Oates, J. A. and Woosley, R. L. (1980) Antiarrhythmic efficacy, pharmacokinetics and safety of N-acetylprocainamide in human subjects: Comparison with procainamide. Am. J. Cardiol. 46, 463 – 468.

56. Stec, G. P., Lertora, J. J. L., Atkinson, A. J., Jr., Nevin, M. J., Kushner, W., Jones, C., Schmid, F. R. and Askenazi, J. (1979) Remission of procainamide-induced lupus erythematosus with N-acetylprocainamide therapy. Ann. Intern. Med. 90, 799 – 801.

57. Alarcon-Segovia, D., Fishbein, E. and Betancourt, V. M. (1969) Antibodies to nucleoprotein and to hydrazide-altered soluble nucleoprotein in tuberculous patients receiving isoniazid. Clin. Exp. Immunol. 5, 429 – 437.

58. Zacest, R. and Koch-Weser, J. (1972) Relation of hydralazine plasma concentration to dosage and hypotensive action. Clin. Pharmacol. Ther. 13, 420 – 425.

58a. Talseth, T. (1977) Kinetics of hydralazine elimination. Clin. Pharmacol. Ther. 21, 715 – 720.

59. Cameron, H. A. and Ramsay, L. E. (1984) The lupus syndrome induced by hydralazine: a common complication with low dose treatment. Br. Med. J. 289, 410 – 412.

60. Russell, G. I., Bing, R. F., Jones, J. A. G., Thurston, H. and Swales, J. D. (1987) Hydralazine

sensitivity: clinical features, autoantibody changes and HLA-DR phenotype. Q. J. Med. 65, 845 – 852.

61. Hughes, G. R. V., Rynes, R. I., Gharavi, A., Ryan, P. F. J., Sewell, J. and Mansilla, R. (1981) The heterogeneity of serologic findings and predisposing host factors in drug-induced lupus erythematosus. Arthritis Rheum. 24, 1070 – 1073.

62. Litwin, A., Adams, L. E., Zimmer, H., Foad, B., Loggie, J. H. M. and Hess, E. V. (1981) Prospective study of immunologic effects of hydralazine in hypertensive patients. Clin. Pharmacol. Ther. 29, 447 – 456.

63. Mansilla-Tinoco, R., Harland, S. J., Ryan, P. J., Bernstein, R. M., Dollery, C. T., Hughes, G. R. V., Bulpitt, C. J., Morgan, A. and Jones, J. M. (1982) Hydralazine, antinuclear antibodies, and the lupus syndrome. Br. Med. J. 284, 936 – 939.

64. Bjorck, S., Svalander, C. and Westberg, G. (1985) Hydralazine-associated glomerulonephritis. Acta Med. Scand. 218, 261 – 269.

65. Naparstek, Y., Kopolovic, J., Tur-Kaspa, R. and Rubinger, D. (1984) Focal glomerulonephritis in the course of hydralazine-induced lupus syndrome. Arthritis Rheum. 27, 822 – 825.

66. Carpenter, J. R., McDuffie, F. C., Sheps, S. G., Spiekerman, R. E., Brumfield, H. and King, R. (1980) Prospective study of immune response to hydralazine and development of antideoxyribonucleoprotein in patients receiving hydralazine. Am. J. Med. 69, 395 – 400.

67. McDuffie, F. C. (1981) Relationship between immune response to hydralazine and to deoxyribonucleoprotein in patients receiving hydralazine. Arthritis Rheum. 24, 1079 – 1081.

68. Hahn, B., Sharp, G. C., Irvin, W. S., Kantor, D. S., Gardner, C., Bagby, B. A., Perry, H. M. and Osterland, C. K. (1972) Immune responses to hydralazine and nuclear antigens in hydralazine-induced lupus erythematosus. Ann. Intern. Med. 76, 365 – 374.

69. Ryan, P. F. J., Hughes, G. R. V., Bernstein, R., Mansilla, R. and Dollery, C. T. (1979) Lymphocytotoxic antibodies in hydralazine-induced lupus erythematosus. Lancet ii, 1248 – 1249.

70. Tan, E. M., Robinson, J. and Robitaille, P. (1976) Studies or antibodies to histones by immunofluorescence. Scand. J. Immunol. 5, 811 – 818.

71. Rubin, R. L., Joslin, F. J. and Tan, E. M. (1982) A solid-phase radioimmunoassay for antihistone antibodies in human sera: comparison with an immunofluorescence assay. Scand. J. Immunol. 15, 63 – 70.

72. Alarcón-Segovia, D., Wakin, K. G., Worthington, J. W. and Wardd, L. E. (1967) Clinical and experimental studies on the hydralazine syndrome and its relationship to systemic lupus erythematosus. Medicine 46, 1 – 33.

73. Batchelor, J. R., Welsh, K. L., Tinoco, R. M., Dollery, C. T., Hughes, G. R. V., Bernstein, R., Ryan, P., Naish, P. F., Aber, G. M., Bing, R. F. and Russell, G. I. (1980) Hydralazine-induced systemic lupus erythematosus: influence of HLA-DR and sex on susceptibility. Lancet i, 1107 – 1109.

74. Harland, S. J., Facchini, V. and Timbrell, J. A. (1980) Hydralazine-induced lupus erythematosus-like syndrome in a patient of the rapid acetylator phenotype. Br. Med. J. 281, 273 – 274.

75. Alarcón-Segovia, D., Fishbein, E. and Alcala, H. (1971) Isoniazid acetylation rate and development of antinuclear antibodies upon isoniazid treatment. Arthritis Rheum. 14, 748 – 752.

76. Reidenberg, M. M., Chase, D. B., Drayer, D. E., Reis, S. and Lorenzo, B. (1984) Development of antinuclear antibody in patients treated with high doses of captopril. Arthritis Rheum. 27, 579 – 581.

77. Baer, A. N., Woosley, R. L. and Pincus, T. (1986) Further evidence for the lack of association between acetylator phenotype and systemic lupus erythematosus. Arthritis Rheum. 29, 508 – 514.

78. Condemi, J. J., Moore-Jones, D., Vaughan, J. H. and Perry, H. M. (1967) Antinuclear antibodies following hydralazine toxicity. N. Engl. J. Med. 276, 486 – 490.

79. Brand, C., Davidson, A., Littlejohn, G. and Ryan, P. (1984) Hydralazine-induced lupus: no

association with HLA-DR4. Lancet i, 462.

80. Tan, E. M. (1974) Drug-induced autoimmune disease. Fed. Proc. 33, 1894 – 1897.

81. Dubroff, L. M. and Reid, R. J., Jr. (1980) Hydralazine-pyrimidine interactions may explain hydralazine-induced lupus erythematosus. Science 208, 404 – 406.

82. Williams, G. M., Mazue, G., McQueen, C. A. and Shimada, T. (1980) Genotoxicity of the antihypertensive drugs hydralazine and dihydralazine. Science 210, 329 – 330.

83. Eldredge, N. T., Robertson, W. V. B. and Miller, III, J. J. (1974) The interaction of lupus-inducing drugs with deoxyribonucleic acid. Clin. Immunol. Immunopathol. 3, 263 – 271.

84. Thomas, T. J. and Messner, R. P. (1986) Effects of lupus-inducing drugs on the B to Z transition of synthetic DNA. Arthritis Rheum. 29, 638 – 645.

85. Gold, E. F., Ben-Efraim, S., Faivisewitz, A., Steiner, Z. and Klajman, A. (1977) Experimental studies on the mechanism of induction of antinuclear antibodies by procainamide. Clin. Immunol. Immunopathol. 7, 176 – 186.

86. Freeman, R. W., Woosley, R. L., Oates, O. A. and Harrison, R. D. (1979) Evidence for biotransformation of procainamide to a reactive metabolite. Toxicol. Appl. Pharmacol. 50, 9 – 16.

87. Freeman, R. W., Uetrecht, J. P., Woosley, R. L. Oates, J. A. and Harbison, R. D. (1981) Covalent binding of procainamide in vitro and in vivo to hepatic protein in mice. Drug Metab. Dispos. 9, 188 – 192.

88. Uetrecht, J. P. (1985) Reactivity and possible significance of hydroxylamine and nitroso metabolites of procainamide. J. Pharmacol. Exp. Ther. 232, 420 – 425.

89. Yamauchi, Y., Litwin, A., Adams, L., Zimmer, H. and Hess, E. V. (1975) Induction of antibodies to nuclear antigens in rabbits by immunization with hydralazine-human serum albumin conjugates. J. Clin. Invest. 56, 958 – 969.

90. Sim, E., Gill, E. W. and Sim, R. B. (1984) Drugs that induce systemic lupus erythematosus inhibit complement component C4. Lancet i, 422 – 424.

91. Sim, E. and Law, S.-K. (1985) Hydralazine binds covalently to complement component C4. Different reactivity of C4A and C4B gene products. FEBS Lett. 184, 323 – 327.

92. Uetrecht, J. P., Sweetman, B. J., Woosley, R. L. and Oates, J. A. (1984) Metabolism of procainamide to a hydroxylamine by rat and human hepatic microsomes. Drug Metab. Dispos. 12, 77 – 81.

93. Budinsky, R. A., Roberts, S. M., Coats, E. A., Adams, L. and Hess, E. V. (1987) The formation of procainamide hydroxylamine by rat and human liver microsomes. Drug Metab. Dispos. 15, 37 – 43.

94. Rubin, R. L., Uetrecht, J. P. and Jones, J. E. (1987) Cytotoxicity of oxidative metabolites of procainamide. J. Pharmacol. Exp. Ther. 242, 833 – 841.

95. Larsson, A. and Reichard, P. (1967) Enzymatic reduction of ribonucleotides. In: J. N. Davidson and W. E. Cohn (Eds.), Progress in Nucleic Acid Research and Molecular Biology. Vol. 7, New York, Academic Press, pp. 303 – 345.

96. Ludden, T. M., McNay, J. L., Shepherd, A. M. M. and Lin, M. S. (1981) Variability of plasma hydralazine concentrations in male hypertensive patients. Arthritis Rheum. 24, 987 – 993.

97. Streeter, A. J. and Timbrell, J. A. (1983) Studies on the in vivo metabolism of hydralazine in the rat. Drug Metab. Dispos. 11, 184 – 189.

98. Whittingham, S., Mackay, I. R., Whitworth, J. A. and Sloman, G. (1972) Antinuclear antibody response to procainamide in man and laboratory animals. Am. Heart J. 84, 228 – 234.

99. Cannat, A. and Seligmann, M. (1968) Induction by isoniazid and hydralazine of antinuclear factors in mice. Clin. Exp. Immunol. 3, 99 – 105.

100. Ten Veen, J. H. and Feltkamp, T. E. W. (1972) Studies on drug induced lupus erythematosus in mice. I. Drug induced antinuclear antibodies (ANA). Clin. Exp. Immunol. 11, 265 – 276.

101. Tannen, R. H. and Weber, W. W. (1980) Antinuclear antibodies related to acetylator phenotype in mice. J. Pharmacol. Exp. Ther. 213, 485 – 490.

102. Roberts, S. M., Budinsky, R. A., Adams, L. E., Litwin, A. and Hess, E. V. (1985) Procainamide acetylation in strains of rat and mouse. Drug Metab. Dispos. 13, 517–519.

103. Freireich, E. J., Gehan, E. A., Rall, D. P., Schmidt, L. H. and Skipper, H. E. (1966) Quantitative comparison of toxicity of anticancer agents in mouse, rat, hamster, dog, monkey and man. Cancer Chemother. Rpts. 50, 219–244.

104. Parker, C. W. (1981) Hapten immunology and allergic reactions in humans. Arthritis Rheum. 24, 1024–1036.

105. Weigle, W. O. (1973) Immunological unresponsiveness. Adv. Immunol. 16, 61–122.

106. Allison, A. C. (1971) Unresponsiveness to self antigens. Lancet ii, 1401–1403.

107. Gleichmann, E., Pals, S. T., Rolink, A. G., Radaskiewicz, T. and Gleichmann, H. (1984) Graft-versus-host reactions: clues to the etiopathology of a spectrum of immunological diseases. Immunol. Today 5, 324–332.

108. Rolink, A. G., Pals, S. T. and Gleichmann, E. (1983) Allosuppressor and allohelper T cells in acute and chronic graft-vs.-host disease. II. F_1 recipients carrying mutations at H-2K and/or I-A. J. Exp. Med. 157, 755–771.

109. Weinstein, A. (1980) Drug-induced lupus erythematosus. Prog. Clin. Immunol. 4, 1–21.

110. Russell, A. S. (1981) Drug-induced autoimmune disease. Clin. Immunol. Allergy 1, 57–76.

111. Nitsche, J. F., Tucker, E. S. III, Sugimoto, S., Vaughan, J. H. and Curd, J. G. (1981) Rocket immunoelectrophoresis for C4 and C4d: a simple sensitive method for detecting complement activation in plasma. Am. J. Clin. Pathol. 76, 679–684.

112. Burlingame, R. W., Love, W. E., Wang, B.-C., Hamlin, R., Xuong, N.-H. and Moudrianakis, E. N. (1985) Crystallographic structure of the octameric histone core of the nucleosome at a resolution of 3.3 A. Science 228, 546–553.

M.E. Kammüller, N. Bloksma and W. Seinen (Eds.)
Autoimmunity and Toxicology
© 1989 Elsevier Science Publishers B.V. (Biomedical Division)

Autoimmune reactions in humans induced by diphenylhydantoin and nitrofurantoin

5

D. ALARCÓN-SEGOVIA and MARTA ALARCÓN-RIQUELME

Department of Immunology and Rheumatology, Instituto Nacional de la Nutrición Salvador Zubirán, México City, Mexico

I. Diphenylhydantoin

Diphenylhydantoin (phenytoin, DPH) is a structural relative of phenobarbital (Fig. 1) used primarily for all types of epilepsy except absence seizures. DPH was synthetized in 1908 by Biltz, but its anticonvulsant activity was not discovered until 1938 [1]. It has been more thoroughly studied in the laboratory and clinic than any other antiepileptic agent. Because of this, extensive and diverse reports are found concerning its toxic effects.

The pharmacokinetic characteristics of DPH are influenced by its limited aqueous solubility and its dose-dependent elimination. It is important to note here that its inactivation by the hepatic microsomal enzyme system is susceptible to inhibition by other drugs. Thus, there is a well-documented increase in the concentration of DPH in plasma when it is concurrently administered with drugs such as chloramphenicol, dicumarol, disulfiram, isoniazid, or certain sulfonamides. A good correlation is usually observed between the total concentration of DPH in plasma and the clinical effect. Toxic effects develop with plasma concentrations above 10 μg/ml. However, adverse reactions have been observed at therapeutic concentrations and these sometimes cannot be related to either dosage or to the duration of treatment. DPH is a weak acid and its absorption after oral ingestion is slow, sometimes variable and incomplete. Peak concentrations after a single dose may occur in plasma as early as 2 h or as late as 6 h after ingestion. It is 90% bound to plasma proteins [2]. However, the degree of protein binding and, therefore, the concentration of drug that is free in plasma, varies from patient to patient. In a study of 25

DIPHENYLHYDANTOIN

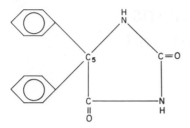

Fig. 1. Chemical structure of diphenylhydantoin.

patients [3] it was found that toxicity correlated well with the concentration of un-bound DPH.

DPH is widely distributed in all tissues and about 2% of it is excreted unchanged in the urine. The rest is metabolized by hepatic microsomal enzymes.

1. ADVERSE REACTIONS: EPIDEMIOLOGY AND PREDISPOSING FACTORS

Untoward effects of DPH are relatively common and quite varied. The main ones are shown in Table 1. Many of these reactions are toxic, particularly those affecting the central nervous system or causing peripheral neuropathy, and they depend heavily on drug concentration, particularly of that unbound to protein. Gingival hyperplasia is quite common, occurring in up to 20% of patients on DPH, par-ticularly in the young ones. It seems to be due to an aberration of connective tissue metabolism which leads to increased collagen deposition locally [4]. Interestingly, this collagen deposition seems to depend on the presence of bacterial plaque on the teeth and does not associate with increased collagen deposition elsewhere, nor with scleroderma. It is possible that local (gingival) fibroblasts are particularly stimulated to form increased amounts of collagen in a manner akin to that postulated for localized forms of scleroderma or clubbing of fingers.

Immunological reactions are also common and varied (Table 2). Some seem to be related to allergy such as various forms of rash, eosinophilia and, perhaps, the Stevens-Johnson syndrome [5]. Others may result from immune complex deposition such as drug-related serum sickness [6], vasculitis [7, 8] or arthritis [9]. Still others seem to result from an immune disregulation affecting cellular immunity that leads to IgA and IgE deficiency, to drug-related lupus syndromes, to the formation of an-tinuclear and other autoantibodies, and to the appearance of lymphomata and pseudolymphomata [10, 11]. Evidence of this immune disregulation caused by DPH includes a decrease in intradermal responses [12 – 14], as well as decreased produc-tion of antibodies to tetanus toxoid and *Salmonella typhi* vaccine when administered to patients [13]. Mononuclear cells from these patients also have decreased

TABLE 1

Adverse reactions to diphenylhydantoin (I)

Central nervous system
  nystagmus
  ataxia
  diplopia
  vertigo
  blurred vision
  mydriasis
  hyperactive tendon reflexes
  behavioral defects
  hyperactivity
  silliness
  confusion
  dullness
  drowsiness
  hallucinations
  peripheral neuropathy

Hematologic
  leukopenia
  thrombocytopenia
  agranulocytosis
  aplastic anemia

Gastrointestinal
  nausea
  vomiting
  epigastric pain
  anorexia

Endocrine
  inhibition of secretion
    of antidiuretic hormone
  hyperglycemia
  glucosuria
  osteomalacia
  gynecomastia

^{3}H-thymidine incorporation upon phytohemagglutinin (PHA) [13] and/or pokeweed mitogen [15] stimulation. These mitogenic responses might be further decreased with the addition of DPH in vitro, but this observation has been contested [13, 16].

Patients receiving DPH have been found to have normal proportion of E rosette-forming (T) lymphocytes and reduced immunoglobulin surface-bearing (B) lymphocytes, whereas those patients on DPH who have antibody deficiencies may have

154

TABLE 2

Adverse reactions to diphenylhydantoin (II)

Immunological reactions
  drug-related serum sickness
  morbilliform rash
  Stevens-Johnson syndrome
  drug-related lupus erythematosus
  hepatic necrosis
  vasculitis
  eosinophilia
  arthritis
  antinuclear antibodies
  IgA deficiency
  IgE deficiency
  lymphocytotoxic antibodies
  serum anticoagulant against factor VIII
  lymphadenopathy
  pseudolymphoma
  angioimmunoblastic lymphadenopathy
  lymphoma
  mycosis fungoides

decreased plaque-forming cells and increased suppressor cell function, as compared to normal subjects as well as to patients on DPH who do not develop immunoglobulin deficits [17 – 19]. Reduced immunoglobulin concentration might also be due to impaired macrophage function as has been found experimentally by means of the polyvinylpyrrolidone-binding tests in mice given DPH [20].

In vitro treatment of neutrophils with DPH also causes reversible inhibition of superoxide anion generation and lysosomal enzyme liberation in a concentration-dependent fashion but this does not inhibit their chemotactic capacity [21]. Subcutaneous injection of DPH into the footpad of mice caused regional lymph node hyperplasia that seemed to be dependent on T lymphocytes [22]. Similar lymph node enlargement took place upon injection of splenic cells from animals receiving DPH or splenic cells treated in vitro with DPH [22]. Pretreatment with intraperitoneal injection of DPH abrogated this lymph node reaction. It was postulated that this response was equivalent to a syngeneic mixed lymphocyte reaction that was somehow favored by DPH [22]. The anticonvulsant itself has not been found to have a mitogenic effect [23].

Appearance of antinuclear antibodies (ANA) without actual occurrence of systemic lupus erythematosus (SLE), as well as the occurrence of full blown drug-related SLE have both been reported [24 – 27]. It is of interest that nearly all anticonvulsants, despite chemical differences, have been reported to cause the development of ANA without clinical manifestations or drug-related SLE. The only exception thus far is sodium valproate [28]. The antigenic specificity of ANA that appear in patients who receive hydantoins (mainly DPH) has been studied and compared to those elicited by other anticonvulsants as well as to those elicited by other lupus-inducing drugs [28, 29]. The main findings are that the most frequent ANA that appear with all anticonvulsants are those directed to soluble nucleoprotein; they are significantly more frequent than are those reacting with particulate nucleoprotein [29] (Table 3). In another study, the main reactivity found was that with particulate nucleoprotein, but soluble nucleoprotein was apparently not studied [30]. The higher prevalence of ANA to soluble nucleoprotein is also apparent with isoniazid, where interaction between the drug and soluble nucleoprotein may take place [31]. Patients on isoniazid do not develop antibodies to DNA whether single- or double-stranded [31]. Contrarily, patients receiving chlorpromazine have ANA to soluble nuclueoprotein less frequently than they do to single-stranded DNA [32] (Table 3). Of the anticonvulsants only DPH and carbamazepine elicit ANA to both double-stranded and single-stranded DNA, and in our study, DPH was the only anticonvulsant that was found to induce ANA to Sm antigen (Table 4) [29]. This is, however, controversial, since Bardana et al., using a different but probably less sensitive method, did not find antibodies to Sm antigen in DPH-treated epileptics [30]. Antibodies to soluble nucleoprotein occur with the same frequency in males and females, whereas antibodies to single- and double-stranded DNA as well as those to the Sm antigen are significantly more frequent in females than in males [29].

In another study 10% of patients on DPH developed ANA de novo when placed on DPH, while another 10% already had ANA prior to the initiation of therapy

TABLE 3

Prevalence of antinuclear antibodies in patients on various anticonvulsants, on chlorpromazine or on isoniazid; comparison to findings in patients with spontaneous SLE and in normal controls

	Positive (percentage)					
	particulate nucleo-protein	soluble nucleo-protein	single-stranded DNA	double-stranded DNA	Sm antigen	any one antigen
Anticonvulsants (170[a])[b]	3	58	22	14	18	69
Chlorpromazine (54)	15	17	30	11	0	39
Isoniazid (214)	35	42	0	0	–	51
SLE (109)	51	48	53	51	39	91
Controls (54)	0	4	0	0	10	12

[a] 142 of the 170 were receiving DPH.
[b] Parentheses indicate number of subjects in each group.

TABLE 4

Prevalence of antinuclear antibodies in patients receiving anticonvulsants

Medication	Positive (percentage)				
	particulate nucleoprotein	soluble nucleoprotein	single-stranded DNA	double-stranded DNA	Sm antigen
Diphenylhydantoin (50)[a]	4	58	18	12	20
Primidone (10)	0	50	0	0	0
Carbamazepine (9)	11	78	11	11	0

[a] Parentheses indicate number of subjects in each group.

[30]. Their specificities could not be determined with the techniques employed. On immunofluorescence they often gave a speckled pattern suggesting reactivity with an extractable nuclear antigen.

Some of the reactivities of ANA which occur in patients who receive anticonvulsants have been ascribed to their pharmacological properties. DPH, for instance, has a direct effect on membrane permeability that could cause leakage of soluble antigens from inside the nucleus [33]. It has also been found to bind to nuclei and ribosomes and has actually been postulated to enter the nucleus, where it is bound to histone or nucleoprotein to subsequently accumulate in ribosomes [33]. The more recently described penetration of ANA into cells could permit their access there [34]. Sex differences in the production of some of the ANA might indicate that what the drug actually might do is to affect immunoregulation, thus permitting the increased appearance of ANA, that are actually natural antibodies [35].

The great majority of the more than 80 cases of anticonvulsant-related lupus that have been reported has been due to DPH [36 – 60]. As opposed to procainamide-induced lupus erythematosus, in which distinct differences with spontaneously-occurring SLE have been noticed [61], patients who develop SLE upon DPH-treatment differ little clinically from those with spontaneous disease. The main problem has been determining if the convulsive disorder that led to the administration of the drug was not actually a manifestation of SLE which may have had its debut with convulsions. Some patients have been described, however, in whom the convulsions could clearly be related to head trauma and who subsequently developed SLE while on hydantoins [62]. Another interesting observation is that of a complete clinical and laboratory remission in most patients on DPH-related SLE in whom the drug was stopped altogether and/or substituted for sodium valproate [28]. The following case report illustrates how DPH-related SLE may disappear completely and permanently after DPH withdrawal.

Case report. In 1962 a 26-year-old woman developed generalized convulsions with an abnormal electroencephalogram. She was placed on primidone which she took until late May 1966, when, because of dizziness, it was changed to DPH, 300 mg/day.

One month later she developed fever, cervical lymphadenopathy and an exanthema that recurred periodically and disappeared with scaling. She was treated with antibiotics without improvement and the fever only relented when given corticosteroids. She remained well but developed signs of hypercortisonism. In mid October, after being in the sun, she developed generalized arthritis. The dose of corticosteroids was increased to 30 mg/day of prednisone with improvement. She, however, developed a light pleuritic pain, and also a sore throat, cutaneous hyperpigmentation and alopecia.

When seen in December 1966 her skin was hyperpigmented and scaly, her throat was reddened, she had a systolic murmur, a left pleural rub with decreased respiratory sounds on both bases, and synovitis of both knees.

Laboratory studies showed a normochromic normocytic anemia with 11.2 g of hemoglobin. She had 3 125 leukocytes with 21% lymphocytes; LE cells and antinuclear antibodies were positive.

The dose of prednisone was left unchanged but DPH was stopped. With it all symptoms, physical signs and laboratory tests improved and the corticosteroids were decreased and later withdrawn. Arthralgias of the knees were the last to disappear 4 months after withdrawal of DPH. For 9 months she continued having occasional arthralgias and pleural pain. There has not been further evidence of SLE and LE cells, and antinuclear antibodies have remained negative until she was last seen in March, 1986.

Comment. This patient illustrates well the clinical picture of DPH-induced SLE that continued symptomatically despite corticosteroid treatment, but disappeared completely and permanently when DPH was withdrawn.

Remission may be so complete that even the study of immunoregulatory circuits, with tests that remain abnormal in patients with idiopathic SLE who have been in remission for years [63], is found to be normal in patients with DPH-induced SLE in remission [64] (Table 5). Such findings would indicate that the alteration caused by DPH that leads to autoantibody production is not permanent, and possibly lasts only while the drug is being given or shortly thereafter. Some of the patients, however, could have an innate predisposition to the development of SLE [61] and could thus continue to have positive ANA and some clinical symptoms after withdrawal of DPH. The following case report may illustrate this.

Case report. A 23-year-old female had been diagnosed as having SLE because of multisystemic disease associated with positive LE cells. She was receiving DPH because of an abnormal EEG found when she was being studied because of psychosis. She had been placed on prednisone at a dose of 30 mg but she continued having arthritis and vasculitis. When we saw her we stopped DPH treatment and began decreasing prednisone. Psychiatric manifestations, however, worsened and the dose of prednisone, which had come down to 7.5 mg/day, was doubled. With this, psychiatric manifestations improved, there was gradual improvement also of arthralgias and vasculitis. She, however continued to have facial erythema upon exposure to sun light.

Although clinical evidence of SLE has only occasionally emerged, she has had on and off positive antinuclear antibodies, DNA uptake and/or low C3 levels. Her psychosis has remained present with features of schizophrenia, and has required continued treatment.

Comment. This patient illustrates the difficulties in establishing the role of DPH in development of SLE. Although the clinical features of SLE became gradually quiescent after DPH withdrawal, antinuclear antibodies have continued to appear

TABLE 5

Immunoregulatory findings in patients with DPH-related SLE; comparison to patients with untreated idiopathic active and inactive SLE and normal controls [64]

Study	Patients			Normal controls (32)
	DPH-related SLE (3)	idiopathic SLE		
		inactive (13)	active (19)	
T_{ar}^{e} cells, %	23.3 ± 1.2[a, b]	9.9 ± 1.0	7.9 ± 0.8	22.8 ± 0.5
T_{γ}^{f} cells, %	12.7 ± 0.9[a, b]	7.4 ± 0.7	6.1 ± 0.3	14.0 ± 2.1
T_{μ}^{f} cells, %	40.6 ± 0.9[a]	40.2 ± 0.6	39.5 ± 0.3	40.2 ± 2.1
Suppression[g]				
Con-A induced	60.3 ± 1.6[a, c]	20.3 ± 1.4	18.8 ± 1.9	74.7 ± 5.5
spontaneous	61.0 ± 1.0[d]	15.9 ± 1.9	1.0 ± 4.9	77.2 ± 4.5
Feedback				
inhibition[h]	71.6 ± 1.3[a, b]	16.2 ± 4.0	16.8 ± 4.6	62.5 ± 4.4

[a] Difference not significant vs. normal controls.
[b] $p < 0.0005$ vs. active or inactive SLE.
[c] $p < 0.025$ vs. active or inactive SLE.
[d] $p < 0.01$ vs. inactive SLE; $p < 0.0005$ vs. active SLE.
[e] T_{ar}, % of total peripheral T cells forming rosettes with autologous erythrocytes, being Fc_{γ} and Fc_{μ} negative.
[f] T_{γ} and T_{μ}, % of total peripheral T cells with Fc_{γ} and Fc_{μ} receptors, respectively, as determined with IgG- or IgM-coated ox erythrocytes.
[g] Inhibition of pokeweed mitogen-induced antibody formation by peripheral blood mononuclear cells upon addition of autologous T cells cultured in the presence or absence of concanavalin A.
[h] Inhibiton of pokeweed mitogen-induced antibody formation by mixtures of autologous peripheral T_{μ} cells, B cells and T_{ar} as compared to mixtures without T_{ar} cells.

sporadically. Psychosis may have been a manifestation of SLE. It would appear that this patient had a mild form of SLE that was worsened by DPH treatment.

2. POSSIBLE MECHANISMS

The mechanism whereby DPH could cause an immune dysregulation leading to autoantibody formation has not been, thus far, unraveled. The hypothesis has been put forward that a graft-versus-host-like reaction occurs by the adherence of DPH to the surface of B lymphocytes where helper T cells recognize them in conjunction with DR antigens [65]. This would cause activation and perhaps differentiation of B cells. Another possibility is that DPH actually caused a T cell disregulation that permitted B cells to produce natural autoantibodies. This would be similar to what has been documented for procainamide [66 – 68], cimetidine [69] and L-canavanine [70], the non protein amino acid present in alfalfa sprouts that has been found capable of inducing SLE in monkeys [71]. Different effects can be observed in different individuals on DPH administration. In some, there would be an immune disregulation leading to a positive net regulation, thus permitting the development of autoantibodies or even autoimmune disease. Continued stimulation could become clonally restricted, leading to lymphatic (B cell) neoplasia. This would be similar to what seems to happen in primary Sjögren's syndrome. In other individuals, DPH could cause an increase in suppressor cell function with a negative net regulation that would cause inhibition of IgA, and/or IgE production. These two modes of action could, however, not be mutually exclusive since it could occur with increased IgA-related suppressor cell function and normal or increased IgG-related suppression, possibly through the role of a T cell subpopulation that participates in this latter function and/or in the IgG switch. The occurrence of autoimmunity-related selective IgA deficiency illustrates the feasibility of such a coexistence.

Because of the afore-mentioned effect of DPH on suppressor cell function that could be capable of inhibiting IgA production, this drug has also recently been advocated for treatment of rheumatoid arthritis [72] where IgA levels are often raised [73]. This peculiar situation, where a drug capable of causing an autoimmune-like disease is used to treat another autoimmune disease, is similar to that of D-penicillamine that can cause a SLE-like disease, as well as myasthenia gravis, but is quite effective in the management of rheumatoid arthritis.

II. Nitrofurantoin

Nitrofurantoin is a synthetic bacteriostatic nitrofuran (Fig. 2) used in the treatment of urinary tract infections. Although most often used for a short term, it is also sometimes used prolongedly in the prevention of recurrent urinary infections. Nitrofurantoin is administered orally since its gastrointestinal absorption is prompt and complete. Elimination occurs through the kidney and is also quite prompt so that antibacterial concentrations are achieved in the urine but not in plasma. Renal

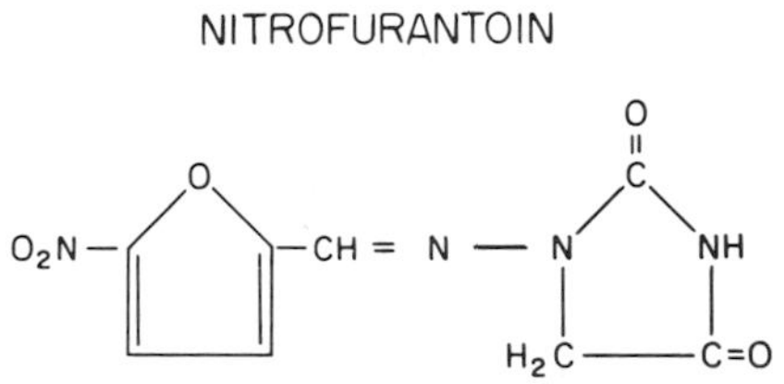

NITROFURANTOIN

Fig. 2. Chemical structure of nitrofurantoin.

failure may increase its toxicity and decrease its efficacy in treating urinary infections.

1. ADVERSE REACTIONS: EPIDEMIOLOGY AND PREDISPOSING FACTORS

Adverse reactions to nitrofurantoin are common since, aside from those due to gastrointestinal intolerance such as nausea, vomiting and/or diarrhea, they constitute up to 12% of all drug reactions registered by the Swedish Adverse Drug Reaction Committee [74]. This frequency in Sweden might indicate either the common use of nitrofurantoin in that country, particularly in chronic form for the prevention of urinary infection, or a particular predisposition by people of Scandinavian extraction to develop these adverse reactions.

Adverse reactions to nitrofurantoin are, in general, considerably more frequent in women (86%), but this might also be due to its more frequent use in females. However, blood dyscrasias occurring as a result of nitrofurantoin are significantly more frequent in men. Reactions are also more frequent in the elderly, perhaps due to decreased renal clearance. However, an older mean age of patients who developed chronic pulmonary reactions (68 years) than of those who developed acute ones (59 years), or of the total group (62 years) [75], might indicate some relationship between some of the reactions to other factors such as involution of immunoregulatory mechanisms.

Relationship of the hemolytic anemia caused by nitrofurantoin with glucose-6-phosphate dehydrogenase deficiency of erythrocytes is well recognized, and causation of chronic active hepatitis by nitrofurantoin is thought to be related to the presence of HLA-B8 antigen [76].

2. DISEASE PATTERNS AND THEIR PATHOLOGY

Adverse reactions to nitrofurantoin have been analyzed in a large Swedish study [74]. Acute pulmonary reactions, probably due to 'hypersensitivity' constitute 43% of all adverse effects. Allergic reactions, comprising cutaneous and anaphylactic manifestations, contribute another 42%. Thus, 85% of reactions to nitrofurantoin seem to be allergic. The remaining 15% are represented by liver disease, (6%), chronic interstitial pneumonitis (5%), blood dyscrasias (2%), and neuropathy (2%). Acute and chronic pulmonary reactions seemed to be different entities. Thus, chronic pulmonary disease was not often preceded by acute pulmonary reactions. In a large study on pulmonary reactions to nitrofurantoin [75], acute pulmonary reactions occurred mainly in patients whose treatment had been planned to be short, whereas the chronic reactions occurred in patients who were on continuous long-term therapy [75]. It therefore resulted that the duration of treatment with nitrofurantoin had a median of 7 days in the acute cases while that of the chronic ones had a median of 17 months. Patients with chronic pulmonary reactions had more often dyspnea, dry cough, fatigue, cyanosis, weight loss, jaundice, elevated liver enzymes, and pulmonary infiltrates on chest roentgenograms, than those with acute reactions. The latter had more often fever, rash, influenza-like symptoms, eosinophilia, and normal roentgenograms.

Hypergammaglobulinemia and antinuclear antibodies occurred in 80% and 60%, respectively, of 20 patients with chronic pulmonary reactions in whom these were studied [75]. Antigenic specificity of such antinuclear antibodies has not been recorded. Most patients who have died with chronic pulmonary reactions to nitrofurantoin have been found to have interstitial pneumonitis and/or pulmonary fibrosis. Association with cirrhosis of the liver was also encountered. One patient who died with an acute reaction, was found to have a desquamative alveolitis [75].

Prompt occurrence of acute pulmonary reactions after initiation of nitrofurantoin, and its association with eosinophilia and skin rash, suggests atopy, and a similarity with extrinsic allergic alveolitis has been proposed. However, immune complex deposition has also been postulated and lymphopenia also occurs [77]. Conversely, association of the chronic form with antinuclear antibodies, with antibodies specific to nitrofurantoin of the IgG class [78], as well as with abnormal lymphocyte transformation tests with nitrofurantoin [78, 79] and with the occurrence of T lymphocyte infiltration [80], all suggest an autoimmune pathogenesis.

Occurrence of lupus-like syndromes related to nitrofurantoin [81, 82], some of which have been associated with a chronic interstitial pneumonitis, support this possibility, as does the association of nitrofurantoin reactions with chronic active hepatitis [83, 84]. Association, in one case, with interstitial cystitis is of interest since an autoimmune pathogenesis has been proposed [85], and its relationship to systemic lupus erythematosus has been documented [86]. In another instance, panniculitis, leukopenia and positive antinuclear antibodies occurred, mimicking lupus profundus (lupus panniculitis), in a patient being treated with nitrofurantoin [87]. Studies on the role of oxidant injury of the parenchymal cells by nitrofurantoin [88] do not exclude the role of an immunoregulatory disturbance in the causation of the adverse immune reactions. Thus, interleukin-1, the monocyte/macrophage cytokine, has been postulated to induce similar oxidant injury through the liberation of prostaglandin-E2 in rheumatoid arthritis [89], an autoimmune disease in which both systemic and local (intraarticular) immune disregulation have been found to occur.

Acknowledgements

Data from our laboratory included here was elicited with support of grants from the Consejo Nacional de Ciencia y Tecnología, the Fondo de Fomento Educativo and the Fondo para Estudios e Investigaciones Ricardo J. Zevada, México.

162

References

1. Merritt, H. H. and Putnam, T. J. (1938) Sodium diphenylhydantoinate in treatment of convulsive disorders. J. Am. Med. Assoc. 111, 1068 – 1073.
2. Booker, H. E. and Darcey, B. (1973) Serum concentrations of diphenylhydantoin and their relationship to clinical intoxication. Epilepsia 14, 177 – 184.
3. Buchtal, F. and Svensmark, O. (1971) Serum concentrations of diphenylhydantoin (phenytoin) and phenobarbital and their relation to therapeutic and toxic effects. Psychiat. Neurol. Neurochir. 74, 117 – 136.
4. Hassell, T. M., Page, R. C., Narayana, A. S. and Cooper C. G. (1976) Diphenylhydantoin (DILANTIN) gingival hyperplasia: drug-induced abnormality of connective tissue. Proc. Natl. Acad. Sci. USA 73, 2909 – 2912.
5. Burge, S. M. and Dawber, R. R. R. (1985) Stevens-Johnson syndrome and toxic epidermal necrolysis in a patient with systemic lupus erythematosus. J. Am. Acad. Dermatol. 13, 665 – 666.
6. Yermakov, V. M., Hithi, I. F. and Sutton, A. L. (1983) Necrotizing vasculitis associated with diphenylhydantoin. Two fatal cases. Hum. Pathol. 14, 182 – 184.
7. Braverman, I. M. and Levin, J. (1963) Dilantin-induced serum sickness. Am. J. Med. 35, 418 – 421.
8. Gaffey, C. M., Chun, B., Harvey, J. C. and Manz, H. J. (1986) Phenytoin-induced systemic granulomatosus vasculitis. Arch. Pathol. Lab. Med. 110, 131 – 135.
9. Stalnikowicz, R., Mosseri, M. and Shalev, O. (1982) Phenytoin-induced arthritis. Neurology 32, 1317 – 1318.
10. Wilden, J. N. and Scott, C. V. (1978) A pseudolymphomatous reaction in soft tissue associated with phenytoin sodium. J. Clin. Pathol. 31, 761 – 764.
11. Rosenthal, C. J., Noguera, C. A., Coppola, A. and Kapelner S. N. (1982) Pseudolymphomata with mycosis fungoids manifestation hyperresponsiveness to diphenylhydantoin and lymphocyte disregulation. Cancer 49, 2305 – 2314.
12. Grob, P. J. and Herold, G. E. (1972) Immunological abnormalities and hydantoins. Br. Med. J. 2, 561 – 563.
13. Sorrell, T. C. and Forbes, I. J. (1975) Depression of immune competence by phenytoin and carbamazepine. Studies in vivo and in vitro. Clin. Exp. Immunol. 20, 273 – 285.
14. Higashi, A., Matsuda, I., Sinosuka, S., Ohtsuka, H., Eudo, F., Maeda, T., Ikeda, T. and Miyoshino, S. (1978) Delayed cutaneous hypersensitivity in children with severe multiple handicaps treated with phenytoin. Eur. J. Pediat. 129, 273 – 278.
15. Menitove, J. E., Rassiga, A. L., McLaren, G. D., Daniel, T. M. and Mahmound, A. A. F. (1981) Antigranulocyte antibodies and deranged immune function associated with phenytoin-induced serum sickness. Am. J. Hematol. 10, 277 – 284.
16. Speier, S., Bronberg, J. M. and Lempert, N. (1981) Phenytoin, methylprednisolone sodium succinate and graft survival. J. Pharmacol. Exp. Ther. 216, 101 – 103.
17. Guerra, I. C., Fawcett, W. A. IV, Redmon, A. H., Lawrence, E. C., Rosenblatt, H. M. and Shearer, W. T. (1986) Permanent intrinsic B cell immunodeficiency caused by phenytoin hypersensitivity. J. Allergy Clin. Immunol. 77, 603 – 607.
18. Dosch, H. M., Jason, J. and Gelfand, E. W. (1982) Transient antibody deficiency and abnormal T suppressor cells induced by phenytoin. N. Engl. J. Med. 306, 406 – 409.
19. Neilan, B. A. and Leppik, I. E. (1980) Phenytoin and formation of T lymphocyte rosettes. Arch. Neurol. 37, 580 – 581.
20. Seager, J., Coovadia, H. M. and Soothill, J. F. (1978) Reduced immunoglobulin concentration and impaired macrophage function in mice due to diphenylhydantoin. Clin. Exp. Immunol. 33, 437 – 440.
21. Webster, R. O., Goldstein, I. M. and Flick, M. R. (1984) Selective inhibition by phenytoin of

chemotactic factor-stimulated neutrophil functions. J. Lab. Clin. Med. 103, 22 – 33.

22. Gleichmann, H. (1981) Studies on the mechanism of drug sensitization: T-cell-dependent popliteal lymph node reaction to diphenylhydantoin. Clin. Immunol. Immunopathol. 18, 203 – 211.

23. MacKinney, A. A. and Booker, H. E. (1972) Diphenylhydantoin effects on human lymphocytes in vitro and in vivo. An hypothesis to explain some drug reactions. Arch. Intern. Med. 129, 988 – 992.

24. Boston, J. W., Tynes, B., Register, H. B., Alford, C. and Holley, H. L. (1962) Systemic lupus erythematosus occurring during anticonvulsant therapy. J. Am. Med. Assoc. 180, 115 – 118.

25. Wilske, K. R., Shalit, L. E., Willkens, R. F. and Decker, J. L. (1965) Findings suggestive of systemic lupus erythematosus in subjects on chronic anticonvulsant therapy. Arthritis Rheum. 8, 260 – 266.

26. Singsen, B. H., Fishman, L. and Manson, V. (1976) Antinuclear antibodies and lupus-like syndromes in children receiving anticonvulsants. Pediatrics 57, 529 – 534.

27. Alarcón-Segovia, D., Fishbein, E., Reyes, P. A., Díes, H. and Shwadsky, S. (1972) Antinuclear antibodies in patients on anticonvulsant therapy. Clin. Exp. Immunol. 12, 39 – 47.

28. Alarcón-Segovia, D. and Kraus, A. (1983) Drug-related lupus syndromes. In: L. Lensberger and M. M. Reidenberg (Eds.), Proceedings of the Second World Conference on Clinical Pharmacology and Therapeutics. Am. Soc. Pharmacol. Exp. Ther., Bethesda, pp. 187, 206.

29. Alarcón-Segovia, D. and Fishbein, E. (1975) Patterns of antinuclear antibodies and lupus-activating drugs. J. Rheumatol. 2, 167 – 171.

30. Bardana, E. J., Gabourel, J. D., Davies, G. H. and Graig, S. (1983) Effects of phenytoin on man's immunity. Evaluation of changes in serum immunoglobulins, complement, and antinuclear antibody. Am. J. Med. 74, 289 – 296.

31. Alarcón-Segovia, D., Fishbein, E. and Betancourt, V. M. (1969) Antibodies to nucleoprotein and to hydrazide-altered soluble nucleoprotein in tuberculosis patients receiving isoniazid. Clin. Exp. Immunol. 5, 429 – 437.

32. Alarcón-Segovia, D., Fishbein, E., Cetina, J. A., Raya, R. J. and Becerra, E. (1973) Antigenic specificity of chlorpromazine-induced antinuclear antibodies. Clin. Exp. Immunol. 15, 543 – 548.

33. Woodbury, D. M. and Kemp, J. W. (1970) Some possible mechanisms of action of antiepileptic drugs. Pharmacopsychiat. Neuropsychopharmacol. 3, 201 – 226.

34. Alarcón-Segovia, D., Ruíz-Argüelles, A. and Fishbein, E. (1978) Antibody to nuclear ribonucleoprotein penetrates live human mononuclear cells through Fc receptors. Nature 271, 271 – 274.

35. Dighiero, G., Lymberi, P., Guilbert, B., Ternynck, T. and Avrameas, S. (1986) Natural autoantibodies constitute a substantial part of normal circulating immunoglobulins Ann. NY Acad. Sci. 475, 135 – 145.

36. Miescher, P. and Delacrétaz, J. (1953) Démonstration d'un phénomène, 'L.E.' positif dans deux cas d'hypersensibilité médicamenteuse. Schweiz. Med. Wochenschr. 83, 536 – 538.

37. Lee, S. L., Rivero, I. and Siegel, M. (1966) Activation of systemic lupus erythematosus by drugs. Arch. Intern. Med. 177, 620 – 626.

38. Lobuglio, A. F. and Jandl, J. M. (1967) The nature of the alfamethyldopa red-cell antibody. N. Engl. J. Med. 276, 658 – 665.

39. Siegel, M., Lee, S. L. and Peress, N. S. (1967) The epidemiology of drug-induced systemic lupus erythematosus. Arthritis Rheum. 10, 407 – 415.

40. Benton, J. W., Tynes, B., Register, H. B. Jr., Alford, C. and Holley, H. L. (1962) Systemic lupus erythematosus occurring during anticonvulsive drug therapy. J. Am. Med. Assoc. 180, 115 – 118.

41. Jacobs, J. C. (1963) Systemic lupus erythematosus in childhood: report of thirty-five cases, with discussion of seven apparently induced by anticonvulsant medication and of prognosis and treat-

ment. Pediatrics 32, 257 – 264.

42. Shulman, L. E. (1963) Inducing agents and relationship to other diseases. Rheumatology (Suppl.) 6, 558 – 571.

43. Rallison, M. L., Carlisle, J. W., Lee, R. E. Jr., Vernier, R. L. and Good, R. A. (1961) Lupus erythematosus and Stevens-Johnson syndrome: occurrence as reaction to anticonvulsant medication. Am. J. Dis. Child. 101, 725 – 738.

44. Alarcón-Segovia, D. (1959) Manifestaciones viscerales del lupus eritematoso diseminado. Thesis. Universidad Nacional Autónoma de México.

45. Alarcón-Segovia, D. and Osmundson, P. J. (1965) Peripheral vascular syndromes associated with systemic lupus erythematosus. Ann. Intern. Med. 62, 907 – 919.

46. Schütz, E. and Frenger, W. (1965) Lupus erythematosus syndrom nach längerer Hydantoin Behandlung. Med. Klin. 60, 537 – 541.

47. Strejcek, J. and Hrbkova, M. (1965) Vztah hydantoinovyak preparatu ke vzniku diseminovaneko erythematodu. Cas. Lek. Cesk. 104, 1158 – 1161.

48. Leövey, A., Petrányi, Gy. and Gyula, S. (1966) Epilepsia, systemás lupus erythematosus és az anticonvulsiv therápia kapscolata. Orv. Hetil. 107, 1785 – 1786.

49. Bréaud, P. and Caviezel, O. (1966) Lupus érythémateux et épilepsie – un cas après traitement à l'hydantoine. Praxis 55, 1095 – 1100.

50. Ruppli, H. and Vossen, R. (1957) Nebenwirkung der Hydantoinkörpertherapie under dem Bilde eines visceralen Lupus erythematosus. Schweiz. Med. Wochenschr. 87, 1555 – 1558.

51. Ahuja, G. K. and Schumacher, G. A. (1966) Drug-induced systemic lupus erythematosus: primidone as a possible cause. J. Am. Med. Assoc. 198, 669 – 671.

52. Livingston, S., Rodríguez, H., Greene, C. A. and Lydia, P. L. (1968) Systemic lupus erythematosus: occurrence in association with ethosuximide therapy. J. Am. Med. Assoc. 204, 731 – 732.

53. Haserick, J. R. (1955) Modern concepts of systemic lupus erythematosus: a review of 126 cases. J. Chron. Dis. 1, 317 – 334.

54. Ortíz-Neu, C. and Leroy, C. (1969) The coincidence of Klinefelter's syndrome and systemic lupus erythematosus. Arthritis Rheum. 12, 241 – 246.

55. Segami, M. I. and Alarcón-Segovia, D. (1977) Systemic lupus erythematosus and Klinefelter syndrome. Arthritis Rheum. 20, 1565 – 1566.

56. Livingston, S., Rodríguez, M., Greene, C. A. and Lydia, P. L. (1968) Systemic lupus erythematosus: occurrence in association with ethosuximide therapy. J. Am. Med. Assoc. 204, 731 – 732.

57. Monnet, P., Salle, B., Poncet, J., Gauthier, J. et al. (1968) Lupus érythémateux disséminé induit par l'ethosuccimide chez une fille de 6 ans. Lyon Med. 220, 467 – 478.

58. Teoh, P. C. and Chan, H. L. (1975) Lupus-scleroderma syndrome induced by ethosuximide. Arch. Dis. Child. 50, 658 – 661.

59. Simpson, J. R. (1966) 'Collagen disease' due to carbamazepine (Tegretol). Br. Med. J. 2, 1434.

60. Takigawa, M., Kanoh, T., Imamura, S. and Takahashi, C. (1976) IgA deficiency and systemic lupus erythematosus. Occurrence in an oriental woman with idiopathic epilepsy. Arch. Dermatol. 112, 845 – 849.

61. Alarcón-Segovia, D. (1969) Drug-induced lupus syndromes. Mayo Clin. Proc. 44, 664 – 681.

62. Lindqvist, T. (1957) Lupus erythematosus disseminatus often administration of mesantoin: report of two cases. Acta Med. Scand. 158, 131 – 138.

63. Ruíz-Argüelles, A., Alarcón-Segovia, D., Llorente, L. and Del Giudice-Knipping, J. (1980) Heterogeneity of the spontaneously expanded and mitogen-induced generation of suppressor cell function of T cells on B cells in systemic lupus erythematosus. Artritis Rheum. 23, 1004 – 1009.

64. Alarcón-Segovia, D. and Palacios, R. (1981) Differences in immunoregulatory T cell circuits

between diphenyl-hydantoin-related and spontaneously occurring systemic lupus erythematosus. Arthritis Rheum. 24, 1086 – 1092.

65. Gleichmann, E. and Gleichmann, H. (1980) Spectrum of diseases caused by alloreactive T cells, mode of sensitization to the drug diphenylhydantoin and possible role of SLE-typical self antigens in B cell triggering. In: R. S. Krakauer and M. K. Cathcart (Eds.), Immunoregulation and Autoimmunity, Elsevier, New York, pp. 73 – 83.

66. Bluestein, H. G., Weisman, M. H., Zvaifler, N. J. and Shapiro, R. F. (1979) Lymphocyte alteration by procainamide: relation to drug-induced lupus erythematosus syndrome. Lancet 2, 816 – 819.

67. Miller, K. B. and Salem, D. (1982) Immunoregulatory abnormalities produced by procainamide. Am. J. Med. 73, 487 – 492.

68. Ochi, T., Goldings, E. A., Lipsky, P. E. and Ziff, M. (1983) Immunomodulatory effect of procainamide in man. Inhibition of human suppressor T-cell activity in vitro. J. Clin. Invest. 71, 36 – 45.

69. Palacios, R. and Alarcón-Segovia, D. (1981) Cimetidine abrogates suppressor T cell function in vitro. Immunol. Lett. 3, 33 – 37.

70. Alcocer-Varela, J., Iglesias, A., Llorente, L. and Alarcón-Segovia, D. (1985) Effects of L-canavanine on T cells may explain the induction of systemic lupus erythematosus by alfalfa. Arthritis Rheum. 28, 52 – 57.

71. Malinow, M. R., Bardana, E. J. Jr., Pirofsky, B., Craig, S. and McLaughlin, P. (1982) Systemic lupus erythematosus-like syndrome in monkeys fed alfalfa sprouts: role of a nonprotein amino acid. Science (Wash. DC) 216, 415 – 417.

72. Richards, I. M., Fraser, S. M., Hinter, J. A. and Capell, H. A. (1987) Comparison of phenytoin and gold as second line drugs in rheumatoid arthritis. Ann. Rheum. Dis. 46, 667 – 669.

73. Stanworth, D. R. (1985) IgA dysfunction in rheumatoid arthritis. Immunol. Today 6, 43 – 45.

74. Holmberg, L., Boman, G., Böttiger, L. E., Eriksson, B., Spross, R. and Wessling, A. (1980) Adverse reactions to nitrofurantoin. Analysis of 921 reports. Am. J. Med. 69, 733 – 738.

75. Holmberg, L. and Boman, G. (1981) Pulmonary reactions to nitrofurantoin. 447 cases reported to the Swedish adverse drug reaction committee 1966 – 1976. Eur. J. Respir. Dis. 62, 180 – 189.

76. Hatoff, D. E., Cohen, M., Schveigert, B. F. and Talbert, W. M. (1979) Nitrofurantoin: another cause of drug induced chronic active hepatitis. A report of a patient with HLA-B8 antigen. Am. J. Med. 67, 117 – 121.

77. Geller, M., Flaherty, D. K., Dickie, H. A. and Reed, C. E. (1977) Lymphopenia in acute nitrofurantoin pleuropulmonary reactions. J. Allergy Clin. Immunol. 58, 445 – 448.

78. Back, O., Liden, S. and Ahlstedt, S. (1977) Adverse reactions to nitrofurantoin in relation to cellular and humoral immune responses. Clin. Exp. Immunol. 28, 400 – 406.

79. Pearsall, H. R., Ewalt, J., Tsoi, M. S., Sumida, S., Backus, D., Winterbauer, R. H., Webb, D. R. and Jones, H. (1974) Nitrofurantoin lung sensitivity: report of a case with prolonged NF lymphocyte sensitivity and interaction of NF-stimulated lymphocytes with alveolar cells. 83, 728 – 737.

80. Brutinel, W. M. and Martin, W. J., II (1986) Chronic nitrofurantoin reaction associated with T-lymphocyte alveolitis. Chest 89, 150 – 152.

81. Back, O., Lundgren, R. and Wunan, L. G. (1974) Nitrofurantoin-induced pulmonary fibrosis and lupus syndrome. Lancet 1, 930.

82. Selross, O. and Edgren, J. (1975) Lupus-like syndrome associated with pulmonary reaction to nitrofurantoin. Report of 3 cases. Acta Med. Scand. 197, 125 – 129.

83. Black, M., Rabin, L. and Schatz, N. (1980) Nitrofurantoin-induced chronic active hepatitis. Ann. Intern. Med. 92, 62 – 64.

84. Tolman, K. G. (1980) Nitrofurantoin and chronic active hepatitis. Ann. Intern. Med. 92, 119 – 120.

85. Shipta, E. A. (1965) Hunner's ulcer (chronic interstitial cystitis). A manifestation of collagen disease. Br. J. Urol. 37, 443 – 449.
86. Alarcón-Segovia, D., Abud-Mendoza, C., Reyes-Gutiérrez, E., Iglesias-Gamarra, A. and Díaz-Jouanen, E. (1984) Involvement of the urinary bladder in systemic lupus erythematosus. A pathologic study. J. Rheumatol. 11, 208 – 210.
87. Sanford, R. G. and Almstead, P. M. (1987) Nitrofurantoin-induced antinuclear antibodies and panniculitis. Arthritis Rheum. 30, 1076 – 1078.
88. Martin, W. J., II (1983) Nitrofurantoin: evidence for the oxidant injury of lung parenchymal cells. Annu. Rev. Respir. Dis. 127, 482 – 486.
89. Alarcón-Riquelme, M. E. and Alarcón-Segovia, D. (1988) Interleuquina-1. Factor multipotencial en patogenia de enfermedad. Dolor e Inflamación (Madrid, España) 1, 95 – 103.

M.E. Kammüller, N. Bloksma and W. Seinen (Eds.)
Autoimmunity and Toxicology
© 1989 Elsevier Science Publishers B.V. (Biomedical Division)

Autoimmune reactions to D-penicillamine

6

PAUL EMERY and GABRIEL S. PANAYI

Rheumatology Research Wing, The Medical School, University of Birmingham, Birmingham B15 2TJ
and Rheumatology Unit, U.M.D.S., Guy's Hospital, London, SE 1 9RT, UK

I. Introduction

In 1943, Abraham et al. identified dimethylcysteine amongst the hydrolysis products of penicillin and gave it the name of D-penicillamine [1]. Structurally D-penicillamine is a sulphhydryl amino acid, differing from cysteine by the substitution of two methyl groups in the beta position (β,β-dimethylcysteine). The ability of this compound to chelate heavy metals was its first property to be recognised and led to its use in the treatment of Wilson's disease [2]. Subsequently, the effectiveness of D-penicillamine in rheumatoid arthritis, the disease for which it is most commonly prescribed, was demonstrated [3]. Since that time D-penicillamine has additionally been used in the therapy of cysteinuria [4], scleroderma [5], primary biliary sclerosis [6] and chronic active hepatitis [7]. In all these diseases, the drug is repeatedly prescribed and it is under these circumstances that the spectrum of drug-induced, immunologically mediated disease occurs.

II. Absorption and pharmacokinetics

Oral administration of a single dose in the fasting state produces levels of D-penicillamine which peak within a few hours and then decline sharply [8]. However, the resulting low levels at 12 hours post dose subsequently decline very slowly, suggesting the presence of at least two pools [9]. D-penicillamine may interact with

dietary constituents especially metals and drugs with clinically important consequences, for example, in four patients toxicity to D-penicillamine occurred when
concurrent iron therapy was ceased [10]. Pharmacokinetic studies have been
hampered by the lack of a satisfactory method of analysis [9, 11, 12]. Estimates of
the amount excreted in urine and faeces vary with the analytical method used [9].
Thus, radioactive analysis using ^{14}C-labelled drug shows a greater recovery than
chemical analysis, probably because some of the metabolic products of D-
penicillamine are chemically non-identifiable. Known metabolites of D-penicillamine include the internal disulphide (D-penicillamine-D-penicillamine), the mixed
disulphide (D-penicillamine cysteine) and S-methyl-D-penicillamine. D-penicillamine
disappears from the serum either irreversibly by predominantly renal excretion or
by a reversible move into the tissue pool. Of an oral dose of D-penicillamine around
two-thirds is absorbed and about one-fifth is converted to S-methyl-D-penicillamine,
which is then either renally excreted or oxidised in the liver. As a consequence of
the formation of mixed disulphides, there is an inverse correlation between the cysteine level in the serum and the dose of D-penicillamine administered [13].

D-penicillamine is taken up into collagen-containing tissues and, to a lesser extent,
into protein-rich tissues [9]. The presence of this tissue pool accounts for the slow
release of the drug. This slow release has been documented both in human and in
animal models, with metabolites of D-penicillamine having been found in the urine
months after cessation of therapy [9].

III. Pharmacology and mode of action

The chemical structure of D-penicillamine determines its pharmacological activities.
The thiol group reacts with disulphide bridges and thus affects biological systems,
whereas both the amino and thiol groups are implicated in heavy metal chelation
[14]. The high affinity of D-penicillamine for these metals results in soluble chelates
that are excreted by the kidney. The interference of D-penicillamine with collagen
cross-linking is more complex. This includes a reversible reaction with aldehyde
groups, necessary for cross-linking, forming a thiazolidine ring, and also irreversible
chelation of Cu, thus inhibiting lysyl oxidase, an enzyme system involved in collagen
synthesis [15]. The binding of Cu may also produce chelates with super oxide
dismutase activity. Another action of D-penicillamine is that of vitamin B6 an-
tagonism [16], but as administration of this vitamin does not influence the clinical
outcome, this action is of doubtful relevance.

However, despite better understanding of its pharmacological activities, the properties responsible for its immunomodulatory role in immune-mediated diseases
such as rheumatoid arthritis (RA) remain unclear. Administration of D-penicillamine to patients with rheumatoid arthritis has been shown to reduce immune complexes in both blood and synovial fluid, but it is not known whether this is a primary

effect. During a favourable therapeutic response there is a gradual fall in erythrocyte sedimentation rate and rheumatoid factor titre over the first 3 – 6 months, similar to that occurring with other disease-modifying drugs. The possible mechanisms of action of D-penicillamine have been examined in numerous studies. In vitro, the drug has been shown to suppress mitogen-driven lymphocyte transformation [17], and a small amount of Cu has been shown to significantly enhance this suppression via a specific action on helper T lymphocytes [18]. Paradoxically, other investigations have found it to be stimulatory [19], transformation of lymphocytes from patients taking D-penicillamine is normal [20, 21], contrasting with the generally reduced cellular immune responses normally seen in patients with RA [22]. This normal cellular immunity probably reflects the general improvement in immunological status that occurs after therapy with D-penicillamine [20, 21].

IV. Disease patterns and epidemiology

D-penicillamine produces adverse reactions in 50 – 70% of patients treated, and this leads to withdrawal of therapy in 26 – 40% of patients [23 – 28] on long-term therapy. It is possible to divide the adverse reactions into two broad overlapping groups. First are those which occur early in treatment and which are thought to be due to a direct toxic effect of the drug. Features of these adverse reactions do not suggest that they have an immunological basis and at present there is no way of predicting the likelihood of such reactions. This early toxicity includes adverse reactions such as rash, dysgeusia (loss of taste), anorexia and other gastro-intestinal tract abnormalities. Certain of these side effects, especially dysgeusia and gastro-intestinal intolerance, are self-limiting and may allow continuation of the therapy. Second, and of particular relevance to this article, are those adverse reactions which are considered to be immunologically based. These reactions occur usually after more prolonged therapy of between 3 and 6 months and include thrombocytopenia, proteinuria and, less frequently, drug-induced autoimmune disorders such as autoimmune skin disorders, systemic lupus erythematosus, myasthenia gravis, polymyositis and others mentioned below. In patients suffering from these drug-induced diseases, there is usually the same association with autoantibodies as that seen in the idiopathic disease, although the specificities of the antibodies may differ in the idiopathic and drug-induced disorders.

1. HAEMATOLOGICAL ABNORMALITIES

Thrombocytopenia, leucopenia and aplastic anaemia have all been observed after therapy with D-penicillamine. Thrombocytopenia is the most common haematological side effect occurring in patients treated with D-penicillamine. In 259 patients studied for 3 years [26], 3% developed thrombocytopenia and 2% leucopenia; in another prospective study of 101 patients [25] studied for just over 1 year, a fall in platelets occurred in 10, and necessitated withdrawal in 5, whereas the corresponding figures for leucopenia were 6 and 4. In a multinational prospective study of 1 491 patients, Kay [29] found that 3% of patients were withdrawn, due to haematological abnormalities, with thrombocytopenia being 'twice as common' as neutropenia. Because of these risks, blood counts are measured regularly and abnormalities spotted early. Normally, no action other than stopping D-penicillamine is required. Experience with sodium aurothiomalate, a drug which produces a spectrum of haematological side effects similar to D-penicillamine, has produced evidence of two separate pathogenic mechanisms for drug-induced thrombocytopenia [24, 30]. The first type has features which suggest a direct toxic action, with the bone marrow showing reduced activity of megakaryocytes. In patients with this type the platelets tend to fall slowly and to levels not below 100×10^9 per litre, provided the gold is discontinued. The second type is characterised by a sudden fall in platelet numbers, the presence of antiplatelet antibodies and normal or increased megakaryocyte activity in the bone marrow. This second type has been shown to occur almost exclusively in patients possessing HLA-DR3 [30]. The possibility that the same pathogenetic mechanisms are operating in D-penicillamine-induced thrombocytopenia is supported by an association with HLA-DR3 and clinical observations which suggest two patterns of thrombocytopenia. Extrapolating from the example of sodium aurothiomalate induced thrombocytopenia, it may be important to clinically distinguish the two types if the immunological associations are to be defined. It is normal policy not to re-challenge patients with D-penicillamine who have had major haematological toxicity but some patients, presumably those with a toxic type of thrombocytopenia, have been successfully re-started on the drug at lower doses.

As mentioned above, the toxic effect of D-penicillamine on white cells is much less common; however, in rare instances, marrow aplasia occurs and cases of fatal aplastic anaemia have been recorded [31]. Eosinophilia occurs occasionally after therapy with D-penicillamine but without a close association with toxicity [32], and isolated cases of thrombotic thrombocytopenia have also been recorded [33].

2. RENAL SIDE EFFECTS

There are a variety of renal toxic effects induced by D-penicillamine. Treatment with D-penicillamine can lead also to microscopic haematuria, but it is rarely severe, and other causes of haematuria need to be excluded [34, 35].

Proteinuria is common in patients taking D-penicillamine for over 6 months [24, 36, 37] and is thought to be due to immune complex deposition in the glomerular basement membrane [36]. The prevalence of proteinuria is probably increased in patients with rheumatoid arthritis in comparison to those with Wilson's disease [39]. It is currently believed that immune complexes form in-situ rather than being filtered from the circulation, as circulating immune complexes have not been found in patients developing D-penicillamine-induced proteinuria [40]. Significant proteinuria occurs in around 20–30% of patients treated with D-penicillamine, the peak incidence occurring at 6–9 months after commencement of therapy [41]. Proteinuria always disappears on withdrawal of the drug, but sometimes improvement is slow whilst continuation of therapy may lead to the nephrotic syndrome. It has been suggested that elevated levels of antigalactosyl antibody reflect renal injury after treatment with D-penicillamine [42].

Histological examination of affected kidneys usually shows glomeruli with only minimal change nephropathy but, occasionally, mesangio-proliferative glomerulonephritis is found. Electron microscopic examination of affected glomeruli, however, has revealed changes which are consistent with the earliest manifestations of membranous glomerulonephritis with subepithelial electron-dense deposits, fusion of epithelial cell foot processes, and evidence of mesangial matrix increase [38]. Immunofluorescence shows evidence of deposits of IgG and C3. Furthermore, re-biopsy after the disappearance of proteinuria has shown histological features consistent with healing membranous glomerulonephritis, and these changes may persist for some time.

An increased risk of D-penicillamine toxicity has been shown with high doses of the drug [41, 44]. In one study, significantly more patients suffered proteinuria in the group treated with 600 mg compared to those receiving 300 mg/day of D-penicillamine [43]. In the majority of studies which addressed the question, proteinuria during a previous course of gold therapy has also been shown to indicate an increased risk of proteinuria on D-penicillamine (vide infra). The explanation for the association probably lies with shared inherited risk factors for toxicity, i.e. HLA-DR3 and poor sulphoxidation (vide infra).

3. LUNG ABNORMALITIES

Lung disorders in patients taking D-penicillamine are rare [45]. However, an unusual complication of rheumatoid arthritis, obliterative bronchiolitis, was noted by Geddes [46] to be increased in frequency and to be more aggressive in nature in patients taking D-penicillamine [47–49]. As well as this different clinical course, which has often proved fatal, a characteristic concentric obliteration of bronchioles has subsequently been noted histologically [47]. Aggressive cytotoxic therapy has been employed and does appear to slow the progression of this severe disease [47]. Obliterative bronchiolitis has also been seen in patients with eosinophilic fasciitis and with Wilson's disease, both of whom had been treated with D-penicillamine.

Diffuse interstitial lung disease has been described following therapy with D-penicillamine with a similar presentation but a lower prevalence to that seen with gold [50, 51]. There has been difficulty distinguishing this from pulmonary haemorrhage [52] occurring either as part of a drug-induced Goodpasture's syndrome or

172

in isolation and this has lead to some confusion [50]. Goodpasture's syndrome, which is characterised by pulmonary haemorrhage and renal failure, is due to an autoantibody directed against glomerular basement membrane. It has been recorded in patients treated with D-penicillamine [53, 54].

4. OTHER AUTOIMMUNE PHENOMENA

There have been numerous uncontrolled reports showing an increase in a variety of autoantibodies and autoimmune diseases in rheumatoid arthritis patients treated with D-penicillamine. The evidence suggests that the immune disorders are secondary to administration of the drug rather than due to clustering of autoimmune diseases in patients with immune dysregulation. Thus, both the disease and the relevant autoantibody disappear on cessation of drug therapy and recur after reintroduction of the drug. Furthermore, these syndromes can occur in patients who do not have an immunologically based disease (e.g. cysteinuria) when treated with D-penicillamine. Finally, in certain cases there is a difference between the genetic background predisposing to the idiopathic and to the drug-induced disorders; this is best documented for myasthenia gravis.

5. AUTOANTIBODY PRODUCTION

In uncontrolled studies, antinuclear antibody has been found in up to 40% of patients with RA treated with D-penicillamine. However, the one controlled study to examine this question prospectively did not find any increased prevalence of these autoantibodies in 140 patients treated with D-penicillamine for a mean of 30 weeks [55]. Other autoantibodies reported to occur after D-penicillamine therapy include insulin antibodies [56, 57], anti-basement membrane antibodies [53] and acetylcholine receptor antibodies [58].

6. SYSTEMIC LUPUS ERYTHEMATOSUS (SLE)

D-penicillamine can give rise to a drug-induced SLE syndrome. This is generally mild and improves on either stopping or lowering the dose of D-penicillamine. Only rarely are steroids required for its treatment. In six patients with rheumatoid arthritis who developed the syndrome, the most common feature was pleurisy, with haematological abnormalities being the next most frequent [59]. Of 120 patients with Wilson's disease treated with D-penicillamine, four patients developed drug-induced SLE, the clinical manifestations being fever, joint pains and serositis [60]. Unlike other drug-induced SLE, that following D-penicillamine administration can have autoantibodies with anti-nuclear binding activity against double-stranded DNA. Hypocomplementemia has also been recorded [61]. Glomerulonephritis and neurological disorders, both normally considered to be confined to idiopathic SLE, have been seen in D-penicillamine-induced SLE. Although immune complex deposition in skin and kidney has been demonstrated in drug-induced SLE, histological distinctions between this disorder and immune complex-mediated disease have been documented [62].

The diagnosis of drug-induced SLE is serological, with all patients possessing antinuclear antibody titres which fall with cessation of drug treatment. The diagnosis should be entertained in all patients who develop antinuclear antibodies with a raised erythrocyte sedimentation rate whilst on D-penicillamine therapy.

7. POLYMYOSITIS/DERMATOMYOSITIS

Polymyositis/dermatomyositis has been reported in a small number of patients treated with D-penicillamine, most of them having seropositive rheumatoid arthritis [63, 64], but cases developing in patients with systemic sclerosis [65], and Wilson's disease [66] have also been recorded. The initial feature was weight loss in about 50% of cases, and other symptoms included the rash of dermatomyositis. Cardiac involvement has been recorded in three cases [67], and was associated with an unfavourable outcome, proving fatal in two of the cases. The diagnosis of D-penicillamine-induced myositis is made by the conventional criteria of elevated muscle enzymes, a characteristic electromyogram and muscle biopsy, together with a temporal association with administration of D-penicillamine. Steroids were given in 50% of cases but without a dramatic effect [64]. In the surviving patients, all symptoms resolved.

8. MYASTHENIA GRAVIS

Myasthenia gravis has been observed in a small proportion of patients with every disease that has been treated with D-penicillamine [68, 69]. In a review of 18 cases, most patients presented with diplopia and or ptosis [68]. Unfortunately, due to delays in diagnosis and presentation, D-penicillamine was continued for a mean of 12 further weeks during which time seven patients progressed to generalised myasthenia. Autoantibodies to the acetylcholine receptor were found in 17 out of 17 cases. Anticholinesterase drugs were required in 12 patients. Cessation of D-penicillamine therapy produced permanent resolution of myasthenic symptoms in all but three cases, two of which were left with ptosis and one with diplopia.

The genetics of this disorder are interesting, as the HLA associations are different for the drug-induced and idiopathic varieties of the disease. The former has an increased prevalence of HLA-DR1 (63% compared to 17% of controls [68]), with no increase in prevalence of HLA-DR3, whereas the reverse applies for the spontaneously occurring disease. The different genetic backgrounds provide further evidence that the two diseases are distinct and that the drug-induced disease is a genuine entity. The auto-antibodies found in the drug-induced and idiopathic disease do have differences of avidity and of light-chain composition [71], and have only limited cross-reactivity unlike the spontaneously occurring forms [69, 70].

9. DERMATOLOGICAL ABNORMALITIES

D-penicillamine is known to induce a syndrome with the clinical, histological and immunological characteristics of pemphigus vulgaris or one of its variants [71 – 76]. Cases appear after a mean treatment period of 11 months and clinically are indistinguishable from the spontaneously occurring disease. As in the latter, circulating anti-epithelial antibodies are found, and immunofluorescence of affected skin shows immunoglobulin and complement deposited in the intercellular substance. Most cases resolve spontaneously, but unusually for drug-induced responses, some cases have been persistent. A fatal outcome has even been recorded [77]. A case of pemphigus has been reported with bound IgG directed against the dermo-epidermal junction (i.e. site of antibody binding normally associated with pemphigoid), but as no subepidermal blistering was seen, it was concluded that the autoantibodies were biologically inactive [78].

D-penicillamine can also cause pseudoxanthoma elasticum [79, 80]. It is thought that this is due to its ability to block aldehyde cross-linking which subsequently affects collagen cross-linking (vide supra).

10. MAMMARY GIGANTISM

Weight gain, hot flushes and mammary gigantism have all been reported after D-penicillamine therapy [81 – 83], suggesting that an alteration either in hormone status or receptor may be involved. Raised prolactin levels have been found in some cases, and responses to danazol (an anterior pituitary suppressant) have been reported [84]. However, in another study a careful search for abnormal hormonal status or receptor levels was unfruitful [85].

V. Factors determining toxicity

1. METABOLIC FACTORS IN D-PENICILLAMINE TOXICITY

The initial failure to find the same association with HLA-DR3 in D-penicillamine-induced toxicity as that seen in gold-induced toxicity, led to the search for additional factors, and in particular whether variations in drug metabolism could determine toxicity.

It is known that polymorphisms exist for certain metabolic pathways and it is believed that these are genetically determined. Such polymorphisms can be assayed using a probe drug. Adverse reactions to these drugs occur predominantly in the minority of individuals who are poor metabolisers of these compounds. Consequently, the risk of side effects can be predicted from a knowledge of the patient's metabolic status. For example, by using a compound such as debrisoquine as a probe drug, the hydroxylation status can be determined [86]. In an individual with impaired hydroxylation, there is an increased risk of toxicity with drugs such as phenformin [87] or perhexiline [88], as these are metabolised by hydroxylation. Similarly, poor acetylators, as determined by the use of sulphonamide as a probe drug, are known to have an increased risk of developing hydralazine-associated side effects [89]. This latter example provides an interaction between three genetically determined factors, a metabolic pathway, the HLA status and the sex of the individual (see also chapters by Rubin, Hein and Weber, and Sim, in this volume).

The demonstration that the capacity to produce sulphoxidation products of carbocysteine (a drug structurally very similar to D-penicillamine) also exhibited skewed distribution in the population [90], led to the examination of the role of sulphoxidation in D-penicillamine-induced toxicity. It was found that the prevalence of toxicity was significantly increased in those patients with impaired sulphoxidation, with normal distribution of sulphoxidation being determined from a previous population study [91]. HLA-DR3 was also found to be significantly associated with the development of adverse reactions, with 12 out of 20 patients possessing this haplotype developing adverse reaction compared to 10 out of 35 without it [92]. There was no association between DR antigen status and sulphoxidation ability. The two risk factors were not additive, and possession of either HLA-DR3 or impaired sulphoxidation produced a much greater risk than the two together.

This is in contrast to the situation which prevails in other drug-induced disorders such as hydralazine-induced lupus where an additive risk for slow acetylation, HLA-DR4 positivity and female sex is found. These results provide evidence for two populations of patients with differing risks of toxicity and, thus, can explain several features of D-penicillamine administration: the difficulty in developing a standardised drug schedule, the dose dependence of toxicity, and the incomplete relationship with gold toxicity. The association between toxicity and impaired sulphoxidation ability has been confirmed [93], and a recent abstract suggests that all patients who develop D-penicillamine-induced myasthenia gravis possess the impaired sulphoxidation phenotype [94].

The mechanism for this association between poor sulphoxidation and toxicity is unknown. However, it has been assumed that, because of the structural similarity between D-penicillamine and carbocysteine, poor sulphoxidation results in the impaired metabolism of D-penicillamine and leads to an increased immunogenicity of either the drug or one of its metabolites, thus producing immunologically mediated side effects. However, it has recently been shown [95, 96] that patients who develop adverse reactions to sodium aurothiomalate, a drug structurally dissimilar to carbocysteine apart from the presence of a thiol group, also have an increased prevalence of impaired sulphoxidation. This suggests that the metabolism of the thiol group alone is likely to be a critical determinant of toxicity. At present, the relationship between HLA status and sulphoxidation status in gold-induced toxicity is unknown. Because of the potential importance of these findings it is essential that the constancy of the sulphoxidation type should be established in disease, during therapy and with ageing.

2. HLA AND D-PENICILLAMINE TOXICITY

Soon after the demonstration of an increased prevalence of the class II antigen HLA-DR4 in patients with rheumatoid arthritis, it was shown that the risk of developing certain immunological adverse reactions after administration of gold was increased in those patients possessing HLA-DR3. Studies [97 – 99] which looked for D-penicillamine-induced toxicity, however, failed to show a significant association with HLA-DR3. This was surprising, as several reports [100 – 102] had suggested that a patient developing toxicity on gold therapy had an increased risk of developing the same toxicity after D-penicillamine treatment, although others have not found this association [103]. The major reason for the failure to show a correlation with HLA-DR3 were the small numbers of patients included in the studies. Subsequently, three studies [86, 92, 104] looking at larger numbers of patients, have found a significant association between HLA-DR3 and D-penicillamine-induced proteinuria. One study found an association between HLA-DR3 and haematological abnormalities [92], as did another group which grouped together adverse reactions to both gold and D-penicillamine. In addition to the association with proteinuria, one group found an association with non-nephrological adverse reactions in patients possessing HLA-B7 and DR2, whilst an Australian group [104] found that A1 and DR4 were associated with D-penicillamine-induced thrombocytopenia, as was the possession of a null allele at the C4B complement locus on chromosome 6 mapping near to the HLA-DR antigen locus.

3. IMMUNOLOGICAL FACTORS IN D-PENICILLAMINE TOXICITY

The mechanisms involved in the various autoimmune phenomena associated with D-penicillamine have been a source of speculation. One theory is that D-penicillamine binds to tissue components, thereby forming a hapten and thus stimulating autoantibody production. Although there is some evidence from animal models to support this [105], it does not account for the diversity of autoantibodies produced. A second hypothesis is that D-penicillamine has an immunomodulatory role allowing release of previously suppressed B cell clones [106]. Finally, it is possible that D-penicillamine may interact with pre-existing antibodies, altering their affinity and even possibly their valency, which by altering the size of the antibody/antigen could lead to immune complex formation [107].

Summary and Conclusions

The relationship of HLA-DR3 and impaired sulphoxidation status to D-penicillamine toxicity is now firmly established. We need to refine and simplify the tests involved so as to use this knowledge for the management of patients being treated with this drug. Parallel with this utilitarian aim, we should ascertain the pathogenetic mechanisms linking the drug, the genetic factors and the development of toxic side-effects.

It is clear that D-penicillamine toxicity is multi-factorial, involving such variables as the dose of the drug, HLA and drug metabolism. Our present knowledge still fails to account for a significant minority of patients who develop side effects but do not possess any of the known risk factors.

References

1. Abraham, E. P., Chain, E., Baker, W. and Robinson, R. (1943) Penicillamine, a characteristic degradation produce of penicillin. Nature 107, 151.
2. Walshe, J. M. (1956) Wilson's disease new oral therapy. Lancet i, 25–26.
3. Jaffe, I. A. (1965) Comparison of the effect of plasmaphoresis and penicillamine on the level of circulating rheumatoid factor. Ann. Rheum. Dis. 22, 71 76.
4. Crawhall, J. C., Scowen, E. F. and Watts, R. W. E. (1963) Effects of penicillamine on cysteinuria. Br. Med. J. 588–590.
5. Steen, V. D., Medsger, T. A. and Rodnan, G. P. (1982) D-penicillamine therapy in progressive systemic sclerosis, a retrospective analysis. Ann. Intern. Med. 97, 652–659.
6. Jain, S., Scheuer, P. J., Samourian, S., McGee, J. O'D. and Sherlock, S. (1977) A controlled trial of D-penicillamine in primary biliary cirrhosis. Lancet i, 831–834.
7. Stern, R. B., Wilkinson, S. P., Howarth, P. J. N. and Williams, R. (1977) Controlled trial of synthetic D-penicillamine in maintenance therapy for active chronic hepatitis. Gut 18, 19–22.
8. Van der Korst, J. K., Van de Stadt, R. J., Muijsers, A. O., Ament, H. J. W. and Henrichs, A. M. A. (1981) Pharmacokinetics of D-penicillamine in rheumatoid arthritis. In: R. N. Maini and H. Berry (Eds.), Modulation of Autoimmunity and Disease, Praeger, Eastbourne.
9. Perrett, D. (1981) Metabolism and pharmacology of D-penicillamine in man. J. Rheumatol., Suppl. 7, 41–50.
10. Harkness, J. A. L. and Blake, D. R. (1982) Penicillamine nephropathy and iron. Lancet ii, 1368–1369.
11. Kucharczyk, N. and Shahinian, S. (1981) An overview of assay methods for D-penicillamine. J. Rheumatol., Suppl. 7, 28–34.
12. Butler, M., Carruthers, G., Harth, M., Freeman, D., Percy, J. and Rabenstein, D. (1982) Pharmokinetics of reduced D-penicillamine in patients with rheumatoid arthritis. Arthritis Rheum. 25, 111–116.
13. Van der Korst, J. K., Muijsers, A. O., Henrichs, A. M. A., Ament, H. J. N. and Van Stadt, R. J. (1979) Blood levels and side effects of D-penicillamine. Agents Actions, Suppl. 5, 159–164.
14. Lyle, W. H. and Kleinman, R. L. (Ed.) (1977) Penicillamine at 21. Its place in therapeutics now. Proc. Roy. Soc. Med., Suppl. 3.
15. Nimni, M. E. (1977) Mechanism of inhibition of collagen cross-binding by D-penicillamine.

Proc. Roy. Soc. Med., Suppl. 3, 65 – 72.

16. Kuchinskas, E. J. and Du Vigneaud, V. (1957) An increased vitamin B6 requirement in the rat on diet containing D-penicillamine. Arch. Biochem. 66, 1.

17. Lipsky, P. E. and Ziff, M., (1980) Inhibition of human helper T cell function in vitro by D-penicillamine. J. Clin. Invest. 65, 1069 – 1076.

18. Lipsky, P. E. and Ziff, M. (1978) The effect of D-penicillamine on mitogen-induced lymphocyte proliferation: synergistic inhibition by D-penicillamine and Cu salts. J. Immunol. 120, 1006.

19. Maini, R. N. and Roffe, L. (1976) D-penicillamine and lymphocyte function in rheumatoid arthritis. In: E. Munthe (Ed.), Penicillamine Research in Rheumatoid Arthritis, Fabritius and Sonner, Oslo.

20. Merryman, P. and Jaffe, I. A. (1978) Effect of penicillamine on the proliferative response of human lymphocytes. Proc. Soc. Exp. Biol. Med. 25, 603.

21. Zuckner, J. Ramsey, R. H., Dorner, R. W. and Gantner, G. E. (1970) D-penicillamine in rheumatoid arthritis. Arthritis Rheum. 13, 131 – 138.

22. Emery, P., Panayi, G. S. and Nouri, A. M. E. (1984) Interleukin-2 reverses deficient cell-mediated immune responses in rheumatoid arthritis. Clin. Exp. Immunol. 57, 123 – 129.

23. Huskisson, E. C., Gibson, T., Balme, H. W., Berry, H., Burry, H. C., Grahame, R., Dudley Hart, F., Henderson, D. R. F. and Wojtulewski, J. A. (1974) Trial comparing D-penicillamine and gold in rheumatoid arthritis. Preliminary report. Ann. Rheum. Dis. 33, 532 – 535.

24. Halverson, P. B., Koxin, F., Bernard, G. C. and Goldman, A. L. (1978) Toxicity of penicillamine. A serious limitation to therapy in rheumatoid arthritis. J. Am. Med. Assoc. 17, 1870 – 1871.

25. Kean, W. F., Dwosh, I. L., Anastassiades, T. P., Ford, P. M. and Kelly, H. G. (1980) The toxicity pattern of D-penicillamine therapy. Arthritis Rheum. 23, 158 – 164.

26. Stein, H. B., Patterson, A. C., Offer, R. C., Atkins, C. J., Teufel, A. and Robinson, H. S. (1980) Adverse effects of D-penicillamine in rheumatoid arthritis. Ann. Intern. Med. 92, 24 – 29.

27. O'Brien, W. M. (1980) Toxicity of D-penicillamine in rheumatoid arthritis. Ann. Intern. Med. 92, 120 – 122.

28. Munthe, E. and Kass, E. (1981) Penicillamine in rheumatoid diseases: a prospective study of tolerance and efficacy. J. Rheumol., Suppl. 7, 161 – 165.

29. Kay, A., (1986) European League against rheumatism study of adverse reactions to D-penicillamine. Br. J. Rheumatol. 25, 193 – 198.

30. Panayi, G. S. (1981) HLA antigens and adverse reactions to anti rheumatic drugs. In: R. N. Maini and H. Berry (Eds.), Modulation of Autoimmunity and Disease: The Penicillamine Experience, Praeger, Eastbourne, pp. 65 – 69.

31. Richards, A. I., Velvin, D. S. and Whitmore, D. N. (1976) Fatal aplastic anaemia and D-penicillamine. Lancet, i, 646 – 647.

32. Smith, D. H., Scott, D. L. and Zaphiropoulos, G. C. (1983) Eosinophilia in D-penicillamine therapy. Ann. Rheum. Dis. 42, 408 – 410.

33. Speth, P. A., Boerbooms, A. M., Holdrinet, R. S., Van de Putte, L. B. and Meyer, J. W. (1982) Thrombotic thrombocytopenic purpura associated with D-penicillamine treatment in rheumatoid arthritis. J. Rheumatol. 9, 812 – 813.

34. White, E. G., Smith, D. H. and Zaphiropoulos, G. C. (1984) Haematuria occurring during antirheumatoid therapy. Br. J. Rheumatol. 23, 57 – 60.

35. Barraclough, D., Cunningham, T. J. and Muriden, K. D. (1981) Microscopic haematuria in patients with rheumatoid arthritis on D-penicillamine. Aust. NZ. J. Med. 11, 706 – 708.

36. Penicillamine nephropathy (editorial) (1981) Br. Med. J. 282, 761 – 762.

37. Crawhall, J. C. (1981) Proteinuria in D-penicillamine-treated rheumatoid arthritis. J. Rheumatol., Suppl. 7, 161 – 163.

38. Dische F. E., Swinson, D. R., Hamilton, E. B. and Parsons, V. (1984) Immunopathology of

penicillamine-induced glomerular disease. J. Rheumatol. 11, 584 – 585.

39. Lyle, W. H. (1979) Penicillamine. In: Clinics in Rheumatic Diseases. W. B. Saunders Co. Ltd., London.

40. Fernandes, L., Vergani, D., Davies, E., Berry, H., Hamilton, E. and Tee, D. (1981) D-penicillamine nephropathy, circulating immune complexes and autoantibodies. In: R. N. Maini and H. Berry (Eds.), Modulation of Autoimmunity and Disease, Praeger, Eastbourne.

41. Stein, H. B., Schroader, M. L. and Dillon, A. M. (1986) Penicillamine induced proteinuria: risk factors. Semin. Arthritis Rheum. 15, 282 – 287.

42. Malaise, M. G., Davin, J. C., Mahieu, P. R. and Franchimont, P. (1986) Elevated antigalactosyl antibody titres reflect renal injury after gold or D-penicillamine in rheumatoid arthritis. Clin. Immunol. Immunopathol. 40, 356 – 364.

43. Nissila, M., Nuotio, P., Von Essen, R. and Makisara, P. (1982) Low dose penicillamine treatment of rheumatoid arthritis. Scand. J. Rheumatol. 11, 161 – 164.

44. Williams, H. J., Ward, J. R., Reading, J. C., Egger, M. J., Grandone, J. T., Samuelson, C. O., Furst, D. E., Sullivan, J. M., Watson, M. A., Guttadauria, M. et al. (1983) Low dose D-penicillamine therapy in rheumatoid arthritis. Arthritis Rheum. 26, 581 – 592.

45. Turner Warwick, M. (1981) Adverse reactions affecting the lung: possible association with D-penicillamine. J. Rheumatol., Suppl. 7, 166 – 168.

46. Geddes, D. M., Corrin, B., Brewerton, D. A., Davies, R. J. and Turner-Warwick, M. (1977) Progressive airway obliteration in adults and its association with rheumatoid disease. Q. J. Med. 184, 427 – 444.

47. Van de Laar, M. A., Westermann, C. J., Wagenaar, S. S. and Dinant, H. J. (1985) Beneficial effect of intravenous cyclophosphamide and oral prednisolone on D-penicillamine associated bronchiolitis obliterans. Arthritis Rheum. 28, 93 – 97.

48. Murphy, K. C., Atkins, C. J., Offer, R. C., Hogg, J. C. and Stein, H. B. (1981) Obliterative bronchiolitis in two rheumatoid arthritis patients treated with penicillamine. Arthritis Rheum. 24, 557 – 560.

49. Penny, W. J., Knight, R. K., Rees, A. M., Thomas, A. L. and Smith, A. P. (1982) Obliterative bronchiolitis in rheumatoid arthritis. Ann. Rheum. Dis. 41, 469 – 472.

50. Scott, D. I., Bradby, G. V., Aitman, T. J., Zaphiropoulos, G. C. and Hawkins, C. F. (1981) Relationship of gold and penicillamine therapy to diffuse interstitial lung disease. Ann. Rheum. Dis. 40, 136 – 141.

51. Bamji, A. and Cooke, N. (1981) Pulmonary damage with gold or penicillamine. Ann. Rheum. Dis. 40, 531.

52. Louie, S., Gamble, C. N. and Cross, C. E. (1986) Penicillamine associated pulmonary haemorrhage. J. Rheumatol. 13, 963 – 966.

53. Sternlieb, I. Bennett, B. and Scheinburg, I. H. (1975) D-penicillamine induced Goodpasture's disease in Wilson's disease. Ann. Intern Med. 82, 673 – 676.

54. Gibson, T., Burry, H. C. and Ogg, C. (1976) Goodpastures syndrome and D-penicillamine. Ann. Intern. Med. 84, 100.

55. Weinstein, A. and Rothfield, N. F. (1986) Lack of induction of antinuclear antibodies by D-penicillamine in rheumatoid arthritis: a controlled study. J. Rheumatol. 13, 308 – 312.

56. Benson, E. A., Healey, L. A. and Barron, E. J. (1985) Insulin antibodies in patients receiving penicillamine. Am. J. Med. 78, 857 – 860.

57. Becker, R. C. and Martin, R. G. (1986) Penicillamine-induced insulin antibodies. Ann. Intern. Med. 104, 127 – 128.

58. Vincent, A. and Newsom Davis, J. (1982) Acetylcholine receptor antibody characteristics in myasthenia gravis. II. Patient with penicillamine-induced myasthenia or idiopathic myasthenia of recent onset. Clin. Exp. Immunol. 49, 266 – 272.

59. Chalmers, A., Thompson, D., Stein, H. E., Reid, G. and Patterson, A. C. (1982) Systemic

lupus erythematosus during penicillamine therapy for rheumatoid arthritis. Ann. Intern. Med. 97, 659 – 663.

60. Walshe, J. M. (1981) Penicillamine and the SLE syndrome. J. Rheumatol., Suppl. 7, 155 – 160.

61. Hughes G. R., Rynes, R. I., Gharavi, A., Ryan, P. F., Sewell, J. and Mansilla, R. (1981) The heterogeneity of serologic findings and predisposing host factors in drug-induced lupus erythematosus. Arthritis Rheum. 24, 1070 – 1073.

62. Walshe, J. M. (1981) Penicillamine-induced SLE. Lancet 2, 1416.

63. Lund, H. I. and Nielsen, M. (1983) Penicillamine-induced dermatomyositis. A case history. Scand. J. Rheumatol. 12, 350 – 352.

64. Halla, J. T., Fallahi, S. and Koopman, W. J. (1984) Penicillamine-induced myositis. Observations and unique features in two patients and review of the literature. Am. J. Med. 4, 719 – 722.

65. Nishikai, M., Tunatu, Y. and Homma, M. (1974) Monoclonal gammopathypenicillamine-induced polymyositis and systemic sclerosis. Arch. Dermatol. 110, 253 – 255.

66. Schraeder, P. L., Peters, H. A. and Dahl, D. S. (1972) Polymyositis and penicillamine. Arch. Neurol. 476 – 477.

67. Doyle, D. R., McCurley, T. L. and Sergent, J. S. (1983) Fatal polymyositis and D-penicillamine-treated rheumatoid arthritis. Ann. Intern. Med. 3, 327 – 330.

68. Delamere, J. P., Jobson, S., Mackintosh, L. P., Wells, L. and Walton, K. W. (1983) Penicillamine-induced myasthenia in rheumatoid arthritis: its clinical and genetic features. Ann. Rheum. Dis. 42, 500 – 504.

69. Dawkins, R. L., Garlepp, M. J., McDonald, B. L., Williamson, J., Zilko, P. J. and Carrano, J. (1981) Myasthenia gravis and D-penicillamine. J. Rheumatol., Suppl. 7, 169 – 174.

70. Garlepp, M. J., Dawkins, R. L. and Christiansen, F. T. (1983) HLA antigens and acetylcholine receptor antibodies in penicillamine-induced myasthenia gravis. Br. Med. J. 286, 338 – 340.

71. Sternlieb, I., Fisher, M. and Scheinberg, I. H. (1981) Penicillamine induced skin lesions. J. Rheumatol. 7, 149 – 154.

72. Santa Cruz, D. J., Prioleau, P. G., Marcus, M. D. and Uitto, J. (1981) Pemphigus-like lesions induced by D-penicillamine. Analysis of clinical histopathological and immunofluorescence features in 34 cases. Am. J. Dermatopathol. 3, 85 – 92.

73. Yung, C. W. and Hambrick, G. W., Jr. (1982) D-penicillamine-induced pemphigus syndrome. J. Am. Acad. Dermatol, 6, 317 – 324.

74. Bailin, P. L. and Matkaluk, R. M. (1982) Cutaneous reactions to rheumatological drugs. Clin. Rheum. Dis. 8, 493 – 516.

75. Levy, R. S., Fisher, M. and Alter, J. N. (1983) Penicillamine review and cutaneous manifestations. J. Am. Acad. Dermatol. 8, 548 – 558.

76. Ho, V., C., Stein, H. B., Ongley, R. A. and McLeod, W. A. (1985) Penicillamine-induced pemphigus. J. Rheumatol. 12, 583 – 586.

77. Kohn, S. R. (1986) Fatal penicillamine-induced pemphigus foliaceus like dermatosis. Arch. Dermatol. 122, 17.

78. Velthuis, P. J., Hendrikse, J. C. and Nefkens, J. J. (1985) Combined features of pemphigus and pemphigoid induced by penicillamine. Br. J. Dermatol. 112, 615 – 619.

79. Light, N., Meyrick Thomas, R. H., Stephens, A., Kirby, J. D., Fryer, P. R. and Avery, N. C. (1986) Collagen and elastin changes in D-penicillamine-induced pseudoxanthoma elasticum-like skin. Br. J. Dermatol. 114, 381 – 388.

80. Meyrick Thomas, R. H. and Kirby, J. D. (1985) Elastosis perforans serpiginosa and pseudoxanthoma elasticum-like skin change due to D-penicillamine. Clin. Exp. Dermatol. 10, 386 – 391.

81. Desai, S. N. (1973) Sudden gigantism of breasts: drug-induced? Br. J. Plast. Surg. 26, 271 – 272.

82. Passas, C. and Weinstein, A. (1978) Breast gigantism with penicillamine therapy. Arthritis Rheum. 21, 167 – 168.

83. Taylor, P. J., Cumming, D. C. and Corenblum, B. (1981) Successful treatment of D-penicillamine-induced breast gigantism with danazol. Br. Med. J. 282, 362 – 363.

84. Rooney, P. J. and Cleland, J. (1981) Successful treatment of D-penicillamine-induced breast gigantism with danazol. Br. Med. J. 282, 1627 – 1628.

85. Finer, N., Emery, P. and Hicks, B. H. (1984) Mammary gigantism and D-penicillamine. Clin. Endocrinol. 21, 219 – 222.

86. Scherak, O., Smolen, J. S., Mayr, W. R., Mayrhofer, F., Kolarz, G. and Thumb, N. J. (1984) HLA antigens and toxicity to gold and penicillamine in rheumatoid arthritis. J. Rheumatol. 11, 610 – 614.

87. Oates, N. S., Shah, R. R., Idle, J. R. and Smith, R. L. (1981) Phenformin-induced lactic acidosis associated with impaired debrisoquine hydroxylation. Lancet 1, 837 – 838.

88. Shah, R. R., Oates, N. S., Idle, J. R. Smith, R. L. and Lockhart, J. D. F. (1982) Impaired oxidation of debrisoquine in patients with perhexiline neuropathy. Br. Med. J. 284, 295 – 299.

89. Batchelor, J. R., Welsh, K. I. and Mansilla Tinoco, R. (1980) Hydralazine-induced systemic lupus erythematosus influence of HLA-DR and sex on susceptibility. Lancet 1, 1107 – 1109.

90. Mitchell, S. C., Waring, R. H. and Haley, C. S. (1984) Genetic aspects of the polymodally distributed sulphoxidation of S-carboxymethyl-L-cysteine in man. Br. J. Clin. Pharmacol. 18, 507 – 521.

91. Waring, R. H. Mitchell, S. C. and Shah, R. R. (1982) Polymorphic sulphoxidation of S-carboxymethyl-L-cysteine in man. Biochem. Pharmacol. 31, 3151 – 3154.

92. Emery, P., Panayi, G. S., Huston, G. Welsh, K. I., Mitchell, S. C., Idle, J. K., Smith, R. L. and Waring, R. H. (1984) D-penicillamine-induced toxicity in rheumatoid arthritis. The role of sulphoxidation status and HLA DR3. J. Rheumatol. 11, 626 – 632.

93. Madhok, R., Thompson, A. and Zoma, A. (1986) The predictive value of sulphoxidation status in D-penicillamine toxicity. Br. J. Rheumatol. 25, 113.

94. Ayesh, R., Scadding, G., Mitchell, S. C., Waring, R. H., Witherington, R. H., Brostoff, J., Newson-Davis, J., Smith, R. H. and Seifert, M. H. (1986) Penicillamine-induced myasthenia gravis and sulphoxidation capacity in rheumatoid arthritis patients. Br. J. Rheumatol. 25, 50.

95. Ayesh, R., Mitchell, S. C. and Waring, R. H. (1987) Sodium aurothiomalate toxicity and sulphoxidation capacity in rheumatoid arthritis patients. Br. J. Rheumatol. 26, 197 – 201.

96. Madhok, R., Capell, H. and Waring, R. (1987) Does sulphoxidation state predict gold toxicity in rheumatoid arthritis? Br. Med. J. 294, 483.

97. Wooley, P. H., Griffin, J., Panayi, G. S., Batchelor, J. R., Welsh, K. I. and Gibson, T. (1980) HLA-DR antigens and toxic reaction to sodium aurothiomalate and D-penicillamine in patients with rheumatoid arthritis. N. Engl. J. Med. 303, 300 – 302.

98. Bardin, T., Dryll, A., Debeyre, N., Ryckewaert, A., Legrand, L., Marcelli, A. and Dausset, J. (1982) HLA system and side effects of gold salts and D-penicillamine treatment of rheumatoid arthritis. Ann. Rheum. Dis. 41, 599 – 601.

99. Dawkins, R. L., Zilko, P. J. and Carrano, J. (1981) Immunobiology of D-penicillamine. J. Rheumatol. 8, 56 – 61.

100. Smith, P. J., Swinburn, W. R., Swinson, D. R. and Stewart, I. M. (1982) Influence of previous gold toxicity on subsequent development of penicillamine toxicity. Br. Med. J. 285, 595 – 596.

101. Dodd, M. J., Griffiths, I. D. and Thompson, M. (1980) Adverse reactions to D-penicillamine after gold toxicity. Br. Med. J. 280, 1498 – 1500.

102. Stein, H. B., Ruedy, J., Atkins, C. J. and Offer, R. C. (1983) Penicillamine compared to previous chrysotherapy in rheumatoid arthritis. J. Rheumatol. 10, 319 – 322.

103. Kean, W. F., Lock, C. J., Howard-Lock, H. E. and Buchanan, W. W. (1982) Prior gold therapy does not influence the adverse effects of D-penicillamine in rheumatoid arthritis. Arthritis Rheum. 25, 917 – 922.

104. Stockman, A., Zilko, P. J., Major, G. A., Tait, B. D., Property, D. N., Mathews, J. D., Hannah,

M. C., McCluskey, J. and Muirden, K. D. (1986) Genetic markers in rheumatoid arthritis relationship to toxicity from D-penicillamine. J. Rheumatol. 13, 269 – 773.

105. Dewdney, J. A. (1979) Drugs as haptens. In: T. J. Turk and D. Parker (Eds.), Drugs and Immune Responsiveness, MacMillan, London.

106. Gleichmann, E. and Gleichmann, H. (1981) Spectrum of disease caused by alloreactive T cells. In: R. S. Krakauer (Ed.), Immunoregulation in Autoimmunity, Elsevier/North-Holland, New York. '

107. Aarden, L. A., Lamaker, F. and De Groot, E. (1977) Immunology of DNA. VI. The effect of mercaptans on IgG and IgM anti dsDNA. J. Immunol. Methods 16, 143 – 146.

M.E. Kammüller, N. Bloksma and W. Seinen (Eds.)
Autoimmunity and Toxicology
© 1989 Elsevier Science Publishers B.V. (Biomedical Division)

Zimeldine: febrile reactions and peripheral neuropathy

7

ANN KRISTOFFERSON[a] and BENGT S. NILSSON[b]

[a] *Research Laboratories, Astra Alab AB, and* [b] *Medical Department, Astra Läkemedel AB, S-151 85 Södertälje, Sweden*

I. Introduction

Zimeldine is an antidepressant drug, which was approved by regulatory authorities in most West European countries during 1981 – 1982 and was introduced for general use in those countries in the spring of 1982.

During the later clinical trials it had been found that approximately 1 – 2% of treated patients had experienced 'flu-like' reactions, consisting of pyrexia, myalgia/arthralgia and increased levels of transaminases.

In the spring of 1983, after approximately 1½ year of general use, corresponding to approximately 200 000 – 250 000 treated patients, reports of cases of peripheral neuropathy started to emerge, in the most serious cases the Guillain-Barré syndrome. The development of neuropathy in those cases had been preceded by symptoms of the above-mentioned febrile reactions. In September 1983, eight cases of Guillain-Barré syndrome in zimeldine-treated patients had been reported to Astra, representing a clear-cut increase over the expected background incidence. In this situation Astra's judgement was: (1) febrile reactions could occur in connection with zimeldine treatment; (2) peripheral neuropathy, in the most serious cases the Guillain-Barré syndrome, was a potential complication of the febrile reactions; (3) both the febrile reactions and neuropathy seemed to occur in an unpredictable manner.

Therefore, despite the documented advantages of zimeldine in comparison with traditional antidepressants, Astra decided to withdraw zimeldine from general use and to stop ongoing clinical trials. The withdrawal was effected on September 19, 1983.

In this chapter we review the characteristics and epidemiology of the febrile reactions and neuropathy and data relevant to the understanding of the underlying mechanisms. As an introductory background we give a brief summary of the most important pharmacologic and clinical properties of the drug.

In the process of analyzing and making judgements of the adverse reaction problems, considerable research efforts were made within Astra, and in collaboration with experts in various fields relevant to the problems. Parts of the results of this work only exists as internal Astra Report documents which were used in decision processes and for submission to drug regulatory authorities. Data from those sources will be cited in this chapter whenever appropriate, and will be referenced as 'Astra, data on file'. In addition, published data relevant to the problem are reviewed.

The current generic name of the substance, which is used throughout this chapter, is zimeldine. We want to point out, however, that the original generic name was zimelidine, and this name is found in some of the older references cited. The name was changed due to the similarity with cimetidine, to avoid risks of confusion in countries where generic prescription is possible.

II. Properties of zimeldine

1. EXPERIMENTAL DATA

Zimeldine (chemical name: (Z)-3-(4-bromophenyl)-*N*-*N*-dimethyl-3-(3-pyridyl)-allylamine dihydrochloride monohydrate; see Fig. 1 for chemical formula; trade marks: Zelmid, Normud, Zelmidine) is an antidepressant drug with predominant activity on reuptake of serotonin (5-HT) (for review, see [1, 2]).

The substance, as judged from various pharmacological systems, has negligible effects on noradrenergic transmission, muscarinic receptors, alpha adrenergic receptors, histamine H_1 and H_2 receptors. Most of the pharmacological effects are exerted by the demethylated metabolite, norzimeldine.

Zimeldine was investigated in a full-scale toxicological program, including acute and subacute toxicity studies in several species, life-time carcinogenicity studies in two species, fertility and teratogenicity studies and mutagenicity studies [3]. In brief, no findings predictive of the adverse reactions encountered in man were made. In most studies, animals given high dose levels (50 – 100 mg/kg, as compared to the human dose level of approximately 3 – 4 mg/kg) had symptoms of appetite loss, weight decrease, aggressiveness etc., probably due to marked effects on the serotonin turnover. In the rat, findings of foam cells in the lungs were made, similar to what has been reported with e.g. brompheniramine, haloperidol and chlorpromazine [4].

In the process of analyzing the adverse reactions, the toxicological data have been repeatedly scrutinized for any signs of reactions or findings relevant to the adverse reactions problems, however with negative results. Therefore, one of the important conclusions from the zimeldine experience has been that 'conventional' toxicological systems are unable to predict adverse reactions of the kind encountered with zimeldine.

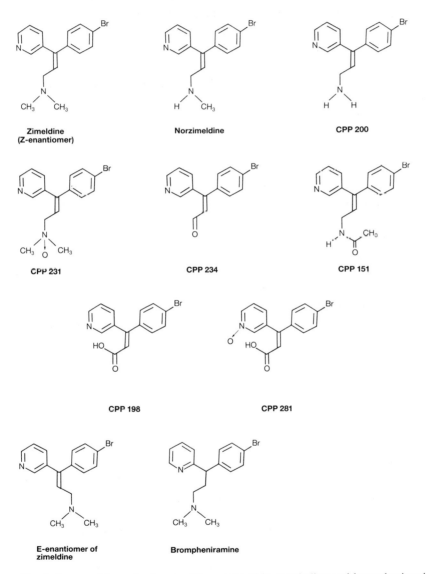

Fig. 1. Structural formulae for zimeldine, some of its metabolites and brompheniramine.

2. PHARMACOKINETICS AND HUMAN PHARMACOLOGY

Zimeldine has relatively uncomplicated pharmacokinetics [5, 6]. Fig. 1 depicts zimeldine and some of the metabolites and related compounds, which have been used in the research concerning the adverse reactions. The most important metabolic route, similar to other antidepressants, is to a demethylated, active metabolite. This metabolite, norzimeldine, exerts most of the pharmacologic activity of the drug, both because it is much more potent as a 5-HT uptake inhibitor than zimeldine itself, and due to a longer plasma half-life (approximately 16 h, vs. 5 h for zimeldine). Standard daily dosage has been 200 mg, normally administered once daily; in the elderly a daily dose of 100 mg has been recommended.

Compared to tricyclic antidepressants, zimeldine has few effects on cardiovascular function [7], few anticholinergic effects and little disturbance of psychomotor function [8].

3. CLINICAL STUDIES

A large program of comparative clinical studies, involving approximately 4 000 patients in trials world-wide, has been performed with zimeldine, using amitriptyline as the main comparative drug, but also including comparisons with a number of other antidepressants such as imipramine, desipramine, maprotiline and others. The results of this program were essentially uniform: the efficacy of zimeldine is comparable to that of conventional antidepressants (see e.g. [9]), whereas the frequency of 'conventional' antidepressant side effects has been lower with zimeldine. One of the latest published clinical studies with zimeldine illustrates typical adverse reaction findings in clinical studies [10]. In this study, which was a randomized, double-blind comparative study with placebo and amitriptyline in a total of 263 patients, withdrawals due to adverse reactions were:

placebo	2/87	(2.3%)
amitriptyline	16/85	(18.8%)
zimeldine	8/91	(8.8%)

The incidence of adverse symptoms was significantly higher with amitriptyline compared to zimeldine for a total of 10 different symptoms. Zimeldine showed a significantly higher incidence compared to placebo for two symptoms: increased sweating and dry mouth. No adverse symptoms occurred more frequently in the zimeldine group than in the amitriptyline group.

In summary, the research and development of zimeldine, for some time, seemed to confirm the 'serotonin hypothesis': that a serotonin-selective antidepressant might be an effective antidepressant with less side-effect problems than conventional antidepressants.

III. Epidemiology and clinical characteristics of febrile reactions

This section, and the following, will deal only with the reactions that have become characteristically associated with zimeldine. As mentioned above, the incidence of other side effects has been notably low. However, similar to the experience with other 5-HT-selective antidepressants, certain patients have experienced nausea and headache, often early in treatment and reversible on dose reduction. Although this has not been conclusively proven, these effects could well be early systemic effects of the serotonin uptake inhibition. Also, apart from skin reactions in connection with the febrile reactions, skin reactions of hypersensitivity type (urticaria, various kinds of exanthemas) seemed to occur fairly frequently, although solid comparative data with other drugs in this respect are not available.

The reported cases of peripheral neuropathy, especially the Guillain-Barré syndrome, were the direct reason for the withdrawal. However, these reactions, as will be discussed below, were intimately associated with generalized symptoms, such as pyrexia, myalgia/arthralgia and liver function disturbance. Therefore, the epidemiology of these febrile reactions will be described first and the cases of neuropathy discussed separately.

1. FINDINGS IN CLINICAL TRIALS

In early clinical trials, single cases of reversible liver function disturbance were observed, sometimes in association with general symptoms such as pyrexia and myalgia/arthralgia. In 1980, a comparative analysis of the incidence of liver function disturbance in the total material of patients treated in clinical trials was per-

TABLE 1

Frequency of liver function disturbance with antidepressants

Drug	Proportion of patients with elevated values of		
	ASAT[a] (GOT)	ALAT[b] (GPT)	ALP[c]
Zimeldine	37/303 = 12.2%	42/295 = 14.2%	38/350 = 10.9%
Amitriptyline	3/49 = 6.1%	9/38 = 23.7%	5/71 = 7.0%
Maprotiline	4/26 = 15.4%	9/45 = 20.0%	4/45 = 8.9%
Desipramine	3/24 = 12.5%	5/24 = 20.8%	7/24 = 29.2%
Imipramine	2/17 = 11.8%	4/17 = 23.5%	2/17 = 11.8%

[a] Aspartate aminotransferase.
[b] Alanine aminotransferase.
[c] Alkaline phosphatase.
(Data, with permission, from Groschinsky-Grind et al., 1980 [11].)

formed [11]. Table 1 illustrates the findings of this analysis, which involved approximately 300 patients treated with zimeldine, 70 on amitriptyline and 20 – 40 patients each on the other drugs.

Later analyses of larger patient materials confirmed these findings, i.e. the incidence of liver function disturbance as such was not higher in zimeldine-treated patients compared to patients treated with other antidepressants. However, cases of febrile symptoms in connection with liver function disturbance were not identified in patients treated with other antidepressants.

It was thus suspected that the febrile reactions with liver function disturbance observed in clinical trials could represent a new type of adverse reaction. Therefore, in the continued clinical research program this problem was the subject of intensive surveillance. Repeated analyses demonstrated the incidence of such reactions to be in the range 1 – 2% of treated patients. The latest analysis of this kind [12] related to a patient population of close to 3 900 patients treated with zimeldine in clinical trials. In this analysis the reactions were subdivided in: (1) typical reactions (fever, pain in muscles and/or joints, increases in transaminase) and (2) incomplete reactions (lacking some of the above features, but still with the suspicion that the reaction belongs to the same category).

This report probably includes a substantial number of cases not related to the treatment (e.g. patients with viral infections), since the ambition in the analysis was to include even cases with only a remote possibility of relation to the treatment. Since it represents the largest material available and has not been published, we will give some details of the analysis below.

(a) Incidence figures

The analysis related to a clinical trial population of 3 843 patients and a Swedish population of patients given zimeldine on special license (named patient basis), amounting to approximately 775 patients. In these patient populations the incidence of febrile reactions was:

clinical trials	89/3 843	= 2.3%
license population	5/775	= 0.6%
total	94/4 618	= 2.0%

Using the FDA algorithm for judging the relation to treatment (from: Excerpt from Procedure Manual for Handling Drug Experience Reports: Glossary, Paper Flow and Algorithms, Reports Evaluation Branch, Division of Drug Experience, Bureau of Drugs, Food and Drug Administration, USA) it was found that the incidence of cases with a definite or probable relation to treatment was 65/4 618 = 1.4%. Approximately half of the patients had typical reactions, the remainder incomplete reactions.

(b) Geographical distribution

Interesting and still unexplained geographical differences in incidence were noted. Table 2 summarizes the data from the most important countries (only clinical trial patients; cases included regardless of the judged relation to treatment).

Some of these differences in incidence could well be explained by differences in medical culture and surveillance. However, the differences between Sweden and UK on the other hand and USA, Canada and Australia on the other, all being countries with highly qualified investigators and efficient surveillance of adverse reactions, are intriguing and still unexplained. A special Astra analysis [13] and published data [14] confirm the high incidence of reactions in Canada.

TABLE 2

Incidence of febrile reactions in clinical trials with zimeldine in various countries

Country	Number of treated patients	Adverse reaction cases	
		number	percentage
Japan	930	0	0
UK + Eire	601	9	1.4
USA	445	22	4.9
Sweden	388	7	1.8
Canada	268	32	11.9
Germany	187	1	0.5
France	183	0	0
Australia + NZ	151	12	7.9
Finland	97	0	0
Belgium	94	0	0
Denmark	53	6	11.3

(Data, with permission, from Nilsson et al., 1983 [12].)

(c) Symptomatology and deviations in laboratory variables

The onset of reactions followed a very characteristic pattern, the majority (68%) occurring within 8–14 days after start of treatment, and only 8% starting later than 29 days after start of treatment.

Among the patients with complete or incomplete reactions, the frequency of the various symptoms involved was, by order of frequency:

pyrexia   84.8%
myalgia   76.1%

headache	73.6%
nausea	50.0%
arthralgia	45.7%
exanthema	26.1%

In patients where liver tests had been performed, the incidence of abnormal variables in connection with the reaction was:

ASAT (GOT)	64.9%
ALAT (GPT)	74.5%
ALP	56.4%

In cases where liver biopsies had been performed, these showed relatively modest changes, mainly of granulomatous type.

The liver test abnormalities were reversed relatively rapidly after stopping treatment, with approximately 80% of values normalized within 2 weeks after the onset of the reaction.

Clinical chemistry data other than liver tests were available only in a minority of the patients. Among these, a tendency to lowering of white blood cells, haemoglobin and thrombocytes was seen.

Anti-nuclear antibodies had been tested in eight patients, with three positive results (titers 1:160 – 1:40). One of these patients was also tested for anti-DNA antibodies, with negative result.

(d) Treatment and outcome of the febrile reactions

In 69 of the 94 patients treatment was discontinued permanently. In 14 patients the treatment was continued without modification and the symptoms subsided. This finding raises two different possibilities. The most conventional interpretation would be that the disappearance of symptoms during continued treatment suggests that the symptoms were unrelated to the zimeldine treatment. The other possibility would be that the nature of the reaction is such that it can subside despite continued treatment.

In seven patients, after stopping treatment, a rechallenge with the original dose was performed, after interruption of the treatment for an average of 11.6 days. In six of those patients this led to a prompt reappearance of the symptoms. In five patients a rechallenge was performed, using a 'titration' schedule, starting with a low dose and then gradually increasing the dosage. In three of the patients this led to a reappearance of the symptoms, whereas the remaining two patients were symptom-free.

In all patients where adequate follow-up data were available, a complete recovery was seen.

2. OTHER REPORTS OF FEBRILE REACTIONS

When zimeldine was in general use, reactions of the kinds described above were reported to the various national adverse reaction reporting schemes. Data from such reports in Sweden and UK have been reviewed [15] and the pattern was quite similar to what had been found in the clinical trials. The incidence of reported adverse reactions in the above-mentioned countries was estimated by Astra to be between 0.3 – 0.4%; however, it is well known that these official adverse reaction reporting systems tend to markedly underestimate the real incidence of adverse reactions.

Single cases of varieties of febrile reactions have been published from Sweden [16 – 18] and also from other countries [19 – 22]. These reports have in many cases tended to focus on the liver function disturbance; however, when the actual case descriptions are scrutinized, the clinical picture shows great similarities to the cases described above.

Cases occurring in clinical trials have also been described in various publications (see e.g. [14, 23 – 25]).

IV. Epidemiology and clinical characteristics of cases of neuropathy

A variety of drugs has been associated with peripheral neuropathy [26]. In most cases the mechanisms are poorly understood. In the case of zimeldine, as will be discussed below, there was a clear-cut increase over the background incidence of the Guillain-Barré syndrome, but also reports of other types of peripheral neuropathy. Since the Guillain-Barré cases are the most well-defined and permit comparisons with known background incidences we will focus the discussion on these cases.

1. BACKGROUND DATA ON THE GUILLAIN-BARRÉ SYNDROME

The Guillain-Barré syndrome is an uncommon disease, with incidence rates in the range 1 – 2 cases/100 000 population/year [27]. By a generally accepted definition [28], clinical features required for diagnosis are: progressive motor weakness of more than one limb and absent tendon reflexes. Among important supportive findings is elevation of spinal fluid protein levels. A variety of factors has been associated with the syndrome, such as infections of various kinds, vaccinations, immunologic diseases, endocrine and metabolic disturbances, chemicals, preceding surgery, etc. (for review, see [29]). The most conclusive association hitherto reported has been with certain vaccine batches used in the 1976 – 1977 influenza vaccination campaign in the USA [30].

Interestingly, the Guillain-Barré syndrome can occur in serum sickness [31] and it is commonly believed that in most cases the development of the syndrome has an immunologic background (see e.g. [32]).

2. THE GUILLAIN-BARRÉ CASES IN ZIMELDINE-TREATED PATIENTS

As mentioned earlier, in August 1983 eight cases of Guillain-Barré syndrome in zimeldine-treated patients were known to Astra, seven of which had occurred in Sweden. Details of these cases were outlined in a document, which formed an important part of the basis for the withdrawal [33]. These cases, and an additional six cases, which were either reported later, or not known to Astra in August 1983, were analyzed by an expert group, gathered by the Swedish Drug Board. This group later published their analysis [34]. Out of the 13 cases in this report, 10 were judged to fulfil the criteria for the Guillain-Barré syndrome and the remaining cases had much in common with the 10 Guillain-Barré cases. The time course was similar to that mentioned above, i.e. in every case the symptoms started within the first month of treatment, and in each case the neurologic symptoms were preceded by a febrile illness. Table 3 summarizes the most important clinical data in this analysis (data reproduced with permission from the authors).

TABLE 3

Characteristics of Guillain-Barré syndrome in zimeldine-treated patients

Case No.	Sex/age	Duration of treatment[a]	Initial symptoms	Neurologic symptoms
1.	F/47	11/14	Fever, myalgia, photophobia	Limb weakness and paraesthesiae; cranial nerve palsies; areflexia arms and legs; respiratory paralysis.
2.	M/61	6/11	Fever, myalgia, headache, nausea	Severe limb weakness, mild sensory loss; cranial nerve palsies; postural hypotension; areflexia arms, legs.
3.	F/81	15/23	Fever, myalgia	Severe leg weakness; sensory loss arms and legs; areflexia legs; plantar response extensor?
4.	M/49	14/26	Fever, myalgia	Severe distal limb weakness, inability to walk unaided; sensory loss arms, legs; facial nerve palsy; areflexia legs.
5.	M/65	17/18	Fever, sore throat, myalgia	Severe leg weakness; sensory loss arms, legs; bladder paresis; areflexia legs.
6.	F/63	9/22	Fever, myalgia, headache	Severe limb weakness; sensory loss arms, legs; ataxia; areflexia arms, legs.

TABLE 3 (*continued*)

Case No.	Sex/age	Duration of treatment[a]	Initial symptoms	Neurologic symptoms
7.	M/72	14/20	Fever, myalgia, nausea	Slight leg weakness; paraesthesiae arms, legs; leg ataxia; areflexia legs.
8.	F/70	14/18	Fever, myalgia, sore throat	Severe leg weakness, slight arm weakness; limb paraesthesiae; leg ataxia; areflexia legs.
9.	M/52	14/27	Fever, nausea	Slight foot weakness, numbness, paraesthesiae feet; facial nerve palsies; areflexia legs.
10.	M/68	9/16	Fever, myalgia	Moderate leg weakness, inability to walk unaided; mild sensory loss, leg ataxia; facial nerve palsies; areflexia legs.
11.	F/52	14/24	Fever, myalgia, exanthema, headache, nausea, conjunctivitis	Sensory loss in trunk, face, tongue; facial nerve palsies; no areflexia.
12.	M/72	8/17	Fever	Severe limb weakness with muscle wasting; sensory loss arms, legs; areflexia arms, legs.
13.	M/68	16/30	Myalgia, fever	Severe limb weakness with muscle wasting; sensory loss legs; painful paraesthesiae legs, hands; areflexia arms, legs.

[a] Days of treatment before initial symptoms/days of treatment before first neurologic symptoms. (Data, with permission, from Fagius et al., 1985 [34].)

3. INCIDENCE – RISK INCREASE

In our own analysis, it was estimated that the seven Guillain-Barré cases reported in Sweden related to a treated population of approximately 75 000 patients, which would point to an incidence of approximately one Guillain-Barré case per 10 000 patients treated. This should be compared to the expected background incidence of approximately one case per 100 000 population and year, i.e. the zimeldine treatment increased the risk to develop Guillain-Barré syndrome by approximately a factor 10. However, the background incidence figures are annual incidences, whereas it should be clear from Table 3 that all Guillain-Barré cases occurred during the first treatment month. Making various assumptions about the risk period and the background incidence, it was calculated that the size of the risk increase (relative risk) was in the range between 56 and 224 (B. Huitfeldt, personal communication).

The independent group cited above [34] used other methods of calculating the relative risk and came to an estimated increase in incidence of the Guillain-Barré syndrome in zimeldine-treated patients as compared to the general population of between 23 and 31.

4. OTHER CASES OF PERIPHERAL NEUROPATHY

In addition to the reports of the Guillain-Barré syndrome, there were reports also about other kinds of neuropathy [33]. In many of these cases the connection with zimeldine treatment was uncertain, and background incidence figures were unobtainable. Four cases of facial (Bell's) palsy were reported, with a time course quite similar to the Guillain-Barré cases. Three patients had entrapment neuropathy (two cases of carpal tunnel syndrome and one case of severe Paget's disease of the neck). One elderly patient developed 'foot drop', one patient an ulnar neuropathy and two sensory neuropathies of the lower limbs.

The report cited above, with the ambition of absolute completeness, also described further cases of possible neurologic symptoms, such as paraesthesiae, headache, extrapyramidal symptoms, etc.; however, most of these cases were not judged to be suggestive of peripheral neuropathy and in many cases the connection between the symptoms and zimeldine treatment was judged uncertain.

Two cases of peripheral neuropathy other than Guillain-Barré have also been published [35].

In summary, it has been well established that zimeldine treatment can be associated with peripheral neuropathy. The evidence, on a single case basis as well as epidemiologically, is convincing in case of the Guillain-Barré syndrome and suggestive in case of certain other kinds of peripheral neuropathy. From the clinical point of view, the development of the Guillain-Barré syndrome of zimeldine-treated patients has been intimately associated with preceding symptoms of febrile reactions of the kind described in the preceding section.

V. Investigations into the pathogenetic mechanisms of adverse reactions

Several hypotheses have been put forward to explain the mechanisms underlying the febrile reactions and the Guillain-Barré syndrome in zimeldine-treated patients. The most important of these hypotheses are: (1) the mechanism is related to the pharmacological action of the drug; (2) the mechanism is related to the formation of a toxic metabolite [14]; (3) the mechanism is related to an immunologic reaction to antigens created in the presence of zimeldine and metabolites.

As research by us and others into the mechanism of the adverse reactions has progressed, the indications for an immunologic mechanism have gradually become strengthened. We have, therefore, focused most of the research efforts towards this possibility. We have, however, considered a number of other possibilities, such as direct toxicity, formation of abnormal metabolites or high drug levels, serotonin-related effects, etc., and will discuss also these possibilities.

The original suspicions of an immunological mechanism were based on the time course and symptomatology of the febrile reactions. Most commonly, 'drug fever' has an immunologic background [36, 37]. Once reports about cases of the Guillain-Barré syndrome started to emerge, the suspicions were strengthened by the fact that the Guillain-Barré syndrome is commonly regarded as having an immunologic background [32], and that the syndrome and other peripheral neuropathies can occur as a complication of a classic immunological disorder − serum sickness [31]. Also, the prompt recurrence of symptoms on rechallenge, in the cases where this was performed, would point strongly in the direction of an immunologic mechanism.

A drug can cause disease via immunologic mechanisms in at least three different ways: (1) the drug or a metabolite may exert toxic effects on immunologic organs, targets or cells; (2) the pharmacological activity of the drug may have a modulatory effect on immune function; and (3) the treatment may induce an immune response to an antigenic determinant created in the presence of the drug or some of its metabolites.

In our experimental as well as clinical research work into the pathogenetic mechanisms we have considered all these possibilities.

In the final part of this section we also describe the findings of a retrospective case-control type of study, where patients who had experienced a febrile reaction were compared with matched controls. The main aim of this study was to investigate whether there existed any difference in background characteristics of the patients with adverse reactions as compared to controls. If such differences existed they could shed further light on the pathogenetic mechanisms of the reactions but also, possibly, be used as predictors for a reaction.

1. TOXICITY OF ZIMELDINE OR METABOLITES TO THE IMMUNE SYSTEM

In the toxicology studies in various species [3], which involved long-term studies with extreme doses, there were no indications of effects on lymphoid organs or clinical signs of immune disturbances. Lüllman et al. found lamellar inclusions in lymphocytes and macrophages from rats treated with zimeldine [4] and similar findings also with chlorpromazine and some other drugs. In this context it is of interest that the cholestatic reactions commonly seen in chlorpromazine-treated patients may well have an immunologic background [38]. However, an investigation of lym-

TABLE 4

Toxicity of zimeldine and some of its metabolites as recorded in cultures of proliferating lymphocytes and growing human embryo cells, Flow 5000

Compound	Lymphocytes		Flow 5000 Cell number
	cell viability	^{3}H-thymidine in-corporation	
	IC$_{50}$ μM	IC$_{50}$ μM	IC$_{50}$ μM
Zimeldine	60 – 120	25 – 60	10 – 100
Norzimeldine	25 – 60	25 – 60	10 – 100
CPP 200	60 – 120	25 – 60	10 – 100
CPP 151	nd	75 – 150	nd
CPP 234	240 – 300	> 100	10 – 100
CPP 231	> 300	> 100	> 100
CPP 281	> 300	> 100	> 100
CPP 198	> 300	> 100	> 100

Lymphocytes, isolated on ficoll paque, were cultivated in the presence of purified protein derivative (PPD) 10 μg/ml and the tested drugs at various concentrations. Cell viability (trypan blue exclusion) and incorporation of tritiated thymidine into cells pulsed for 4 h were recorded after 5 days. Cultures of Flow 5000 were run for 48 h in the presence of the drugs, whereafter the number of cells were recorded. At this time control cultures had passed on average 1.5 cell cycles. Results are given as the interval of concentration where 50% inhibition was recorded (IC$_{50}$).
nd, not done.

phocytes in zimeldine-treated patients did not reveal any changes of the type seen by Lüllman et al. [3].

We also studied the toxicity of zimeldine and some of its metabolites (see Fig. 1) in cell cultures, using human peripheral blood mononuclear cells and human embryo cells Flow 5000 (Table 4). Zimeldine and the metabolites studied inhibited cellular proliferation at similar concentrations in both cell types used [39]. A sharp dose-response curve was recorded for the most cytotoxic compounds, i.e. norzimeldine, CPP 200, zimeldine and CPP 151, here listed according to their relative toxicity. At concentrations of 10 μM no inhibitory effects were seen. Thus, IC$_{50}$ values for cytotoxic effects were considerably higher than plasma concentrations after ordinary clinical dosage, which normally are in the range below 1 μM [5].

Thus, it seems improbable that a direct toxic mechanism on the immune system would be involved in the adverse reactions.

2. IMMUNOMODULATORY EFFECTS OF SEROTONIN

Zimeldine has been shown to reduce serotoninergic transmission [2] and to diminish levels of serotonin in platelets [40]. However, it is also conceivable that zimeldine,

TABLE 5

In vivo studies where zimeldine and norzimeldine were not found to exert immunomodulatory activity [47]

Animal	Antigen	Treatment	Immune response
Mice CBA	PO-BGG 0.5 μg s.c. neck	Zimeldine or nor- zimeldine 2 × 10 μmol/kg s.c. neck	Serum antibodies IgM, IgG (ELISA) IgE (PCA rats)
	day 0 – 4	day 0 – 10	day 14
Rats Sprague Dawley	PO-BGG 25 μg s.c. neck	Zimeldine or nor- zimeldine 2 × 10 μmol/kg s.c. neck	Serum antibodies IgG, IgM (ELISA)
	day 0 – 2	day 0 – 10	day 14
Mice CBA	Picryl chloride 0.5% abdomen, hind paws day 1 1%, ear day 6	Zimeldine 2 × 10 μmol/kg s.c. neck day 0 – 5	Ear swelling day 7
Mice CBA	Picryl chloride 0.5% abdomen, hind paws day 0 1%, ear day 6	Zimeldine or nor- zimeldine 10 μmol/kg, p.o. − 1 h, + 4 h (day 6)	Ear swelling day 7
Mice CBA	Picryl chloride 0.5% abdomen, hind paws day 14 1%, ear day 21	Zimeldine or nor- zimeldine 50 μmol/kg s.c., neck day 0 – 21	Serum antibodies IgG (ELISA, TNP-HSA) day 22, 28 Ear swelling day 22
Rats Sprague Dawley	PO-BGG 20 μg in Evans blue i.v. 72 h after passive sensitization	Zimeldine or nor- zimeldine 10 μmol/kg p.o. 2 h before elici- tation	PCA (IgE-containing PO-antiserum)

through cellular uptake inhibition, could give rise to locally increased concentrations of serotonin. Therefore, the pharmacological effect of zimeldine could be dual − either an increase or a decrease in triggering of serotonin-modulated targets.

The effects of serotonin on immune function have not been thoroughly studied, but it is known that pharmacological enhancement of 5-HT metabolism suppresses, e.g. antibody formation and graft rejections in vivo (reviewed in [41, 42]). This effect is thought to be mediated peripherally rather than centrally [43]. Serotonin has been shown to induce production of monocyte chemotactic factor [44], and macrophages have been shown to have an active serotonin uptake system [45]. Serotonin has also been shown to affect vascular permeability and to be involved in delayed type hypersensitivity responses in mice [46].

To investigate any possible immunomodulatory effects of zimeldine, we studied the influence of zimeldine and norzimeldine on antibody responses in mice and rats, delayed type hypersensitivity in mice, and passive cutaneous anaphylaxis (PCA) in rats ([47], Table 5). Neither substance, at a daily dose of 2×10 μmol/kg had any influence on IgE, IgG or IgM antibody responses to penicilloylated bovine gammaglobulin (PO-BGG). Induction and elicitation of delayed type hypersensitivity to picryl chloride in CBA mice was not influenced. Zimeldine or norzimeldine (10 μmol/kg) given orally 2 h before elicitation of passive cutaneous anaphylaxis in rats did not affect the titers recorded, while amitriptyline and mianserin at the same dose level were shown to exert an inhibitory effect [47]. Similarly, Henderson et al. [48] could not demonstrate any immunomodulatory effects of zimeldine or paroxetine, another 5-HT reuptake inhibitor. In their studies, the two drugs did not affect the development of anti-SRBC antibody secreting cells or mitogen-induced proliferation in vitro using spleen cells from treated $(C_{57}BL_{10} \times DBA_2)F_1$ mice. In experiments with peritoneal macrophages, treatment of mice with zimeldine (25 mg $\cdot$ kg^{-1} $\cdot$ day^{-1}) did not affect ex vivo capacity of peritoneal macrophages to form monolayers or the capacity of muramyl dipeptide activated macrophages to phagocytose sheep erythrocytes [48].

3. IMMUNOLOGIC RESPONSE TO ZIMELDINE AND ZIMELDINE-DERIVED STRUCTURES

As pointed out previously, the clinical characteristics of the adverse reactions to zimeldine, and the prompt recurrence of symptoms upon rechallenge with the drug, point to the possibility of an immune response to the drug or to antigens created in the presence of the drug. It has recently been hypothesized that such an event may also lead to a state of autoimmunity [49]. One of the suggested possibilities implies that haptens bound to autologous proteins may stimulate hapten-specific T cells to provide help to B cells binding to the carrier and thereby induce production of autoantibodies, giving rise to a graft-versus-host-like disease.

(a) Experimental studies of the immunogenic potential of zimeldine

Although evidence exists for immunogenicity of zimeldine in man, we also investigated the immunogenic potential in experimental systems.

(i) Binding to macromolecules. For a low molecular weight substance like zimeldine, covalent binding to macromolecules has generally been considered as a prerequisite for immunogenicity [50 – 54]. Zimeldine has a poor protein reactivity. Henderson et al. [48] could not demonstrate binding to either primary amino groups of human serum albumin or cystein thiol groups. However, it has been shown that low molecular weight substances can form reactive intermediary metabolites, via biotransformation in the liver [55], gut [56] or skin [57]. Such reactive metabolites may be able to conjugate to proteins and thus form immunogens.

Even if covalent coupling has been the major concept to explain sensitization to drugs, little evidence is actually available on this point in man [58]. It is plausible that the most important criterion for immunogenicity of haptens is not the capacity to bind covalently to proteins but rather the overall stability of the hapten protein complex [59]. In some cases multiple salt linkages appear sufficient to induce an immune response. Acid polymers like nucleic acids and oligonucleotides can be made immunogenic by complexing with basic protein carriers such as methylated bovine serum albumin [60, 61]. Since zimeldine has amphiphilic properties, it is conceivable that the compound may interact directly on the phospholipid bilayer of cell membranes, or after accumulation within lysosomes create an immunogenic determinant in association with other membrane determinants. Such a hypothesis would be supported by the findings of lamellar inclusions in lymphocytes and macrophages in the rat [4]. These inclusions are believed to be due to complex formation between cationic amphiphilic drugs and certain polar lipids [62].

Whatever the mechanism of formation of a complex between a drug and macromolecules may be, it is difficult to predict the antigenic specificity resulting from such binding. This may be one of the major reasons why tests for specific antibodies in patients hypersensitive to drugs have had such limited success.

In summary, zimeldine and the metabolites identified do not have a strong protein reactivity and would thus not conventionally be expected to behave as strong immunogens. However, an unidentified reactive metabolite or efficient protein association via other mechanisms could create sufficiently effective antigen presentation for an immune reaction to be initiated.

(ii) Immune responses to zimeldine conjugates. When attempting to induce experimental immune responses to zimeldine, we used a traditional approach, coupling the succinylated derivative of norzimeldine to carbodiimide-activated bovine gamma globulin (BGG) and human serum albumin (HSA) [63]. Sprague Dawley rats were immunized with norzimeldine succinic acid amide-BGG (Norzim-BGG) in

Freunds complete adjuvant. A hapten-specific IgG and IgM antibody response developed, as measured with ELISA technique, using HSA as carrier for conjugated norzimeldine [47]. Hapten inhibition studies showed equal inhibitory capacity for zimeldine and norzimeldine, indicating that the induced immune response was directed towards structures common for both compounds (Fig. 2). Although the rat strain used readily developed antibodies to conjugated norzimeldine, we were unable to demonstrate antibodies to Norzim-HSA in sera from rats after dietary administration of zimeldine for 3 months.

Norzim-HSA was also used in an attempt to demonstrate antibodies to zimeldine in allergic employees and hypersensitive patients (see below for further comments about these individuals). IgG antibodies binding to Norzim-HSA were found in sera from both categories investigated, but antibodies were also found to a similar extent in sera of individuals never exposed to zimeldine [39] (Table 6). Allergic employees, hypersensitive patients and unexposed controls were all found to respond to Norzim-HSA in lymphocyte transformation test (LTT; see further below about details of the technique), but this ability was not found related to LTT responsiveness to zimeldine or norzimeldine (unpublished results). Furthermore, zimeldine treatment and febrile reactions in hypersensitive patients did not affect the serum levels of Norzim-HSA-binding antibodies (Table 6).

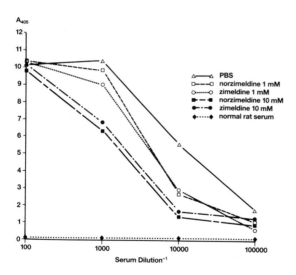

Fig. 2. IgG antibodies against conjugated norzimeldine in serially diluted serum, pooled from five rats immunized with Norzim-BGG in Freunds complete adjuvant, as analysed with ELISA using Norzim-HSA as antigen. The antisera were serially diluted in phosphate-buffered saline (PSB) containing 20% normal rat serum. Zimeldine and norzimeldine were equally efficient to inhibit binding of antibodies, when added to diluted antiserum 30 min before start of incubation in antigen-coated tubes. The amount of antibodies bound is given as optical density recorded at A_{405}.

TABLE 6

IgG antibodies to Norzim-HSA in sera from hypersensitive patients, allergic employees and unexposed controls analysed with ELISA

		Prior to exposure				After febrile or allergic reaction			
		(serum dilution)$^{-1}$				(serum dilution)$^{-1}$			
		20	40	100	1000	20	40	100	1000
Hypersensitive patients	1	0.78	0.46	0.05	0.03	0.78	0.46	0.25	0.18
	2	0.38	0.21	0.19	0.13	0.53	0.20	0.16	0.12
	3	1.80	1.17	0.76	0.25	1.74	1.12	0.69	0.20
	4	1.28	1.08	0.67	0.27	1.29	1.06	0.61	0.19
	5	1.31	0.65	0.43	0.18	1.62	0.90	0.51	0.16
	6	0.93	0.70	0.33	0.12	0.82	0.43	0.30	0.06
	7					1.49	0.60	0.33	0.21
	8					1.64	1.17	0.60	0.15
Unexposed controls	1	1.57	1.19	0.79	0.34				
	2	0.83	0.67	0.36	0.17				
	3	1.26	1.27	0.85	0.36				
	4	0.93	0.73	0.34	0.26				
	5	1.03	0.74	0.46	0.24				
Allergic employees	1					1.66	0.70	0.47	0.15
	2					1.30	0.48	0.30	0.05

Sera from hypersensitive patients were prepared before start of treatment and within 2 weeks after development of febrile reactions. IgG antibody values are given as optical density A_{405}.

We, therefore, conclude that the antigenic determinant created in Norzim-HSA, although capable of inducing a hapten-specific immune response in animals, is probably not relevant for the adverse reactions seen in man.

(iii) Epicutaneous sensitization. Epicutaneous sensitization has so far been the most successful tool to demonstrate immunogenic capacity of low molecular weight compounds. We failed to demonstrate a sensitizing capacity of zimeldine using the Magnusson-Kligman guinea pig sensitization test [64, 65]. One reason for this could be that only low concentrations of the compound could be used in the initial sensitization, since zimeldine, being a dihydrochloride is locally irritating.

Henderson et al. [48] found zimeldine to be a weak to moderate sensitizer in Dunkin-Hartley guinea pigs, using a modified split adjuvant contact sensitivity test [66]. It is notable that they were unable to demonstrate antibodies to Norzim-ovalbumin in sensitized guinea pigs. Their results are in agreement with our results in hypersensitive patients and employees with occupational allergy to zimeldine, where immunological reactivity to Norzim-HSA was found to be unrelated to exposure or sensitization to zimeldine. This supports the notion that the antigenic determinants created by coupling norzimeldine to proteins by conventional methods may lack relevance for immune responses to zimeldine in man.

(iiii) Results with the popliteal lymph node assay. Thomas et al. have studied zimeldine and related compounds using the popliteal lymph node assay (C. Thomas, personal communication). In the popliteal lymph node (PLN) assay, drugs like diphenylhydantoin (DPH) and D-penicillamine have been shown to induce a pathology showing similarities to graft-versus-host reactions [67, 68]. Both these drugs are known to induce adverse effects of suspected immunologic origin and with clinical similarities to the febrile reactions seen with zimeldine. Furthermore, DPH-specific lymphoproliferation in vitro has been demonstrated in several patients sensitized to the drug [69].

Using the PLN assay in mice, Thomas et al. found zimeldine, norzimeldine and the E-enantiomer of zimeldine to be potent inducers of lymph node enlargment, while CPP 200 and brompheniramine were less potent and CPP 198 inactive (see Fig. 1 for formulae). Zimeldine, norzimeldine and the E-enantiomer of zimeldine, but not CPP 200 and brompheniramine, were potent inducers of a prolonged IgG antibody response. Since none of the compounds were found to be mitogenic in vitro, the results indicate that proliferation as well as antibody production are due to a specific immunological mechanism. However, the specificity of the induced IgG antibody response remains to be determined.

These findings, together with the previous ones with the PLN assay, may indicate that this assay could be used for predictions about potential immunological problems with new drugs.

(b) Immunogenic potential of zimeldine in man

The capacity of zimeldine to induce an immunological response in exposed humans is obvious from the finding that three employees at Astra have developed allergy to the compound. After occupational exposure in the production unit or development of pharmaceutical preparations of zimeldine, these individuals all exhibited symptoms of rhinitis, excema and swelling of eye lids. Two of the individuals were skin tested with zimeldine. Both had a positive patch test to zimeldine and one of them tested with prick test was positive to zimeldine also in this test. All three gave a positive response to zimeldine in the lymphocyte transformation test, while five control individuals, three of which had been working with zimeldine, all were negative in the LTT [70]. The lymphocyte proliferative responses to zimeldine were recorded both as increases in lymphocyte incorporation of ^{3}H-thymidine and as induced blastogenesis in May-Grünwald-Giemsa-stained smears (Fig. 3).

These individuals offered an opportunity to study the specificity of the immune response to zimeldine in man. Apart from zimeldine, lymphocytes from the allergic individuals were challenged with the E-enantiomer and seven of the metabolites (see Fig. 1) identified in zimeldine-treated patients [6, 71]. These studies demonstrated that the allergenic structure involved comprised the allyl amine part of zimeldine [70] (Fig. 3). Thus, zimeldine induced the strongest responses, the Z- and E-

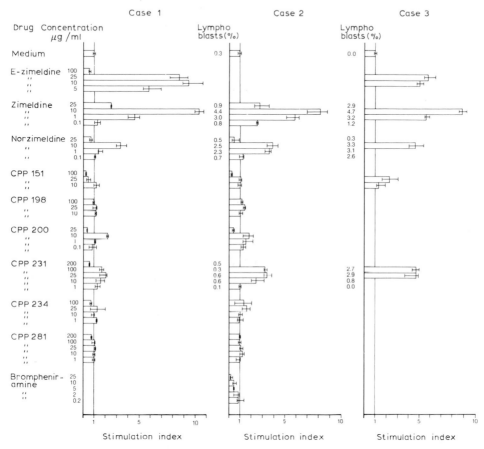

Fig. 3. Lymphoproliferative responses to zimeldine and related structures recorded for three allergic employees in LTT. Mononuclear cells were isolated from defibrinated peripheral blood and 10^6 cells incubated for 5 days in the presence of various concentrations of the compounds diluted in RPMI 1640. After washing, May-Grünwald-Giemsa stained smears were prepared and 10^5 cells were added in triplicates onto microplates and incubation was carried on for another 4 h in the presence of tritiated thymidine. The amount of incorporated ^{3}H-thymidine was recorded after harvesting cells on filter discs. Results are presented as mean and max.-min. of stimulation index (SI) of two or three cultures run in parallel.

$$SI = \frac{\text{cpm in culture cultivated with drug}}{\text{cpm in culture cultivated with medium}}$$

The percentage of lymphoblasts was calculated in May-Grünwald-Giemsa stained smears.

204

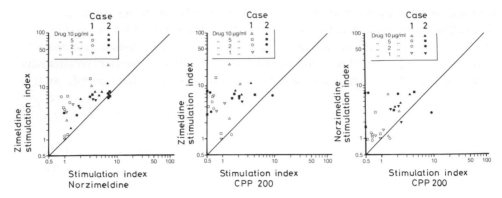

Fig. 4. The reproducibility in relative potency of zimeldine, norzimeldine and CPP 200 to trigger LTT responses in two allergic employees tested at six different occasions over a period of 2 years after terminated exposure. For methods, see Fig. 3.

enantiomers both being potent. Norzimeldine was more potent than the primary amine (CPP 200) and N-oxide (CPP 231) of zimeldine. Metabolites where the nitrogen of the allyl amine chain had been lost did not induce lymphocyte proliferation. Brompheniramine showed no cross-reactivity with zimeldine. Since the magnitude of LTT responses is known to show a great variability between test and sampling occasions [72], two of the allergic employees were repeatedly tested to establish their relative responsiveness to zimeldine, norzimeldine and CPP 200 in LTT. Although a considerable variability in magnitude of LTT responses was recorded between test occasions, the relative potency of the compounds was found to be consistent (Fig. 4).

None of the compounds tested was found to be mitogenic or to potentiate PPD-induced proliferative responses in lymphocytes from normal donors. However, it is notable that the peak responses in the LTT of allergic employees were recorded at concentrations close to those causing inhibition of PPD responses in lymphocytes from normal donors.

We found no relationship between the potency of the compounds to induce lymphocyte proliferation and their potency regarding 5-HT uptake inhibition. In this respect, norzimeldine is more potent than zimeldine and the E-enantiomer of zimeldine is far less active than the clinically used Z-enantiomer [73].

On the other hand, the relative potency of zimeldine and metabolites to elicit LTT responses in allergic employees corresponded well to their relative capacity to induce IgG antibody production in the popliteal lymph node assay in mice (see above).

(c) LTT responses in patients with febrile reactions and/or neuropathy

Having found that individuals sensitized by occupational exposure to zimeldine gave a positive response in the LTT, we used this test to investigate, in retrospect, patients who had gone through a febrile reaction [74]. The patients investigated, as well as the controls, took part in a retrospective case-control study [75] described later in this section.

A total of 55 patients was investigated, 27 controls who had been treated with zimeldine without developing any adverse reaction and 28 patients with a documented febrile reaction, three of which had developed a Guillain-Barré syndrome. Data concerning zimeldine therapy and timing of adverse reactions are given in Table 7.

Zimeldine and the two metabolites tested (norzimeldine and CPP 200) were found to induce proliferative responses (measured as increase in ^{3}H-thymidine incorporation) in lymphocyte cultures from patients who had experienced febrile reactions (Fig. 5). Patients classified as having suffered from a severe febrile reaction showed the most marked responses in LTT. Responses of low magnitude were recorded also for a small number of the controls. Compared to the responses in the allergic employees, the responses in the patients were lower (cf. Fig. 3). Interestingly, the relative potency of the various compounds tested differed between the two groups (Fig. 4). In the allergic employees zimeldine was most potent, whereas in patients norzimeldine was significantly more potent ($p < 0.01$, Wilcoxon rank sum test).

These results demonstrate that zimeldine-treated patients who have gone through

TABLE 7

Zimeldine therapy and timing of febrile reactions in patients investigated for lymphoproliferative responses to zimeldine in vitro

	Patients		Controls
	Hypersensitivity reactions		
	severe	mild + moderate	
Number of cases	16	12	27
Treatment with zimeldine:			
mg/day (mean ± SD)	230 ± 50	217 ± 39	209 ± 44
patients with lower initial dose	6	5	7
days of treatment (median)	17	17	214
days of treatment (min.-max.)	10 – 56	12 – 264	34 – 1689
Start of febrile reaction:			
days of treatment (median)	12	12	–
days of treatment (min.-max.)	8 – 20	7 – 19	–
Interval last dose-LTT:			
days (median)	659	595	550
days (min.-max.)	263 – 1313	278 – 1242	0 – 1270

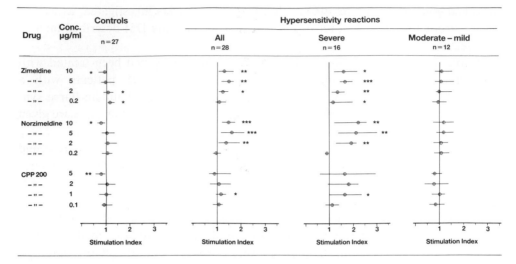

Fig. 5. Lymphoproliferative responses to zimeldine, norzimeldine and CPP 200 in hypersensitive and control patients assayed as increase in ^{3}H-thymidine incorporation in lymphocyte cultures after 5 days of culture in the presence of drug. For each patient stimulation index (SI) was calculated from

$$SI = \frac{\text{median of cpm in 3 cultures cultivated with drug}}{\text{median of cpm in 5 cultures cultivated with medium}}$$

Results are presented as medians of SI for the various groups of patients with 89 – 96% non-parametric confidence intervals. Significantly increased (decreased) responses are indicated by * ($p < 0.05$), ** ($p < 0.01$) and *** ($p < 0.001$).

a febrile reaction have memory cells reactive to the drug. The magnitude of the in vitro response is correlated to the severity of the reaction.

Although the positive LTT responses in patients who had gone through a febrile reaction can not be regarded as conclusive evidence for an underlying immunologic mechanism, we feel that these findings point strongly in that direction.

4. CHARACTERISTICS OF PATIENTS WITH FEBRILE REACTIONS – A CASE-CONTROL STUDY

Based on the hypothesis that the febrile reactions and neuropathy encountered in zimeldine-treated patients had an immunologic background, we speculated that those patients who developed such reactions could represent a particularly susceptible group of individuals. Therefore, a case-control type of study was set up, where patients who had gone through a febrile reaction were investigated and compared to matched controls [75, 76].

The most important method used in the study was a careful interview with each patient and control, about details in their psychiatric illness, previous medical history, medications and certain other variables. As cited above, an investigation of lymphocyte reactivity was also performed in most of the patients and controls, and in addition investigations of the HLA antigen characteristics were performed. Finally, in a small number of the patients certain pharmacologic variables were investigated.

A total of 35 cases (patients who had gone through a febrile reaction) and 51 matched controls (zimeldine-treated patients who had not developed an adverse reaction) took part in the study, which was retrospective. In most cases the investigations took place approximately 1–2 years after the adverse reaction. The groups were well matched with regard to age, sex, weight and height.

(a) Results of interviews – medical background characteristics

In brief, only one major difference between the groups was found, namely that the proportion who had undergone psychotropic drug treatment during the 2 years preceding the zimeldine treatment was higher (67%) in the controls than in the cases (26%). For the other variables included in the interview no differences were found between the groups. These variables were: the indications for treatment, dosage of zimeldine, previous psychiatric history, previous medical history, presence of allergy to other drugs or food, use of alcohol and tobacco, food habits, previous anaesthesia or blood transfusion, history of diseases in the family.

Thus, within the limitations of the interview method, no important differences between the groups could be demonstrated, i.e. no clinically useful predictor could be identified.

(b) HLA antigen determinations

Low molecular weight compounds have been claimed to bind directly to HLA-coded structures on the surface of mononuclear cells, and induction of immunity to a compound would thereby be genetically restricted at this level [49]. For certain diseases, a well-documented relationship to HLA haplotype exists [77]. Also for some drug-induced disorders a similar relationship has been established, e.g. for hypersensitivity to gold or D-penicillamine in the tratment of rheumatoid arthritis [78] and hydralazine-induced systemic lupus erythematosus [79].

However, we found no difference in the panel of tested HLA A, B, C and DR haplotypes between the cases and the controls [80]. Thus, lymphoproliferative responses to zimeldine in vitro were not found to be related to HLA-type. This is in agreement with the other findings of the case-control study, i.e. that no features, except the adverse reaction, could be found that distinguished the adverse reaction patients from treated individuals who had not developed such a reaction.

(c) Pharmacologic investigations in adverse reaction patients

We also investigated, in pilot scale, whether the adverse reaction patients had any distinguishing pharmacologic features (unpublished data). We could not demonstrate any distinct abnormalities in hydroxylation capacity, and both slow and fast acetylators were found. Serotonin concentrations in thrombocytes showed no abnormalities.

Previous investigations in adverse reaction patients had shown that these had plasma concentrations within the normal range, except for some elevations during the actual reaction period, which were judged to be due to a concomitant elevation of alpha$_1$-acid glycoprotein (K.-G. Jostell, personal communication).

VI. Summarizing discussion

It is our considered opinion, based on the research performed by us and others, that the febrile reactions and neuropathies seen in patients treated with zimeldine have been caused by an immunologic reaction directed against antigens related to zimeldine or some of its metabolites. After having discussed alternative possibilities, we will briefly summarize and discuss the evidence speaking in favour of this kind of mechanism.

The main alternative explanation that has been considered during the research work has been that the adverse reactions have been caused by a pharmacologic or toxic effect. Investigators in Canada, who observed quite a high incidence of adverse reactions in their patients, have argued for such a pathogenetic mechanism [14].

The main arguments in favour of a pharmacologic or toxic mechanism are: (a) zimeldine represents a new pharmacologic principle − 5-HT uptake inhibition − which could give rise to unexpected effects; (b) zimeldine is a new molecule, with a potential for unknown toxic effects; and (c) in certain clinical studies, where a relatively high daily dose (300 mg) was used, a high proportion of patients showed adverse reactions [14].

We feel, however, that the arguments speaking against a pharmacologic or toxic mechanism are convincing. The most important of those arguments are:

(a) Normally, pharmacologic or toxic effects would be dose-dependent and thus the cumulative dose important for the development of adverse reactions. This has not been the case with zimeldine; the adverse reactions in a limited number of patients have developed after relatively short periods of treatment. Great numbers of patients have been treated over prolonged periods, without developing adverse reactions. Very high doses (many patients on 400 mg daily, a limited number up to 1 200 mg daily) have been used, without problems of the type discussed in this chapter.

(b) There have been no indications for abnormal plasma concentrations of the parent compound or metabolites in patients with reactions. A group of patients of very old age (above 80 years) was treated with a relatively high dose (200 mg) and had high plasma concentration of norzimeldine without developing adverse reactions [81].

(c) Compounds with a similar pharmacologic mechanism (e.g. fluoxetine and fluvoxamine) have been used in large numbers of patients without causing adverse reactions of the type seen with zimeldine. Fluoxetine has been used without problems in patients who previously had developed adverse reactions during treatment with zimeldine [82].

(d) A major experimental program of pharmacology and toxicology studies, in several animal species, including life-time studies in two species, has failed to demonstrate any findings similar to those seen in man.

The major findings, supporting an immunologic mechanism are:
(a) Zimeldine can be immunogenic, as demonstrated in experimental systems and through occupational allergy in employees, verified by skin testing and in vitro lymphocyte transformation tests (LTT).

(b) The clinical characteristics of the febrile reactions both concerning symptomatology and time course show considerable similarity to well-documented immunologic states, e.g. serum sickness, and to other drug-induced disorders known to be of immunologic origin.

(c) Febrile reactions to zimeldine have been demonstrated to recur promptly on rechallenge with the drug.

(d) The Guillain-Barré syndrome is generally thought to have an immunologic background.

(e) Patients who have gone through adverse reactions have been demonstrated to have memory cells with immunologic specificity directed towards antigens related to zimeldine and metabolites.

Concerning the specificity of the postulated immune response, we found that the antigenic determinant created by covalent binding of the allyl amine part of the zimeldine molecule to protein carriers is not relevant for sensitization to zimeldine. Specificity studies with LTT in hypersensive patients and allergic employees showed that small alterations in the allyl amine part of the zimeldine molecule affected the ability to trigger memory cells. These results could reflect different abilities of compounds to form hapten-carrier linkage, but could also be caused by actual differences in the antigenic determinants recognized by memory cells. The failure to demonstrate HLA haplotype as a factor of importance for developing febrile reactions and LTT responses to zimeldine indicates that differences between HLA-coded molecules reflected in the studied panel of antibodies against HLA A, B, C and DR antigens are not critical for antigen formation or triggering of febrile reactions or LTT responses to zimeldine.

210

The fact that zimeldine consistently gave rise to responses in the LTT shows that metabolic processes in liver, gut or skin are not a prerequisite for triggering of memory cells. If this also is true for the processing and presentation of antigenic structures responsible for sensitization is unknown. Pilot studies of the stability of zimeldine and norzimeldine in lymphocyte cultures did not show any metabolic breakdown during the 5-day incubation period (unpublished results) and, thus, did not reveal that metabolic breakdown of zimeldine played a part in the process of lymphocyte stimulation.

In summary, patients treated with a new 5-HT reuptake inhibitor – zimeldine – developed febrile reactions and in rare cases peripheral neuropathy, including the Guillain-Barré syndrome. Available evidence suggests that the underlying mechanism has been an immunological reaction directed towards antigens related to zimeldine.

References

1. Heel, R. C., Morley, P. A., Brogden, R. N., Carmine, A. A., Speight, T. M. and Avery G. S. (1982) Zimeldine: a review of its pharmacological properties and therapeutic efficacy in depressive illness. Drugs 24, 169 – 206.
2. Ögren, S. O., Ross, S. B., Hall, H., Holm, A. C. and Renyi, A. L. (1981) The pharmacology of zimeldine: a 5-HT selective reuptake inhibitor. Acta Psychiat. Scand. 63, Suppl. 290, 127 – 151.
3. Malmfors, T. (1983) Toxicological studies on zimeldine. Acta Pharm. Suec. 20, 295 – 310.
4. Bockhardt, H. and Lüllman-Rauch, R. (1980) Zimeldine-induced lipidosis in rats. Acta Pharmacol. Toxicol. 47, 45 – 48.
5. Lundström, J. (1981) Summary of human-pharmacokinetical data. Astra, data on file.
6. Lundström, J., Högberg, T., Gostonyi, T. and de Paulis, T. (1981) Metabolism of zimeldine in rat, dog and man. Arzneimittelforsch. 31, 486 – 494.
7. Pottage, A. and Grind, M. (1982) Cardiovascular effects of zimeldine. Acta Psychiat. Scand. 68, Suppl. 308, 125 – 130.
8. Seppälä, T. and Linnoila, M. (1983) Effects of zimeldine and other antidepressants on skilled performance: a comprehensive review. Acta Psychiat. Scand. 68, Suppl. 308, 135 – 140.
9. Huitfeldt, B. and Montgomery, S. A. (1983) Comparison between zimeldine and amitriptyline of efficacy and adverse symptoms – a combined analysis of four British trials in depression. Acta Psychiat. Scand. 68, Suppl. 308, 55 – 69.
10. Claghorn, J., Gershon, S. and Goldstein, B. J. (1983) Zimeldine tolerability in comparison to amitriptyline and placebo: findings from a multicentre trial. Acta Psychiat. Scand. 68, Suppl. 308, 104 – 114.
11. Groschinsky-Grind, M., Cott, J. and Nilsson, B. S. (1980) Influence of antidepressive drugs on liver function. Astra Report 805-04 A 201-2. Astra, data on file.
12. Nilsson, B. S., Grind, M., Lundberg, G., Huitfeldt, B., Jozwiak, H. and Pihl, M.-L. (1983) Hypersensitivity reactions during treatment with zimeldine. Observations on a 'drug-fever'-like syndrome occurring in a major clinical research program. Astra Report 805-04 AC062-1. Astra, data on file.
13. Matsos, G. (1983) Adverse reactions reported during zimeldine treatment of 212 depressed patients. Astra Report 805-04 AC 068-2. Astra, data on file.
14. Langlois, R., Cournoyer, G., De Montigny, C. and Caille G. (1985) High incidence of

multisystemic reactions to zimeldine. Eur. J. Clin. Pharmacol. 28, 67 – 71.

15. Nilsson, B. S. (1983) Adverse reactions in connection with zimeldine treatment – a review. Acta Psychiat. Scand. 68, Suppl. 308, 115 – 119.

16. Paulsen, O., Nilsson, L. M., Sellin, M., Österlind, A., Lundgren, M. and Fahlesson, P. (1983) Huvudvärk, muskelvärk och leverpåverkan – ny sjukdomsbild vid zimeldinbehandling. (Translation: Headache, myalgia and liver disturbance – new disease picture in zimeldine treatment). Läkartidningen (J. Swed. Med. Assoc.) 80, 31.

17. Ursing, B. and Persson, M.-H. (1983) Zimeldinbehandlade patienter fick feber och störd leverfunktion. (Translation: Zimeldine-treated patients developed pyrexia and disturbed liver function). Läkartidningen 80, 32.

18. Sköld, A., Lindholm, C.-G. and Karlsson, R. (1983) Ytterligare ett fall av zimeldinbiverkan. (Translation: A further case of adverse reaction to zimeldine). Läkartidningen 80, 1715.

19. Sommerville, L. S., McClaren, E. H., Campbell, L. M. and Watson, J. M. (1982) Severe headache and disturbed liver function during treatment with zimelidine. Br. Med. J. 285, 1009.

20. Simpson, G. K. and Davidson, N. M. (1983) Possible hepatotoxicity of zimelidine. Br. Med. J. 287, 1181.

21. Sawyer, C. N., Cleary, J. and Gabriel, R. (1983) Possible hepatotoxicity of zimelidine. Br. Med. J. 287, 1555.

22. Pomara, N., Coffman, K. L., Bush, D. F. and Gershon, S. (1984) Myalgia and elevation in muscle creatine phosphokinase during zimeldine treatment. J. Clin. Psychopharmacol. 4, 220 – 222.

23. Burrows, G. D., Norman, T. R., Marriott, P. F. and Davies, B. (1983) Zimeldine in depressive illness – efficacy and safety data. Acta Psychiat. Scand. Suppl. 308, 31 – 40.

24. Hiramatsu, K. I., Takahashi, R., Mori, A., Inoue, R., Kazamatsuri, H., Murasaki, M. and Sakuma, A. (1983) A multicentre double-blind comparative trial of zimeldine and imipramine in primary major depressive disorders. Acta Psychiat. Scand. 68, Suppl. 308, 41 – 54.

25. Larsen, F. W. and Hansen, C. E. (1984) Zimeldine versus amitriptyline in endogenous depression. A double-blind study with special reference to effects on liver function. Acta Psychiat. Scand. 69, 343 – 349.

26. Foster, J. B. and Stewart-Wynne, E. G. (1981) Neurological disorders. In: D. M. Davies (Ed.), Textbook of Adverse Drug Reactions, Oxford University Press, Oxford, pp. 436 – 448.

27. Schoenburg, B. S. (1978) Epidemiology of Guillain-Barré syndrome. Adv. Neurol. 19, 249 – 260.

28. National Institutes of Health (1978) Diagnostic criterions for Guillain-Barré. J. Am. Med. Assoc. 240, 1709 – 1710.

29. Leneman, F. (1966) The Guillain-Barré syndrome. Arch. Int. Med. 118, 139 – 144.

30. Schonberger, L. B., Bregman, D. J., Sullivan-Bolyai, J. Z., Keenlyside, R. A., Ziegler, D. W., Retailliau, H. F., Eddins, D. L. and Eddins, D. L. (1979) Guillain-Barré syndrome following vaccination in the national influenza immunization program. An.. J. Med. 110, 105 – 110, 105 – 123.

31. Arnason, B. G. W. (1975) Neuropathy of serum sickness. In: P. J. Dyck, P. K. Thomas and E. H. Lambert (Eds.), Peripheral Neuropathy, W. B. Saunders, Philadelphia, pp. 1104 – 1109.

32. Fink, J. N. and Arnason, B. G. W. (1982) Immunological aspects of neurological and neuromuscular diseases. J. Am. Med. Assoc. 248, 2710 – 2715.

33. Nilsson, B. S., Lundberg, G. and Pottage, A. (1983) Reports of neuropathy in patients treated with zimeldine. Astra Report 805-04 AC 071-1. Astra, data on file.

34. Fagius, J., Osterman, P.-O., Sidén, Å. and Wiholm, B.-E. (1985) Guillain-Barré syndrome following zimeldine treatment. J. Neurol. Neurosurg. Psychiat. 48, 65 – 69.

35. Dexter, S. L. (1984) Zimeldine induced neuropathies. Hum. Toxicol. 3, 141 – 143.

36. Lipsky, B. A. and Hirschmann, J. V. (1981) Drug fever. J. Am. Med. Assoc. 245, 851 – 854.

37. Townsend, Y. and Cranston, W. I. (1981) Disorders of temperature regulation. In: D. M. Davies (Ed.), Textbook of Adverse Drug Reaction, Oxford University Press, Oxford, pp. 597 – 601.

38. Mullock, B. M., Hall, D. E., Shaw, L. J. and Hinton, R. H. (1983) Immune responses to chlorpromazine in rats. Detection and relation to hepatoxicity. Biochem. Pharmacol. 32, 18, 2733 – 2738.

39. Kristofferson, A., Andersson, M. and Sohl Åkerlund, A. (1983) Investigations of immunological reactivity to zimeldine in sera and lymphocytes of patients with hypersensitivity reactions. A preliminary report. Astra Report 805-04 AF 58-1. Astra, data on file.

40. Ross, S. B., Aperia, J., Beck-Friis, S., Jansa, L., Wetterberg, L. and Åberg, A. (1980) Inhibition of 5-hydroxytryptamine uptake in human platelets by antidepressant agents in vivo. Psychopharmacology, 67, 1 – 7.

41. Maestroni, G. J. M. and Pierpaoli, W. (1981) Pharmacologic control of hormonally mediated immune response. In: R. Ader (Ed.), Psychoneuroimmunology, Academic Press, New York, pp. 405 – 428.

42. Walker, R. F. and Codd, E. E. (1985) Neuroimmunomodulatory interactions of norepinephrine and serotonin. J. Neuroimmunol. 10, 41 – 58.

43. Jackson, J. C., Cross, R. J., Walker, R. F., Markesbery, W. R., Brooks, W. H. and Roszman, T. L. (1985) Influence of serotonin on the immune response. Immunology 54, 505 – 512.

44. Foon, K. A., Wahl, S. M., Oppenheim, J. J. and Rosenstreich, D. L. (1976) Serotonin-induced production of a monocyte chemotactic factor by human peripheral blood leucocytes. J. Immunol. 117, 5, 1545 – 1552.

45. Rozman, T. L. and Brooks, W. H. (1985) Neural modulation of immune function. J. Neuroimmunol. 10, 59 – 69.

46. Askenase, P. W. (1977) Role of basophils, mast cells, and vasoamines in hypersensitivity reactions with delayed time course. In: P. Kallos, B. H. Waksman and A. L. de Weck (Eds.), Progress in Allergy, Vol. 23, Karger, Basel, pp. 199 – 320.

47. Kristofferson, A., Hall, E. and Sohl Åkerlund, A. (1983) Investigations of the immunogenic and immunomodulatory potency of zimeldine in animals. A preliminary report. Astra Report 805-04 AF 57-1. Astra, data on file.

48. Henderson, D. C., Edwards, R. G., Weston, B. J. and Dewdney, J. M. (1988) Immunological studies on paroxetine, a novel antidepressant drug. Int. J. Immunopharmacol. 10, 361 – 367.

49. Gleichmann, E., Pals, S. T., Rolink, A. G., Radaszkiewicz, T. and Gleichmann, H. (1984) Graft-versus-host reactions: clues to the etiopathological spectrum of immunological diseases. Immunol. Today 5, 324 – 332.

50. Landsteiner, K. and Jacob, J. (1936) Sensitization of animals with simple chemical compounds, II. J. Exp. Med. 64, 625 – 639.

51. Eisen, H. N., Orris, L. and Belman, S. (1959) Elicitation of delayed allergic skin reactions with haptens: the dependence of elicitation on hapten combination with protein, J. Exp. Med. 95, 473 – 487.

52. Van Arsdel, P. P. (1978) Adverse drug reactions. In: E. Middelton, C. E. Reed and E. S. Ellis (Eds,), Allergy, Principles and Practice, Mosby, St. Louis, pp. 1133 – 1158.

53. Parker, C. W. (1981) Hapten immunology and allergic reactions in humans. Arthritis Rheum. 24, 1024 – 1036.

54. Bundgaard, H. (1984) Immunochemical mechanisms involved in allergic reactions to chemicals: an overview. Arch. Pharm. Chem. Sci. 12, 103 – 109.

55. Gillete, J. R., Mitchell, J. R. and Brodie, B. B. (1974) Biochemical mechanisms of drug toxicity, Annu. Rev. Pharmacol. 14, 271 – 288.

56. Wu, C. and Matthews, K. P. (1986) Generation of drug metabolite antigenicity in intestinal mucosa. Immunopharmacology. 12, 53 – 58.

57. Pannatier, A., Jenner, P., Testa, B. and Etter, J. C. (1978) The skin as a drug-metabolizing organ. Drug Metab. Rev. 8, 319 – 343.

58. Park, B. K., Coleman, J. W. and Kitteringham, N. R. (1987) Drug disposition and drug hypersensitivity. Biochem. Pharmacol. 36, 5, 581 – 590.

59. Parker, C. W. (1972) Allergic drug responses: mechanisms and unsolved problems. In: L. Golberg (Ed.), CRC Crit. Rev. Toxicol. 1, 261 – 281.

60. Plescia, O. J., Palczuck, N. C., Braun, W. and Cora-Figueroa, E. (1965) Antibodies to DNA and a synthetic polydeoxyribonucleotide produced by oligodeoxyribonucleotides. Science 148, 1102 – 1103.

61. Plescia, O. J., Palczuck, N. C. and Cora-Figueroa, E. (1965) Production of antibodies to soluable RNA (S-RNA). Proc. Natl. Acad. Sci. USA 54, 1281 – 1285.

62. Lüllman, H., Lüllman-Rauch, R. and Wassermann, O. (1978) Lipidosis induced by amphiphilic cationic drugs. Biochem. Pharmacol. 27, 1103 – 1108.

63. Kamel, R. S., Landon, J. and Smith, D. S. (1979) Novel ^{125}I-labelled nortriptyline derivatives and their use in liquid-phase or magnetizable solid-phase second antibody radioimmunoassays. Clin. Chem. 25, 1997 – 2002.

64. Magnusson, B. and Kligman, A. M. (1970) Allergic contact dermatitis in the guinea pig. Identifications of contact allergens. C. C. Thomas Publ., Springfield, IL.

65. Astra Toxicology Laboratories, Södertälje, Sweden, (1979) Allergenicity of zimeldine hydrochloride and tocainide hydrochloride measured by the Magnusson-Kligman guinea pig maximization test. Astra Report 805-04 T984. Astra, data on file.

66. Maguire, H. C. (1975) Estimation of the allergenicity of prospective human contact sensitizers in the guinea pig. In: H. I. Maibach (Ed.), Animal Models in Dermatology, Churchill Livingstone, Edinburgh, pp. 67 – 75.

67. Gleichmann, H. (1981) Studies on the mechanism of drug senstization: T-cell-dependent popliteal lymph node reaction to dephenylhydantoin. Clin. Immunol. Immunopathol. 18, 203 – 211.

68. Hurtenbach, U., Gleichmann, H., Nagata, N. and Gleichmann, E. (1987) Immunity to D-penicillamine: genetic, cellular and chemical requirements for induction of popliteal lymph node enlargement in the mouse. J. Immunol. 139, 2, 411 – 416.

69. Rosenthal, C. J., Noguera, C. A., Coppola, A. and Kapelner, S. N. (1982) Pseudolymphoma with mycosis fungoides manifestations, hyperresponsiveness to diphenylhydantoin, and lymphocyte disregulation. Cancer 49, 2305 – 2314.

70. Kristofferson, A., Sohl Åkerlund, A., Olin, B. and Sjöström, B. (1986) In vitro lymphocyte proliferative responses in employees with occupational allergy to zimeldine. Reproducibility, specificity and effects of monocyte depletion. Astra Report 805-04 AF 108-1. Astra, data on file.

71. Lundström, J. Data to be published.

72. Sabbe, L. J. M., De Bode, L. and Van Rood, J. J. (1983) Analysis of variability in lymphocyte transformation tests. J. Immunol. Methods 57, 21 – 32.

73. Ross, S. B. (1984) Antidepressant drugs: (Z)- and (E)-isomers. In: D.F. Smith (Ed.), CRC Handbook of Stereoisomers: Drugs in Psychopharmacology, CRC Press, Inc. Boca Raton, Florida, pp. 241 – 253.

74. Kristofferson, A., Nilsson, B. S., Sohl Åkerlund, A., Hall, E., Sjöström, B., Bengtsson, B.-O., Jozwiak, H. and Ogenstad, S. (1985) Zimeldine and metabolites induce ^{3}H-thymidine incorporation in lymphocyte cultures from patients where hypersensitivity reactions developed during zimeldine therapy. Astra Report 805-04 AF 102-1. Astra, data on file.

75. Bengtsson, B.-O., Nilsson, B. S., Jozwiak, H., Wiholm, B.-E. and Wålinder, J. (1985) Characteristics of patients with 'hypersensitivity' reactions to zimeldine. A case-control study. Astra Report 84-ZI01. Astra, data on file.

76. Bengtsson, B.-O. et al. Data to be published.

77. Rosenbaum, J. T. and Engelman E. G. (1982) Histocompatibility antigens and disease suscep-
    tibility. In: J. J. Twomey (Ed.), The Pathophysiology of Human Immunologic Disorders, Urban
    and Schwarzenberg, Baltimore-Munich, pp. 51 – 62.
78. Wooley, P. H., Griffen, J: Panayi, G. S., Batchelor, J. R., Welsh, K. I. and Gibson, T. H.
    (1980) HLA-DR antigens and toxic reaction to sodium aurothiomalate and D-penicillamine in pa-
    tients with reumatoid arthritis. N. Engl. J. Med. 303, 300 – 302.
79. Batchelor, J. R., Welsh, K. I. Mansilla-Tinoco, R., Dollery, C. T., Hughes, G. R. V., Bernstein,
    R., Ryan, P., Maish, P. F., Aber, G. M., Bing, R. F. and Russel, G. I. (1980) Hydralazine-
    induced systemic lupus erythematosus: influence of HLA-DR and sex on susceptibility. Lancet 1,
    1107 – 1109.
80. Bengtsson, B.-O., Holmlund, G., Joswiak, H., Kristofferson, A., Lindahl, P., Lindblom, B.,
    Nilsson, B. S., Wiholm, B.-E. and Wålinder, J. (1988) HLA-typing of zimeldine-treated
    psychiatric patients with and without febrile reactions. In manuscript.
81. Dehlin, O., Björnson, G., Lundström, J. and Nörgård, J. (1984) Zimeldine to geriatric patients
    in once daily dosage. A pharmacokinetic and clinical study. Acta Psychiat. Scand. 69, 103 – 111.
82. Chouinard, G. and Jones B. (1984) No crossover of hypersensitivity between zimelidine and
    fluoxetine, letter. Can. Med. Assoc. J. 131, 1190.

M.E. Kammüller, N. Bloksma and W. Seinen (Eds.)
Autoimmunity and Toxicology
© 1989 Elsevier Science Publishers B.V. (Biomedical Division)

Halothane hepatitis – an example of possibly immune-mediated hepatotoxicity

8

JAMES NEUBERGER

The Liver Unit, The Queen Elizabeth Hospital, Edgbaston, Birmingham B15 2TH, UK

I. Introduction

Halothane (1-bromo-1-chloro-2,2,2-trifluoroethane) is a volatile halogenated hydrocarbon which was developed by Raventos in the 1950s as an anaesthetic agent. Its rapidly increasing use during the 1960s reflected the many advantages this agent had over other volatile agents: its use could easily be taught and the ready availability of calibrated vaporisers allowed for easy and sensitive control of administration. Few interactions with other drugs were noted and side effects, such as cardiorespiratory depression, could readily be identified and corrected. Numerous retrospective and prospective studies had attested the safety and efficacy of halothane so that in the early 1970s, halothane was the most popular agent for general anaesthesia. However, during the 1960s, isolated case reports began to appear of unexplained liver damage following halothane anaesthesia and this led, in 1966, to the large-scale retrospective National Halothane Study [7]. Since that time, the association between halothane exposure and the development of liver damage has been gradually accepted, although this occurred after much and often acrimonious discussion between hepatologists and anaesthetists. Interest has now centred on the mechanism of the liver damage and this will be the basis for discussion in this chapter.

II. Clinical features of halothane hepatitis

In the absence of any other generally recognised definition, halothane hepatitis will, in this context, be arbitrarily defined as the appearance of otherwise unexplained liver damage occurring within 28 days of halothane exposure in a patient with previously normal liver function. The causes of liver dysfunction seen post-operatively are many (Table 1) and it will be seen therefore, that in the absence of any widely available diagnostic test for the disease, the diagnosis remains one of exclusion. While many of the causes of liver dysfunction post-operatively listed in Table 1 can be excluded either on clinical or serological grounds, it must be pointed out that there still remains no histological test for diagnosis of non-A, non-B viral hepatitis.

The spectrum of liver damage that may follow halothane anaesthesia varies from the minor increases in concentration of serum aminotransferases to the rarer instances of fulminant hepatic failure. It is still not clear whether these conditions represent two different pathogenic forms of liver damage, or whether they represent extreme ends of a spectrum. Nevertheless, some authors have categorised halothane hepatitis into two forms: type I representing the mild form of halothane hepatitis and type II the severe form often associated with fulminant hepatic failure [1, 2].

TABLE 1

Causes of post-operative jaundice

Pre-hepatic
  blood transfusion
  haemolytic anaemia
  resorption of blood
  Gilberts syndrome

Hepatic
  shock
  infection (general)
  drugs including halothane
  pre-existing liver disease
  hepatitis due to viruses (HAV, HBV, non-A, non-B, CMV, EBV)
  post-operative intra-hepatic cholestasis

Post-hepatic
  cholestasis
  bile duct damage
  pancreatitis

1. TYPE I HALOTHANE HEPATITIS

Less severe reactions following halothane have been well defined in a number of well-controlled prospective studies, the conclusions from each being similar in that halothane exposure is frequently followed by minor elevations of serum aminotransferase levels [3 – 7]. This elevation is not accompanied in the majority of cases by any clinical illness. The study from Oxford [5] showed that elevated serum transaminases were seen more often following halothane exposure than with other anaesthetics. In two of the patients with high serum transaminases, liver biopsy showed appearances of a focal hepatitis. Essentially similar results were shown from a study in Southampton by Wright and colleagues [4]. However, one additional finding from this study was that abnormal liver function tests may not be detectable until the second post-operative week. This observation has important implications for other studies where liver function tests had only been performed for the first 7 days after halothane exposure. Both studies suggested that the incidence of abnormal liver tests following halothane is about 1 in 5. An additional point from the Southampton study suggested that re-exposure to halothane in a patient who had already exhibited minor derangement of liver function was not necessarily followed by repeat elevation of repeat liver function tests. The Belfast study [6] produced similar findings and in none of these three series was there any case of fulminant hepatic failure. Fulminant hepatic failure is defined as the onset of encephalopathy occurring within 8 weeks of jaundice in patients with a previously normal liver. A more recent study by Allan and colleagues [2] used an alternative marker of liver damage, glutathione-S-transferase (GST). This enzyme is distributed primarily in centrilobular hepatocytes and may be a more sensitive index of acute liver cell damage. The authors studied three groups of patients: two groups were given halothane, one in 30% oxygen and the other group in 100% oxygen. The control group were given isoflurane in 30% oxygen (Table 2). The results showed that minor liver damage, as evidenced by elevation of serum GST levels, were found in one-third of the patients given halothane under low oxygen tensions, in one-quarter of the patients given halothane under higher oxygen tensions and in none of the pa-

TABLE 2

Percentage of incidence of raised glutathione S-transferase (GST) levels after anaesthesia

GST	Halothane 30% oxygen (n = 37)	Halothane 100% oxygen (n = 17)	Isoflurane (n = 17)
Normal < 4 µg/l	65	76	100
Raised > 4 µg/l	35	24	0

(From Allan et al. [2], with permission.)

tients exposed to isoflurane. Thus, there seems little doubt that halothane itself may be associated with evidence of direct hepatotoxicity.

2. TYPE II HALOTHANE HEPATITIS

This form of halothane hepatitis is characterised by severe disturbance of liver function and in many cases is associated with fulminant hepatic failure. The retrospective study performed in the United States by the National Halothane Study [7] examined the causes of massive liver cell necrosis following anaesthesia in 856 000 patients anaesthetised between 1959 and 1962. Of these patients, 82 cases of massive liver cell necrosis were identified, and in all but nine instances defined factors such as pre-existing liver disease, sepsis, shock or heart failure could account for the hepatitis. Of the remaining patients, seven had received halothane anaesthesia and one each ethylene and cyclopropane. Thus, the incidence of massive liver cell necrosis following halothane anaesthesia was estimated to be of the order of 1 in 35 000 (7 cases in 255 000). In those patients who had received more than one halothane exposure within a 1-month period, the incidence of massive liver cell necrosis was higher, at approximately 1 in 3 700. This retrospective study has been criticised on a number of points. Nevertheless, two broad conclusions can be drawn from the study: firstly that halothane hepatitis is very uncommon. Secondly, the incidence of halothane hepatitis is higher in patients who have been exposed to halothane on more than one occasion. An alternative way of examining the association between halothane anaesthesia and hepatitis is to identify the possible aetiological factors in patients dying with fulminant hepatic failure. The largest of these studies is that of Trey [8], who examined the cause of death in 150 patients with fulminant hepatic failure. Of these patients, 41 had died following surgery and in all but six, patients had received halothane. Of these 35 cases, 27 had received halothane on more than one occasion.

In the UK, fulminant hepatic failure is most commonly seen following Paracetamol overdose and after viral infection (usually with hepatitis A, B or the presumed non-A, non-B viruses), each accounting for about 45% of all cases [9]. The third most common cause is halothane hepatitis, which accounts for about 5% of cases. Thus, halothane is the most common iatrogenic cause of fulminant hepatic failure and is seen more than 10 times more commonly than liver failure from all other drugs together.

3. OTHER FEATURES OF HALOTHANE HEPATITIS

Analysis of the major published reports [1, 8, 10 – 17] of the clinical and histological features of 690 patients with halothane hepatitis is given in Table 3. Not all of the features listed were reported in all these instances, but the characteristic features of the syndrome is the high female to male ratio, the finding that over three-quarters of the patients had been exposed to halothane on more than one occasion, and the high mortality. Although some reports have drawn attention to the increased incidence of allergy to other drugs in such patients, this suggestion must be treated with some caution; firstly, one report [18] has shown a similar incidence of drug allergy in the general anaesthetic population and secondly, the basis for the diagnosis of drug allergy is rarely defined. Other reports have drawn attention to the increased incidence of obesity in such patients, but again, obesity is rarely defined and the author is unaware of any survey of obesity in the anaesthetic population at risk. Other features of halothane hepatitis include a peripheral eosinophilia and the presence in serum of autoantibodies. The spectrum of autoantibodies in such patients is diverse ([19], Table 4), although the characteristic autoantibodies associated with the condition are liver kidney microsomal antibodies type I. These antibodies probably react with the cytochrome *P450* which metabolises halothane. Other abnormalities include an increased incidence of circulating immune complexes, as detected by the C1q assay [20] (a feature not found in direct toxic liver injury).

Whether there is any genetic component with a tendency to develop halothane hepatitis, remains unclear. Hoft and colleagues [21] described severe hepatic necrosis after halothane anaesthesia occurring in three pairs of closely related

TABLE 3

Features of halothane hepatitis

Female:male	1.6:1
Previous halothane exposures	78%
Drug allergy	15%
Peripheral eosinophilia	21%
Autoantibodies	29%

TABLE 4

Serum autoantibodies in halothane hepatitis

	Homberg et al. ($n = 6$)	Neuberger et al. ($n = 20$)
Anti-nuclear	1	0
Anti-smooth muscle	1	4
Anti-LKM[a]	2	4

[a] Liver-kidney microsomal.
(From Homberg et al. [19] and Neuberger (unpublished).)

220

women, all with a common Mexican Indian or Mexican Spanish background. Furthermore, Farrell [22] and co-workers showed that patients with halothane hepatitis have lymphocytes which are more susceptible to a metabolite of phenytoin; this lymphocyte sensitivity was also reported in the relatives of the patients. Evidence for an association of any HLA phenotypes with halothane anaesthesia is conflicting. Eade [23] was unable to identify any specific HLA phenotype with the condition, although the fact that the patient group he was studying was of mixed ethnic background may have masked such an association. A study from Otsuka [24] looked at HLA class I and class II antigens in 38 Japanese patients who had developed and recovered from halothane hepatitis. Patients were divided into two sub-groups, those with and those without jaundice. Their results are summarised in Table 5. The DR2 phenotype was found in over half the patients with jaundice, compared with one-third of the healthy controls and this was significant at the 0.025 level. Furthermore, the haplotype frequency of Aw24, Bw52 and DR2 was high in the patients with jaundice. These results must be interpreted with caution, since in only six patients was hepatitis A viral infection excluded and hepatitis B viral infection was excluded by the absence of hepatitis B surface antigen; however, recent acute infection with the hepatitis B virus can only be excluded by the absence of IgM anti-HBc in serum. Furthermore, in over half the patients there was no previous history of halothane exposure, thus the accuracy of the diagnosis must remain in some doubt. Finally, no statistical correction was made for the number of antigens tested.

The most recent large-scale series of patients with halothane hepatitis was that reported from Kings College Hospital [25]. Analysis of the 40 patients with halothane hepatitis examined in the 3 years 1983 – 5 is summarised in Table 6, which shows a number of the features of halothane hepatitis. There is a wide range of ages

TABLE 5

HLA antigens in Japanese patients

	% Distribution of halothane hepatitis		Healthy controls (n = 1 234)
	with jaundice (n = 24)	without jaundice (n = 14)	
A2	33[a]	64[a]	41
AW24	67[a]	36[a]	60
BW44	21[a]	50[a]	13
BW52	42[a]	7[a]	23
DR2	58[a]	7	34[b]

[a] $p < 0.05$, halothane hepatitis jaundice vs. no jaundice.
[b] $p < 0.25$, halothane hepatitis jaundice vs. control.
(From Otsuka et al. [24], with permission.)

TABLE 6

Clinical features of 39 patients with presumed halothane hepatitis, whose sera were tested 1983 – 1985

	With encephalopathy		Without encephalopathy ($n = 23$)
	Grade III/IV ($n = 12$)	Grade I/II ($n = 4$)	
Age (years)	58	52	59
range	(3 – 75)	(1 – 75)	(1 – 68)
Sex ratio (F:M)	10:2	4:0	19:4
Type of operation (major:minor)	7:5	2:2	15:8
Numbers of previous anaesthesias	3	4	2
	(1 – 5)	(3 – 6)	(1 – 8)
Intervals between last anaesthesia	6 wk	7 yr	1 yr
	(17 d – 12 yr)	(5 mo – 12 yr)	(5 wk – 13 yr)
Previous documented halothane reactions	3 (25%)	4 (100%)	6 (26%)
Interval, final anaesthesia to jaundice (days)	7	7	9
	(1 – 28)	(7 – 10)	(1 – 23)
Peak AST concn (i.u.l^{-1})	900	828	1086
	(294 – 3 279)	(794 – 2 616)	(442 – 4 000)

of patients affected, although the median is 55 years, six were aged between 1 and 20 years; there was a female preponderance and all patients had had previous anaesthesia, although in not all cases was the anaesthetic regime known. The Table also emphasises that all patients with halothane hepatitis had received more than one halothane anaesthetic and in 11 of the 40 patients there was a previous adverse reaction documented to halothane. Survival in those with grade III to IV hepatic encephalopathy was nil in that series. The type of operation and length of anaesthesia was found to be unrelated to the probability and severity of developing halothane hepatitis.

Whether halothane hepatitis occurs in patients who have not been previously exposed to halothane remains a matter of controversy and clearly it is of major importance in the arguments concerning immunological mechanisms in the pathogenesis of the disease. Some reports have suggested that halothane hepatitis may occur in the absence of previous exposure to halothane [26]. These reports must be treated with some caution since in our experience at least, all patients who have developed halothane hepatitis have had previous anaesthesia on at least one prior occasion. Recent studies [27, 28] have shown that enough halothane may contaminate the tubing of the anaesthetic equipment, so that when a presumed non-halothane anaesthetic is given, enough of the halothane may be leached off the tubing of the equipment so as to sensitise the patient.

III. Halothane hepatitis − an immune-mediated reaction

From the clinical features of halothane hepatitis listed above, it is clear that the severe form of halothane hepatitis fits in with the criteria for an immune-mediated reaction. The disease is rare, is not dose-related and is associated with features of immunological disturbance in a proportion of patients, notably circulating immune complexes, peripheral eosinophilia and organ non-specific autoantibodies.

There is little doubt in the animal models that halothane may be directly hepatotoxic. It is probably that this direct hepatotoxicity accounts for the frequent but mild elevations of liver enzymes as discussed in the type I halothane hepatitis reactions. Since the purpose of this chapter is to discuss the immunological aspects of the disease, no further discussion will be made, but the reader is referred to various reviews on the subject [29, 30].

1. SENSITISATION TO HALOTHANE-ALTERED LIVER CELL COMPONENTS

Initial studies to seek evidence of sensitisation to halothane itself produced conflicting results. Using blast cell transformation or leucocyte migration inhibition, conflicting results were obtained when halothane itself was used as an antigen [31 − 34]. Although in part the discrepancy between results may be a consequence of the different concentrations of halothane used, an alternative explanation was that halothane itself may not be the target antigen. Indeed, as halothane itself is a small molecule, it may act as a hapten itself or alternatively a metabolite, either itself or as hapten may act as antigen.

Because of the problems of selecting the appropriate antigen for in vitro testing, Vergani and colleagues adopted an alternative approach [35]. Rabbits were exposed to halothane by inhalational anaesthesia for 45 min and allowed to recover for 18 h before the livers were removed and used as antigenic preparations. Depending on the assay used (see below), mechanically or collagenase-digested isolated hepatocytes or homogenate of liver was used. The interval between anaesthesia and killing was to allow any antigen to develop. Initial studies used leucocyte migration inhibition assay and sensitisation was shown in 8 of 12 patients with presumed halothane hepatitis (Fig. 1). This showed that peripheral blood cells from some of the patients were sensitised to halothane-altered cells, not control liver cells. These studies provided the first clear-cut evidence of lymphocyte sensitisation specifically to halothane-altered liver cell components.

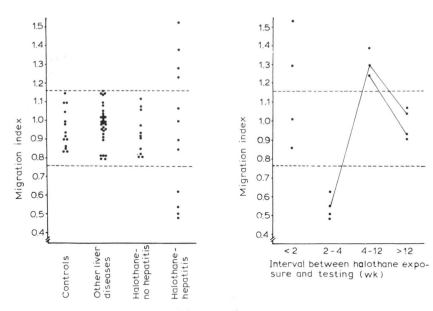

Fig. 1. Leucocyte migration test results using liver homogenate from halothane-treated rabbits and the relation between the migration index and the interval between halothane exposure and testing. (Reproduced with permission from the Lancet, from Vergani et al. [35], with permission.)

To look for the presence of circulating antibodies to these at yet undefined halothane-altered components, two techniques were used: indirect immunofluorescence and antibody-dependent cell-mediated cytotoxicity (ADCC) [36]. In the former, hepatocytes were isolated from halothane pre-treated or control rabbits by mechanical dissection; the isolated hepatocytes incubated with serum to be tested and the presence of antibody-coated target cells detected using fluorescein-labelled second antibody. Using serum that had been absorbed with normal hepatocytes to remove any antibodies reacting with normal liver cell components, it was shown that in patients with halothane hepatitis, there was a characteristic granular pattern of fluorescence. In nearly all cases the use of selective second antibodies showed that the halothane antibodies were of the IgG class. Furthermore, the prolonged incubation of these antibody-coated hepatocytes showed the phenomenon of capping-migration of fluorescein-labelled antibody to one pole of the cell; this finding indicates that the antibody/antigen complex is likely to be on the surface membrane of the hepatocyte and the antigen may therefore be a target for immune damage in vivo.

Using the ADCC reaction, hepatocytes were isolated by collagenase digestion and incubated with patient serum. The antibody-coated target cells are detected by the ability of a sub-population of lymphocytes from normal individuals (K cells) to bind to and lyse these cells. Significantly increased cytotoxicity to halothane hepatocytes was induced only by sera from patients with halothane hepatitis and in none of the sera in any of the control groups. Patients with the type I halothane hepatitis (minor abnormalities of liver function tests following halothane anaesthesia), did not have such antibody detectable in the serum. Sera which grew significant cytotoxicity to halothane pre-treated hepatocytes did not induce such cytotoxicity to the normal hepatocytes (Fig. 2).

ADCC experiments suffer from a number of potential criticisms. Although the specificity of the assay has been validated by blocking and absorption studies, there remain a number of problems: firstly, the assay is cumbersome and expensive to perform. Secondly, adherent hepatocytes are counted manually and, although the assay is performed with the observer being blind as to the nature of the serum, there is potential for observer bias. Finally the end point of the assay, namely adherence of the hepatocytes to the tissue culture plastic wells, is far from physiological, and thus interpretation of the results is limited. In order to overcome these objections, an enzyme-linked immunosorbent assay (ELISA) was developed [37]. The principles of the assay are simple; absorbed serum is incubated with microsomal protein derived from the liver of either halothane pre-treated or control rabbits. The antibody reacting with the antigen is detected using a peroxidase-labelled second antibody. The amount of antibody present is proportional to the optical density of the products

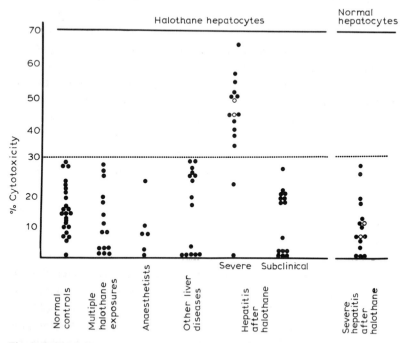

Fig. 2. Induced cytotoxicity of normal lymphocytes to rabbit hepatocytes from halothane-pretreated and normal rabbits. The dotted line represents the upper limit of normal and the open circles represent patients occupationally exposed to halothane. (Reproduced from New Engl. J. Med. [36], with permission.)

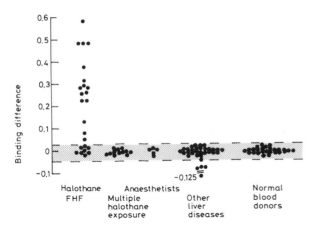

Fig. 3. ELISA results showing the binding differences induced by sera from patients with halothane hepatitis and other conditions. The shaded area indicates the normal range. FHF, fulminant hepatic failure. A490 diff is defined as the difference in optical density (A_{490}) induced to the ELISA by serum reacting with halothane and control homogenate. (Reproduced from J. Immunol. Method [37], with permission.)

of the peroxidase-catalysed reaction. Since it was not possible completely to absorb out all antibody activity reacting with normal rabbit microsomal protein, the amount of halothane antibody present in serum was calculated by subtracting the optical density (A_{490}) obtained with serum incubated with the halothane pre-treated liver from the optical density obtained using the same serum, but reacted with control liver. The results which are shown in Fig. 3 confirm previous results, namely halothane-related antibodies are detectable in most, but not all, sera of patients with halothane hepatitis. Thus, the specificity of the antibody is such that it may be of diagnostic value, although absence of the antibody does not preclude the diagnosis and levels in serum do not reflect disease severity (Table 7). The involvement of the antibody in the pathogenesis of the liver damage cannot be deduced from such experiments.

2. IDENTIFICATION OF ANTIGEN

The presence of the specific halothane-related antibodies in the patients with halothane hepatitis indicates that the administration of halothane is associated with the generation of an antigen. Theoretically this could either be due to a direct interaction between halothane and liver cell membrane or else arises as a consequence of halothane metabolism. It has long been recognised that halothane is metabolised in the liver by the cytochrome *P450* mixed function oxidase system, through at least two different pathways, oxidative and reductive [3]. The preferential route of metabolism is determined by the prevalent oxygen tension and the relative activities

TABLE 7

Incidence and amount of halothane antibodies in 39 patients with halothane hepatitis

	With encephalopathy		Without encephalopathy ($n = 23$)
	Grade III/IV ($n = 12$)	Grade I/II ($n = 4$)	
Halothane antibodies			
incidence	8 (67%)	4 (100%)	16 (70%)
median A_{490} diff[a]	0.235	0.156	0.223
	(0.050 – 0.551)	(0.151 – 0.488)	(0.053 – 0.653)
Interval halothane exposure to testing (days)			
median	28	29	26
range	(4 – 67)	(21 – 49)	(11 – 77)

[a] A_{490} diff was defined as the difference in optical density (A_{490}) induced by serum of patients reacting with halothane and control liver homogenate.

of the constituent *P450* isoenzymes. At the oxygen tension prevailing during anaesthesia, halothane is metabolised in man through both oxidative and reductive routes. The oxidative route, which is preferentially stimulated at high oxygen tensions and by enzyme pretreatment with inducers such as 3-methylcholanthrene, is associated with the generation of trifluoroacetic acid, whereas the reductive route, preferentially stimulated by low oxygen tensions and enzyme inducers such as phenobarbitone, is associated with cleavage of fluoride from the halothane molecule. In both routes there is generation of reactive metabolites which bind to cellular macromolecules, both proteins and lipids.

That halothane antigens are not generated as direct interaction between the anaesthetic itself and the cellular membrane is suggested by a number of observations: firstly, the time course of halothane antigen generation suggests halothane antigen expression or rabbit hepatocyte, is not detectable for at least 2 h after halothane administration and is maximal at 12 h (unpublished data). Secondly, it has been shown that oxidative metabolism of halothane is associated with generation of the antigen [38]. Rabbits were given halothane under high or low oxygen tensions, with or without enzyme pre-treatment with phenobarbitone or 3-methylcholanthrene. The liver cells were isolated and used in the antibody-dependent cell-mediated cytotoxicity assay; the use of sera known to contain halothane antibodies could therefore be used to detect antigens on the membrane.

To characterise these antigens further in molecular terms, Kenna has used halothane antibodies in the serum of patients with halothane hepatitis as specific probes to look for antigenic polypeptides in rabbit liver subcellular liver fractions using immunoblotting techniques [39]. Subcellular fractions were solubilised in SDS in both reducing and non-reducing conditions. SDS-polyacrylamide gel elec- trophoresis was performed on a linear gradient resolving gel. Resolved polypeptides were transferred electrophoretically to nitrocellulose. Nitrocellulose strips were in- cubated with patient serum and after further washing were incubated with peroxidase-conjugated antihuman IgG. Peroxidase activity was then determined colorimetrically. These experiments (Fig. 4) showed that three polypeptide antigens of M_r 100 000, 76 000 and 57 000 were expressed in liver fractions from animals sacrificed 16 h after exposure to 1% halothane in oxygen. Using differential and sucrose density centrifugation to isolate subcellular fractions, it was shown that an- tigens were present in a microsomal subfraction relatively enriched in glucose-6- phosphatase activity, and therefore presumably derived from endoplasmic reticulum. While it was noted that all three antigens were invariably expressed in the liver of all rabbits exposed to halothane, not all serum contained antibodies to all antigenic polypeptides. Thus, antibodies were present in a total of 19 of 24 sera analysed, and four distinct patterns of antibody specificity were observed; seven pa- tients had antibodies to the 100 000 and 76 000 antigens, seven had antibodies to the 100 000 alone, three patients to the 76 000 alone and two patients to the 57 000

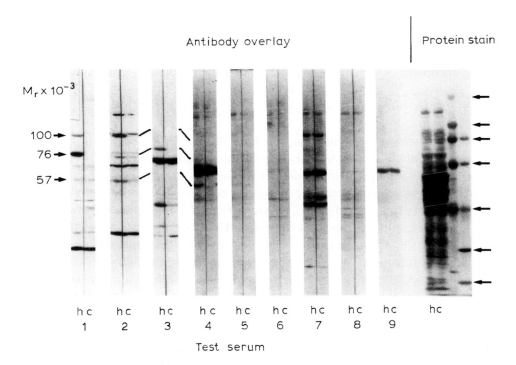

Fig. 4. Immunoblotting showing binding of patient sera to liver homogenates obtained from halothane- treated (h) and control (c) rabbit. The protein stain and molecular weight markers are showing weight rate. (Reproduced with permission from J. Pharmacol. Exp. Ther. [39].)

alone. The reason for the heterogeneity in antibody specificity in the serum is not clear.

The finding that antigens are present predominantly in the microsomal fraction is in confirmation with the concept outlined earlier that the antigen arises as a consequence of metabolism of halothane in the microsomal fraction of the cell. It is, therefore, possible that there is covalent binding of a reactive metabolite to a subcellular macromolecule and this is subsequently expressed on the cell surface of the membrane.

Additional studies from Satoh [40, 41] have shown that an antibody specific for the trifluoroacetyl (TFA) group can be produced and this has been used to demonstrate the presence of new antigenic sites consisting of TFA-conjugated macromolecules on hepatocytes from rats exposed to halothane. Subsequent immunoblotting studies showed that, in rats previously treated with phenobarbitone, the major protein labelled after halothane administration was a phenobarbitone-induced form of cytochrome *P450* with an apparent molecular weight of 54 000. Further studies showed that a protein of apparent molecular weight of 59 000 was also labelled. This was thought to be possibly another cytochrome *P450* isozyme which was expressed more in uninduced halothane pre-treated rats.

Nonetheless, although these experiments have identified three antigenic polypeptides recognised by antibodies in patients with halothane hepatitis, the exact nature of these antigens still remains to be resolved. Preliminary studies have suggested that these are not intrinsic membrane proteins; it is not yet established whether, for example, halothane or a metabolite is a component of these antigens.

3. HALOTHANE ANTIGEN IN MAN

Studies of halothane metabolism in man have shown that the drug is metabolised in man in a fashion similar to that observed in rats and rabbits.

Initial studies were performed using Alexander cells, which are a human-derived hepatocellular carcinoma cell line. Like all cells maintained in culture, drug metabolising activity is rapidly lost. To overcome this problem, the Alexander cells were incubated with an extra-cellular NADPH-generating system together with halothane for 1 h; after allowing 18 h for generation of the antigen in vitro, these cells were used as targets to look for the appearance of the antigen. The results showed there was the typical granular immunofluorescent pattern on the surface of the membrane of the hepatocytes. Both halothane exposure and the presence of a NADPH-generating system were required for generation of the antigen. In subsequent experiments we were able to study liver that was taken from patients dying from non-hepatic causes following anaesthesia. The liver was taken immediately post mortem and frozen. The liver was subsequently homogenised and used in the immunoblotting experiments as described above. We were unable to detect halothane-related antigen in three patients who had died within 24 h after anaesthesia with non-halothane agents even though all had halothane antibodies in serum, but antigens were present in both liver samples from patients dying within the same period of time after halothane anaesthesia (Kenna and Neuberger, unpublished). We were also able to study liver from three patients dying with halothane hepatitis and in whom the halothane antibody was present in the serum. In none of these cases was the halothane antigen detectable in the liver sample.

Thus, these limited human experiments would appear to support the animal data; human hepatocytes are capable of generating halothane-related liver cell antigen and indeed the antigen appears to be generated in all patients exposed to halothane. Therefore, susceptibility to halothane hepatitis is likely to lie more in the response to the antigen rather than in the generation of the antigen. This situation is analogous to that with hepatitis B viral infection. Hepatitis B virus is not cytopathic, but infection with the virus is associated with the appearance of the core antigen on the surface of the infected liver cells. The immune attack is directed to the core antigen: where there is an impaired immune response, for example in patients receiving immunosuppressive drugs or with renal failure, there is failure to clear the virus and chronic infection results; in contrast, where there is an exaggerated immune response, fulminant hepatic failure often results.

IV. Mechanism of halothane hepatitis

If halothane hepatitis does represent an immune-mediated disease, there are several possible mechanisms whereby halothane exposure may lead to hepatotoxicity. One possibility is that halothane exposure may lead to a breakdown in tolerance. As indicated in earlier chapters, there exists a full repertoire of helper cells which are auto-reactive. These auto-reactive T cells are normally held in check by the suppressor cells. If halothane were able to inhibit non-specifically T cell suppressor activity, then an immune-mediated response would ensue to auto-antigens. This hypothesis has been shown to operate in the case of α-methyldopa-associated liver damage [42]. Global reduction in suppressor cell function would be anticipated to result in the appearance of organ non-specific auto-antibodies and this has been shown with halothane hepatitis. Additionally, both the stress of surgery and anaesthetics themselves may be associated with reduction in suppressor cell function [43]. Our own studies, using a concanavalin A induced suppressor cell functional assay on pokeweed mitogen stimulated cells, have confirmed these findings. Lymphocytes were taken from normal individuals and exposed to 1% halothane in vitro. The effect of concanavalin A induced lymphocyte suppression on pokeweed mitogen induced production of IgG was then studied and compared with the suppressor cell function in the absence of halothane exposure. The results (Fig. 5) showed that in half of the normal subjects studied halothane exposure was associated with significant reduction of suppressor T cell function.

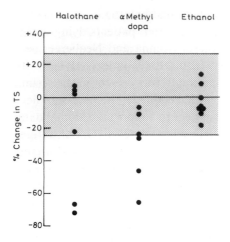

Fig. 5. The effect of pre-incubation of lymphocytes with halothane, α-methyldopa and ethanol on Con A induced total cell suppressor function. The dotted line shows the normal limits. TS, suppressor T cells.

However, despite these findings it is unlikely that this represents the mechanism of halothane hepatitis, since if there was a generalised disturbance of immune regulation, then it is probable that halothane exposure would be associated with damage of other organs in addition to the liver. However, halothane is metabolised primarily in the liver and this appearance of the halothane antigen on the liver cell surface may therefore target the immune response to the liver. Against this argument is the rapid turnover of membrane proteins which is usually a matter of hours, whereas evidence of liver dysfunction may not become apparent until 3 or more weeks after halothane exposure.

An alternative hypothesis, therefore, is that generation of the halothane antigens results in the breakdown of tolerance and thus provokes an auto-immune disease directed to the liver. In support of this hypothesis is the high incidence of antibodies to normal liver cell proteins (Fig. 6). Serum from patients with halothane hepatitis was incubated with normal and halothane-pre-treated hepatocytes, with and without absorption by normal hepatocytes. Using antibody-dependent cell-mediated cytotoxicity, it was shown that the majority of patients with halothane hepatitis have significant amounts of antibodies reacting with normal liver cell determinants. Nevertheless, these results must be treated with some caution as comparable antibodies can occasionally be detected in the serum of patients with liver damage from direct toxicity, such as paracetamol overdose.

A further criticism of this approach is the finding that halothane antibodies are detectable in the serum of only the 75% of patients with halothane hepatitis. While it may be that some of the seronegative patients are not suffering from halothane hepatitis, but from other causes of liver damage, another possibility is that the antibodies are present in too low titre or are present in immune complexes, which have

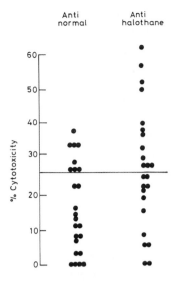

Fig. 6. Percentage of cytotoxicity induced by serum from patients with halothane hepatitis to halothane-pretreated and normal liver cells.

been shown to be present in patients with halothane hepatitis. In order to address this question, we have incubated lymphocytes isolated from patients with halothane hepatitis in vitro for 7 days in the absence of specific stimulation with antigen or mitogen. Using lymphocyte assays from ten patients with halothane hepatitis, it was found that two of the seronegative patients had lymphocytes which in vitro were producing halothane antibody (Kenna and Neuberger unpublished). Thus, in some cases of patients with halothane hepatitis antibody is being generated, but not detectable in the serum.

V. Animal models

As indicated in other chapters, animal models of immune-mediated liver damage are difficult to reproduce. In an attempt to develop an animal model of hepatitis, rabbits were immunised with hepatocytes isolated from litter mates previously exposed to halothane. Immunisation consisted of two intraperitoneal injections of 10^9 cells. This immunisation resulted in the generation of antibodies to both normal and halothane-related liver cell determinants as detected both by immunofluorescence and by direct cytotoxicity (Fig. 7). Exposure of these immunised rabbits to halothane resulted in the disappearance of the halothane-related antibody from the serum. This is presumably due to its reaction with the liver cell membrane halothane-related antigen. However, we were unable to prove this, since immunisation with the halothane hepatocytes induced the presence of antibodies on the recipient hepatocytes. Although we were able to show that both rabbit and human hepatocytes were directly cytotoxic in vitro to these antibody-coated hepatocytes, we were unable to detect any serological or histological evidence of liver damage [44]. Thus, if immune mechanisms are involved in the pathogenesis of halothane hepatitis, other factors must be implicated, and these factors may be related to the adverse host immune response.

An alternative approach was adopted by Gandolfi's group [45]. Previous studies from that group had shown that rabbits exposed to halothane on repeated occasions in high oxygen tensions, produced an antibody that cross-reacts with a trifluoroacetyl moiety of trifluoroacetic acid conjugated with rabbit serum albumin (RSA). Generation of this halothane antigen was dependent on exposure to halothane under high oxygen tensions, since only minimal antibody was found in rabbits exposed to halothane under low oxygen tensions. Furthermore, halothane exposure of rabbits specifically immunised with the TFA-RSA complex induced a secondary antibody response to that immunogen. Rabbits, whether exposed, immunised or not with TFA-RSA, will produce antibodies of varying specificity after multiple halothane exposure. Thus, the evidence from their work suggests that the predominance of the metabolic intermediate, the ensuing immunogen and the subsequent antibody response are highly dependent upon the oxygen tension during the halothane administration. The successive exposures could potentially generate many different immunogens, and these antibodies may be responsible for initiating or

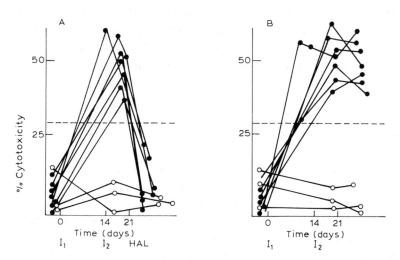

Fig. 7. Percentage of cytotoxicity of human lymphocytes induced by serum from rabbits immunized with halothane (●) or control hepatocytes (○) at times I_1 and I_2 to halothane hepatocytes. I_1 and I_2 represent the two immunisation drugs, at day 0 and 14, respectively. Animals whose sera are represented in A were exposed to halothane (HAL) on day 21. (Reproduced from Int. J. Immunopharmacol. [44], with permission.)

perpetuating halothane-induced liver damage, but futher studies are required to evaluate this.

VI. Conclusion

Many of the clinical and serological features of patients with halothane hepatitis suggest that the severe form of liver damage is an adverse reaction which has many features of an immune-mediated syndrome. Studies have shown that such patients have a high incidence of antibodies to both normal liver components and specifically to halothane-related antigens. These antigens, which have not yet been fully defined, are associated with metabolism of halothane by the oxidative route, and occur in both laboratory animals and in man.

It remains to be clearly demonstrated whether these halothane-isolated antibodies are involved in the pathogenesis of halothane hepatitis. There are certain pointers which suggest that this may be the case: firstly, as discussed above, the 'halothane' antibodies can induce lymphocytes from normal individuals to become cytotoxic to antibody-coated hepatocytes. Secondly, it is unlikely that the appearance of these antibodies is merely secondary to a toxic effect of liver damage. IgG class antibodies are detected very early on in the illness. Although switching from IgM to IgG production can occur very quickly, it is more likely that the appearance of early IgG antibodies reflects previous sensitisation. Additionally in patients who, following halothane anaesthesia, have developed severe liver damage from other causes (such as hepatitis A viral infection or malignant infiltration of the liver), it has not been possible to demonstrate the halothane antibodies. Finally, in patients with liver failure from a direct hepatotoxic drug, acetaminophen, it has not been possible to demonstrate analogous antibodies. As with most instances of unpredictable drug reactions, it has not been possible to provide a convincing animal model of halothane hepatitis. Thus, it remains to be conclusively shown that the liver damage following halothane anaesthesia is an immune-mediated event. However, the many clinical and immunological features suggest that immune mechanisms are involved in this drug reaction, and further work is required to identify the exact nature of the antigens and those factors which determine the immune response to novel, drug-induced antigens; this should allow elucidation of the mechanism of this condition.

Acknowledgement

I am grateful to Miss J. Ariss and Miss J. Wormington for secretarial assistance.

References

1. Neuberger, J. M. and Williams, R. (1984) Halothane anaesthesia and liver damage. Br. Med. J. 289, 1136–1139.
2. Allan, L. G., Hussey, A. J., Howie, J., Beckett, G. J., Smith, A. F., Haynes, J. D. and Drummond, G. B. (1987) Hepatic glutathione S-transferase release after halothane anaesthesia. Lancet i, 771–774.
3. Stock, J. G. L. and Strunin, L. (1985) Unexplained hepatitis following halothane. Anesthesiology 63, 424–439.
4. Wright, R., Chisholm, M., Lloyd, B., Edwards, J. C., Eade, O. E., Hawksley, M., Moles, T. M. and Gardner, M. (1975) A controlled prospective study of the effect on liver function of multiple exposures to halothane. Lancet i, 821–823.
5. Trowell, J., Peto, R. and Crampton Smith, A. (1975) Controlled trial of repeated halothane anaesthetics in patients with carcinoma of the uterine cervix treated with radium. Lancet i, 821–824.
6. Fee, J. P. H., Black, J. W., Dundee, J. W., McIlroy, D. A., Johnston, H. L., Johnston, S. B., Black, I. H. C., McNeill, D. W., Doggart, J. R., Merrett, J. D. I., McDonald, J. R., Bradley, D. S. G., Haire, M. and McMillan, S. A. (1979) A prospective study of liver enzyme and other changes following repeated administration of halothane and enflurane. Br. J. Anaesth. 51, 1133–1141.
7. National Halothane Study (1966) Summary of the National Halothane Study: possible association between halothane anaesthesia and postoperative hepatic necrosis. J. Am. Med. Assoc. 1977, 121–134.
8. Trey, C., Lipworth, L., Chalmers, T. C., Davidson, C. S., Gottlieb, L. S., Popper, H. and Saunders, S. J. (1968) Fulminant hepatic failure: presumable contribution by halothane. N. Engl. J. Med. 279, 798–801.
9. Gimson, A. E. S. and Williams, R. (1983) Acute hepatic failure. In: A. C. Thomas and R. N. M. MacSween (Eds.), Recent Advances in Hepatology, Vol. 1, Churchill Livingstone, Edinburgh, pp. 57–70.
10. Klion, F. M., Schaffner, F. and Popper, H. (1969) Hepatitis after exposure to halothane. Ann. Intern. Med. 71, 467–477.
11. Inman, W. H. W. and Mushin, W. W. (1977) Jaundice after repeated exposure to halothane. Br. Med. J. i, 5–10.
12. Inman, W. H. W. and Mushin, W. W. (1978) Jaundice after repeated exposure to halothane. Br. Med. J. ii, 1455–1456.
13. Walton, B., Simpson, B. R., Strunin, L., Doniach, D., Perrin, J. and Appleyard, A. J. (1976) Unexplained hepatitis following halothane. Br. Med. J. i, 1171–1173.
14. Klion, F. M., Schaffner, F. and Popper, H. (1969) Hepatitis after exposure to halothane. Ann. Intern. Med. 71, 467–477.
15. Reed, N. and Williams, R. (1972) Halothane hepatitis as seen by the physician. Br. J. Anaesth. 44, 935–936.
16. Moult, P. J. A. and Sherlock, S. (1975) Halothane-related hepatitis. Quart. J. Med. 44, 99–114.
17. Bottinger, L. E., Dalen, E. and Hallen, B. (1976) Halothane-induced liver damage: an analysis of the material reported to the Swedish Adverse Drug Reaction Committee 1966–1973. Acta Anaesthesiol. Scand. 20, 40–46.
18. Fee, J. P. H., McDonald, J. R., Clarke, R. S. J., Dundee, J. W. and Pal, P. K. (1978) The incidence of atopy and allergy in 10 000 pre-anaesthetic patients. Br. J. Anaesth. 50, 74.
19. Homberg, J. C., Abuaf, N., Helmy-Khalil, S., Biour, M., Poupon, R., Islam, S., Darnis, F., Levy, V. G., Opolon, P. and Beaugrand, M. (1985) Drug-induced hepatitis associated with anticytoplasmic autoantibodies. Hepatology 5, 722–727.

20. Canalese, J., Wyker, J., Vergani, D., Eddleston, A. L. W. R. and Williams, R. (1981) Calculating immune complexes in patients with fulminant hepatic failure. Gut 22, 845 – 848.

21. Hoft, R. H., Bunker, J. P., Goodman, H. and Gregory, P. B. (1981) Halothane hepatitis in three pairs of closely related women. N. Engl. J. Med. 304, 1023 – 1024.

22. Farrell, G., Prendergast, D. and Murray, M. (1985) Halothane hepatitis: detection of a constitutional susceptibility factor. N. Engl. J. Med. 313, 1310 – 1314.

23. Eade, O. E., Krawitt, E. L., Grice, D., Wright, R. and Trowell, J. (1978) HLA antigens and halothane hepatitis. Lancet 2, 1384 – 1385.

24. Otsuka, S., Yamamoto, M., Kasuya, S., Ohtomo, H., Yamamoto, Y., Yoshida, T. O. and Atala, T. (1985) HLA antigens in patients with unexplained hepatitis following halothane anaesthesia. Acta Anaesthesiol. Scand. 29, 497 – 501.

25. Kenna, J. G., Neuberger, J. and Williams, R. (1987) Specific antibodies to halothane induced liver antigen in halothane associated hepatitis. Br. J. Anaesth. 59, 1286 – 1290.

26. MacKay, I. R. (1985) Induction by drugs of hepatitis and auto-antibodies to cell organelles: significance and interpretation. Hepatology 5, 904 – 906.

27. Varma, R. R., Whitesell, R. C. and Iskandarani, M. M. (1985) Halothane hepatitis without halothane: role of inapparent circuit contamination and its prevention. Hepatology 5, 1159 – 1162.

28. Conn, H. O. and Skornicki, J. (1985) Halothane hepatitis sans halothane. Hepatology 5, 1238 – 1240.

29. Lind, R. C., Gandolfi, A. J., Sipes, I. G., Brown, B. R. and Waters, S. J. (1986) Oxygen concentration required for reductive defluorination of halothane by rat hepatic microsomal. Anaesth. Analg. 65, 835 – 895.

30. Gelman, S. (1986) Halothane hepatotoxicity – again. Anaesth. Analg. 65, 831 – 834.

31. Paronetto, F. and Popper, H. (1970) Lymphocyte stimulation induced by halothane in patients with hepatitis following exposure to halothane. N. Engl. J. Med. 283, 277 – 280.

32. Walton, B., Dumonde, D. C., Williams, C., Jones, D., Strunin, J. M., Layton, J. M., Strunin, L. and Simpson, R. (1973) Lymphocyte transformation: absence of increased responses in alleged halothane jaundice. J. Am. Med. Assoc. 225, 494 – 498.

33. Walton, B., Hamblin, A., Dumonde, D. C. and Simpson, R. (1974) Lymphocyte transformation: absence of cellular hyper-sensitivity in patients with unexplained jaundice following halothane. Anaesthesioly 44, 391 – 397.

34. Moult, P. J. A., Adjukiewicz, A. B., Gaylarde, P. M., Sarkany, I. and Sherlock, S. (1975) Lymphocyte transformation in halothane related hepatitis. Br. Med. J. ii, 69 – 70.

35. Vergani, D., Eddleston, A., Tsantoulas, D., Davis, M. and Williams, R. (1978) Sensitisation to halothane-altered liver components in severe hepatic necrosis after halothane anaesthesia. Lancet, i, 801 – 803.

36. Vergani, D., Mieli Vergani, G., Alberti, A. Neuberger, J., Eddleston, A., Davis, M. and Williams, R. (1980) Antibodies to the surface of halothane-altered rabbit hepatocytes in patients with severe halothane-associated hepatitis. N. Engl. J. Med. 303, 66 – 71.

37. Kenna, J. G., Neuberger, J. M. and Williams, R. (1984) An enzyme-linked immunosorbent assay for detection of antibodies against halothane-altered hepatocyte antigens. J. Immunol. Meth. 75, 3 – 14.

38. Neuberger, J., Mieli Vergani, G., Tredger, J. M., Davis, M. and Williams, R. (1981) Oxidative metabolism of halothane in the production of altered hepatocyte membrane antigens in acute halothane-induced necrosis. Gut 22, 669 – 672.

39. Kenna, J. G., Neuberger, J. and Williams, R. (1987) Identification by immunoblotting of three halothane-induced liver microsomal polypeptide antigens. J. Pharmacol. Exp. Ther. 242, 733 – 740.

40. Satoh, H., Fukuda, Y., Anderson, D. K., Ferrans, V. J., Gillette, J. R. and Pohl, L. R.

236

(1985) Immunological studies on the mechanism of halothane-induced hepatotoxicity: immunohistochemical evidence of trifluoroacetylated hepatocytes. J. Pharmacol. Exp. Ther. 233, 857 – 862.

41. Satoh, H., Gillette, J. R., Davies, H. W., Schulick, R. and Pohl, L. R. (1985) Immunochemical evidence of trifluoroacetylated cytochrome P-450 in the liver of halothane-treated rats. Mol. Pharmacol. 28, 468 – 474.

42. Kirtland, H., Daniel, M. D., Mohler, N. and Horwitz, D. A. (1980) Methyl dopa inhibition of suppressor lymphocyte function. N. Engl. J. Med. 302, 825 – 831.

43. Watkins, J. and Salo, M. (1982) Trauma, stress and immunity in anaesthesia and surgery. Butterworths, London.

44. Neuberger, J., Kenna, J. G. and Williams, R. (1987) Halothane hepatitis: attempt to develop an animal model. Int. J. Immunopharmacol. 9, 125 – 131.

45. Callis, A. H., Brooks, S. D., Rota, T. P., Gandolfi, A. J. and Brown, B. R. (1987) Characteristics of a halothane-induced humoral immune response in rabbits. Clin. Exp. Immunol. 67, 343 – 351.

SECTION IV

Properties of immunomodulating drugs and chemicals

M.E. Kammüller, N. Bloksma and W. Seinen (Eds.)
Autoimmunity and Toxicology
© 1989 Elsevier Science Publishers B.V. (Biomedical Division)

Metabolism of procainamide, hydralazine, and isoniazid in relation to autoimmune(-like) reactions

9

DAVID W. HEIN* and WENDELL W. WEBER

Departments of Pharmacology, The Morehouse School of Medicine, Atlanta, Georgia and The University of Michigan, Ann Arbor, MI, USA

I. Introduction

Soon after the introduction of procainamide, hydralazine and isoniazid into clinical therapy, reports of autoimmune-like reactions were observed with each of them [1 – 4]. As reviewed by Uetrecht and Woosley [5], and in the following two chapters, investigators have sought to discover common denominators between the various drugs that induce adverse autoimmune-like reactions. A prominent relationship between procainamide, hydralazine, and isoniazid is that they are each a primary arylamine or hydrazine chemical subject to metabolic biotransformations by both acetylation and oxidation pathways. In the biotransformation of each drug, acetylation appears to compete with oxidation. Furthermore, in each case, oxidation pathways generate reactive electrophilic intermediates that bind covalently to cellular nucleic acids and other macromolecules, while conversely, N-acetylation pathways generate stable products that undergo urinary excretion.

Of particular importance in this regard is the existence of a hereditary acetylation polymorphism in man and other mammalian species. As recently reviewed [6, 7], individuals can be identified as rapid, intermediate, or slow acetylator phenotypes. The frequency of each phenotype varies racially and geographically, but most populations of North America and Europe are about equally divided between rapid

---

* Correspondence: Dr. David W. Hein, Department of Pharmacology, The Morehouse School of Medicine, 720 Westview Drive, Atlanta, GA 30310-1495, USA.

and slow acetylators [6, 7]. The acetylator phenotype is inherited by simple autosomal Mendelian inheritance of two codominant alleles at a single gene locus. The acetylation capacity in vivo is reflected in the catalytic activity of cytosolic N-acetyltransferase enzyme(s) [6, 7]. As discussed more fully in the later sections of this chapter, slow acetylators more frequently suffer autoimmune (lupus)-like reactions from procainamide, hydralazine, and isoniazid. Additionally, associations between slow acetylator phenotype and idiopathic lupus have also been suggested [8], although several studies have failed to confirm this association (reviewed in [6, 7]).

Arylamines and hydrazines in general require metabolic activation to highly reactive electrophiles in order to inflict the toxic manifestations attributable to them. The most thoroughly investigated include the metabolic activation of arylamine carcinogens such as 2-aminofluorene to induce DNA adducts, DNA damage, mutagenesis and carcinogenesis. Slow acetylator phenotype is also a recognized predisposing factor to the incidence of bladder cancer following exposure to arylamine carcinogens [6, 7]. Thus, there are strong suggestions that the metabolic activation pathways important in the initiation of cancer may be pertinent to the induction of autoimmune-like disorders. As discussed in this chapter, N-hydroxylation to a N-hydroxyarylamine intermediate appears to be critical in the initiation of arylamine-induced genotoxicity and procainamide-induced autoimmune toxicity. Recent studies have demonstrated the identity of arylamine N-acetyltransferase and N-hydroxyarylamine O-acetyltransferase enzymes [9, 10] and have provided evidence for common genetic control in hamsters (Fig. 1) and humans (Fig. 2).

Several important generalizations about the metabolic activation of arylamine carcinogens have been reported [13 – 15]. Acetylated and non-acetylated C-8 and N-2

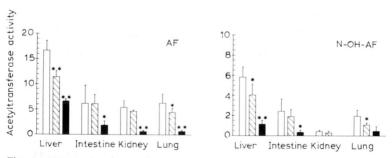

Fig. 1. Acetyl coenzyme A dependent 2-aminofluorene (AF) N-acetyltransferase and N-hydroxy-2-aminofluorene (N-OH-AF) O-acetyltransferase activities in hamster tissue cytosols. AF N-acetyltransferase activity in nmol acetylated per min per mg protein and N-OH-AF O-acetyltransferase activity in nmol bound per 15 min per mg DNA/mg protein are plotted on the ordinates for various inbred hamster tissue cytosols. □, Bio. 87.20 homozygous rapid acetylator hamsters, ■, Bio. 82.73/H homozygous slow acetylator hamsters, and ▨, (Bio. 87.20 × Bio. 82.73/H) F_1 heterozygous acetylator progeny. Significant acetylator gene dose-responses are shown for both activities in each tissue (*, $p < 0.05$; **, $p < 0.01$). (Adapted from Hein et al., 1987 [11].)

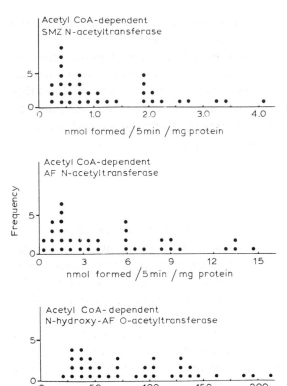

Fig. 2. Distribution of acetyl coenzyme A dependent sulfamethazine (SMZ), and 2-aminofluorene (AF) *N*-acetyltransferase and *N*-hydroxy-2-aminofluorene (N-hydroxy-AF) *O*-acetyltransferase in human liver cytosols. (Reproduced with permission from Flammang et al., 1987 [12].)

adducts of guanine are generated in target and non-target tissues that correlate with short-term assays of mutagenicity and carcinogenicity. The adducts and their effects are heterogeneous across tissues, in large part due to the heterogeneous concentrations of reactive metabolites generated. These concentration differences are secondary to pharmacokinetic differences in disposition and to enzymatic differences in activation as well as deactivation pathways that are subject to genetic variability.

Although the pathogenesis of arylamine-induced lupus is less understood, recent studies have reported the presence of IgG antiguanosine antibodies in idiopathic [16] and procainamide-induced [17] lupus. Comparisons of the antibodies in the sera of patients with drug-induced lupus showed that the IgG antiguanosine antibodies were more associated with the autoimmune symptomatology than were antinuclear and IgG antibodies to single-stranded DNA. In addition, the titer of IgG antiguanosine antibodies decreased after discontinuation of procainamide therapy, providing further support for a strong association between IgG antiguanosine antibodies and the major clinical manifestations of procainamide-induced lupus.

Thus, there is some evidence to support common mechanisms for the pathogenesis of lupus and neoplasia from arylamines. Metabolic activation (oxidation) of arylamines (e.g. procainamide) may generate reactive electrophiles that form DNA adducts. The DNA adducts can initiate mutagenic and carcinogenic events or alternatively may serve as antigen for the production of antibodies and the immunotoxic symptomatology of drug-induced lupus.

II. Metabolism of procainamide

The clinical pharmacokinetics of procainamide in man has been reviewed elsewhere [18]. Over half of administered procainamide is excreted in the urine unchanged, while the rest is metabolized. The primary metabolite is N-acetylprocainamide. The acetylation of procainamide is of interest because of the well-documented N-acetylation polymorphism expressed in humans and other mammalian species [6, 7]. In addition to N-acetylprocainamide, additional metabolites that have been identified in humans include p-aminobenzoic acid and its acetylated derivative N-acetyl-p-aminobenzoic acid [19] and desethylprocainamide and its acetylated derivative N-acetyldesethylprocainamide [20 – 22]. Three additional metabolites, N-acetyl-3-hydroxyprocainamide, N-acetylprocainamide-N-oxide, and N-acetylaminohippuric acid have also been identified in a rat perfusion model [23].

Three of the metabolites are products of N-acetylation reactions. The total urinary excretion of N-acetyl-p-aminobenzoic acid is equivalent in rapid and slow acetylators [19] consistent with its monomorphic acetylation by human liver N-acetyltransferase in vitro [24, 25]. The disposition of desethylprocainamide and its N-acetyl metabolite is more complex however. Kinetic studies suggest that the formation of N-acetyldesethylprocainamide occurs via dealkylation of procainamide to desethylprocainamide, followed by N-acetylation [21, 22]. After properly compensating for acetylator phenotype-related differences in urinary N-acetylprocainamide to procainamide ratios, the excretion levels of N-acetyldesethylprocainamide were consistent with polymorphic N-acetylation of desethylprocainamide [21, 22]. The significance of the polymorphic N-acetylation of desethylprocainamide with respect to therapeutic activity or induction of systemic lupus erythematosus (SLE) is unknown.

The N-acetylation of procainamide to N-acetylprocainamide, and its relation to the hereditary N-acetylation polymorphism has received the greatest attention in human and animal studies. The N-acetylation of procainamide in vivo has been reported as monomorphic in rats [26] and mice [26, 27]. The N-acetylation of procainamide in vitro was found to be monomorphic in rat liver [26] and mouse liver [26, 27], but polymorphic in rabbit liver [28] and mouse blood lysates [27]. The

N-acetylation of procainamide by hamster liver is complex. Although N-acetylation of procainamide by crude hamster cytosol preparations is monomorphic [29], two N-acetyltransferase isozymes, differing in chromatographic properties and genetic control have been isolated from hamster liver [30, 31, 11]. As shown in Fig. 3, the N-acetylation of procainamide by one N-acetyltransferase isozyme is controlled by the acetylator gene whereas a second N-acetyltransferase isozyme catalyzes at rates independent of acetylator genotype.

In humans the role of acetylator phenotype in the N-acetylation of procainamide has been the subject of numerous studies [32 – 34, 19, 35 – 39]. Significantly higher urinary excretion levels of N-acetylprocainamide have been observed in rapid acetylators compared to slow acetylators following single or multiple doses of procainamide [33 – 35, 19, 39]. The most striking example was reported following single ingestion of 50 mg procainamide in 33 healthy persons [34]. The urinary excretion

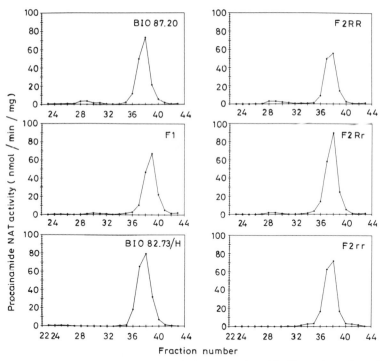

Fig. 3. Separation and identification of two procainamide N-acetyltransferase isozymes in hamster liver cytosol following ion-exchange chromatography. The faster eluting isozyme (ca. fraction 29) is acetylator genotype dependent (polymorphic), with highest activity in homozygous rapid acetylator (RR) Bio. 87.20 and (Bio. 87.20 × Bio. 82.73/H) F_2 progeny (top panels), intermediate activity in heterozygous acetylator (Rr) (Bio. 87.20 × Bio. 82.73/H) F_1 and F_2 progeny (middle panels), and lowest activity in homozygous slow acetylator (rr) Bio. 82.73/H and (Bio. 87.20 × Bio. 82.73/H) F_2 progeny (lower panels). The slower eluting isozyme (ca. fraction 38) is acetylator genotype independent (monomorphic) in the same animals. (Adapted from Hein et al., 1985 [30].)

TABLE 1

Clearance values for subjects receiving procainamide orally

Patient	Plasma $\frac{\text{NAPA}}{\text{PA}}$[a]	Urinary $\frac{\text{NAPA}}{\text{PA}}$[b]	Renal clearance[c] (ml/min)		Renal clearance Creatinine clearance	
			NAPA	PA	NAPA	PA
Slow acetylators						
1	0.75	0.41	75.3	133	1.1	1.9
2	0.56	0.63	–	–	–	–
3	0.57	0.51	75.1	112	1.2	1.8
4	0.63	0.55	69.9	75.6	1.2	1.3
5	0.65	0.35	23.5[d]	42.8	1.1	1.9
6	0.50	0.19	135	360	1.7	4.6
Mean ± SD	0.61 ± 0.09[e]	0.44 ± 0.16[f]	75.8 ± 39.6[g]	145 ± 125[g]	1.3 ± 0.3[g]	2.3 ± 1.3[g]
Rapid acetylators						
7	2.0	17.9	95.1	10.6	0.59	0.07
8	0.96	0.33	85.3	226	1.4	3.8
9	1.0	0.67	39.2	55.6	0.82	1.2
10	2.3	1.0	45.2	111	1.2	3.0
11	2.3	1.1	–	–	–	–
12	1.4	0.68	122	246	1.3	2.6
13	2.4	0.81	93.0	235	0.68	1.7
14	2.0	1.5	50.7	61.1	1.9	2.3
Mean ± SD	1.8 ± 0.59	3.0 ± 6.0	75.8 ± 31.1	135 ± 99	1.1 ± 0.5	2.1 ± 1.2

[a] 3 h after dose. Abbreviations: PA, procainamide; NAPA, N-acetylprocainamide.

[b] Urine was collected 1.5–3 h after last dose.

[c] Renal clearance = $\dfrac{\text{amount excreted in urine } 1.5\text{–}3 \text{ h after last dose}/90 \text{ min}}{\text{average plasma levels } 1.5 \text{ and } 3 \text{ h after last dose}}$.

[d] Since this patient had an incomplete urine collection, these values are artificially low. However, the other derived values for this patient in this Table are accurate.

[e] $p < 0.001$.

[f] $p = 0.01$.

[g] No significant difference between rapid and slow acetylators.

(Adapted from Reidenberg et al., 1975 [32], with permission.)

of N-acetylprocainamide in these individuals measured 19% in rapid acetylators versus 9% in slow acetylators ($p < 0.001$). Similarly, as shown in Table 1, Reidenberg and coworkers clearly observed phenotype-related excretion of N-acetylprocainamide. Individuals with N-acetylprocainamide/procainamide ratios less than 0.85 appeared to be slow acetylators whereas those with ratios greater than 0.95 appeared to be rapid acetylators. The clearance of N-acetylprocainamide was about half that of procainamide, but no differences associated with acetylator phenotype were noted in the renal clearance of procainamide or N-acetylprocainamide (Table 1). The renal clearance of procainamide ranged from 179–660 ml/min [18] indicating active tubular secretion. Because of its high dependence on renal function, steady state N-acetylprocainamide/procainamide ratios in plasma and urine do not reflect acetylator status as well as other drugs subject to N-acetylation such as isoniazid and hydralazine (see below). Thus, plasma half-lives for procainamide disappearance either do not differ between rapid and slow acetylators [35, 36] or differ only slightly [19].

A consequence of the major role of renal excretion in procainamide elimination is that the role of acetylator phenotype in the frequency of procainamide-induced lupus is less convincing than with hydralazine-induced lupus and/or formation of antinuclear antibodies [39–42]. However, studies by Woosley and colleagues convincingly demonstrate that although both rapid and slow acetylators develop antinuclear antibodies during procainamide therapy, nevertheless, the rate at which procainamide induces antinuclear antibodies (Fig. 4) and the lupus syndrome (Fig. 5) is significantly higher in slow acetylators than in rapid acetylators.

The findings of Woosley and coworkers are consistent with the more striking results in hydralazine-induced lupus (see Section III in this chapter) that indicate that N-acetylation of procainamide serves as a protection mechanism, and further

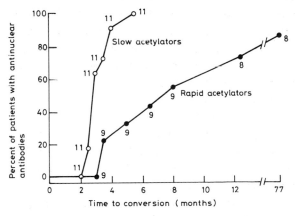

Fig. 4. The development of procainamide-induced antinuclear antibodies in human slow acetylators (○) and rapid acetylators (●) with time. The number of patients followed is indicated at each point. (Reproduced with permission from Woosley et al., 1978 [43].)

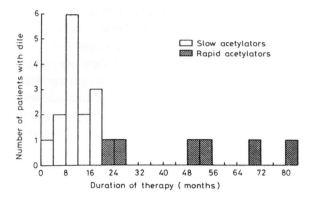

Fig. 5. Histogram showing the relationship between acetylator phenotype and the rate of development of procainamide-induced lupus. DILE, drug-induced lupus erythematosus. (Reproduced with permission from Woosley et al., 1978 [43].)

that the induction of antinuclear antibodies and the lupus syndrome are mediated via either the parent amine, or more likely a non-acetylated metabolite derived from procainamide. Additional evidence for this hypothesis is provided by observations that antiarrhythmic therapy with N-acetylprocainamide does not appear to induce the lupus syndrome [44 – 47].

The definite mechanism by which procainamide induces the lupus syndrome is not known, but several studies suggest that it is mediated via an oxidized metabolite(s) (Fig. 6). Freeman and coworkers showed that procainamide, but not N-acetylprocainamide, was activated by microsomal monooxygenase(s) to reactive metabolite(s) as measured by a positive Ames test [48] and by covalent binding to hepatic microsomal protein [49]. In further studies, the same group showed monooxygenase-mediated metabolic activation of procainamide in both rat and human microsomal preparations [50], and this finding has been confirmed by others [51]. Uetrecht has provided additional studies to support the mechanism proposed in Fig. 6. N-hydroxyprocainamide bound covalently to microsomal protein to a much greater degree than procainamide and, in contrast to the monooxygenase requirement for procainamide binding, no metabolic activation was required [52]. Uetrecht showed that N-hydroxyprocainamide binding occurred via non-enzymatic conversion to nitrosoprocainamide [52] and the two reactive species may exist in chemical equilibrium. Although the nitrosoprocainamide bound covalently to albumin, histone protein, and DNA, the reactivity towards DNA was much less than towards protein [52]. As discussed more fully by Rubin (Chapter 4), most antinuclear antibodies in procainamide-induced lupus have been found to bind to histone protein [53, 54]. Thus, the formation of nitroso-procainamide-histone protein adducts is consistent with clinical observations, and supports the hypothesis that nitrosoprocainamide acts as a hapten to induce antibodies that cross-react with native histone protein [52].

Rubin and coworkers [55] have shown that *N*-hydroxyprocainamide/nitrosoprocainamide is highly toxic to lymphocytes. Uetrecht et al. [56] demonstrated activation of procainamide by activated neutrophils and mononuclear leukocytes to cytotoxic products, and the predominant metabolite was *N*-hydroxyprocainamide.

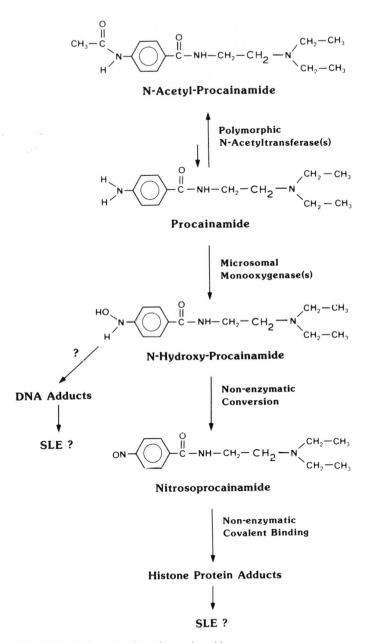

Fig. 6. Metabolic activation of procainamide.

248

Based on these data, Uetrecht and coworkers [56] propose that formation of these reactive oxidative metabolites on the surface of activated monocytes may facilitate reactions with class II major histocompatibility glycoproteins or other membrane structures providing a stimulus for antibody production and other manifestations of procainamide-induced lupus. It should be noted, however, that recent studies report that the major manifestations of procainamide-induced lupus associate most strongly with IgG antiguanosine antibodies [17]. The hypothesis that procainamide and other arylamines have a direct effect on the immune system [8] seems less likely, but the two theories are not mutually exclusive. In support of the latter theory, Tannen and Weber [27] reported that procainamide tended to suppress antinuclear antibody formation in rapid acetylator C57BL/6J inbred mice but enhanced it in slow acetylator A/J inbred mice. However, procainamide also suppressed antinuclear antibody formation in slow acetylator F_2 and backcross progeny of the two strains [27].

Although nitrosoprocainamide binds primarily to histone protein and not DNA [52], it is possible that metabolic activation of the N-hydroxyprocainamide to produce DNA adducts may be mediated via another manner. As recently reviewed [57], many carcinogenic arylamines such as N-hydroxy-2-aminofluorene and N-hydroxy-3,2'-dimethyl-4-aminobiphenyl undergo acetyl coenzyme A dependent O-acetylation to N-acetoxy esters which form electrophiles that spontaneously bind covalently to DNA. As suggested in Fig. 7, the enzymatic catalysis for N-hydroxyarylamine O-acetylation may be the same as for arylamine N-acetylation (reviewed in [57]). One might speculate that polymorphic O-acetylation of N-hydroxyprocainamide can

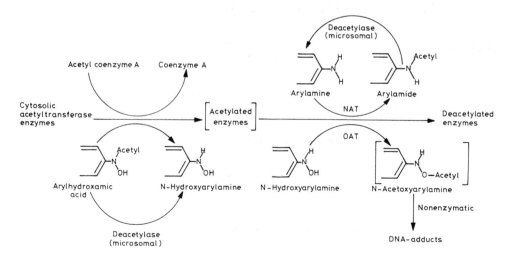

Fig. 7. Inter-relationships of acetyl transfer in the metabolism of arylamines. Evidence suggests the arylamine N-acetyltransferase (NAT) and N-hydroxyarylamine O-acetyltransferase (OAT) activities are catalyzed by common enzyme(s).

generate DNA adducts, perhaps binding to guanosine to generate IgG antiguanosine antibodies. In light of the recent strong associations between the toxic manifestations of procainamide-induced lupus and IgG antiguanosine antibodies, this hypothesis warrants investigation.

III. Metabolism of hydralazine

The clinical pharmacokinetics of hydralazine in humans has been reviewed [58]. Shortly after its introduction as an antihypertensive agent, hydralazine was shown to be rapidly and extensively metabolized in humans [2], and was shown to be metabolized in vitro at higher rates by rapid acetylator liver biopsy homogenates than by slow acetylator homogenates [59] suggesting that N-acetylation was involved in the metabolic pathway. A study by Perry and coworkers in 1970 [60] reported that 12 patients who developed hydralazine-induced lupus, all were slow acetylators. Since this initial report, other investigations have confirmed the original observation that hydralazine-induced lupus occurs almost exclusively (83 of 88 total patients) in slow acetylators [61 – 64].

The critical importance of acetylator status on the induction of lupus by hydralazine spurred a number of investigations on hydralazine metabolism. Two reports in the early 70's [65, 66] measured plasma hydralazine disappearance in rapid and slow acetylators. Reidenberg et al. [66] observed that the hydralazine plasma half-lives did not differ between rapid and slow acetylator phenotypes and that hydralazine plasma concentration following i.v. administration also did not differ [66]. However, both studies showed that plasma concentrations of hydralazine were lower in rapid acetylators than in slow acetylators following oral administration of hydralazine [65, 66], suggesting a major role for acetylation during first pass through the intestinal wall and liver during absorption, but a considerably smaller role for acetylation in hydralazine elimination from the plasma. Subsequently, newer analytical methodologies have been developed to account for the instability of hydralazine and its metabolites (reviewed in [58]), but similar findings regarding the role of acetylator status on hydralazine metabolism have been reported by numerous investigators [58, 64, 67 – 74]. The more predominant role for acetylator phenotype on hydralazine elimination after oral administration versus i.v. administration is illustrated in Fig. 8.

The overall metabolism of hydralazine is not completely understood, but its complexity is readily apparent (Fig. 9). As shown in Table 2, the urinary excretion of a number of metabolites varies with acetylator status. Thus, metabolic ratios of N-acetylhydrazinophthalazinone/hydralazine hydrazones (NAcHPZ/HH), N-acetylhydrazinophthalazinone/phthalazinone (NAcHPZ/PZ), triazolophthalazine/hydralazine hydrazones (TP/HH), and phthalazinone/triazolophthalazine (PZ/TP) all reflect acetylator status (Table 2) following oral administration of

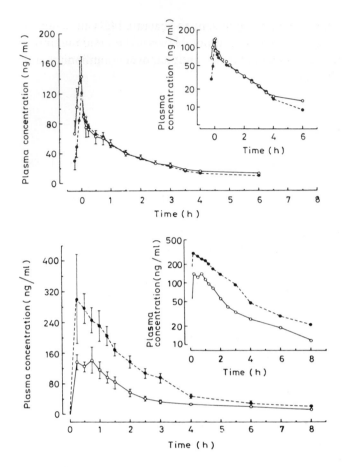

Fig. 8. Time-course of plasma drug concentration in human rapid acetylators (○) and slow acetylators (●) following slow intravenous infusion of 20 mg hydralazine hydrochloride (upper panel) and oral ingestion of 100 mg hydralazine hydrochloride (lower panel). Each point represents the mean ± SEM of five subjects. The insets show semilogarithmic plots of the mean data. (Reproduced, with permission, from Shen et al., 1980 [74].)

hydralazine. Metabolism of hydralazine to HH is more predominant after i.v. administration, in part accounting for the less significant role of acetylator status in hydralazine elimination following i.v. administration (Fig. 8).

Two acetylation pathways have been postulated in hydralazine metabolism. As shown in Fig. 9, hydralazine can undergo acetylation both prior to oxidation and following oxidation of 4-hydrazinophthalazine-1-one (HPZ). Although the overall metabolism of hydralazine is complicated and not eludicated fully, it is readily apparent that the N-acetylation polymorphism plays an important role. As shown in Table 2, slow acetylators excrete higher urinary levels of HH, PZ, and hydrazine (HZ) than rapid acetylators, but lower urinary levels of 3-hydroxymethyltriazolo-

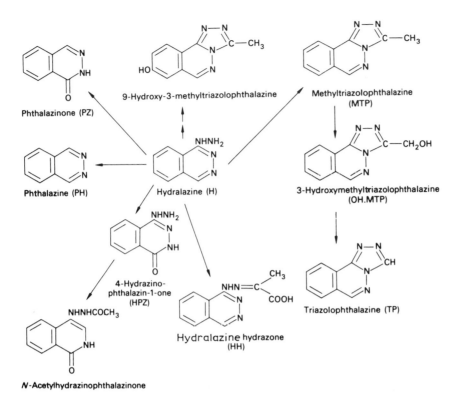

Fig. 9. Metabolism of hydralazine. (Reproduced, with permission, from Facchini and Timbrell, 1981 [68].)

phthalazine (OH.MTP), NAcHPZ, and TP than rapid acetylators. Thus, it is clear that slow acetylators divert more hydralazine via some oxidation pathways than do rapid acetylators and that this phenotypic low acetylation capacity predisposes individuals to hydralazine-induced lupus.

Timbrell and colleagues [64] also examined hydralazine metabolism in hydralazine-lupus patients compared to controls. As shown in Table 2, the only significant difference between slow acetylator control and lupus patients was a higher excretion of TP in lupus patients. The implications of this are unclear however, as the higher excretion of TP in rapid acetylators does not predispose them to hydralazine-lupus. The metabolic profile of a rapid acetylator patient who developed hydralazine-lupus as reported by Timbrell et al. [64] may be particularly enlightening. As shown in Table 2, although the excretion of both NAcHPZ and OH.MTP were in the range of rapid acetylator controls, the excretion of PZ, HZ, and HH were greater, and the excretion of PZ was lower, than rapid acetylator controls. In some instances, the levels were closer to those seen in slow acetylators. Timbrell et al. [64] suggest that this rapid acetylator lupus patient has certain similarities in

252

TABLE 2

Hydralazine metabolism in rapid and slow acetylator control and hydralazine-induced lupus patients (Table values represent mean ± SD)

Percent dose urinary metabolites

Patient	(n)	Acetylator phenotype	HH	MTP	OH.MTP	TP	PZ	NAcHPZ	HZ	Total[f]
Control	(8)	slow	5.3 ± 5.6	3.2 ± 1.1	3.8 ± 1.8	0.8 ± 0.7	7.1 ± 3.4	11.4 ± 5.7	1.2 ± 0.5[b]	32.2 ± 7.4
Lupus	(5)	slow	3.6 ± 3.9	3.2 ± 1.7[a]	3.4 ± 1.9	2.2 ± 0.9[c]	10.1 ± 9.1	14.0 ± 9.9[a]	0.2 ± 0.5[a]	35.7 ± 17.4[c]
Control	(9)	rapid	1.2 ± 0.9	3.6 ± 1.5	13.3 ± 4.7	2.2 ± 0.9	3.4 ± 1.8	24.6 ± 17.7[d]	0.2 ± 0.4[b]	48.1 ± 22.1[d]
Lupus	(1)	rapid	3.3	5.5	12.3	0.9	11.9	21.7	1.84	55.6

Urinary metabolite ratios

Patient	(n)	Acetylator phenotype	OH.MTP/HH	NAcHPZ/HH	PZ/TP	TP/HH
Control	(8)	slow	1.35 ± 0.82	3.67 ± 2.56	10.25 ± 11.5	0.24 ± 0.22
Lupus	(5)	slow	1.42 ± 0.76	6.73 ± 4.46[a]	15.49 ± 26.9	0.71 ± 0.52
Control	(9)	rapid	12.93 ± 5.43	21.67 ± 9.55[d]	2.75 ± 3.48	2.27 ± 1.41
Lupus	(1)	rapid	3.73	6.58	13.22	0.27

[a] $n = 4$.
[b] $n = 5$.
[c] $n = 3$.
[d] $n = 8$.
[e] $p < 0.01$.
[f] Excluding HZ.
(Reproduced, with permission, from Timbrell et al., 1984 [64].)

hydralazine metabolism with patients of the slow acetylator phenotype. Furthermore, Timbrell et al. [64] found that PZ represented a metabolite that was excreted at higher levels in lupus patients than controls in both acetylator phenotypes (Table 2), suggesting an important role of PZ in the metabolic activation of hydralazine to immunotoxic metabolites. Hydrazine is another metabolite of some interest. As shown in Table 2, although the excretion levels are very low, they are nonetheless higher in slow acetylator controls than in rapid acetylator controls. Surprisingly, its excretion was very low in the slow acetylator lupus patients, but comparatively very high in the rapid acetylator lupus patient (Table 2). The significance of this finding is not known.

The molecular mechanism for hydralazine-induced lupus is not understood. Early studies in this decade showed that hydralazine could interact directly with pyrimidine bases in DNA, a reaction accelerated by exposure to UV light [75]. Subsequent studies confirmed the binding of hydralazine to DNA [76] and further showed that hydralazine was a direct acting mutagen in bacterial systems [77]. McQueen et al. [78] studied the genotoxicity of hydralazine in hepatocyte primary cultures isolated from rapid and slow acetylator rabbits. Higher rates of hydralazine-induced unscheduled DNA repair, indicative of DNA damage, were found in slow acetylator than in rapid acetylator hepatocytes, suggesting that metabolic activation of hydralazine via non-acetylation pathways was important in the generation of the genotoxic intermediate(s). The predominant role of acetylator status on the incidence of hydralazine-induced lupus further supports this hypothesis.

Although the oxidative metabolism of hydralazine is incompletely understood, several studies suggest that oxidative pathway(s) are involved in the activation of hydralazine to reactive intermediates believed to be responsible for hydralazine-induced lupus. Streeter and Timbrell have investigated the metabolism of hydralazine in rats both in vivo [79] and in vitro [80, 81]. These investigators observed substantial differences between the in vivo and in vitro metabolism in the rat, and further that the in vivo metabolism of hydralazine differed considerably between rats and humans [79].

Nevertheless, multiple studies [80–82] have now consistently shown that hydralazine is metabolized by microsomal enzymes to a metabolite(s) that binds covalently to cellular macromolecules. The metabolic activation requires oxygen and NADPH, and is inhibited by carbon monoxide [80]. Phenobarbital pretreatment fails to increase the binding whereas pretreatment with 3-methylcholanthrene does slightly, which suggests the involvement of specific cytochrome *P450* monooxygenase isozymes [80]. Based on further studies, Streeter and Timbrell [81] and LaCagnin et al. [82] have postulated possible metabolic pathways for the generation of the reactive species. Streeter and Timbrell [81] propose hydroxylation of the hydrazine moiety followed by loss of water and N_2 to form the reactive phthalazinyl free radical. Alternatively, LaCagnin and coworkers [82] propose one electron oxidative cleavage of the hydrazine moiety giving rise to both the nitrogen-centered phthalazinylhydrazyl free radical and the carbon-centered phthalazinyl free radical. Evidence for both types of free radicals has been provided by Sinha and coworkers [76, 83 – 85]. LaCagnin and coworkers [82] further suggest a combination of the two radicals to form a dimerization product, followed by enzymatic oxidation to a nitroso intermediate, followed by break down to nitrite and a putative amine dimer metabolite [82].

Thus, although much remains to be elucidated with respect to the complex metabolism of hydralazine, it appears that the formation of reactive free radicals catalyzed by oxidative pathways that compete with acetylation is involved in the biochemical mechanism of hydralazine-induced lupus.

IV. Metabolism of isoniazid

Prolonged ingestion of isoniazid can induce premonitory signs of lupus (i.e., production of antinuclear antibodies), although the incidence is lower than with hydralazine and procainamide. Approximately 20% of tuberculosis patients treated with isoniazid develop antinuclear antibodies [86 – 88]. One study reported that four of five patients with isoniazid-lupus were slow acetylators [89], whereas another study found that the induction of antinuclear antibodies from isoniazid was unassociated with acetylator phenotype [88].

The molecular basis for isoniazid-induced lupus has not been reported to any appreciable extent. Rather, the metabolism of isoniazid has been investigated in relation to its activation to intermediates capable of causing liver necrosis, because of the appreciable risk of hepatotoxicity [90]. One might speculate, however, that metabolic activation of isoniazid to reactive intermediates is involved in the pathogenesis of isoniazid-induced lupus, analogous to that for procainamide and hydralazine.

The clinical pharmacokinetics of isoniazid in humans has been reviewed [91]. Isoniazid is rapidly and completely absorbed and appreciable first pass metabolism is observed. This may be due to acetylation of isoniazid by the mucosal cells of the gut, the main site of isoniazid absorption. Following oral administration, the major urinary metabolites are isoniazid, pyruvic acid hydrazone, α-ketoglutaric acid hydrazone, acetylisoniazid, isonicotinic acid, isonicotinyl glycine, acetylhydrazine, and diacetylhydrazine. As shown in Fig. 10, two steps in the metabolic pathway are catalyzed by polymorphic N-acetyltransferase(s) accounting for the apparent first-order rate constant differences between rapid and slow acetylators for the acetylation of isoniazid to acetylisoniazid, and of acetylhydrazine to diacetylhydrazine (Table 3). Evidence from rapid and slow acetylator rabbits strongly suggests that the N-acetylation of isoniazid and acetylhydrazine are catalyzed by a common polymorphic N-acetyltransferase (Fig. 11). Investigations in the rapid and slow acetylator

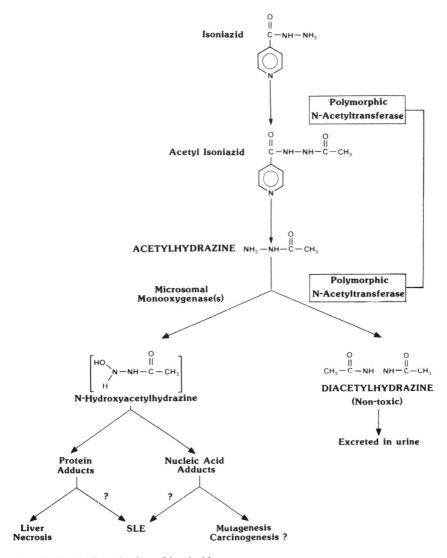

Fig. 10. Metabolic activation of isoniazid.

hamster (Fig. 12) and mouse [94] show that the N-acetylation of isoniazid can be catalyzed by acetylator genotype-independent (monomorphic) *N*-acetyltransferase(s) in addition to acetylator genotype-dependent (polymorphic) *N*-acetyltransferase(s). The implications of these results in hamster and mouse with respect to humans are unclear, and require further study.

Although the metabolic pathways necessary for the induction of isoniazid-lupus have not been elucidated, other studies have reported the putative mechanisms required to activate isoniazid to reactive metabolites capable of producing

256

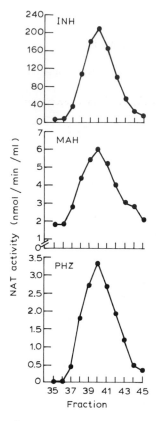

Fig. 11. Co-purification of homozygous rapid acetylator rabbit liver isoniazid (INH), monoacetylhydrazine (MAH) and phenelzine (PHZ) N-acetyltransferase activities through gel filtration chromatography. (Reproduced, with permission, from Hein and Weber, 1982 [93].)

macromolecular adducts (Fig. 10). Nelson and coworkers [95] showed that isoniazid is activated to (a) highly reactive electrophiles by cytochrome *P450* monooxygenase(s) in rat and human microsomes, and that the covalent binding of these metabolites to liver macromolecules paralleled hepatic cellular necrosis. They further found, as shown in Fig. 10, that the reactive metabolite arose from the acetylhydrazine moiety [96]. Since greater amounts of acetylisoniazid are formed in rapid than slow acetylators, it follows that greater amounts of the proximate electrophilic intermediate acetylhydrazine are also formed in rapid than in slow acetylators (Table 4). This observation might suggest that greater quantities of reactive electrophiles would be formed in rapid acetylators, and hence a higher likelihood of isoniazid-lupus. However, as shown in Fig. 10, acetylhydrazine is also polymorphically N-acetylated (Table 3) to the non-toxic and stable diacetylhydrazine metabolite excreted in the urine [92, 97]. Thus, rapid acetylators not only form greater quantities of acetylhydrazine than slow acetylators, but also detoxify

TABLE 3

Apparent first-order rate constants for elimination of isoniazid and its metabolites in urine

Compound	Dose (mg)	Process	First-order rate constant (min^{-1})	
			slow acetylator	rapid acetylator
Isoniazid	250	Acetylation[a]	0.0018	0.0065
	900	Hydrolysis to acetylisoniazid		
Acetylisoniazid	500	Excretion	0.0023	0.0018
		Hydrolysis to acetylisoniazid	0.0011	0.0015
Isonicotinic acid	25	Excretion	0.0080	0.0082
	25	Conjugation with glycine	0.0060	0.0065
Acetylhydrazine	74	Excretion and hydrazone formation	0.00033	0.00033
	74	Acetylation[a]	0.00083	0.0038
Diacetylhydrazine	116	Excretion	0.0017	0.0020

[a] Polymorphic acetylation steps.
(Modified from Ellard and Gammon, 1976 [92].)

TABLE 4

Microsomal metabolism of acetylhydrazine in humans administered isoniazid

Metabolite	Mean % of 300 mg oral dose isoniazid	
	rapid acetylators	slow acetylators
Acetylisoniazid (excreted)	46.3 ± 22.4	28.9 ± 1.7
Acetylisoniazid (formed)	87.4[a]	54.5[a]
Acetylhydrazine (excreted)	1.8 ± 0.4	2.5 ± 0.5
Acetylhydrazine (formed)	41.1[a]	25.6[a]
Diacetylhydrazine (excreted)	23.0 ± 2.0	4.9 ± 0.9
Acetylhydrazine and diacetylhydrazine (excreted)	24.9 ± 2.1	7.5 ± 0.5
Acetylhydrazine metabolized through microsomal pathway	16.3[a]	18.2[a]

[a] Calculated estimates.
(Data adapted from Timbrell et al., 1977 [97].)

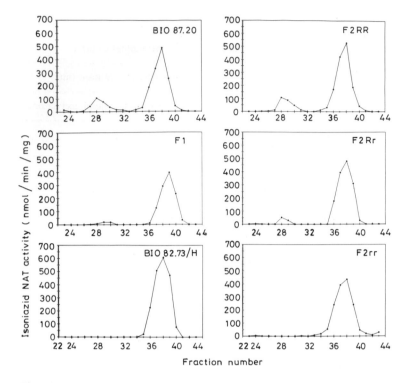

Fig. 12. Separation and identification of two isoniazid N-acetyltransferase isozymes in hamster liver cytosol following ion-exchange chromatography. The genetic control of the two isozymes is as described in the legend to Fig. 3. (Adapted from Hein et al., 1985 [30].)

more of it to diacetylhydrazine as well. Based upon these measurements, Timbrell and coworkers calculated that the amount of acetylhydrazine that could undergo metabolic oxidation to electrophilic intermediates should be similar in rapid and slow acetylators (Table 4).

Since isoniazid and acetylhydrazine undergo N-acetylation via a common enzyme (Fig. 11), it is possible that inhibitory interactions between them could shunt the metabolism through the oxidative pathways leading to generation of electrophiles (Fig. 10). From rat studies, Timbrell and Wright [98] have suggested that the predominant interaction following normal therapeutic doses of isoniazid in humans would be isoniazid inhibition of acetylhydrazine N-acetylation. Inasmuch as higher levels of isoniazid remain for longer periods of time in slow acetylators (Table 4), one could propose that slow acetylators would have comparatively greater inhibition of acetylhydrazine N-acetylation, and hence greater shunting through oxidative pathways to generate reactive intermediates. Lauterberg et al. [99] have reported human pharmacokinetic data that support this hypothesis, suggesting that slow acetylators have particularly high metabolic activation via the oxidative pathways following larger doses (e.g. 10 mg/kg) of isoniazid.

A further consideration is the possibility that *N*-hydroxyacetylhydrazine could undergo genetically polymorphic O-acetylation, although no evidence for this has been reported. Thus, the role of acetylator status on the generation of reactive intermediates, and presumably on isoniazid-lupus are complex and incompletely understood.

Recent studies by Lauterberg and colleagues have shed some light on this matter. The plasma concentrations of isoniazid, acetylisoniazid, acetylhydrazine, and diacetylhydrazine were measured in healthy subjects following the ingestion of 300 mg isoniazid. They confirmed that rapid acetylators generated more acetylisoniazid and acetylhydrazine than slow acetylators, but that the total exposure to acetylhydrazine was similar in the two phenotypes because of the polymorphic N-acetylation of acetylhydrazine to diacetylhydrazine [99, 100]. These investigators also measured the exhalation of $^{14}CO_2$ following the ingestion of isoniazid and ^{14}C-acetylisoniazid, and showed that the exhalation of $^{14}CO_2$ originated from the metabolism of acetylhydrazine, thus providing a measure of metabolism through the oxidative pathway [100]. The cumulative exhalation of $^{14}CO_2$ was higher in slow acetylators than in rapid acetylators suggesting greater exposure to the oxidative reactive metabolites in the slow acetylator phenotype, particularly in the very slow acetylator individual [100]. Thus, although the clinical implications of this data are usually applied towards the incidence of hepatotoxicity, nevertheless, these data are consistent with the reported higher risk of isoniazid-lupus in slow acetylators [89] and are pertinent to the extent that the pathogenesis of isoniazid-lupus includes formation of macromolecular adducts derived from oxidative reactive intermediates (Fig. 10). Recent studies have reported the formation and persistence of isoniazid-DNA adducts in mouse tissues [101].

Finally, free hydrazine has been detected in the plasma [102] and urine [103] of patients ingesting isoniazid. Evidence has been reported to support the formation of hydrazine radicals ($H_2\dot{N}NH$) from hydrazine [104] and accumulations of hydrazine have been noted in slow acetylators [103]. The significance of these findings to isoniazid-lupus remain unknown at this time.

V. Summary

Numerous drugs are capable of providing an autoimmune-like disorder resembling lupus erythematosus. Many of these drugs contain a primary (unsubstituted) amine group. The most important of these are the aromatic amines such as procainamide and the hydrazines such as hydralazine. The precise mechanism by which these drugs produce this disorder is not entirely understood. Hereditary differences in acetylation capacity is acknowledged as an important determinant of susceptibility to this disorder and genetically slow acetylator individuals are significantly more susceptible to drug-induced lupus that rapid acetylator individuals. Studies of the molecular basis for this disorder strongly suggest that it may be mediated through reactive intermediates of oxidative metabolites which involve hydroxylamines of these drugs or chemical species that are in equilibrium with the hydroxylamines.

Acknowledgements

The authors are supported in part by USPHS Grants CA-34627, RR-08248, GM-27028, and CA-39018. The assistance of Ronald J. Ferguson, Vereen Williams, Esther Otu, Joseph N. Miceli, and James Perry in the construction of the chapter was greatly appreciated. We also thank Jack Uetrecht for sharing manuscripts with us prior to publication.

References

1. Morrow, J. D., Schroeder, H. A. and Perry, H. M. (1953) Studies in the control of hypertension by hyplex. II. Toxic reactions and side effects. Circulation 8, 829 – 839.
2. Perry, H. M., Schroeder, H. A., Goldstein, G. S. and Menhard, E. M. (1954) Studies on the control of hypertension by hypen. III. Pharmacological and chemical observations on 1-hydrazinophthalazine. Am. J. Med. Sci. 228, 396 – 404.
3. Ladd, A. T. (1962) Procainamide-induced lupus erythematosus. N. Engl. J. Med. 267, 1357 – 1358.
4. Zingale, S. B., Minzer, L., Rosenberg, B. and Lee, S. L. (1963) Drug-induced lupus-like syndrome. Arch. Intern. Med. 112, 63 – 66.
5. Uetrecht, J. A. and Woosley, R. L. (1981) Acetylator phenotype and lupus erythematosus. Clin. Pharmacokinet. 6, 118 – 134.
6. Weber, W. W. and Hein, D. W. (1985) N-Acetylation pharmacogenetics. Pharmacol. Rev. 37, 25 – 79.
7. Weber, W. W. (1987) The Acetylator Genes and Drug Response. Oxford University Press, New York.
8. Reidenberg, M. M. (1983) Aromatic amines and the pathogenesis of lupus erythematosus. Am. J. Med. 75, 1037 – 1042.
9. Saito, K., Shinohara, A., Kamataki, T. and Kato, R. (1986) N-hydroxyarylamine O-acetyltransferase in hamster liver: identity with arylhydroxamic acid N,O-acetyltransferase and arylamine N-acetyltransferase. J. Biochem, 99, 1689 – 1697.
10. Mattano, S., Land, S., King, C., and Weber, W, (1988) Purification of hepatic arylamine N-acetyltransferase from rapid and slow acetylator mice: identity with arylhydroxamic acid N,O-acyltransferase. In: C. King, D. Schuetzle, and L. Romano (Eds.). Carcinogenic and Mutagenic Responses to Aromatic Amines and Nitroarenes, Elsevier, New York, pp. 155 – 160.
11. Hein, D. W., Flammang, T. J., Kirlin, W. G., Trinidad, A. and Ogolla, F. (1987) Acetylator genotype-dependent metabolic activation of carcinogenic N-hydroxyarylamines by S-acetyl coenzyme A dependent enzymes of inbred hamster tissue cytosols: relationship to arylamine N-acetyltransferase. Carcinogenesis 8, 1767 – 1774.
12. Flammang, T. J., Yamazoe, Y., Guengerich, F. P. and Kadlubar, F. F. (1987) The S.-acetyl coenzyme A dependent metabolic activation of the carcinogen N-hydroxy-2-aminofluorene and its relationship to the aromatic amine N-acetyltransferase phenotype. Carcinogenesis 8, 1967 – 1970.

13. Beland, F. A. and Kadlubar, F. F. (1985) Formation and persistence of arylamine-DNA adducts in vivo. Environ. Health Persp. 62, 19 – 30.

14. Neumann, H. G. (1986) The role of DNA damage in chemical carcinogenesis of aromatic amines. J. Cancer Res. Clin. Oncol. 112, 100 – 106.

15. Kadlubar, F. F. (1987) Metabolism and DNA binding of carcinogenic aromatic amines. ISI Atlas of Science: Pharmacology 1, 129 – 132.

16. Weisbart, R. H., Garrett, R. A., Liebling, M. R., Barnett, E. V., Paulus, H. E. and Katz, D. H. (1983) Specificity of anti-nucleoside antibodies in systemic lupus erythematosus. Clin. Immun. Immunopathol. 27, 403 – 411.

17. Weisbart, R. H., Yee, W. S., Colburn, K. K., Whang, S. H., Heng, M. K. and Boucek, J. (1986) Antiguanosine antibodies: a new marker for procainamide-induced systemic lupus erythematosus. Ann. Intern. Med. 104, 310 – 313.

18. Karlsson, E. (1978) Clinical pharmacokinetics of procainamide. Clin. Pharmacokinet. 3, 97 – 107.

19. DuSouich, P. and Erill, S. (1976) Patterns of acetylation of procainamide and procainamide-derived p-aminobenzoic acid in man. Eur. J. Clin. Pharmacol. 10, 283 – 287.

20. Dreyfuss, J., Bigger, J. T., Cohen, A. I. and Schreiber, E. C. (1972) Metabolism of procainamide in rhesus monkey and man. Clin. Pharmacol. Ther. 13, 366 – 371.

21. Ruo, T. I., Morita, Y., Atkinson, A. J., Henthorn, T. and Thenot, J. P. (1981) Plasma concentrations of desethyl N-acetylprocainamide in patients treated with procainamide and N-acetylprocainamide. Ther. Drug Monit. 3, 231 – 237.

22. Ruo, T. I., Morita, Y., Atkinson, A. J., Henthorn, T. and Thenot, J. P. (1981) Identification of desethyl procainamide in patients: a new metabolite of procainamide. J. Pharmacol. Exp. Ther. 216, 357 – 362.

23. Uetrecht, J. P., Woosley, R. L., Freeman, R. W., Sweetman, B. J. and Oates, J. A. (1981) Metabolism of procainamide in the perfused rat liver. Drug Metab. Dispos. 9, 183 – 187.

24. Hein, D. W., Hirata, M. and Weber, W. W. (1981) An enzyme marker to ensure reliable determinations of human isoniazid acetylator phenotype in vitro. Pharmacology 23, 203 – 210.

25. Glowinski, I. B., Radtke, H. E. and Weber, W. W. (1978) Genetic variation in N-acetylation of carcinogenic arylamines by human and rabbit liver. Mol. Pharmacol. 14, 940 – 949.

26. Roberts, S. M., Budinsky, R. A., Adams, L. E., Litwin, A. and Hess, E. V. (1985) Procainamide acetylation in strains of rat and mouse. Drug Metab. Dispos. 13, 517 – 519.

27. Tannen, R. H. and Weber, W. W. (1980) Antinuclear antibodies related to acetylator phenotype in mice. J. Pharmacol. Exp. Ther. 213, 485 – 490.

28. Hein, D. W., Smolen, T. N., Fox, R. R. and Weber, W. W. (1982) Identification of genetically homozygous rapid and slow acetylators of drugs and environmental carcinogens among established inbred rabbit strains. J. Pharmacol. Exp. Ther. 223, 40 – 44.

29. Hein, D. W., Omichinski, J. G., Brewer, J. A. and Weber, W. W. (1982) A unique pharmacogenetic expression of the N-acetylation polymorphism in the inbred hamster. J. Pharmacol. Exp. Ther. 220, 8 – 15.

30. Hein, D. W., Kirlin, W. G., Ferguson, R. J. and Weber, W. W. (1985) Biochemical investigation of the basis for the genetic N-acetylation polymorphism in the inbred hamster. J. Pharmacol. Exp. Ther. 234, 358 – 364.

31. Hein, D. W., Kirlin, W. G., Ogolla, F., Trinidad, A., Thompson, L. K. and Ferguson, R. J. (1986) The role of acetylator genotype on hepatic and extrahepatic acetylation, deacetylation, and sulfation of 2-aminofluorene, 2-acetylaminofluorene and N-hydroxy-acetylaminoflurene in the inbred hamster. Drug Metab. Dispos. 14, 566 – 573.

32. Reidenberg, M. M., Drayer, D. E., Levy, M. and Warner, E. (1975) Polymorphic acetylation of procainamide in man. Clin. Pharmacol. Ther. 17, 722 – 730.

33. Gibson, T. P., Matuski, J., Matusik, E., Nelson, H. A., Wilkinson, J. and Briggs, N.

262

A. (1975) Acetylation of procainamide in man and its relationship to isoniazid acetylation phenotype. Clin. Pharmacol. Ther. 17, 395 – 399.

34. Kalsson, E. and Molin, L. (1975) Polymorphic acetylation of procainamide in healthy subjects. Acta Med. Scand. 197, 299 – 302.

35. Frislid, K., Berg, M., Hansteen, V. and Lunde, P. K. M. (1976) Comparison of the acetylation of the procainamide and sulfadimidine in man. Eur. J. Clin. Pharmacol. 9, 433 – 438.

36. Giardina, E. V., Stein, R. M. and Bigger, J. T. (1977) The relationship between the metabolism of procainamide and sulfamethazine. Circulation 55, 388 – 394.

37. DuSouich, P. and Erill, S. (1977) Metabolism of procainamide and p-aminobenzoic acid in patients with chronic liver disease. Clin. Pharmacol. Ther. 22, 588 – 595.

38. DuSouich, P. and Erill, S. (1978) Metabolism of procainamide in patients with chronic heart failure, chronic respiratory failure and chronic renal failure. Eur. J. Clin. Pharmacol. 14, 21 – 27.

39. Ylitalo, P., Ruosteenoja, R., Leskinen, O. and Metsa-Ketela, T. (1983) Significance of acetylator phenotype in pharmacokinetics and adverse effects of procainamide. Eur. J. Clin. Pharmacol. 25, 791 – 795.

40. Davies, D. M., Beedie, M. A. and Rawlins, M. D. (1975) Antinuclear antibodies during procainamide treatment and drug acetylation. Br. Med. J. 3, 682 – 683.

41. Henningsen, N. C., Cederberg, A., Hanson, A. and Johansson, B. W. (1975) Effects of long-term treatment with procainamide. Acta Med. Scand. 198, 475 – 482.

42. Sonnhag, C., Karlsson, E. and Hed, J. (1979) Procainamide-induced lupus erythematosus-like syndrome in relation to acetylator phenotype and plasma levels of procainamide. Acta Med. Scand. 206, 245 – 251.

43. Woosley, R. L., Drayer, D. E., Reidenberg, M. M., Nies, A. S., Carr, K. and Oates, J. A. (1978) Effect of acetylator phenotype on the rate at which procainamide induces antinuclear antibodies and the lupus syndrome. N. Engl. J. Med. 298, 1157 – 1159.

44. Lahita, R., Kluger, J., Drayer, D. E., Koffler, D. and Reidenberg, M. M. (1979) Antibodies to nuclear antigens in patients treated with procainamide or acetylprocainamide. N. Engl. J. Med. 301, 1382 – 1385.

45. Roden, D. M., Reele, S. B., Higgins, S. B., Wilkinson, G. R., Smith, R. F., Oates, J. A. and Woosley, R. L. (1980) Antiarrhythmic efficacy, pharmacokinetics, and safety of N-acetylprocainamide in human subjects: comparisons with procainamide. Am. J. Cardiol. 46, 463 – 468.

46. Kluger, J., Drayer, D. E., Reidenberg, M. M. and Lahita, R. (1981) Acetylprocainamide therapy in patients with previous procainamide-induced lupus syndrome. Ann. Intern. Med. 95, 18 – 23.

47. Atkinson, A. J., Lertora, J. L., Kushner, W., Chao, G. C. and Nevin, M. J. (1983) Efficacy and safety of N-acetylprocainamide in long-term treatment of ventricular arrhythmias. Clin. Pharmacol. Ther. 33, 565 – 576.

48. Freeman, R. W., Woosley, R. L., Oates, J. A. and Harbison, R. D. (1979) Evidence for the biotransformation of procainamide to a reactive metabolite. Toxicol. Appl. Pharmacol. 50, 9 – 16.

49. Freeman, R. W., Uetrecht, J. P., Woosley, R. L., Oates, J. A. and Harbison, R. D. (1981) Covalent binding of procainamide in vitro and in vivo to hepatic protein in mice. Drug Metab. Dispos. 9, 188 – 192.

50. Uetrecht, J. P., Sweetman, B. J., Woosley, R. L. and Oates, J. A. (1983) Metabolism of procainamide to a hydroxylamine by rat and human hepatic microsomes. Drug Metab. Dispos. 12, 75 – 81.

51. Budinsky, R. A., Roberts, S. M., Coats, E. A., Adams, L. and Hess, E. (1987) The formation of procainamide hydroxylamine by rat and human liver microsomes. Drug Metab. Dispos. 15, 37 – 43.

52. Uetrecht, J. P. (1985) Reactivity and possible significance of hydroxylamine and nitroso

metabolites of procainamide. J. Pharmacol. Exp. Ther. 232, 420 – 425.

53. Fritzler, M. J. and Tan, E. M. (1978) Antibodies to histones in drug-induced and idiopathic lupus erythematosus. J. Clin. Invest. 62, 560 – 567.

54. Portanova, J. P., Rubin, R. L., Joslin, F. G., Agnello, V.D. and Tan, E. M. (1982) Reactivity of anti-histone antibodies induced by procainamide and hydralazine. Clin. Immunol. Immunopathol. 25, 67 – 79.

55. Rubin, R. L., Uetrecht, J. P. and Jones, J. E. (1987) Cytotoxicity of oxidative metabolites of procainamide. J. Pharmacol. Exp. Ther. 242, 833 – 841.

56. Uetrecht, J., Zahid, N. and Rubin, R. (1988) Metabolism of procainamide to a hydroxylamine by human neutrophils and mononuclear leukocytes. Chem. Res. Toxicol. 1, 74 – 78.

57. Hein, D. W. (1988) Acetylator genotype and arylamine-induced carcinogenesis. Biochim. Biophysica Acta, 948, 37 – 66.

58. Ludden, T. M., McNay, J. L., Shepherd, A. M. M. and Lin, M. S. (1982) Clinical pharmacokinetics of hydralazine. Clin. Pharmacokinet. 7, 185 – 205.

59. Evans, D. A. P. and White, T. A. (1964) Human acetylation polymorphism. J. Lab. Clin. Med. 63, 394 – 403.

60. Perry, H. M., Tan, E. M., Carmody, S. and Sakamota, A. (1970) Relationship of acetyl transferase activity to antinuclear antibodies and toxic symptoms in hypertensive patients treated with hydralazine. J. Lab. Clin. Med. 76, 114 – 125.

61. Perry, H. M. (1973) Late toxicity to hydralazine resembling systemic lupus erythematosus or rheumatoid arthritis. Am. J. Med. 54, 58 – 72.

62. Strandberg, I., Boman, G., Hassler, I. and Sjöqvist, F. (1976) Acetylator phenotype in patients with hydralazine-induced lupoid syndrome. Acta Med. Scand. 1, 269 – 274.

63. Batchelor, J. R., Welsh, K. I., Mansilla-Tinoco, R., Dollery, C. T., Hughes, G. R. V., Bernstein, R., Ryan, P., Naish, P. F., Aber, G. M., Bing, R. F. and Russell, G. I. (1980) Hydralazine-induced systemic lupus erythematosus: influence of HLA-DR and sex on susceptibility. Lancet 1, 1107 – 1109.

64. Timbrell, J. A., Facchini, V., Harland, S. J. and Mansilla-Tinoco, R. (1984) Hydralazine-induced lupus: is there a toxic metabolic pathway? Eur. J. Clin. Pharmacol. 27, 555 – 559.

65. Zacest, R. and Koch-Weser, J. (1972) Relation of hydralazine plasma concentration to dosage and hypotensive action. Clin. Pharmacol. Ther. 13, 420 – 425.

66. Reidenberg, M. M., Drayer, D., DeMarco, A. L. and Bello, C. T. (1973) Hydralazine elimination in man. Clin. Pharmacol. Ther. 14, 970 – 977.

67. Timbrell, J. A., Harland, S. J. and Facchini, V. (1980) Polymorphic acetylation of hydralazine. Clin. Pharmacol. Ther. 28, 350 – 355.

68. Facchini, V. and Timbrell, J. A. (1981) Further evidence for an acetylator phenotype difference in the metabolism of hydralazine in man. Br. J. Clin. Pharmacol. 11, 345 – 351.

69. Schmid, K., Kung, W., Riess, W., Dollery, C. T. and Harland, S. J. (1981) Metabolism of hydralazine in man. Arzneim.-Forsch. 31, 1143 – 1147.

70. Timbrell, J. A., Harland, S. J. and Facchini, V. (1981) Effect of dose on acetylator phenotype distribution of hydralazine. Clin. Pharmacol. Ther. 29, 337 – 343.

71. Reece, P. A., Cozamanis, I. and Zacest, R. (1980) Kinetics of hydralazine and its main metabolites in slow and fast acetylators. Clin. Pharmacol. Ther. 28, 769 – 778.

72. Shepherd, A. M. M., McNay, J. L., Ludden, T. M., Lin, M. S. and Musgrave, G. (1981) Plasma concentration and acetylator phenotype determine response to oral hydralazine. Hypertension 3, 580 – 585.

73. Shepherd, A. M. M., Irvine, N. A., Ludden, T. M., Lin, M. S. and McNay, J. L. (1984) Effect of oral dose size on hydralazine kinetics and vasodepressor response. Clin. Pharmacol. Ther. 36, 595 – 600.

74. Shen, D. D., Hosler, J. P., Schroder, R. L. and Azarnoff, D. L. (1980) Pharmacokinetics of

hydralazine and its acid-labile hydrazone metabolites in relation to acetylator phenotype. J. Pharmacokinet. Biopharm. 8, 53 – 68.

75. Dubroff, L. W. and Reid, R. J. Jr., (1980) Hydralazine-pyrimidine interactions may explain hydralazine-induced lupus erythematosus. Science 208, 404 – 406.

76. Sinha, B. K. and Patterson, M. A. (1983) Free radical metabolism of hydralazine binding and degradation of nucleic acids. Biochem. Pharmacol. 32, 3279 – 3284.

77. Williams, G. M., Mazue, G., McQueen, C. M. and Shimada, T. (1980) Genotoxicity of the antihypertensive drugs hydralazine and dihydralazine. Science 210, 329 – 330.

78. McQueen, C. A., Maslansky, C. J., Glowinski, I. B., Crescenzi, S. B., Weber, W. W. and Williams, G. M. (1982) Relationship between the genetically determined acetylator phenotype and DNA damage induced by hydralazine and 2-aminofluorene in cultured rabbit hepatocytes. Proc. Natl. Acad. Sci. USA 79, 1269 – 1272.

79. Streeter, A. J. and Timbrell, J. A. (1983) Studies on the in vivo metabolism of hydralazine in the rat. Drug Metab. Dispos. 11, 184 – 189.

80. Streeter, A. J. and Timbrell, J. A. (1983) Enzyme-mediated covalent binding of hydralazine to rat liver microsomes. Drug Metab. Dispos. 11, 179 – 183.

81. Streeter, A. J. and Timbrell, J. A. (1985) The in vitro metabolism of hydralazine. Drug Metab. Dispos. 13, 255 – 259.

82. LaCagnin, L. B., Colby, H. D. and O'Donnell, J. P. (1986) The oxidative metabolism of hydralazine by rat liver microsomes. Drug Metab. Dispos. 14, 549 – 554.

83. Sinha, B. K. and Motten, A. G. (1982) Oxidative metabolism of hydralazine: evidence for nitrogen centered radicals formation. Biochem. Biophys. Res. Commun. 105, 1044 – 1051.

84. Sinha, B. K. (1983) Enzymatic activation of hydrazine derivatives: a spin-trapping study. J. Biol. Chem. 258, 796 – 801.

85. Kalyanaraman, B. and Sinha, B. K. (1985) Free radical-mediated activation of hydrazine derivatives. Environ. Health Persp. 64, 179 – 184.

86. Cannat, A. and Seligmann, M. (1968) Induction by isoniazid and hydralazine of antinuclear factors in mice. Clin. Exp. Immunol. 20, 99 – 105.

87. Alarcon-Segovia, D., Fishbein, E. and Betancourt, V. M. (1969) Antibodies to nucleoprotein in tuberculous patients receiving isoniazid. Clin. Exp. Immunol. 5, 429 – 437.

88. Evans, D. A. P., Bullen, M. F., Houston, J., Hopkins, C. A., and Vetters, J. M. (1972) Antinuclear factor in rapid and slow acetylator patients treated with isoniazid. J. Med. Genet. 9, 53 – 56.

89. Godeau, P., Aubert, M., Imbert, J. C. and Herreman, G. (1973) Lupus érythémateux disséminé et taux d'isoniazide actif. Ann. Med. Intern. 124, 181 – 186.

90. Maddrey, W. C. and Boinott, J. K. (1973) Isoniazid hepatitis. Ann. Intern. Med. 79, 1 – 12.

91. Weber, W. W. and Hein, D. W. (1979) Clinical pharmacokinetics of isoniazid. Clin. Pharmacokinet. 4, 401 – 422.

92. Ellard, G. A. and Gammon, P. T. (1976) Pharmacokinetics of isoniazid metabolism in man. J. Pharmacokinet. Biopharm. 4, 83 – 133.

93. Hein, D. W. and Weber, W. W. (1982) Polymorphic N-acetylation of phenelzine and monoacetylhydrazine by highly purified rabbit liver isoniazid N-acetyltransferase. Drug Metab. Dispos. 10, 225 – 229.

94. Hein, D. W., Trinidad, A., Yerokun, T., Ferguson, R. J., Kirlin, W. G. and Weber, W. W. (1988) Genetic control of acetyl coenzyme A dependent arylamine N-acetyltransferase, hydrazine N-acetyltransferase, and N-hydroxyarylamine O-acetyltransferase enzymes in C57BL/6J, A/J, $AC57F_1$, and the rapid and slow acetylator A.B6 and B6.A congenic inbred mouse. Drug Metab. Dispos. 16, 341 – 347.

95. Nelson, S. D., Mitchell, J. R., Timbrell, J. A., Snodgrass, W. R. and Corcoran, G. B. (1976) Isoniazid and iproniazid: activation of metabolites to toxic intermediates in man and rat. Science 193, 901 – 903.

96. Timbrell, J. A., Mitchell, J. R., Snodgrass, W. R. and Nelson, S. D. (1980) Isoniazid hepatotoxicity: the relationship between covalent binding and metabolism in vivo. J. Pharmacol. Exp. Ther. 213, 364 – 369.

97. Timbrell, J. A., Wright, J. M. and Baillie, T. A. (1977) Monoacetylhydrazine as a metabolite of isoniazid in man. Clin. Pharmacol. Ther. 22, 602 – 608.

98. Timbrell, J. A. and Wright, J. M. (1979) Studies on the effects of isoniazid on acetylhydrazine metabolism in vivo and in vitro. Drug Metab. Dispos. 7, 237 – 240.

99. Lauterberg, B. H., Smith, C. V., Todd, E. L. and Mitchell, J. R. (1985) Pharmacokinetics of the toxic hydrazino metabolites formed from isoniazid in humans. J. Pharmacol. Exp. Ther. 235, 566 – 570.

100. Lauterberg, B. H., Smith, C. V., Todd, E. L. and Mitchell, J. R. (1985) Oxidation of hydrazine metabolites formed from isoniazid. Clin. Pharmacol. Ther. 38, 566 – 571.

101. Maru, G. B., Bhide, S., Jaffhill, R. and O'Connor, P. J. (1987) Formation and persistence of isoniazid-DNA adducts in mouse tissue. Hum. Toxicol. 6, 153 – 158.

102. Noda, A., Goromaru, T., Matsuyama, K., Sogabe, K., Hsu, K.-Y., and Iguchi, S. (1978) Quantitative determination of hydrazine derived from isoniazid in patients, I. J. Pharmacobiodyn. 1, 132 – 141.

103. Timbrell, J. A. and Harland, S. J. (1979) Identification and quantitation of hydrazine in the urine of patients treated with hydralazine. Clin. Pharmacol. Ther. 26, 81 – 88.

104. Noda, A., Noda, K., Ohno, T., Sendo, A., Misaka, A., Kanazawa, Y., Isobe, R. and Hirata, M. (1986) Spin trapping of a free radical intermediate formed during microsomal metabolism of hydrazine. Biochem. Biophys. Res. Commun. 133, 1086 – 1091.

M.E. Kammüller, N. Bloksma and W. Seinen (Eds.)
Autoimmunity and Toxicology
© *1989 Elsevier Science Publishers B.V. (Biomedical Division)*

Drug interactions with complement components in relation to the induction of autoimmune(-like) reactions

10

E. SIM

Department of Pharmacology, University of Oxford, South Parks Road, Oxford, OX1 3QT, UK

I. Introduction

The complement system, which consists of around 20 proteins in the blood, acts as a link between specific recognition of foreign antigens and the means of destroying these antigens. The complement system is often referred to as the major effector mechanism of humoral immune defence. It is convenient, when considering the role of complement, to divide antigens into two types − cellular and non-cellular. The interaction of the complement system with those groups of antigens is summarised in Fig. 1.

For cellular antigens complexed with antibody or for bacteria, the complement system causes lysis of these cells. For non-cellular antigens, complement causes solubilisation of preformed complexes with antibody *in vitro* [1], although *in vivo* inhibition of precipitation of immune complexes is likely to be more important [2]. Phagocytosis of both non-cellular and cellular antigens is promoted by complement, and this action of complement is termed opsonisation.

Complement is triggered via a recognition component followed by sequentially activated proteases, and there are two ways in which this can occur (for review see [3]). The two activation routes are known as the classical and alternative pathways and they have different recognition components. The recognition component of the classical pathway is C1q which binds to the Fc portion of antibody, after it has bound to antigen, and thereby promotes activation of the first serine proteases, C1r

268

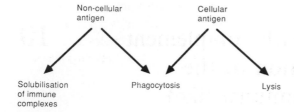

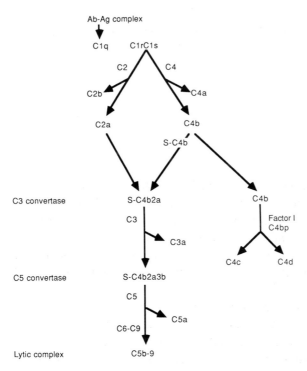

Fig. 1. The roles of the complement system. The central event in each case is covalent binding of C3b. Complement activation by either the classical or alternative pathways can be triggered by antibody-antigen complexes or sometimes by antigen alone. Activation without the need for antibody usually occurs with large particulate antigens, e.g. micro-organisms.

Fig. 2. Activation of the classical pathway. C1q recognises antibody in an immune complex and this leads sequentially to activation of serine proteases C1r and C1s. C1s cleaves C4 and C2, fragments C4b and C2a form the C3 convertase of the classical pathway (C4b2a) if the C4b becomes covalently bound via the thioester site to a surface (S). C4b in the fluid phase is rapidly degraded to C4c and C4d by factor I and its cofactor C4b-binding protein (C4bp). The control proteins also act on surface-bound C4b. C3b, produced by the classical pathway convertase, can participate in the alternative pathway (see Fig. 3), and can form a C5 convertase of the classical pathway (C4b2aC3b). C5b acts as a focus for the lytic assembly. C3, C4 and C5 are all structurally related but C5 has no internal thioester. C3a, C4a and C5a are anaphylatoxins. C5a is also chemotactic.

and C1s (Fig. 2). The recognition mechanism of the alternative pathway is not well defined but it is known that a range of materials, e.g. yeast cell walls, parasites, bacterial lipopolysaccharide, in addition to antibody-antigen complexes, can activate the alternative pathway, probably through protection of the key enzyme, C3 convertase, from degradation [4] (Fig. 3).

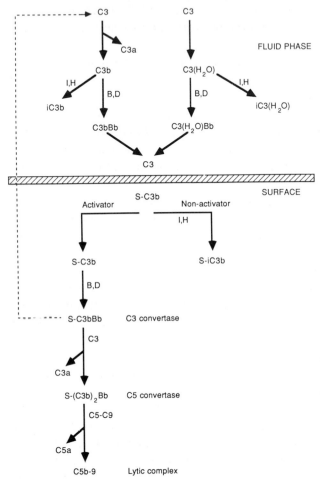

Fig. 3. The alternative pathway of complement. Initiation results from spontaneous hydrolysis of the thioester site in C3 to produce 'C3b-like C3' ($C3H_2O$). The resulting C3 convertase [($C3H_2O$)Bb] catalyses production of C3b which may become covalently bound to a surface on exposure of the reactive thioester group. The thioester in C3b which does not react with a surface, is hydrolysed to form C3b in the fluid phase. Fluid phase C3b will either be degraded by factor I and factor H to form iC3b, or else will form a fluid phase C3 convertase (C3bBb). The C3b which becomes bound to a surface (S-C3b) will either be degraded by factor I and factor H to S-iC3b if the surface is not an alternate pathway activator, or if the surface is an activator, a solid phase C3 convertase (S-C3bBb) will be formed. S-C3bBb cleaves more fluid phase C3 and so is an amplification mechanism for C3b deposition. It also acts as the focus for C5b production and subsequent assembly of the lytic complex. (After Pangburn and Müller-Eberhard, 1983 [76].)

For both of these activation routes, the outcome is the same. Complex enzymes called C3 convertases are produced which cleave C3, the major complement protein, to C3b. C3b is of particular importance because it becomes covalently bound to the surface which activated complement. C3b bound in this way (a) acts as a focus for C5b production and subsequent assembly of the lytic pathway components (C5-C9); (b) acts as a label for recognition by phagocytic cells via C3 receptors; and (c) disrupts the antibody-antigen lattice, preventing formation of large insoluble aggregates ('solubilisation'; Fig. 1).

Therefore, C3b deposition (covalent binding) is crucial in determining the fate of immune complexes (immune complex handling), since it is involved in both phagocytosis and control of immune complex size. Any reduction in C3b binding to immune complexes is likely to result in decreased phagocytosis and solubilisation of non-cellular immune complexes with the outcome that larger complexes persist for longer in the circulation. Such a situation is likely to promote deposition of immune complexes particularly in small blood vessels, as is found in systemic lupus erythematosus.

Idiopathic systemic lupus erythematosus (SLE) is a condition in which immune complexes containing non-cellular antigens become deposited at inappropriate sites in the body and the disease can be considered as a disorder of immune complex handling [5]. Evidence for the importance of the complement system in clearance of non-cellular antigens such as are found in SLE, is provided by patients with deficiencies of components C1, C4 and C2 of the classical pathway. These individuals are at increased risk of suffering from idiopathic systemic lupus erythematosus [6]. Since the autoimmune-like side effects of hydralazine, isoniazid, and procainamide resemble SLE in that antinuclear antibodies are found together with tissue deposition of immune complexes, it seemed plausible at the outset of the work which will be described that these drugs could interact with the early components of complement to interfere with immune complex clearance.

The C3 convertases of the classical and alternative pathways (C4b2a and C3bBb, respectively), each consist of a serine protease (activated C2 or factor B) which is only active when bound to a regulatory component, either C4b or C3b. This represents the major amplification stage of the complement sequence, since C3b acts as the regulatory subunit of the alternative pathway C3 convertase and so can catalyse its own production. The control protease, factor I, and its cofactor, factor H, act to cleave C3b to iC3b which can no longer participate in the complement cascade (Fig. 3). These control proteins are important physiologically and if factor I is removed from serum, then the normal 'tick-over' of activation of the alternative pathway which occurs continuously at a low level [4] will lead to complete conversion of serum C3 to C3b.

The protein structure and molecular biology of many of the complement proteins is well understood [7]. The reactivity of the related proteins C4 and C3 is important for consideration of the interactions of drugs which induce SLE-like symptoms as a toxic side effect.

Complement components C4 and C3 (Fig. 4) are each activated by proteolysis of a single bond producing a polypeptide of 8 000 molecular weight (C3a or C4a) and the remainder of the protein is termed C3b or C4b. In C3 and C4 there is an internal thioester group between a cysteine and a glutamyl residue (Fig. 5) (for review see [8]). The thioester is buried within the protein until it is activated to produce 'a' and 'b' fragments. Immediately after activation of C4 by C1s in an immune complex, the thioester group becomes accessible and highly reactive in C4b. The activated thioester will react within 100 μs to form a covalent bond with any adjacent nucleophilic groups. This is summarised in Fig. 6. If the group to which the activated C4b or C3b binds covalently is on the surface of an immune complex then the bound complement protein participates in the continuation of the complement sequence on the surface of the immune complex. However, only around 10% of C4b

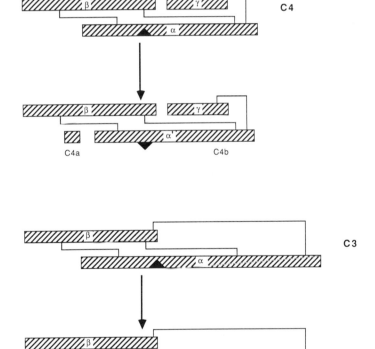

Fig. 4. Protein structure of C4 and C3. C4 consists of three polypeptide chains and C3 consists of two polypeptide chains linked by disulphide bridges. Activation fragments C4a and C3a each with a molecular weight of 8 000 are released from the amino terminus of the α chain. The thioester site, which becomes exposed on activation, is shown as a spike.

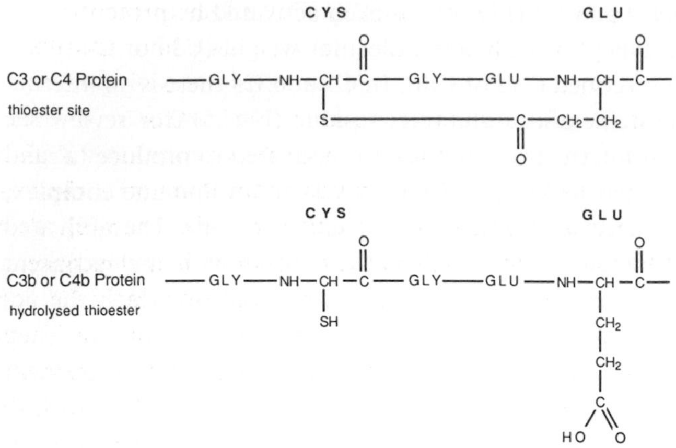

272

CYS

GLU

C3 or C4 Protein —GLY—NH—CH—C—GLY—GLU—NH—CH—C—

thioester site

Fig. 5. The sequence of the thioester site in C3 and C4. The sequence of the pentapeptide forming the thioester in C3 and C4 is shown.

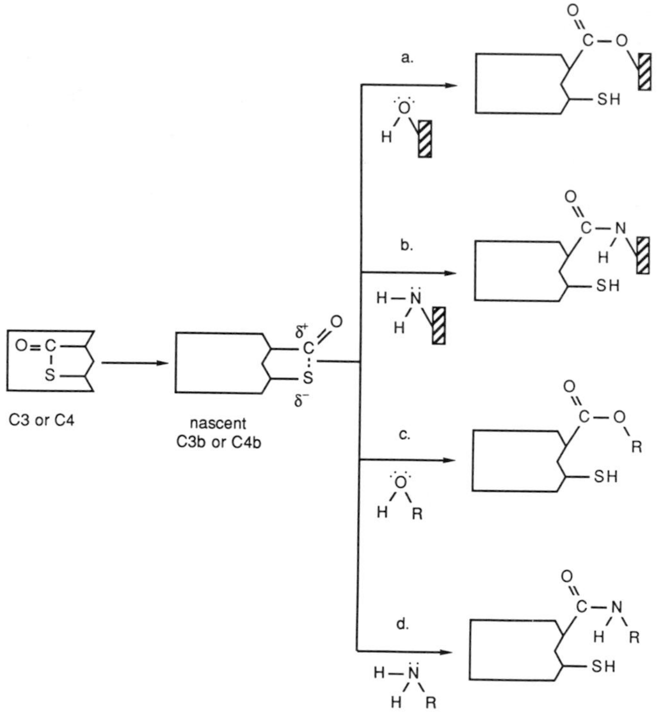

CYS

GLU

C3b or C4b Protein —GLY—NH—CH—C—GLY—GLU—NH—CH—C—

hydrolysed thioester

a.

b.

O=C
S

C3 or C4

nascent
C3b or C4b

c.

d.

Fig. 6. The covalent binding reaction of C3 and C4. C4 is activated by C1s and C3 is activated by C3 convertase. C3b or C4b in the nascent state has a half-life of 100 μs before it is hydrolysed [9]. During this time it can bind covalently to complement activating surfaces (hatched areas) by either ester (a) or amide (b) bonds. Fluid phase hydroxyl (c) or amino (d) groups compete for binding to the surface. If the hydroxyl group (c) comes from water then C3b or C4b with a hydrolysed thioester is produced. Reaction of hydralazine with C4 during activation occurs through route d.

or C3b which is activated becomes covalently bound to the surface of the immune complex in this way [9] (routes a and b, Fig. 6). The majority of activated C4b or C3b reacts with water, and C4b or C3b in which the active site thioester is hydrolysed (route c, Fig. 6), floats away in solution unable to participate further in the complement sequence on the activating surface. Other nucleophiles in solution will also react with activated C4b or C3b (route d, Fig. 6). In this case, the thioester is cleaved and the nucleophile itself becomes covalently bound to the carbonyl group [9]. This modified C4b or C3b is also unable to participate in the continuation of the complement sequence on the immune complex. Any inhibition by nucleophiles of C4b or C3b binding to the immune complex surface would result in inhibition of amplification of activation of the complement sequence on the surface of the immune complex.

The covalent binding of C3b to immune complexes was initially discovered using red blood cells as antigens [10], and these studies have been extended to binding of C4b and C3b to immune complexes with non-cellular antigens [11, 12]. The thioester site in C3 and C4 is buried in the native proteins and exposure of the thioester site on activation of C4 or C3 occurs as a result of proteolysis of a bond distant in primary sequence from the thioester site (see [13] for review). However, structural modification of these proteins can occur such that the thioester site is exposed without prior proteolysis (Fig. 7). The thioester exposed in this way has been shown to react with water [8] or with nucleophiles [14].

If the polypeptide chain of C3 is intact but the thioester is hydrolysed (C3b-like C3), the protein, although it cannot bind to immune complexes, can form part of

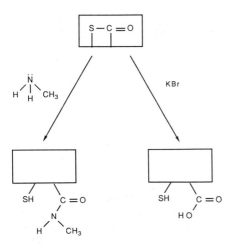

Fig. 7. Production of 'C3b-like C3' and 'C4b-like C4'. Chaotropic agents e.g. KBr, interact with C3 or C4 and cause a conformational change such that, with the polypeptide still intact, the thioester site becomes exposed and hydrolysed. High concentrations of small nucleophiles (e.g. 200 mM methylamine, pH 9) can also react with the buried thioester.

a C3 convertase in the fluid phase (Figs. 3 and 7). So if sufficient 'C3b-like C3' is generated, it can act as a fluid-phase complement activator [15, 16]. Fluid-phase complement activation is not a major problem under normal circumstances. C3b which is generated in plasma as a normal consequence of complement activation, is degraded rapidly to iC3b which is inactive in C3 convertase formation. However, in pathological conditions, e.g. deficiency of factor I or factor H [4], or inhibition of factor I, uncontrolled C3 activation can occur.

To recap, two distinct reactivities of the active site of C3 and C4 are important for interaction with xenobiotics.

(a) In the case of low concentrations of most nucleophiles, interaction can only occur when the nucleophile is present during activation of C4 or C3. The thioester is rendered accessible to interaction with nucleophiles as a result of conformational change after proteolytic cleavage of C4 or C3 by the appropriate enzyme.

(b) The other aspect involves interaction with nucleophiles without proteolytic cleavage of the native molecule (Fig. 7). Low molecular weight nucleophiles present at high concentrations (e.g. 200 mM methylamine, pH 9), can penetrate into the buried thioester site and react with it. Conformational change of the native C3 or C4 molecules occurs on incubation with chaotropic agents (e.g. KBr) such that the active site thioester becomes exposed and susceptible to hydrolysis. The resulting C3 and C4 with the thioester cleaved are termed 'C3b-like C3' and 'C4b-like C4',

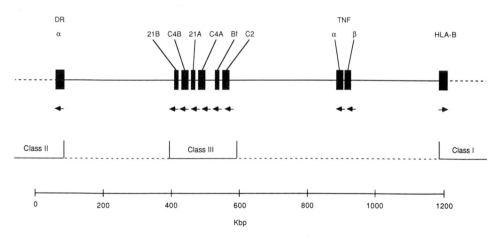

Fig. 8. HLA class III region. The HLA class III region on the short arm of human chromosome 6 has been positioned between the class I region HLA-B and the class II region HLA-DR α chain genes. Complement factor B (Bf) of the alternative pathway, C2, C4A and C4B are indicated. The steroid 21 hydroxylase A pseudogene (21A) and the steroid 21 hydroxylase B gene (21B) are very close to C4A and C4B, respectively. The number of copies of C4A and C4B genes depends on the HLA haplotype, but the most common arrangement is one copy of C4A and one copy of C4B per chromosome. The tumour necrosis factor (TNF) genes are also shown. The direction of the genes is indicated by arrows and the distances are in kilobasepairs (Kbp) [79].

respectively, because they have structural and functional properties resembling C3b or C4b in the fluid phase (Figs. 3 and 7).

These two aspects of C3 and C4 reactivity form the basis for the autoimmune-like reactions which will be discussed in this chapter – drug-induced SLE and hypersensitivity [17].

One other important question is genetic variation amongst individuals such that only a proportion of patients develop a toxic reaction. Complement component C4 is highly polymorphic, and as a 'target' molecule this polymorphism may be important in immunotoxicity. C4 is encoded in the major histocompatibility complex at two highly polymorphic loci termed C4A and C4B [13] (Fig. 8). There are at least 35 different C4 variants (e.g. C4A6 or C4B1): the products of different possible alleles at both loci. Normal individuals have four C4 genes, two each of C4A and of C4B, but null alleles with no functional gene products occur in 25% of individuals and multiple copies of either the A or the B gene (as a result of gene duplication) are also found [13]. The gene products of the C4A locus and the C4B locus have been the subject of intense investigation. It has been known for many years that the reactivities, in terms of haemolytic efficiency of the A and B gene products, are different. The origin of the difference in haemolytic activities of the C4A

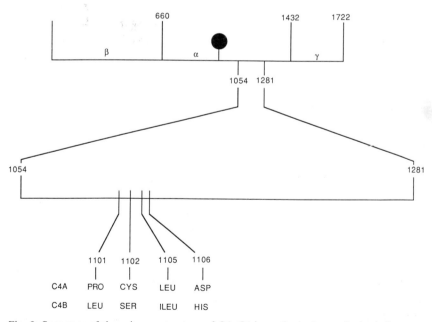

Fig. 9. Summary of the primary structure of C4. C4 is synthesised as a single chain precursor of 1 722 amino acids and the numbers refer to the amino acid position in the single chain form. The α, β and γ chains are indicated. The thioester site is marked by a lollipop. The polymorphic region of the sequence of the chain is expanded. Within this region residues 1 101 – 1 106 contain the C4A- or C4B-specific sequences.

and C4B gene products is now known to be a result of different covalent binding properties of the C4A and C4B proteins after activation [18, 19], although there are only four type-specific amino acid differences between C4A and C4B out of 1 722 amino acid residues (Fig. 9) [20, 21]. Both gene products have the same activation mechanism and reactive thioester binding site. However, the carbonyl group of the thioester of C4A is more reactive with nitrogen nucleophiles, while the carbonyl group of the thioester of C4B is more readily attacked by hydroxyl groups [18, 19]. The increased haemolytic activity of C4B is due to the abundance of hydroxyl groups from cell surface carbohydrate on the surface of the red cell as antigen in the complement-activating complex (see Fig. 6, route a). The increased reactivity of C4A with amino groups (Fig. 6, routes b and d) has raised the possibility that the C4A protein is more important in handling immune complexes with protein as antigen, e.g. histones, whereas C4B might be more important with cellular antigens, e.g. bacteria [22]. The four A- or B-specific amino acid residues are distant in primary sequence from the thioester site (Fig. 9), but these regions of the protein must be adjacent in overall three-dimensional structure (see [13] for review).

It has been observed [23] that idiopathic SLE is associated with a non-functioning or null C4A gene at one or both C4A loci.* This may be a clinical manifestation of a reduced ability to cope with immune complexes containing non-cellular antigens, since it has been observed that individuals with only one functional C4A gene have less C4A protein than those with two functional C4A genes [24]. Those with no functional C4A genes have no C4A protein. The C4 type of an individual could also contribute to development of drug-induced SLE.

II. Hypersensitivity reactions

1. RADIOGRAPHIC CONTRAST MEDIA

Following injection of iodinated radiographic contrast media (RCM), in a small proportion of individuals, adverse effects are produced [25]. These immediate symptoms range from nausea, headache and urticaria, to severe oedema, asthma and hypotensive shock [25]. The reactions seem unlikely to be accounted for by antibody production, and adverse effects have been associated with complement activation [26] leading to histamine release. It has been shown that a wide range of contrast media, particularly the protein-binding RCM used to visualise the liver (hepatotropic), cause hydrolysis of the thioester in C3 and C4 without proteolysis of the polypeptide chains [27] (Fig. 7). C3 with the thioester cleaved in this way

---

*C4A and C4B are different gene products whereas C4a and C4b are activation fragments of C4. The terms 'C4 gene' and 'C4 locus' are used interchangeably.

(C3b-like C3) has been shown to participate in formation of a fluid-phase C3 convertase of the alternative pathway (C3bBb) (Fig. 3). This complex enzyme will trigger subsequent activation of C3 by proteolytic cleavage, which results in amplification of the complement cascade and generation of the peptides C3a and C5a. High concentrations of RCM are injected clinically (0.2 – 1 M), and the concentration at the site of injection is likely to cause hydrolysis of the thioester in C3 and C4, since it has been observed that less than 1% of C3 activity remains after treatment of serum with 25 mM adipiodone, a hepatotropic RCM.

Not all radiographic contrast media promote activation of the complement cascade in this way. It has been observed that metrizamide [27] is less effective in mediating hydrolysis of the thioester in C3 and C4. However, it does inhibit the action of factor I which is responsible for controlling the amplification of the complement cascade (Fig. 3) by converting C3b to iC3b. This removal of the usual inhibition allows the normal 'tick-over' of complement activation to proceed to amplification and generation of anaphylatoxins.

There has been no investigation of the reason for the variation in susceptibility of individuals to RCM hypersensitivity. Since the severe anaphylactic symptoms only occur in 1% of individuals, it is clear that additional factors, either genetic or environmental, contribute to the development of this immunotoxic reaction.

2. OTHER DRUGS

It has been shown that penicillins, to which many individuals experience allergic reactions, bind to proteins to form immunogenic penicilloyl derivatives [28]. It has also been observed that penicillins will induce hydrolysis of the thioester in C3 and C4 [29] (Fig. 7). Since high concentrations of these antibiotics are required (40 mM oxacillin converts 50% of C3 to 'C3b-like C3'), the effect is unlikely to be important clinically in the majority of penicillin allergy cases.

Sulphonamides, bacteriostatic agents, also cause production of 'C3b-like C3' and 'C4b-like C4' but more than 50 mM sulphisomidine is required for 50% conversion of C3. Certain sulphhydryl drugs including captopril, an antihypertensive, N-acetyl cysteine, a mucolytic agent, and penicillamine, an anti-arthritic, are associated with toxic effects resembling immediate hypersensitivity. Although disulphide bridging of captopril to plasma proteins has been observed [30], it has been difficult to detect antibodies against these sulphhydryl drugs as haptens [30, 31]. It has been found that these sulphhydryl drugs cause activation of the alternative pathway of complement [31]. This effect has been traced to inhibition of the control protein, factor I, and so the result is similar to that observed with the RCM, metrizamide (see above). Activation of the alternative pathway by sulphhydryl drugs occurs at around 5 – 10 mM [31]. These concentrations of sulphhydryl drugs are unlikely to be reached clinically, although local high concentrations might be possible.

However, drug treatment of individuals receiving radiographic contrast media

278

should be taken into consideration, since a combination of drugs, each with the potential to activate the alternative pathway, could act synergistically to promote anaphylaxis [17], e.g. giving RCM to patients receiving captopril.

III. Drug-induced SLE

Drugs which induce SLE as a toxic side effect are very varied [32] (Table 1), indicating that the toxicity is not pharmacological in origin. The drugs inducing SLE will be considered as three groups: (1) hydralazine and isoniazid; (2) procainamide and other aromatic amines; (3) penicillamine; and then (4) individual variation in predisposition to drug-induced SLE will be discussed.

1. HYDRALAZINE AND ISONIAZID

During investigation of the reactivity of the thioester group in C3, it was observed that phenylhydrazine is an inhibitor of the covalent binding reaction of C3 when present during activation of C3 [9]. Phenylhydrazine, like both hydralazine and isoniazid, is a monosubstituted hydrazine (Fig. 10). Therefore, in order to investigate the effects of these drugs on the covalent binding reaction of C3 and C4, model systems were established using appropriate activating enzymes bound to Sepharose as a combined activating and binding surface. For C3, trypsin attached to Sepharose [9] will cleave C3 to C3b without further degradation, if incubation is carried out at 20°C. The Sepharose acts as a surface rich in OH groups to which the activated C3b binds covalently (Fig. 6, route a).

For C4 activation, pure human C1s attached to Sepharose is a specific combined binding and activating surface [33]. Inhibition of binding of radiolabelled C3 or C4 was measured in the presence of drugs or metabolites. The results are illustrated in Table 2. Hydralazine and isoniazid both inhibit the covalent binding of C4 to Sepharose-C1s, at a similar concentration to phenylhydrazine. Inhibition of C3 binding is less marked, 50% inhibition occurs at around 2 mM. This is consistent with the clinical observation that C3-deficient individuals suffer from recurrent infections rather than from immune complex disease [6] i.e. inhibition of C4 is likely to contribute more than inhibition of C3 to problems in immune complex handling.

Clinically, for hydralazine [34] and also for isoniazid, there is an inverse association between ability to metabolise the drug and induction of the toxic reaction. These drugs are both metabolised by N-acetylation. The enzyme which catalyses acetylation of the hydrazine group is polymorphic [36], and individuals who develop SLE are found to express the slow acetylator phenotype which supports the suggestion that the acetylated metabolite is not the toxic agent. The acetylated metabolite of isoniazid is N-acetylisoniazid, whereas acetylated hydralazine undergoes cyclisation [37] and methyltriazolophthalazine (MTP) is found in urine. Neither

TABLE 1

Drugs implicated in drug-induced immune complex disease

antiarrhythmic	PROCAINAMIDE	quinidine
anticonvulsant	ethosuximide methoin phenytoin primidone troxidone	carbamazepine phenturide
antihypertensive	HYDRALAZINE	guanoxan methyldopa reserpine
antiinfective	ISONIAZID	griseofulvin nitrofurantoin penicillin sodium aminosalicylate (PAS) streptomycin sulphonamides tetracycline
antithyroid	thiouracils	methimazole
β-adrenoceptor blockers	PRACTOLOL	acebutol labetal pindolol
miscellaneous	chlorpromazine PENICILLAMINE	ambenonium chloride allopurinol chlorprothixene gold salts lithium methysergide oral contraceptives oxyphenbutazone

Those for which there are many reports are in the middle column. Those in capital letters are where there is a certain association. (After Davies, 1985 [32].)

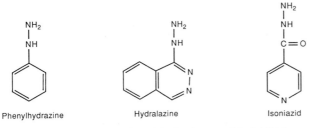

Phenylhydrazine   Hydralazine   Isoniazid

Fig. 10. Structures of substituted hydrazines used in inhibition studies.

TABLE 2

Effect of drugs and metabolites on the covalent binding reaction of C3 and C4

Compound	Concentration (mM) giving 50% inhibition of covalent binding	
	C3	C4
Hydrazine	ND	0.5
Phenylhydrazine	ND	0.88
N-acetyl phenylhydrazine	ND	No inhibition at 20 mM
Hydralazine	2.3	0.84
Methyl triazolophthalazine	ND	No inhibition at 10 mM
Isoniazid	3.6	1.05
N-acetylisoniazid	ND	10% inhibition at 50 mM
Procainamide	14.4	17.5
N-acetyl procainamide	28.4	37.6
Hydroxylamine procainamide	1.7	1.4
Desethyl procainamide	ND	> 20
Practolol	29.2	25.6
Deacetylated practolol	> 10	ND
Hydroxylamine practolol	1.2	1.3

The concentration (mM) of drug or metabolite required to give 50% inhibition of binding of ^{125}I-labelled C3 to Sepharose-trypsin or of ^{125}I-labelled C4 to Sepharose-Cls are shown as determined by Sim et al. [33,78]. ND, not done.

acetylisoniazid nor MTP inhibits the covalent binding of C4 over the same concentration range as the parent drugs (Table 2, Fig. 11).

In order to determine whether hydralazine inhibits C4 binding by the mechanism predicted in Fig. 6, route d, C4 was activated with Cls in the fluid phase in the presence of ^{14}C-hydralazine [38]. The results are shown in Fig. 12. In the presence

Fig. 12. Covalent binding of ^{14}C-hydralazine or ^{14}C-phenylhydrazine to human C4. Pure human C4 was incubated with ^{14}C-hydralazine or ^{14}C-phenylhydrazine in the presence of pure human Cls or with buffer alone as described in [38]. SDS-polyacrylamide gel electropheresis was carried out and an autoradiograph is shown. The positions of the α, β and γ chains of C4 and of the α chain of C4b are shown.

Track 1	[125]IC4 as standard
Track 2	[125]IC4 + Cls as standard
Track 3	C4 + Cls + ^{14}C-hydralazine
Track 4	C4 + phosphate-buffered saline + ^{14}C-hydralazine
Track 5	C4 + Cls + ^{14}C-phenylhydrazine

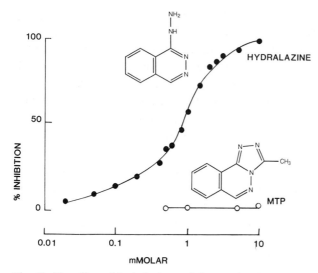

Fig. 11. The effect of hydralazine and the acetylated metabolite, methyltriazolophthalazine (MTP) on the covalent binding of ^{125}I-C4 to Sepharose C1s. The degree of inhibition was determined as described in [33].

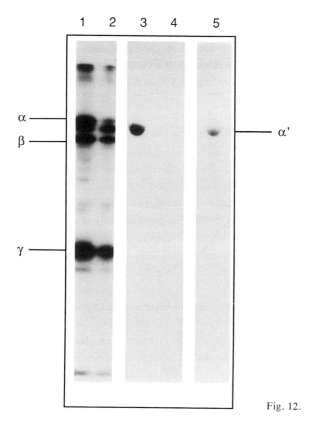

Fig. 12.

of C1s, hydralazine binds to the α' chain of C4b containing the thioester grouping (track 3) whereas in the absence of C1s, hydralazine does not bind to C4. Therefore, these results suggest that hydralazine itself binds directly to C4b thus preventing C4b from interacting covalently with a physiological target, e.g. immune complexes. The concentrations of hydralazine which have been reported in plasma (1 μM) are after short-term oral dosage [39], whereas hydralazine-SLE does not develop until 100 g of the drug has been ingested [40] and accumulation of the drug is likely to occur, although no direct measurement of plasma hydralazine concentration has been made under these conditions. For isoniazid, recorded plasma concentrations [41] would produce 10% inhibition of C4 binding. It may be that continuous low level inhibition of C4 binding finally results in SLE. However, it must be stressed that hydralazine and isoniazid are only inhibitory during C4 activation by immune complexes (Fig. 6) and so no reduction in plasma C4 levels would be expected.

2. PROCAINAMIDE AND PRACTOLOL

Procainamide is an aromatic amine and it is also metabolised by N-acetylation [42] (Fig. 13). Both fast and slow acetylators develop anti-nuclear antibodies, although they take longer to develop in rapid acetylators. It has been suggested in other studies [43 – 45], that an oxidised metabolite of procainamide – e.g. the hydroxylamine metabolite or the nitroso metabolite – may be the toxic agent in drug-induced SLE and that slow acetylators produce more of the oxidised metabolite. In experiments to look at inhibition of covalent binding of C4 or C3 to a complement-

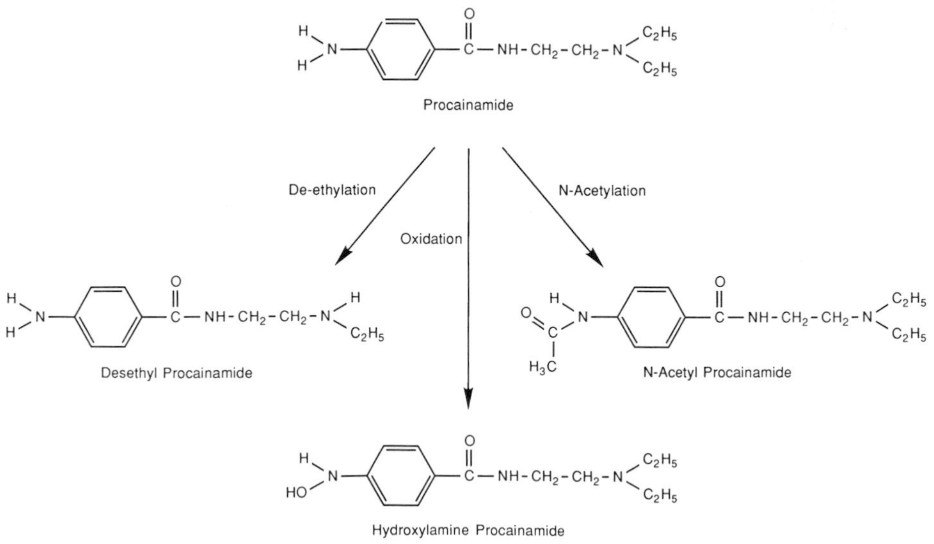

Fig. 13. Generation of procainamide metabolites.

activating surface, it has been found that, although procainamide itself is a poor inhibitor, the hydroxylamine metabolite is inhibitory with 50% inhibition at around 1 mM (Table 2). *N*-acetyl-procainamide is an extremely poor inhibitor of C4 and C3 binding, and it has been observed that administration of *N*-acetylprocainamide as an antiarrhythmic agent does not produce either antinuclear antibodies or SLE in patients [46]. Other aromatic amines induce SLE [47] and it has been found that there is a linear relationship between nucleophilicity and inhibitory potency in nucleophiles in inhibiting C3 binding to Sepharose-trypsin when over 2 000 compounds were tested [48]. For C4, although only a few compounds were tested, there is a general trend suggesting that more nucleophilic compounds are more inhibitory [49]. Hydroxylamines are strong nucleophiles and it seems likely that N-oxidation of aromatic amines could lead to production of a hydroxylamine to inhibit C3 and C4 deposition on immune complexes and, thus, lead to inhibition of normal immune complex clearance. The important question is whether these hydroxylamine metabolites reach high enough concentrations in vivo and this question remains to be answered. To date, there has been much speculation [46] as to the immunotoxic role of such an aromatic hydroxylamine. Inhibition of the covalent binding reaction of C4 and C3, which can be explained at the molecular level, provides the first example where inhibition by such an aromatic hydroxylamine would lead to problems with immune complex handling such as are found in SLE.

Practolol, a cardio-selective β-antagonist, is an *N*-acetyl aromatic amine (Fig. 14)

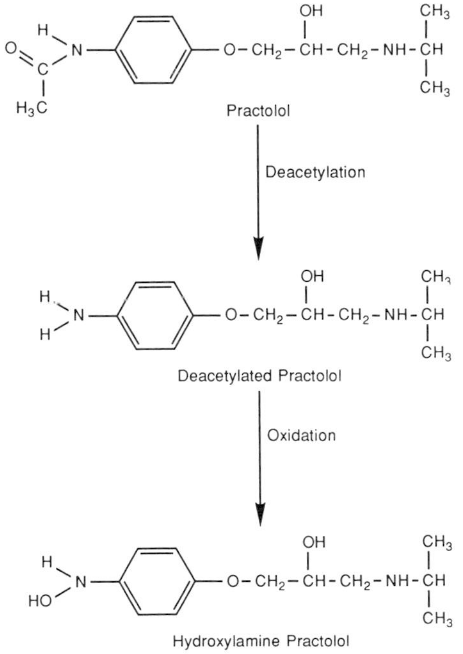

Fig. 14. Possible generation of practolol metabolites.

286

cainamide that the ability to carry out N-acetylation is important in determining susceptibility to drug-induced SLE.

Immunotoxic effects with penicillamine are more common and in one particular study, 36% of patients suffered adverse symptoms [68]. The importance of poly-morphism in drug metabolism in determining whether an individual suffers from pe-nicillamine immunotoxicity is suggested by results showing that poor sulphoxidisers are found at higher frequency in the group showing toxic effects [68]. This is con-sistent with the observation that penicillamine itself inhibits C4 binding to immune complexes (see Section II.3 of this chapter above).

However, it is clear that multiple factors are involved in determining which indivi-duals suffer toxic side effects. For hydralazine-induced SLE, lower levels of red blood cell immune adherence receptors which are receptors for C3b (CRI) have been found in patients suffering the toxic side effect compared to controls [69], and this is likely to be an additional predisposing factor (Fig. 17).

C4 as the target molecule is also polymorphic and C4A is more susceptible to inhi-bition by hydralazine than is C4B [38]. This is as would be expected from the greater reactivity of C4A, compared to C4B, with nitrogen nucleophiles.

For penicillamine, it has also been observed that the covalent binding reaction of C4A, is inhibited to a greater extent than C4B (Fig. 16). Although the amino acid differences between C4A and C4B include a *cys/ser* interchange (Fig. 9), it seems unlikely that interaction of penicillamine with the allotype-specific *cys* residue of C4A is the cause of the difference in reactivity. It is more likely that the thioester itself is more reactive with penicillamine in C4A. Covalent binding of ^{35}S-cysteine (as a penicillamine analogue) to C4 on activation has been observed, and it is not released by addition of another sulphhydryl compound [62], indicating that penicil-lamine does not react with C4 as a mixed disulphide. It has been noted repeatedly that penicillamine SLE-like toxicity is associated with the HLA antigen, DR3 [68,

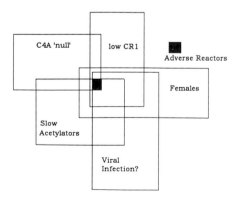

Fig. 17. Schematic diagram of multiple factors likely to be important in patients who develop hydralazine-induced SLE. Only in patients with all predisposing factors will hydralazine-induced SLE be observed.

70]. This is within a population of rheumatoid arthritics who have an increase in the HLA antigen DR4 compared with normals [71]. The DR3 antigen is found in linkage disequilibrium in a group of HLA antigens which includes a null allele at the C4A locus [72]. These individuals with less C4A than normal would be at increased risk of toxic side effects if the C4A gene product were inhibited by penicillamine.

With regard to the role of penicillamine as an anti-arthritic drug, it has been suggested that the C4A gene product is likely to be more important in handling non-cellular immune complexes [19]. In rheumatoid arthritis, immune complexes with IgG and rheumatoid factor are common. Inhibition of C4A binding to these complexes could act to minimise the release of active complement fragments (such as C3b as an opsonin, and C5a as a chemotactic factor) and, thus, reduce infiltration of polymorphs into joints. A balance between beneficial inhibition of C4A and inhibition of C4A leading to immunotoxicity will depend on the genetic make-up of the individual and the environmental circumstances in which penicillamine therapy is given.

In a clinical study to look at histocompatibility types of hydralazine patients, an increase in frequency of C4A null genes was found compared with a normal population [73]. However, it must be stressed that the immunotoxic effect is a result of a variety of overlapping factors, as illustrated in Fig. 17. One environmental factor − exposure to drugs − is obvious, but other environmental factors may also be important, e.g. subclinical viral infection. Accidental exposure to a nucleophile could also be involved, since it has been observed that exposure to hydrazine in the workplace can give rise to SLE-like effects [74] and hydrazine is a potent inhibitor of C4 covalent binding [33]. However, in view of the predominance of slow acetylators in hydralazine-induced SLE cases [34], this pharmacogenetic factor is probably of over-riding importance in predisposition to hydralazine-SLE. For penicillamine, and procainamide lupus, it is not yet possible to say what constitutes the major predisposing factor.

Acknowledgements

The work described has been supported by the Wellcome Trust, Arthritis and Rheumatism Council and by I.C.I.

I should like to thank Bob Sim, Richard Batchelor, Alister Dodds, Alex Law and Edward Gill for scientific collaboration and helpful discussions. I also wish to express my gratitude to all who have worked in the laboratory since the commencement of this work and especially to Michelle Wood. I thank Jan Elgar for speedy preparation of the manuscript and two wee friends, Grace and Francis, for keeping each other busy at the appropriate time.

References

1. Czop, J. and Nussenzweig, V. (1976) Studies on the mechanism of solubilisation of immune precipitates in serum. J. Exp. Med. 143, 615 – 630.
2. Schifferli, J. A., Bartolotti, S. R. and Peters, D. K. (1980) Inhibition of precipitation by complement. Clin. Exp. Immunol. 42, 387 – 393.
3. Whaley, K. (1987) The complement system. In: K. Whaley (Ed.), Complement in Health and Disease, MTP Press, Lancaster, pp. 1 – 35.
4. Lachmann, P. J. (1979) Complement. In: P. D. Sela (Ed.), The Antigens, Vol. V, Academic Press, New York, pp. 312 – 316.
5. Schifferli, J. A. and Peters, D. K. (1983) Complement, the immune complex lattice and pathophysiology of complement-deficiency syndromes. Lancet 2, 957 – 959.
6. Lachmann, P. J. (1984) Inherited complement deficiencies. Phil. Trans. Roy. Soc. Lond. B. 306, 419 – 430.
7. Campbell, R. D., Law, S. K. A., Reid, K. B. M. and Sim, R. B. (1988) Structure, origins and regulation of the complement genes. Annu. Rev. Immunol. 6, 161 – 195.
8. Janatova, J. (1983) The third (C3) and the fourth (C4) components of complement: labile binding site and covalent bond formation. Ann. NY Acad. Sci. 421, 218 – 234.
9. Sim, R. B., Twose, T. M., Paterson, D. S. and Sim, E. (1981) The covalent binding reaction of complement component C3. Biochem. J. 193, 115 – 127.
10. Law, S. K. A. and Levine, R. P. (1977) Interaction between the third complement protein and the cell surface. Proc. Natl. Acad. Sci. USA 74, 2701 – 2705.
11. Campbell, R. D., Dodds, A. W. and Porter, R. R. (1980) The binding of human complement component C4 to antibody-antigen aggregates. Biochem. J. 189, 67 – 80.
12. Gadd, K. J. and Reid, K. B. M. (1981) The binding of complement component C3 to antibody-antigen aggregates after activation of the alternate pathway in human serum. Biochem. J. 195, 471 – 480.
13. Sim, E. and Dodds, A. W. (1987) The fourth component of human complement – towards understanding an enigma of variations. In: K. Whaley (Ed.), Complement in Health and Disease, MTP Press, Lancaster, pp. 99 – 124.
14. Law, S. K. A. (1983) Non-enzymic activation of the covalent binding reaction of the complement protein C3. Biochem. J. 211, 381 – 389.
15. Von Zabern, I., Nolte, R. and Vogt, W. (1981) Treatment of human complement components C4 and C3 with amines or chaotropic ions. Scand. J. Immunol. 13, 413 – 431.
16. Pangburn, M. K. and Müller-Eberhard, H. J. (1983) Initiation of the alternative complement pathway due to spontaneous hydrolysis of the thiol ester of C3. Ann. NY Acad. Sci. 421, 291 – 298.
17. Vogt, W. (1985) Drugs and the complement system. Trends Pharmacol. Sci. 6, 114 – 119.
18. Isenman, D. E. and Young, J. R. (1984) The molecular basis for the difference in immune haemolysis activity of the Chido and Rodgers isotypes of human complement component C4. J. Immunol. 132, 3019 – 3027.
19. Law, S. K. A., Dodds, A. W. and Porter, R. R. (1984) A comparison of the properties of two classes, C4A and C4B, of the human complement component C4. EMBO J. 3, 1819 – 1823.
20. Yu, C. Y., Belt, K. T., Giles, C. M., Campbell, R. D. and Porter, R. R. (1986) Structural basis of the polymorphism of human complement components C4A and C4B. EMBO J. 5, 2873 – 2881.
21. Dodds, A. W., Law, S. K. A. and Porter, R. R. (1986) The purification and properties of some less common allotypes of the fourth component of human complement. Immunogenetics 24, 279 – 285.
22. Porter, R. R. (1985) The complement components coded in the major histocompatibility complex and their biological activities. Immunol. Rev. 87, 7 – 17.

289

23. Fielder, A. H., Walport, M. J., Batchelor, J. R., Rynes, R. I., Black, C. M., Dodi, I. A. and Hughes, G. R. V. (1983) Family studies of the major histocompatibility complex in patients with systemic lupus erythematosus. Br. Med. J. 286, 425 – 428.
24. Holme, E., Cross, S. J., Veitch, D., O'Neill, G. J. and Whaley, K. (1988) Quantitation of human C4A and C4B in serum and plasma by enzyme-linked immunoadsorbant assay. Immunogenetics 27, 295 – 299.
25. Shehadi, W. H. (1975) Adverse reactions to intravascularly administered contrast media. Am. J. Roentgenol. 124, 145 – 152.
26. Long, J. H., Lasser, E. C. and Kolb, W. P. (1976) Activation of the complement system by X-ray contrast media. Invest. Radiol. 11, 303 – 308.
27. Zabern, I. von., Przyklenk, H., Vogt, W. and Sachsenheimer, W. (1983) Effect of radiographic contrast media on complement components C3 and C4: generation of C3b-like C3 and C4b-like C4. Int. J. Immunopharmacol. 5, 503 – 513.
28. Parker, C. W. (1982) Allergic reactions in man. Pharmacol. Rev. 34, 85 – 104.
29. Von Zabern, I., Przyklenk, H., Nolte, R. and Vogt, W. (1984) Effect of different penicillin derivatives on complement components in human serum. Int. Arch. Allergy Appl. Immunol. 75, 164 – 172.
30. Park, B. K., Grabowski, P. S., Young, J. H. K. and Breckenridge, A. M. (1982) Drug protein conjugates. A study of the covalent binding of ^{14}C-captopril to plasma proteins in the rat. Biochem. Pharmacol. 31, 1755 – 1760.
31. Von Zabern, I. and Nolte, R. (1987) Activation of the alternative pathway of human complement by sulfhydryl compounds of analytic and therapeutic use. Int. Arch. Allergy Appl. Imun. 84, 178 – 184.
32. Davies, D. M. (1985) In: Textbook of Adverse Drug Reactions, 2nd edn. Oxford University Press, Oxford, pp. 412 – 419.
33. Sim, E., Gill, E. W. and Sim, R. B. (1984) Drugs that induce systemic lupus erythematosus inhibit complement component C4. Lancet ii, 422 – 424.
34. Perry, H. M., Tan, E. M., Carmody, S. and Sakamoto, A. (1970) Relationship of acetyl transferase activity to anti-nuclear antibodies and toxic symptoms in hypertensive patients treated with hydralazine. J. Lab. Clin. Med. 76, 114 – 125.
35. Godeau, P., Aukert, M., Imbert, J.-C. and Herreman, G. (1974) Lupus érythémateaux disséminé et taux d'isoniazide actif. Ann. Med. Intern. 124, 181 – 186.
36. Weber, W. W. and Hein, D. W. (1985) N-acetylation pharmacogenetics. Pharmacol. Rev. 37, 25 – 77.
37. Timbrell, J. A., Harland, S. J. and Facchini, V. (1980) Polymorphic acetylation of hydralazine. Clin. Pharmacol. Ther. 28, 350 – 355.
38. Sim, E. and Law, S. K. A. (1985) Hydralazine binds covalently to complement component C4. FEBS Lett. 184, 323 – 327.
39. Ludden, T. M., McNay, J. L., Shepherd, A. M. M. and Lim, M. S. (1981) Clinical pharmacokinetics of hydralazine. Clin. Pharmacol. Ther. 7, 185 – 205.
40. Hughes, G. R. V. (1979) Connective Tissue Diseases. Blackwell Scientific, Oxford, p. 44.
41. Sadee, W. and Beelen, G. C. M. (1980) Isoniazid. In: W. Sadee and S. C. M. Beelen (Eds.), Drug Level Monitoring. Wiley, London, pp. 284 – 292.
42. Drayer, D. E. and Reidenberg, M. M. (1977) Clinical consequences of polymorphic acetylation of basic drugs. Clin. Pharmacol. Ther. 22, 251 – 258.
43. Uetrecht, J. P., Sweetman, B. J., Woosley, R. L. and Oates, J. A. (1984) Metabolism of procainamide to a hydroxylamine by rat and human hepatic microsomes. Drug Metab. Dispos. 12, 77 – 81.
44. Uetrecht, J. P. (1985) Reactivity and possible significance of hydroxylamine and nitroso metabolites of procainamide. J. Pharmacol. Exp. Ther. 232, 420 – 425.

45. Budinsky, R. A., Roberts, S. M., Coats, E. A., Adams, L. and Hess, E. V. (1987) The formation of procainamide hydroxylamine by rat and human liver microsomes. Drug Metab. Dispos. 15, 37 – 43.

46. Reidenberg, M. M. (1983) Aromatic amines and the pathogenesis of lupus erythematosus. Am. J. Med. 75, 1037 – 1042.

47. Reidenberg, M. M. (1981) Chemical induction of systemic lupus erythematosus and lupus-like illness. Arthritis Rheum. 24, 1004 – 1008.

48. Twose, T. M., Sim, R. B. and Paterson, D. S. (1980) Covalent binding reaction of complement component C3. 4th International Congress of Immunology, Paris. Abstract No. 15.1.22.

49. Jones, A. J. (1985) Inhibition of the fourth component of human complement by nucleophiles. Chemistry, part II, Thesis, Oxford University, Oxford.

50. Raftery, E. B. and Denman, A. M. (1973) Systemic lupus erythematosus syndrome induced by practolol. Br. Med. J. 2, 452 – 455.

51. Wright, P. (1975) Untoward effects associated with practolol administration: oculomucocutaneous syndrome. Br. Med. J. 1, 595 – 598.

52. Nichols, J. T. (1976) Adverse effects of practolol. Ann. Clin. Res. 8, 229 – 231.

53. Amos, H. E., Brigden, W. D. B. and McKerron, R. A. (1975) Untoward effects associated with practolol: demonstration of antibody binding to epithelial tissue. Br. Med. J. 1, 598 – 600.

54. Amos, H. E., Lake, B. G. and Artis, J. (1978) Possible role of antibody specific for a practolol metabolite in the pathogenesis of the oculomucocutaneous syndrome. Br. Med. J. 1, 402 – 404.

55. Orten, T. C. and Lavery, C. (1981) Practolol metabolism. III. Irreversible binding of ^{14}C-practolol metabolite(s) to mammalian liver microsomes. J. Pharmacol. Exp. Ther. 219, 207 – 212.

56. Rosenbaum, S. E., Lindup, W. E. and Orten, T. C. (1986) Practolol: aspects of its metabolism and ocular binding in the hamster. Xenobiotica 16, 567 – 573.

57. Rosenbaum, S. E., Lindup, W. E. and Orten, T. C. (1985) Practolol and its metabolites: tissue localisation and retention in the hamster. J. Pharmacol. Exp. Ther. 234, 485 – 489.

58. Aarden, L. A., Lakmaker, F. and De Groot, E. (1977) Immunology of DNA. VI. The effect of mercaptans on IgG and IgM anti-ds DNA. J. Immunol. Meth. 16, 143 – 151.

59. Werrick, R., Merryman, P., Jaffe, I. and Ziff, M. (1983) IgG and IgM rheumatoid factors in rheumatoid arthritis. Arthritis Rheum. 26, 593 – 598.

60. Mellbye, O. J. and Munthe, E. (1977) Effect of penicillamine on complement in vitro and in vivo. Ann. Rheum. Dis. 36, 453 – 458.

61. Sim, E., Goldin, A., Wood, M. and Jones, A. (1987) The effect of penicillamine on complement component C4. Hum. Toxicol. 6, 424 – 425.

62. Sim, E., Goldin, A. and Dodds, A. W. Interaction of penicillamine with C4A and C4B allotypes of complement component C4. Immunopharmacology, submitted for publication.

63. Howard-Lock, H. E., Lock, C. J. L., Mewa, A. and Kean, W. F. (1986) D-penicillamine: chemistry and clinical use in rheumatic disease. Sem. Arth. Rheum. 15, 261 – 281.

64. Muijsers, A. O., Van de Stadt, R. J., Henricks, A. M. A. and Van der Korst, J. K. (1979) Determination of D-penicillamine in serum and urine of patients with rheumatoid arthritis. Clin. Chim. Acta. 94, 173 – 180.

65. Perret, D. (1981) The metabolism and pharmacology of D-penicillamine in man. J. Rheumatol. Suppl. 7, 41 – 50.

66. Feltkamp, T. E. W. (1981) Autoantibodies and autoimmunity induced by penicillamine therapy for rheumatoid arthritis. In: R. N. Miani and H. Berry (Eds.), Modulation of Autoantibodies and Disease – the Penicillamine Experience. Praeger, New York, pp. 45 – 50.

67. Ramsay, L. E., Silas, J. and Freestone, S. (1982) Hydralazine antinuclear antibodies and the lupus syndrome. Br. Med. J. 284, 1711.

68. Emery, P., Panayi, G. S., Husten, G., Welsh, K. I., Mitchell, S. C., Shah, R. R., Idle, J. R., Smith, R. L. and Waring, R. H. (1984) D-penicillamine induced toxicity in rheumatoid arthritis:

the role of sulphoxidation status and HLA-DR3. J. Rheumatol. 11, 626 – 632.

69. Mitchell, J. A., Batchelor, J. R., Chapel, H., Spiers, C. N. and Sim, E. (1987) Erythrocyte complement receptor type I (CRI) expression and circulating immune complex levels in hydralazine-induced SLE. Clin. Exp. Immunol. 68, 446 – 456.

70. Scherak, O., Smolen, J. S., Mayr, W. R., Mayrhofer, F., Kolarz, G. and Thumb, N. J. (1984) HLA antigens and toxicity to gold and penicillamine in rheumatoid arthritis. J. Rheumatol. 11, 610 – 614.

71. Dawkins, R. L., Christiansen, F. T., Kay, P. H., Garlepp, M., McCluskey, J., Hollingsworth, P. N. and Zilko, P. J. (1983) Disease associations with complotypes, supratypes and haplotypes. Immunol. Rev. 70, 5 – 22.

72. Awdeh, Z. L., Raum, D., Yunis, E. J. and Alper, C. A. (1983) Extended HLA/complement allele haplotypes: evidence for a T/t-like complex in man. Proc. Natl. Acad. Sci. USA 80, 259 – 263.

73. Batchelor, J. R., Fielder, A. H. L., Hing, S., Dodi, I. A., Spiers, C., Hughes, G. R. V., Bernstein, R., Malasit, P., Isenberg, D. A., Snaith, M., Chapel, H. and Sim, E. (1985) Class III HLA genes and SLE. In: M. Feldmann and A. McMichael (Eds.), Proc. of 6th Immune Response Gene Conference. Humana Press, Clifton, NJ, pp. 87 – 91.

74. Durant, P. J. and Harris, R. A. (1980) Hydrazine and lupus. N. Engl. J. Med. 303, 584 – 585.

75. Domdey, H., Wiebauer, K., Kazmaier, M., Muller, V., Odink, K. and Fey, G. (1982) Characterisation of the mRNA and cloned cDNA specifying the third component of mouse complement. Proc. Natl. Acad. Sci. USA 79, 7619 – 7623.

76. Pangburn, M. K. and Müller-Eberhard, H. G. (1983) The alternative pathway of complement. Springer Sem. Immunopathol. 6, 185 – 214.

77. Sim, E., Dodds, A. W., Wood, M. and Sim, R. B. (1986) Rapid purification of C4 from individual donors. Biochem. Soc. Trans. 14, 77 – 78.

78. Sim, E., Stanley, L., Gill, E. W. and Jones, A. (1988) Metabolites of procainamide and practolol inhibit complement components C3 and C4. Biochem. J. 251, 323 – 326.

79. Trowsdale, J. and Campbell, R. D. (1988) Physical map of the human HLA region. Immunol. Today 9, 34 – 35.

M.E. Kammüller, N. Bloksma and W. Seinen (Eds.)
Autoimmunity and Toxicology
©1989 Elsevier Science Publishers B.V. (Biomedical Division)

Immunomodulating properties of amphiphilic agents

11

LUUK A. TH. HILGERS[a], GUY J.W.J. ZIGTERMAN[b] and HARM SNIPPE[c]

[a] *Duphar BV, Animal Health Division, R & D, Department of Veterinary Vaccines, P.O.B. 2, 1380 AA Weesp, The Netherlands,* [b] *Intervet International BV, P.O.B. 31, 5830 AA Boxmeer, The Netherlands, and* [c] *Laboratory for Microbiology, State University of Utrecht, Catharijnesingel 59, 3511 GG Utrecht, The Netherlands*

I. Introduction

A great number of microbial and synthetic compounds are capable of modifying immunological reactions, which means that they can stimulate or suppress specific immune responses or non-specific resistance. The chemical nature of these so-called immunomodifiers [1 – 3] varies from rather simple (chemically well-defined) compounds to extremely complex (undefined or poorly-defined) substances. Several groups of immunomodifiers can be distinguished as there are polyanions, surfactants, adsorbents, etc. In this chapter, we consider the stimulatory effects of a group of synthetic compounds namely surfactants, on specific immune responses. A relationship between immunostimulatory action of these compounds and physico-chemical properties is sought as it may contribute to the assessment of possible detrimental effects of other surfactants.

Surfactants are among the most widely used chemicals known. Almost every one is exposed to these products every day via food, personal-care and laundry products. The total amount of surfactants produced and sold in the USA in 1980 was about two and a half million tons and they include a wide variety of chemical compounds [4]. Under conditions of normal use, surfactants are not hazardous to men, although irritation of skin and eyes occurs incidentally. More serious than irritation is the capacity of these products to elicitate or promote hypersensitivity (allergic) reactions. In animal models, many surfactants have been shown to enhance the immune response to a given antigen (Table 1).

TABLE 1

Surface-active immunoadjuvants classified on base of their charge

Adjuvant	References
Negatively-charged surfactants	
synthetic sulpholipopolysaccharides	[5]
lipid A	[6, 7]
Positively-charged surfactants	
monoalkylamine	[8]
dialkylamine	[8]
dialkyldimethylamine (e.g. DDA)	[8 – 15]
dialkyldiamine (e.g. avridine)	[8, 16]
Non-ionic surfactants	
non-ionic block polymers (e.g. L121, L101)	[17 – 25]
saponin (Quil A)	[26 – 28]
retinol and retinoids	[29 – 32]
synthetic lipopolysaccharides	[5]
sorbitan monooleate	[8]
polyoxyethylene sorbitan monooleate	[8]
trehalose dimycolate and derivatives	[33 – 36]
maltose tetrapalmitate	[37 – 40]
lysolecithins	[41]
Amphoteric surfactants	
acyl-L-tyrosine	[42, 43]
acyltripeptide (e.g. FK-156, FK-565)	[44 – 47]
tripalmitoylpentapeptide	[48, 49]
lipophilic muramylpeptides	[50]
Miscellaneous	
liposomes	[51 – 53]
emulsions	[54]

II. Physicochemical properties of surfactants

Surfactants contain both lipophilic and hydrophilic moieties [4, 55]. The molecular structure has a profound effect on the surface activity. In general, the hydrophobic part of surfactants consists of linear or branched carbon chains which may be interrupted by oxygen, a benzene ring, amide, or other chemical groups and which may contain double bounds. Furthermore, the carbon chain may carry substituents, mostly halogens. Non-branched non-interrupted alkyl groups contain 12 to 20 carbon atoms. The hydrophilic, water-solubilizing groups of anionic surfactants are either carboxylates, sulphonates or phosphates. Positively charged surfactants are

TABLE 2

HLB value of surfactants in relation to their solubility in water and applications [4, 55]

HLB range	Solubility in water	Application
< 3	no dispersibility	spreading agent
3 – 6	poor dispersibility	water-in-oil emulsion
6 – 8	milky dispersion	wetting agent
8 – 10	stable milky dispersion	oil-in water emulsion
10 – 13	translucent to clear dispersion	oil-in water emulsion
> 13	clear solution	solubilization/detergent

The HLB value can be assessed by using one of the following formulas: HLB $= 20 (1 - S/A)$, where S is the saponification number of the ester and A is the acid number of separated acid, or HLB $= E/5$, where E is the weight percentage ethyleneoxide content.

soluble in water due to the presence of amine or ammonium groups. Hydroxyl and oxyethylene groups are the hydrophilic groups of non-ionic surfactants. The number of oxyethylene units of a polyoxyethylene chain varies from 1 to 20.

Surfactants are soluble in at least one phase of a mixture of polar and apolar liquids. Due to the presence of chemical groups with tendencies to solubilize in either a polar or an apolar solvent, the surfactants concentrate at the interface between two phases. A high interface/bulk partition coefficient indicates high surface activity and a high critical micelle concentration. Increase of the hydrophobicity by increasing the length of the carbon chain or by decreasing the charge, will promote the surface activity. As a consequence, non-ionic surfactants are about a hundred times more surface active than ionic surfactants of similar molecular structure. Molecular modifications such as the addition of double bonds, branching of the chain, and addition of charged groups reduce the degree of hydrophobic interaction. As a consequence, the solubility in water is increased and surface activity is decreased. The surface activity of an agent can be expressed by the hydrophilic-lipophilic balance (HLB) which represents the ratio of the tendencies to solubilize in either water or an organic apolar solvent (Table 2).

III. Immunostimulation by cationic lipophilic amines

Gall [8] tested a large number of surface active agents on their immunostimulatory activity. Among those agents there were various lipophilic amines with considerable adjuvant activity for the humoral immune response to tetanus toxoid in guinea pigs. The active agents are cationic surfactants containing long aliphatic chains. The adjuvant activity of the monoalkyl- and dialkylamines depended on the length of the alkyl chains. The minimal number of carbon atoms of the alkyl chains was 12 and optimal effects were obtained by chains of 18 or 20 carbon atoms. The presence of a benzyl group instead of an alkyl group lowered the activity. The quaternary amine dimethyldioctadecylammonium bromide (DDA; Fig. 1) proved to be a very potent adjuvant for humoral and cellular responses to various antigens [8 – 15].

DDA is a positively charged lipophilic quaternary amine with a molecular weight of 631. It is poorly soluble in water. By heating or ultrasonic treatment, it forms an opalescent solution which flocculates after standing at room temperature within a few days. The lipophilicity of DDA is indicated by partition between water and chloroform phase, since more than 90% is recovered from the chloroform phase [12].

DDA stimulates the immune response to various thymus-dependent but not to thymus-independent antigens in different mammals [8 – 15]. It induced protective immunity to bacterial and viral infections. The adjuvant effect depends on the route of administration. Antibody responses are augmented when DDA and antigen are injected intraperitoneally [9]. Subcutaneous or intracutaneous injection of DDA with antigen failed to induce antibody formation but instead sensitized animals for cellular immunity, notably delayed-type hypersensitivity [13, 14]. Increase of the immune response is probably the result of various effects of DDA on both the antigen and components of the host immune system. There are several lines of evidence indicating that interaction of DDA with antigens is crucial in immunostimulation [11, 56]. DDA can bind to protein and cellular antigens via hydrophobic or electrostatic interaction. These antigens become more lipophilic and more immunogenic. The covalent attachment of lipids to a protein antigen has similar effects on the immunogenicity of the antigen especially when cellular immune responses are involved [57, 58]. The necessity of DDA to form complexes with the antigen has been studied with the monovalent lipophilic antigen A-PE which is 3-(*p*-azobenezenearsonate)-*N*-acetyl derivative coupled to phosphatidylethanolamine [11]. A-PE forms stable insoluble complexes with DDA. The formation of these complexes can be hindered by addition of a blocking agent. Complexed A-PE induced delayed type hypersensitivity in contrast to free, uncoupled A-PE [11]. Apparently, physical interaction of this antigen and adjuvant is important.

Besides binding to antigens, DDA evokes various biological reactions in the host. Intraperitoneal injection of DDA elicits an inflammatory response characterized by the influx of polymorphonuclear and mononuclear phagocytes [59] and by the appearance of serum amyloid protein P in serum (data not published). Furthermore,

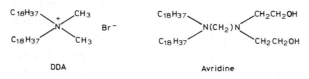

Fig. 1. Chemical structure of dimethyldioctadecylammonium bromide (DDA) and avridine.

DDA affects the trapping of both antigens and lymphocytes, and handling of antigen by antigen-presenting cells [59, 60].

The lipophilic amine N,N-dioctadecyl-N',N'-bis(2-hydroxyethyl)-propanediamine (also called CP-20,961 or avridine; Fig. 1) is closely related to DDA in physicochemical and immunomodulatory respect [16]. Like DDA, the lipophilic diamine avridine contains two long alkyl chains. It is a strong adjuvant for viral, bacterial and parasitic antigens [16]. The adjuvant profile of avridine is very similar to that of DDA. In contrast to DDA, however, avridine is a very potent interferon inducer [61].

IV. Immunostimulation by non-ionic block polymers (NBPs)

The group of NBPs (pluronic polyols manufactured by BASF Wyandotte) includes a number of chemically related compounds which differ in physical properties such as solubility in water, surface activity, HLB value, etc. NBPs are copolymers of hydrophilic polyoxyethylene (POE) and hydrophobic polyoxypropylene (POP). They differ in molecular weight, percentage POE and the mode of linkage of POE and POP-groups. The molecular weight of NBPs with adjuvant activity varies from 2 000 to 8 000 and the percentage POE varies from 10 to 80, but in most cases these values varies between 10 and 20. The molecules have a linear or branched structure with either POE or POP ends (Fig. 2). Several NBPs combined with an oil-in-water

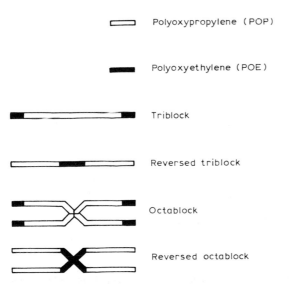

Fig. 2. Schematic representation of linear (triblock and reversed triblock) and branched (octablock and reversed octablock) NBPs comprising polyoxyethylene (POE, black) and polyoxypropylene (POP, white) polymers.

emulsion, demonstrated adjuvanticity for the humoral immune response to BSA in mice [20, 21]. Both linear and branched NBPs with central hydrophobic POP polymers and HLB values of less than 2 displayed considerable adjuvanticity for the antibody response to BSA [20, 21]. Adjuvanticity activity decreased with increase of the percentage of POE or decrease of the molecular weight.

All adjuvant active NBPs are poorly soluble in water and form different types of aggregates in saline. Those NBPs that are strong adjuvants for antibody responses to BSA form fibers in aqueous solutions, while most of the other polymers form smooth spherical masses resembling oil droplets [22, 23]. This suggests that the copolymers with adjuvant activity form typical surfaces which are relatively hydrophilic.

The NBPs were used in combination with an oil-in-water emulsion. As a result of the presence of hydrophobic and hydrophilic parts, NBPs may reside at the interface separating the oil and water phases [17, 18, 22, 23], and form a hydrophilic monolayer surrounding the oil-droplets. This hydrophilic structure promotes the retention of protein antigens on the oil droplet. It is also capable of binding other proteins such as the third component of complement, fibrinogen, etc. Binding of complement components may result in the activation of the complement system leading to the generation of chemotactic compounds and opsonisation of the oil droplets [22]. Furthermore, linear and branched NBPs inhibited the uptake of an-

TABLE 3

Adjuvant activity of various non-ionic block polymers for the humoral response to four antigens[a]

Adjuvant type		HLB[b]	Structure[b]	Stimulation of antibody response to			
				BSA[c]	J-BSA	HS-BSA	J-PE
L81	triblock	2.0	spherical drops	no	moderate	no	strong
L101	triblock	1.0	fibres	moderate	moderate	moderate	moderate
L121	triblock	0.5	fibres	moderate	moderate	moderate	moderate
31R1	reversed triblock	1.7	spherical drops	no	strong	no	strong
T1101	octablock	2.0	oily fibres	moderate	moderate	moderate	poor
T1501	octablock	1.0	fibres	strong	moderate	moderate	strong

[a]The NBP were immobilized on oil droplets and mixed with the antigens BSA, J-BSA and HS-BSA. J-PE was incorporated in liposomes and mixed with NBPs. Mice were injected intraperitoneally and antibody titres were measured in serum.
[b]HLB values and structure of the NBP were obtained from [22].
[c]BSA, bovine serum albumin; J-BSA, dinitrophenyl-alanyl-alanyl-glycine (J) coupled to BSA (J: BSA ratio is 22); J-PE, J-phosphatidylethanolamine incorporated in liposomes; HS-BSA, hexasaccharide fragment of the capsular polysaccharide of *Streptococcus pneumoniae* type 3, coupled to BSA (HS: BSA ratio is 7).

tigen by peritoneal phagocytes in vitro and in vivo [25]. These effects on complement activation and antigen uptake by phagocytes modulate antigen handling, processing and presentation and, consequently, the immune response.

In addition to the effect on the immune response to BSA, adjuvant activity of NBPs for the antibody response to various other antigens were investigated [25, 62]. Distinct profiles of adjuvanticity were observed for the antigens tested (Table 3). The immune response to a certain antigen was stimulated by a given NBP while that to another antigen was not affected. The ability to form fibers in aqueous solutions corresponded quite well with the adjuvanticity for the humoral response to BSA and HS-BSA but not with that against J-BSA and J-PE liposomes (Table 3). The introduction of hapten 'J' (dinitrophenyl-alanyl-alanyl-glycine) into the BSA molecule gives an antigen which is less sensitive to the adjuvanticity of fiber-forming NBPs but more sensitive to the activity of NBPs with a linear structure and a central hydrophilic POE polymer. J-PE liposomes are sensitive to various types of NBPs.

Adjuvanticity of NBPs depends on physicochemical properties of both NBPs and antigen. Apparently, several mechanisms are involved in the stimulation of antibody responses by NBPs. Under restricted conditions a correlationship can been found between adjuvant activity and physicochemical characteristics.

V. Immunostimulation by sulpholipopolysaccharides (SLPs)

SLPs were constructed and synthesized [5] with reference to the observation that combination of lipophilic adjuvants and the polyanionic adjuvant dextran sulphate resulted in synergistic enhancement of the humoral immune response to sheep red blood cells (SRBC [63, 64]). In SLPs, the synthetic polysaccharide Ficoll is used as a backbone. Ficoll is a copolymer of saccharose and epichlorohydrine and contains about 2 000 monosaccharide units per molecule. Different SLPs can be synthesized by varying the number of sulphate and lipid groups and the chain length of the conjugated lipid. The conjugation of sulphate and lipid groups to Ficoll is non-specific, as no preference for a particular hydroxyl-group exists. Consequently, the sulphate and lipid groups are distributed randomly over the molecule and only a gross formula of each SLP can be given. Comparison of the adjuvanticity of these compounds for various antigens enabled us to determine the effect of presence of negatively charged and hydrophobic groups in the SLPs.

Unsubstituted Ficoll did not stimulate the humoral immune response to SRBC after injection in mice, but sulphated Ficoll did. Adjuvant activity increased with increasing numbers of sulphate groups. At a ratio of about 0.6 sulphate groups per monosaccharide unit an optimum was reached. Similar observations have been reported for other sulphated polymers as there are dextran sulphate, polyethylene sulphate, etc. [65]. Conjugates of Ficoll and palmitoyl chains displayed also significant adjuvanticity at a minimal ratio of 0.8 lipid groups per monosaccharide unit.

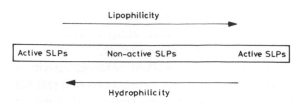

Fig. 3. Schematic representation of the correlationship between hydrophilicity/lipophilicity ratio of SLPs and adjuvant activity for humoral immune response to SRBC injected simultaneously with the SLPs in mice. The hydrophilicity reflects the sulphate content.

Remarkable effects were seen when both sulphate and lipid groups were present on the same molecule. The introduction of lipids into conjugates with moderate or high sulphate contents resulted in strong decrease or even complete annihilation of the adjuvant activity of these compounds. In concert, the adjuvanticity of lipidated Ficoll was reduced by the introduction of sulphate groups. The decrease of the adjuvanticity of lipid derivatives depended on the number of introduced sulphate groups and on the chain length of the conjugated lipids. Low numbers of sulphate groups already reduced the adjuvanticity of lauroyl (a chain of 12 carbon atoms) conjugates, while increasing quantities of sulphates were required for conjugates with longer lipid tails. In sum, strongly negatively charged polysaccharides and strongly hydrophobic polysaccharides display adjuvanticity for SRBC (Fig. 3). Negatively charged sulphate groups and hydrophobic lipid groups counteract each other.

When dinitrophenylated bovine serum albumin (DNP-BSA) was used as antigen, the correlation between the physicochemical properties and adjuvanticity of SLPs described above, appeared to be different. All SLPs with a minimal number of lipid groups augmented the anti-DNP antibody response to DNP-BSA, independent of the number of sulphate groups. Even conjugates with high sulphate and high lipid contents enhanced the response to DNP-BSA significantly (data not published). Furthermore, conjugates which were not effective when injected simultaneously with the antigen, demonstrated significant adjuvanticity when injected 6 h prior to immunization. Apparently, SLPs induce a state of high responsiveness during which increased responses to a given antigen can be generated. Such a high responsiveness has been described also for other agents such as DDA [9], dextran sulphate [9] and non-ionic block polymers [24, 25]. This indicates that SLPs have effects on components of the host immune system and that these effects play a crucial role in the adjuvant activity.

In conclusion, a significant relationship between the composition of SLPs and adjuvanticity could be observed under certain circumstances, but different patterns were seen when the immunization conditions (such as type of antigen and interval between adjuvant and antigen injection) were altered.

VI. General conclusions and Discussion

In the literature, a wide range of compounds has been described with the capacity to enhance specific immune responses to antigens. In this chapter, a relationship was sought between chemical and physical characteristics on one hand, and immunostimulatory potentials on the other. If such a relationship exists, it will increase our alertness to immunomodulatory potentials of new compounds on base of their chemical structure or physicochemical properties. Such a relationship, however, is difficult to make for the following four reasons. Firstly, the mechanisms regulating qualitative and quantitative aspects of the immune response are hardly understood. Secondly, a wide variety of biological and immunological processes is involved in the induction of immunity and is sensitive to extrinsic interference by immunomodulators. Thirdly, the immunomodulators known have multiple rather than a single effect on the immune system. Fourthly, immunostimulatory activity does not only depend on the adjuvant but also on several other factors, e.g. type of antigen, animal species, route and time of administration, dose of antigen and adjuvant, etc.

The adjuvant activity of three types of surfactants are discussed, namely cationic lipophilic amines, anionic sulpholipopolysaccharides, and non-ionic blockpolymers of polyoxyethylene and polyoxypropylene. These surfactants are chemically well-defined and physical properties are at least partially known.

The surfactants with adjuvant activity have distinct hydrophobic and hydrophilic structures. Most of them are non-ionic while only a few are negatively or positively charged (Table 1). The hydrophobic moieties of these adjuvants are either polyoxypropylene, an aliphatic (alkyl, acyl, acoyl, acyloxyacoyl) or an aromatic (benzyl) group. Hydrophobicity of the molecule increases with increasing numbers of lipophilic groups and lengths of the carbon chains but decreases when the carbon chains are interrupted by oxygen or when hydroxyl groups are added. The adjuvanticity of aliphatic compounds increases with increasing length of the carbon chain. The latter observation was made for different types of surface active adjuvants: SLPs [5], alkylamines [8], lysolecithins [41], alkyl-L-tyrosine analogs [42,43], alkyltripeptides [44,45], esters of fatty acids [66], liposomes containing dialkylphosphatidylcholine derivatives [67], etc. The minimal number of carbon atoms of the carbon chain is about 12 and an optimum is reached at 18 or 20 carbon atoms. The replacement of an alkyl group by a benzyl group decreases the adjuvanticity. Primary, secondary and tertiary amines are equally effective while quaternary ammonium salts are more effective.

The hydrophilic part of surface active adjuvants is an amine in cationic, a sulphate, phosphate or carboxyl group in anionic and hydroxyl or oxyethylene in non-ionic surfactants. Amphoteric adjuvants mostly contain amine and carboxyl groups. The hydrophilic groups are often configurated in sugar moieties such as sorbitan, glucose, glucosamine, galactose, mannose, maltose, saccharose, trehalose, muramic acid, etc.

Counteraction of negatively charged and lipophilic groups of adjuvant active surfactants was observed in a number of cases, e.g. SLPs and haptenated liposomes with negatively charged lipids [67]. In addition, positively charged liposomes have shown to be better adjuvants than neutrally or negatively charged liposomes [53]. The presence of negatively charged groups in surface active agents does not always reduce the adjuvanticity. The bacterial lipid A demonstrated optimal adjuvanticity when two phosphate groups were present. Analogs with a single phosphate group displayed significantly less activity, while derivatives without phosphate groups contained no adjuvant activity at all [6]. Therefore, it was concluded that a relationship between adjuvanticity and physicochemical properties exists, but that this relationship is only valid under particular circumstances.

Surfactants are often used in combination with an oil-in-water emulsion. The ability of a surfactant to reside at the surface of the oil droplets is probably important to its biological effects. Protein antigens adsorb onto the oil surface and adopt a conformation which is distinct from that in aqueous solutions. This adsorption is irreversible and improves the stability of the emulsion [55]. The protein may denature followed by a more effective presentation to the host immune system. Correspondingly, adsorption of protein antigens to the surface of a liposomal membrane promotes their immunogenicity [52]. Antigen but also components of the host may adsorb to the oil droplets of an oil-in-water emulsion. Binding of fibrinogen and complement components have been suggested to play a role in the adjuvanticity of oil-in-water emulsions [22,25,36].

Most surfactants with strong adjuvanticity are poorly soluble in water as there are DDA, avridine, trehalose dimycolate, lipophilic SLPs, and a number of NBPs. They form insoluble particles or fibers in aqueous solution. The use of a vehicle such as oil droplets or liposomes may increase the efficacy of these immunostimulators. The immobilization of a surface-active adjuvant on latex particles has been proven to be very effective for trehalose dimycolate [36]. This suggests that the formation of a monolayer of surfactant molecules is crucial to the adjuvant effect.

The immunomodulatory potentials of a compound may be either advantageous or disadvantageous to the animal, depending on the point of view of the examiner. The capacity of an agent to stimulate humoral and cellular immune responses can be utilized in vaccine development. Suppression of desired immune responses and stimulation of responses against self components (autoimmunity) or against other antigens (allergy) are examples of adverse immunomodulatory (immunotoxic) activity. In principle, immunoadjuvants are administered in conjunction with an antigen. Stimulation of the immune response is the result of interaction of the immunoadjuvant with the antigen or with components of the host immune system. Both mechanisms implicate certain risks. Interaction may not only occur with the antigen but also with structures of the host which may become immunogenic. On the other hand, improved immunoresponsiveness of the host may be accompanied by increased reactivity against self (autoimmunity) and non-self (allergy) structures. Immunomodulatory action is not restricted to antigens mixed with the adjuvant. It has been demonstrated that immune responses to antigens injected before or after adjuvant administration and antigens injected into a different physiological compartment are affected also [68]. These potential effects of adjuvants may lead to undesired immunotoxic reactions.

Finally, it is concluded that a relationship between physicochemical properties and immunostimulatory activity of surfactants can be observed under strict experimental conditions. A general relationship, however, is not detected as adjuvanticity depends upon many factors as there are type of antigen, time and route of administration, dose of adjuvant and antigen, animal species, immune status of the host, etc.

References

1. Borek, F. (1977) Adjuvants. In: M. Sela (Ed.), The Antigen, Vol. 4, Academic Press, New York, pp. 374 – 428.
2. Whitehouse, M. W. (1977) The chemical nature of adjuvants. In: L. E. Glynn and M. W. Steward (Eds.), Immunochemistry. An Advanced Textbook. John Wiley and Sons, New York, pp. 572 – 601.
3. World Health Organization (1976) Immunological adjuvants. World Health Organization Technical Report Series No. 595, WHO, Geneva, Switzerland.
4. Cahn, A. and Lynn, J. L., Jr. (1983) Surfactants and detersive systems. In: H.F. Mark, D. F. Othmer, C. G. Overberger and G. T. Seaborg (Eds.), Encyclopedia of Chemical Technology, Vol. 22, John Wiley and Sons, New York, pp. 332 – 432.
5. Hilgers, L. A. Th., Snippe, H., Jansze, M. and Willers, J. M. N. (1987) Synthetic (sulfo-)(lipo-)-polysaccharides: novel adjuvants for humoral immune responses. Immunology 60, 141 – 146.
6. Kotani, S., Takada, H., Tsujimoto, M., Ogawa, T., Takahashi, T., Ikeda, T., Otsuka, K., Shimauchi, H., Kasai, N., Mashimo, K., Nagao, S., Tanaka, A., Tanaka, S., Harada, K., Nagaki, K., Kitamura, H., Shiba, T., Kusumoto, S., Imoto, M. and Yoshimura, H. (1985) Synthetic lipid A with endotoxic and related biological activities comparable to those of a natural lipid A from an *Escherichia coli* re-mutant. Infect. Immun. 49, 225 – 237.
7. Kumazawa, Y., Matsuura, M., Nakatsuru-Watanabe, Y., Fukumoto, M., Nishimura, C., Hooma, Y.J., Inage, M., Kusumoto, S. and Shiba, T. (1984) Mitogenic and polyclonal B cell activation activities of synthetic lipid A analogues. Eur. J. Immunol. 14, 109 – 121.
8. Gall, D. (1966) The adjuvant activity of aliphatic nitrogenous bases. Immunology 11, 369 – 386.
9. Hilgers, L. A. Th., Snippe, H., Jansze, M. and Willers, J. M. N. (1984) Immunomodulating properties of two synthetic adjuvants; dependence upon type of antigen, dose and time of administration. Cell. Immunol. 86, 393 – 401.
10. Hilgers, L. A. Th., Snippe, H., Jansze, M. and Willers, J. M. N. (1986) Synergistic effects of synthetic adjuvants on the humoral response. Int. Arch. Allergy Appl. Immunol. 79, 392 – 396.
11. Hilgers, L. A. Th., Snippe, H., Van Vliet, K. E., Jansze, M. and Willers, J. M. N. (1984) Suppression of the cellular adjuvanticity of quaternary amines by a polyanion. Int. Arch. Allergy Appl. Immunol. 80, 320 – 325.
12. Prager, M. D. (1985) DDA as an immunologic adjuvant. Kodak Laboratory Chemicals Bull. 56, 1 – 4.

13. Snippe, H., Belder, M. and Willers, J. M. N. (1977) Dimethyldioctadecylammonium bromide as adjuvant for delayed type hypersensitivity in mice. Immunology, 33, 931 – 936.
14. Snippe, H., de Reuver, M. J., Strickland, F., Willers, J. M. N. and Hunter, R. L. (1981) Adjuvant effect of nonionic block polymer surfactants in humoral and cellular immunity. Int. Arch. Allergy Appl. Immunol 65, 390 – 398.
15. Willers, J. M. N., Bloksma, N., Van der Meer, C., Snippe, H., Van Dijk, H., De Reuver, M. J. and Hofhuis, F. M. A. (1979) Regulation of the immune response by macrophages. Antonie van Leeuwenhoek 45, 41 – 48.
16. Jensen, K. E. (1986) Synthetic adjuvants: avridine and other interferon inducers. In: R. M. Nervig, P. M. Gouch, M. L. Kaeberle and C. A. Whetstone (Eds.), Advances in Carriers and Adjuvants for Veterinary Biologics. Iowa State University Press, Ames, Iowa, pp. 79 – 89.
17. Allison, A. C. and Byars, N. E. (1986) An adjuvant formulation that selectively elicits the formation of antibodies of protective isotypes and of cell-mediated immunity. J. Immunol. Meth. 95, 157 – 168.
18. Byars, N. E. and Allison, A. C. (1987) Adjuvant formulation for use in vaccines to elicit both cell-mediated and humoral immunity. Vaccine 5, 223 – 231.
19. Allison, A. C. (1987) Vaccine technology: Adjuvants for increased efficacy. Bio/technology 10, 1041 – 1044.
20. Hunter, R. L., Strickland, F. and Kezdy, F. (1981) The adjuvant activity of nonionic block polymer surfactants. I. The role of the hydrophile-lipophile balance. J. Immunol. 127, 1244 – 1250.
21. Hunter, R. L. and Bennett, B. (1984) The adjuvant activity of nonionic block polymer surfactants. II. Antibody formation and inflammation related to the structure of triblock and octablock copolymers. J. Immunol. 133, 3167 – 3175.
22. Hunter, R. L. and Bennett, B. (1986) The adjuvant activity of nonionic block polymer surfactants. III. Characterization of selected biological active surfaces. Scand. J. Immunol. 23, 287 – 300.
23. Hunter, R. L. and Bennett, B. (1986) Structural basis of the activity of surface active surfactants. In: R. M. Nervig, P. M. Gouch, M. L. Kaeberle and C. A. Whetstone (Eds.), Advances in Carriers and Adjuvants for Veterinary Biologics. Iowa State University Press, Ames, Iowa, pp. 61 – 70.
24. Zigterman, G. J. W. J., Snippe, H., Jansze, M. and Willers, J. M. N. (1987) Adjuvant effects of nonionic block polymers surfactants on liposome-induced humoral immune response. J. Immunol. 138, 220 – 225.
25. Zigterman, J. W. J. (1988) Nonionic block polymer surfactants enhance vaccine efficacy. Thesis, State University of Utrecht, Utrecht, The Netherlands.
26. Bomford, R (1984) Relative adjuvant efficacy of Al(OH)$_3$) and saponin is related to the immunogenicity of the antigen. Int. Arch. Allergy Appl. Immunol. 75, 280 – 282.
27. Morein, B., Sundquist, B., Hoglund, S., Dalsgaard, K. and Osterhaus, A. (1984) Iscom, a novel structure for antigenic presentation of membrane proteins from enveloped viruses. Nature (Lond.) 308, 457 – 459.
28. Scott, M. T., Goss-Sampson, M. and Bomford, R. (1985) Adjuvant activity of saponin: antigen localization studies. Int. Arch. Allergy Appl. Immunol. 77, 409 – 412.
29. Jurin, M. and Tannock, I. F. (1972) Influence of vitamin A on immunological response. Immunology 23, 283 – 289.
30. Cohen, B. E. and Cohen, I. K. (1973) Vitamin A: adjuvant and steroid antagonist in the immune response. J. Immunol. 111, 1376 – 1380.
31. Dresser, D. W. (1968) Adjuvanticity of vitamin A. Nature (Lond.) 217, 527 – 529.
32. Spitznagel, J. K. and Allison, A. C. (1970) Mode of action of adjuvants: retinol and other lysosome-labilizing agents as adjuvants. J. Immunol. 104, 119 – 127.
33. Numata, F. N., Nishimura, K., Ishida, H., Ukei, Tone, Y., Ishihara, C., Saiki, I., Sekikawa, I. and Azuma, I. (1985) Lethal and adjuvant activities of cord factor (trehalose-6,6′-dimycolate)

and synthetic analogs in mice. Chem. Pharm. Bull. 33, 4544 – 4555.

34. Parant, M., Audibert, F., Parant, F., Chedid, L., Soler, E., Polonsky, J. and Lederer, E. (1978) Nonspecific immunostimulant activities of synthetic trehalose-6,6′-diesters (lower homologs of cord factor). Infect. Immun. 20, 12 – 19.

35. Retzinger, G. S., Meredith, S. C., Takayama, K., Hunter, R. L. and Kezdy, F. J. (1981) The role of surface in the biological activities of trehalose-6,6′-dimycolate. Surface properties and development of a model. J. Biol. Chem. 256, 8208 – 8216.

36. Retzinger, G. S., Meredith, S. C., Hunter, R. L., Takayama, K. and Kezdy, F. J. (1982) Identification of the physiologically active state of the mycobacterial glycolipid trehalose-6,6′-dimycolate and the role of fibrinogen in the biological activities of trehalose-6,6′-dimycolate monolayers. J. Immunol. 129, 735 – 744.

37. Nigam, V. N., Bonaventure, J., Chopra, C. and Brailovski, C. A. (1982) Effects of structural variations in synthetic glycolipids upon mitogenicity for spleen lymphocytes, adjuvant for humoral immune response and on anti-tumour potentials. Br. J. Canc. 46, 782 – 783.

38. Behling, U. H., Cambell, B., Chang, C. -M., Rumpf, C. and Nowotny, A. (1976) Synthetic glycolipid adjuvants. J. Immunol. 177. 847 – 851.

39. Bonaventure, J., Nigam, V. N. and Brailovsky, C. A. (1984) In vitro spleen cell proliferation following in vivo treatment with a synthetic glycolipid or lipid A in three mouse strains. Int. J. Immunopharmacol. 6, 259 – 267.

40. Rosenstreich, D. L., Asselineau, J., Mergenhagen, S. E. and Nowotny, A. (1974) A synthetic glycolipid with B-cell mitogen activity. J. Exp. Med. 140, 1404 – 1408.

41. Arnold, B., Miller, J. F. A. P. and Weltzien, H. U. (1979) Lysolecithin analogs as adjuvants in delayed-type hypersensitivity in mice. I. Characterization of the adjuvant effect. Eur. J. Immunol. 9, 363 – 366.

42. Landi, S., Penney, C. L., Shah, P., Hart, F., Campbell, J. B. and Cucakovich, N. (1986) Adjuvanticity of stearyl tyrosine on inactivated poliovirus vaccine. Vaccine 4, 99 – 104.

43. Wheeler, A. W., Whittal, V., Spackman, D. M. and Moran, D. M. (1984) Adjuvant properties of hydrophobic derivatives prepared from L-tyrosine. Int. Arch. Allergy Appl. Immunol. 75, 29 – 299.

44. Kitaura, Y., Takeno, H., Okada, S., Nakaguchi, O., Hemmi, K., Mine, Y., Mori, J. and Hashimoto, M. (1982) Synthesis and immunostimulating activity of FK-156 analogues: fatty acid derivatives of N-[N′-(γ-D-glutamyl)-L-lysyl]-D-alanine. Chem. Pharm. Bull. 30, 3065 – 3068.

45. Takeno, H., Okada, S., Yonishi, S., Hemmi, K., Nakaguchi, O., Kitaura, Y. and Hashimoto, M. (1984) Studies of structure activity relationship of FK-156, an immunostimulating peptide, and related compounds. II. Synthesis of N′-(γ-D-glutamyl)-2L, 2′-D-diaminopimelic acid as the minimal essential structure of FK-156. Chem. Pharm. Bull. 32, 2932 – 2941.

46. Okada, S., Takeno, H., Hemmi, K., Kitaura, Y. and Hashimoto, M. (1985) Synthesis and adjuvant activity of FK-156 analogues: acyl derivatives of N-[N′-(L-alanyl-γ-D-glutamyl)-2L, 2′-D-diamino-l-pimeloyl] glycine. Chem. Pharm. Bull. 33, 889 – 892.

47. Takeno, H., Okada, S., Hemmi, K., Aranti, M., Kitaura, Y. and Hashimoto, M. (1984) Studies of structure activity relationship of FK-156, an immunostimulating peptide, and related compounds. I. Synthesis of stereoisomeric analogues of FK-156. Chem. Pharm. Bull. 32, 2925 – 2931.

48. Bessler, W. G., Cox, M., Lex, A., Suhr, B., Wiesmüller, K. -H. and Jung, G. (1985) Synthetic lipopeptide analogs of bacterial lipoprotein are potent polyclonal activators for murine B lymphocytes. J. Immunol. 135, 1900 – 1905.

49. Lex, A., Weismüller, K. -H., Jung, G. and Bessler, W. G. (1986) A synthetic analogue of Escherichia coli lipoprotein, tripalmitoyl pentapeptide, constitutes a potent immune adjuvant. J. Immunol. 137, 2676 – 2681.

50. Kotani, S., Tsujimoto, M., Koga, T., Nagao, S., Tanaka, A. and Kawata, S. (1986) Chemical

structure and biological activity relationship of bacterial cell walls and muramyl peptides. Fed. Proc. 45, 2534 – 2540.

51. Bakouche, O. and Gerlier, D. (1986) Enhancement of immunogenicity of tumour virus antigen by liposomes: the effect of lipid composition. Immunology 58, 507 – 513.

52. Gregoriadis, G., Davis, D. and Davies, A. (1987) Liposomes as immunological adjuvants: antigen incorporation studies. Vaccine 5, 145 – 151.

53. Latif, N. and Bachhawat, B. K. (1984) The effect of surface charges of liposomes in immunopotentiation. Biosci. Rep. 4, 99 – 107.

54. Woodard, L. F. and Jasman, R. L. (1985) Stable oil-in-water emulsions: preparation and use as vaccine vehicles for lipophilic adjuvants. Vaccine 3, 137 – 144.

55. Griffin, W. C. (1979) Emulsions. In: H. F. Mark, D. F. Othmer, C. G. Overberger and G. T. Seaborg (Eds.), Encyclopedia of Chemical Technology, Vol. 8, John Wiley and Sons, New York, pp. 900 – 930.

56. Baechtel, F. S. and Prager, M. D. (1982) Interaction of antigens with dimethyldioctadecylammonium bromide, a chemically defined biological response modifier. Cancer Res. 42, 4959 – 4963.

57. Coon, J. and Hunter, R. (1973) Selective induction of delayed hypersensitivity by a lipid conjugated protein antigen which is localized in thymus dependent lymphoid tissue. J. Immunol. 110, 183 – 190.

58. Dailey, M. O. and Hunter, R. L. (1974) The role of lipid in the induction of hapten-specific delayed hypersensitivity and contact sensitivity. J. Immunol. 112, 1526 – 1534.

59. Hilgers, L. A. Th. (1985) Immunomodulating properties of synthetic adjuvants. Thesis, State University of Utrecht, Utrecht, The Netherlands, pp. 29 – 42.

60. Bloksma, N., De Reuver, M. J. and Willers, J. M. N. (1983) Impaired macrophage functions as a possible basis of immunomodification by microbial agents, tilorone and dimethyldioctadecylammonium bromide. Antonie van Leeuwenhoek 49, 13 – 22.

61. Kraaijeveld, C. A., Snippe, H., Harmsen, T. and Benaissa-Trouw, B. (1982) Enhancement of delayed-type hypersensitivity and induction of interferon by the lipophilic agent DDA and CP-20,961. Cell. Immunol. 74, 277 – 283.

62. Zigterman, G. J. W. J., Snippe, H., Jansze, M., Ernste, E. B. H. W., De Reuver, M. J. and Willers, J. M. N. (1988) Non-ionic block polymers (NBPS) as adjuvants for future vaccines. Adv. Biosci., in press.

63. Hilgers, L. A. Th., Snippe, H., Jansze, M. and Willers, J. M. N. (1985) Combination of two synthetic adjuvants: synergistic effects of a surfactant and a polyanion on the humoral immune response. Cell. Immunol. 92, 203 – 209.

64. Hilgers, L. A. Th., Snippe, H., Jansze, M. and Willers, J. M. N. (1986) Synergistic effects of synthetic adjuvants on the humoral response. Int. Arch. Allergy Appl. Immunol. 79, 392 – 396.

65. Bradfield, J. W. B., Souhami, R. L. and Addison, I. E. (1974) The mechanism of the adjuvant effect of dextran sulphate. Immunology 26, 383 – 392.

66. Bomford, R. (1981) The adjuvant activity of fatty acid esters. The role of acyl chain length and degree of saturation. Immunology 44, 187 – 192.

67. Van Houte, A. J., Snippe, H., Peulen, G. T. M. and Willers, J. M. N. (1979) Characterization of the immunogenic properties of haptenated liposomal membrane in mice. V. Effect of membrane composition on humoral and cellular immunogenicity. Immunology 44, 561 – 568.

68. Hilgers, L. A. Th., Snippe, H., Jansze, M. and Willers, J. M. N. (1986) Route dependent immunomodulation: local stimulation by a surfactant and systemic stimulation by a polyanion. Int. Arch. Allergy Appl. Immunol. 79, 388 – 391.

SECTION V

Experimental approaches to asess the potential of chemicals to induce autoimmune(-like) diseases

M.E. Kammüller, N. Bloksma and W. Seinen (Eds.)
Autoimmunity and Toxicology
© *1989 Elsevier Science Publishers B.V. (Biomedical Division)*

Propylthiouracil-induced immune-mediated disease syndrome in the cat: a novel animal model for a drug-induced lupus-like disease

12

DAVID P. AUCOIN

North Carolina State University, School of Veterinary Medicine, Raleigh, NC 27606, USA

I. Introduction

Peterson was the first to note that some cats receiving propylthiouracil (PTU) for the treatment of hyperthyroidism developed antinuclear antibodies (ANA) and an immune-mediated disease syndrome (IMDS) similar to that seen in humans with systemic lupus erythematosus (SLE) [1]. Subsequent to this finding, my colleagues and I have induced this disease in more than 50% of normal mongrel cats receiving 150 mg of PTU daily for 8 weeks [2–4]. The IMDS is characterized by anorexia, lymphadenopathy, weight loss and fever, with formation of autoantibodies against red blood cells (RBCs), nuclear and cytoplasmic cell components. In man, granulocytopenia, thrombocytopenia, polyarthritis, vasculitis, skin rashes, fever and ANA are rare but recognized complications of PTU therapy [29–33]. Hemolytic anemia has not been described. The mechanism for this drug-induced immune-mediated disease is not known and has not been studied in any detail, due to its low frequency of occurrence. However, research into the mechanism of PTU-induced IMDS in cats has been ongoing in my laboratory for 3 years and has been focused into four primary areas.

First, what is the relationship between PTU's structural composition and the induction of disease? The induction of ANA and IMDS is dependent on the free sulfhydryl group on PTU [1]. The sulfhydryl group could be acting non-specifically such that any SH-containing compound in equimolar amounts could duplicate its

effect. Alternatively, a SH-dependent action, specific to PTU and other antithyroidal compounds, is required for the induction of this IMDS.

Second, is the duration of drug exposure needed to induce the disease upon
rechallenge and which are the dose-dependent requirements of its induction? One
hypothesis for the mechanism of PTU-induced IMDS is that it results from an immune disregulating action of PTU. An alternative hypothesis is that a normal immune system is responding to a foreign antigen (i.e. hapten-mediated event). If an
allergic reaction is responsible for this disease, then multiple exposures to the drug
should induce disease much sooner than the initial induction time, and would be expected to require less drug.

The third area of research interest involves the disposition of PTU in the cat. Not
all the cats receiving PTU develop ANA and IMDS. It is possible that a difference
in disposition between responder and non-responder cats could account for susceptibility to, or protection from, PTU-induced IMDS.

Finally, the specificity of the ANA is being determined to facilitate the understanding of possible mechanisms underlying autoantibody production and their role in
the production of clinical disease.

II. Induction of PTU-induced IMDS

1. STRUCTURE-ACTIVITY RELATIONSHIP

PTU is one of a family of thioureylene compounds which have found clinical usefulness in human and veterinary medicine in the medical treatment of
hyperthyroidism [5, 6]. Common to all thioureylenes is their thioamide group
$$\begin{matrix} S \\ \| \end{matrix}$$
$(-N-C-N)$ which is critical for their antithyroid activity. Methimazole (MMI) is
another more potent thioureylene, with an imidazole ring containing the thioamide
group rather than a purine configuration, as in PTU (Fig. 1). These compounds inhibit thyroxine (T4) production by competitive inhibition of the enzyme thyroid
peroxidase, thereby preventing organification of iodine into the tyrosyl residue of
thyroglobulin [7]. PTU and MMI are substrates for and, thus, inhibitors of other
cellular peroxidase enzymes such as the myeloperoxidases of neutrophilic or
monocytic phagocytes [8, 9]. PTU and MMI undergo oxidative desulfuration in the
process forming the sulfinic and sulfonic reactive oxidative metabolites (Fig. 1)
[10 – 12].

Thioureylenes also undergo S-oxidation by flavin-containing monooxygenases
and possibly from cytochrome *P450* producing these same reactive intermediates.
Not surprisingly, PTU and MMI have been shown to inhibit the activity of these
enzymes in vitro [13, 14]. Removal or methylation of the SH-group on any of the

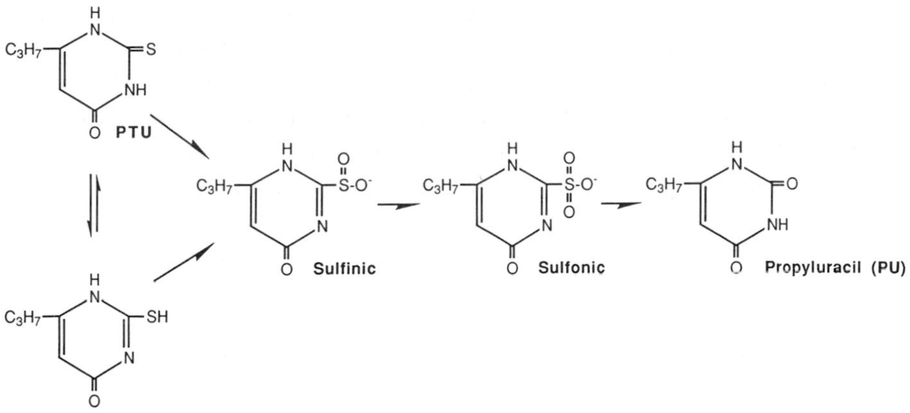

Fig. 1. Oxidative desulfuration of thioureylenes, such as PTU and MMI, occurs via peroxidases, flavin-containing monooxygenases, and possibly cytochrome *P450* enzymes. The sulfinic and sulfonic oxidative intermediates are unstable and progress to the desulfurated end product by non-enzymatic hydrolysis. PTU tautomerises between the sulfone and the sulfhydryl configuration, depending upon the pH. At a physiological pH of 7.4, it is probable that it is mostly a sulfhydryl-containing compound.

antithyroidal compounds destroys their antiperoxidase and presumably their monooxygenase enzyme inhibiting activity [10].

To determine the importance of the sulfhydryl group in the induction of disease and to gain insight into the possible mechanisms of action, we discontinued PTU during nine episodes of PTU-induced IMD in seven cats, and started propyluracil (PU), the desulfurated end product of PTU metabolism. Resolution of both clinical and serologic signs of disease occurred in seven of the nine cases within 1 – 3 weeks (2.1 ± 0.4). The time for disease resolution was similar to discontinuing the PTU alone [1].

Thus, the mechanism of ANA and disease induction is dependent on a free sulfhydryl group and may involve either a non-specific SH- effect, such as a reduction-oxidation reaction, or one or more of the specific SH-dependent actions of the thioureylenes.

To separate these two possibilities, PTU was replaced by captopril, another sulfhydryl-containing drug implicated in producing ANA and a drug-induced lupus-like syndrome in man [15, 16]. However, this compound is neither a substrate for, nor an inhibitor of peroxidase or oxidative microsomal enzymes [17]. Four cats which had previously been treated with PTU, developing ANA and IMDS, were treated with 150 mg of captopril during an 8-week study. Of the four cats used, three had developed ANA and IMDS on two prior occasions and one had been induced for times. The cats had not received PTU for 3 months and were free of disease and ANA for 2 months. After 8 weeks of 150 mg/day of captopril, all cats remained healthy and ANA-negative.

MMI has been reported to produce ANA, but no clinical signs of disease, in hyperthyroid cats [18]. MMI is a more potent antithyroid drug than PTU, requiring just 1/10th of the PTU dose or 15 mg to decrease T4 concentrations. Overall, of the cats followed over the 1-year study, 20% (22 out of 109) developed ANA titers, and of those cats treated longer than 6 months, 36% had ANA titers. An explanation as to why MMI, unlike PTU, produces ANA but not disease, is unclear and its disposition in the cat unknown. However, their mechanisms of antithyroid activity are similar, varying only in potency. The frequency and dose-dependent nature of MMI-induced ANA in normal cats are currently under investigation and, once established, should prove an exciting model of two drugs inducing autoantibodies but only one of them producing clinical disease. The model should help explain the role of ANA in the induction of drug-induced IMDS.

Therefore, with the failure of equimolar doses of captopril to produce ANA and/or IMDS, and with the clinical evidence that MMI, like PTU induces ANA, it can be postulated that the mechanism for PTU-induced IMDS involves a specific SH-dependent action of the drug. This action may involve inhibition of peroxidase or oxygenase enzymes and/or formation of reactive oxidative metabolites which themselves modulate a cellular process involved in immune regulation.

2. DURATION OF DRUG EXPOSURE AND DOSE-DEPENDENCY FOR INDUCTION

The duration of drug administration before the development of a positive Coombs' test or ANA in the 17 of 31 cats tested to date ranges from 2 to 10 weeks (mean ± SEM = 4.1 ± 0.9), with clinical signs, if any, occurring a few weeks later (6.8 ± 0.9) ([1], unpublished data). Following cessation of PTU administration, the clinical and serological signs of disease resolve within 1 to 4 weeks (1.5 ± 0.8) ([1], unpublished data). Four cats, rechallenged with PTU a total of nine times, developed serological signs of disease within 2.5 ± 0.7 weeks, with clinical signs occurring almost simultaneously (2.6 ± 0.7 weeks) [1].

Fig. 2 shows the time course for one cat and indicates that, although the course is shorter upon subsequent challenges, it is not consistently shorter with each successive challenge. Also, the time for disease induction is still weeks, and not days, as might be expected in an amnestic allergic response.

The hypothesis is that the induction of ANA and IMDS is a function of some PTU action, and not a mere haptenic response. Therefore, the same four cats used in the captopril study were rechallenged with a smaller (12.5 mg/day) dose of PTU, to determine if induction of ANA and IMDS was due to a dose-dependent action of PTU [19].

After 8 weeks of receiving the smaller dose all four cats remained clinically and serologically normal. One month later they were given the standard induction dose of 150 mg/day and all four developed IMDS within 3 weeks [19].

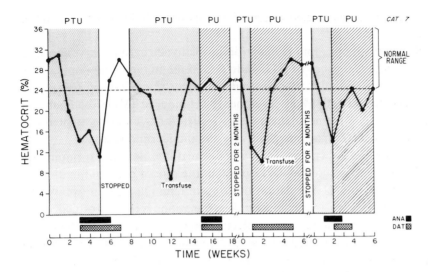

Fig. 2. Effect of repeated challenges of 150 mg/day of PTU on the hematocrit, and the production of a positive direct antiglobulin test (DAT) and antinuclear antibody (ANA) in a cat. The resolution of disease during propyluracil (PU) administration is also shown. The subsequent rechallenges required a shorter time to disease induction as noted by both a decrease in hematocrit and formation of anti-RBC antibodies (as determined by the DAT) and ANA. However, induction still required more than a week, and the fourth induction period was longer than the third rechallenge treatment period.

These findings support our hypothesis that a dosage-dependent action of PTU is required for disease induction, which, coupled with the structure-activity relationship for disease induction, further supports the theory that a specific SH-dependent action of PTU is involved in the pathogenesis of this drug-induced IMDS.

III. Pharmacology of PTU

1. DISPOSITION OF PTU IN THE CAT

To determine whether or not a difference in the disposition of PTU was correlated with the production of ANA and/or disease, both oral and intravenous pharmacokinetic disposition studies were conducted.

Studies were performed initially on hyperthyroid cats, since the disease was initially seen in this population [20]. Not unexpectedly, following a 50-mg i.v. dose of PTU the rate of drug clearance in this group was twice as fast (5.7 vs. 2.7 ml · kg^{-1} · min^{-1}), and the elimination half-lives just half as long compared to the normal control cats (77 vs. 156 min). The reason for the accelerated clearance is unknown but it is probably related to an increase in PTU metabolism, since ac-

Jerry M. Smith, Ph.D., D.A.B.T.
12560 Coopers Lane
Worton, MD 21678
Phone/Fax (410)778-5863

celerated hepatic metabolism has been seen with other drugs in hyperthyroid human patients [21].

The correlation of a more rapid elimination in the hyperthyroid cat vs. normals is compatible with the frequency of PTU-induced disease in these two populations. In the initial description of this disease syndrome only 8% (9 out of 105) of the hyperthyroid cats treated with PTU developed PTU-induced IMDS, compared to a rate of more than 50% for normal cats [1, 2]. Therefore, it was postulated that length of exposure to PTU may correlate with the induction of disease.

To investigate this possibility a study was performed in a normal cat population to determine if there was a bimodal distribution in the rate of drug elimination for PTU in cats, as there is for N-acetylation of drugs in man [22, 23]. In twenty-four cats intravenous and oral pharmacokinetic determinations were performed on sequential days. PTU was prepared for i.v. injection and each cat received 50 mg over 2 min through the femoral vein. Blood was collected at 5, 15, 30, 60, 180, 300 and 480 min following injection. The next day each cat received a 50-mg tablet of PTU orally, and blood was collected at 30, 60, 120, 180, 360, 720 min and 24 h.

PTU concentrations were determined by HPLC [2] and the decreases in serum concentrations were fit to an 1-compartment open pharmacokinetic model of the form $C_p = Ae^{-kt}$, where C_p is the concentration of the drug at time t, A is the concentration at time zero, and k is the elimination rate constant. An initial exponential curve stripping program was used to generate parameter estimates for the final solution which uses a non-linear least squares regression program (SAS-NONLIN) [24]. Parameters derived were then used to calculate the central volume of distribution (V_d), the total body clearance (CL_{tb}) and the elimination half-life ($T_{1/2}$).

Table 1 shows the kinetic parameters for both i.v. and oral PTU disposition. The similarity between these values reflects rapid and complete absorption (> 95% based on area-under-the-curve ratios). Fig. 3 graphically shows the distribution in

TABLE 1

Kinetic parameters following a singe 50 mg intravenous (i.v.) or oral dose of PTU in normal cats

	K (per h)	V_d (l/kg)	$T_{1/2}$ (min)	CL_{tb} (ml · kg^{-1} · min^{-1})
i.v.	0.369 ± 0.020	0.511 ± 0.019	123.4 ± 9.6	3.29 ± 0.22
Oral	0.310 ± 0.029	0.543 ± 0.085	141.9 ± 10.8	2.64 ± 0.90

Values were determined by fitting the decline in serum concentrations over time to a monoexponential function, $C_p = Ae^{-kt}$, where C_p is the drug concentration at time t, A is the concentration at time zero, and k is the elimination rate constant. Kinetic parameters were determined using standard formula. V_d, central volume of distribution; CL_{tb}, total body clearance rate.
Data are reported as mean ± standard error of the mean (SEM).

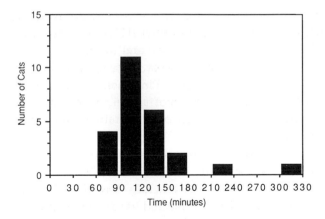

Fig. 3. Frequency histogram of PTU elimination half-lives in cats: 25 normal cats of both sexes and under 1 year of age were giving a 50-mg intravenous bolus of PTU, and multiple blood samples were collected over 8 h. Elimination half-life was determined for each cat after fitting the data to a monoexponential decay curve. Cats were grouped based on half-life on PTU in intervals of 30 min. Only one significant outlier existed in this population of cats. This indicates that the elimination of PTU is fairly homogenous in a normal cat population.

elimination half-lives in these 24 cats, with 22 being clustered around the mean and 2 lying outside this cluster.

This preliminary data does not support a significant bimodal distribution in PTU elimination. However, more cats will have to be used to increase the sensitivity of detecting a lower frequency distribution pattern that 50 : 50 as seen with N-acetylation phenotypes in humans [23].

It is interesting to note that the cat with the longest elimination half-life (313 min) developed the highest titer of ANA and the most extensive lymphadenopathy of the 24 cats tested. However, within the clustered half-lives, no correlation between mean ANA titers or development of IMDS and longer half-lives could be demonstrated (unpublished data).

2. METABOLISM

Perhaps the magnitude of production of a particular metabolite, rather than gross differences in elimination rates makes some cats more susceptible to PTU-induced IMDS. Since the SH-group is essential for PTU activity, it could be postulated that cats with more extensive S-methylation or S-oxidative capacity may be protected from PTU-induced IMD. An alternative hypothesis is that the reactive metabolites of S-oxidation are involved in the induction of disease and cats with more extensive oxidative capacity may be more vulnerable to developing PTU-induced IMDS. In man and the rat, the majority of PTU is excreted either as the unchanged parent compound or as the S-glucuronide metabolite [5, 25]. The end product of oxidative desulfuration, PU, and the methylated metabolite (S-methyl PTU) have also been identified as smaller but significant components in rat bile and urine.

The metabolic fate of PTU is probably different in the cat, since glucuronidation is extremely slow compared with other species [26]. This lack of glucuronyl transferase activity results in a lengthening of duration of action, increased pharmacological response and heightened toxicity of many other metabolized drugs in cats including aspirin and acetaminophen [27].

Preliminary urine metabolite studies have been conducted on four cats after both i.v. and oral doses of 50 mg of PTU. Surprisingly, PTU accounted for 5–8% of the total dose recovered in the urine, while PU was generally less than 1% (unpublished data). S-methyl PTU was detected in cat urine and its identity confirmed by HPLC-mass spectroscopy. Its quantity could not be determined due to the lack of an analytical standard. However, this finding indicated that a genetically controlled enzyme responsible for S-methylation of thiopurines, thiol methyltransferase, is present in the cat and its relative activity between responders and nonresponders may be important [28].

The preliminary findings may reflect a number of possible explanations which are being investigated – the first being assay inaccuracy. The stability of PTU in the normally found acidic (pH = 5) cat urine was determined in vitro by incubating PTU-spiked urine at 37°C for 6 and 12 h. No loss of PTU or PU was noted (unpublished data). The second possible explanation is the fact that significant biliary secretion of PTU occurs in the cat and that the majority of PTU was eliminated by that route. A third explanation is that PTU does undergo conjugation with an amino acid such as glycine prior to elimination, and finally, cats may employ a unique metabolic pathway for thiopurine elimination resulting in, as yet, unidentified metabolites. Radiolabeled PTU metabolism studies addressing these possibilities are in progress.

PTU has been reported to cause a constellation of clinical disease in man, including granulocytopenia, thrombocytopenia, polyarthritis, vasculitis, skin rashes and fever, as well as inducing ANA titers [29–33]. However, the incidence of these cases is low when compared to the extensive use of this drug.

The higher frequency of IMDS seen in cats with PTU compared to man where this drug is routinely used in toxic nodular goiter patients, may be attributable to two factors. First, PTU peak concentrations in the cat after the standard induction dose of 150 mg are $20-25$ μg/ml, whereas in man, after a standard 300-mg dose, concentrations are less than 5 μg/ml [3, 5]. Empirical dose titration studies showed that most cats required 150 mg/day of PTU, which is $5-6$ times the human dose. Second, its disposition in man is similar to that seen in the hyperthyroid cat, where the incidence of disease is much lower than in normal cats and where the elimination half-life is similar to that of hyperthyroid humans [5].

These differences in disposition may be responsible for the difference in disease frequency, or the cat may be genetically more prone to develop drug-induced IMDS due to its unique handling of drugs. The cats' lack of glucuronidation forces them to utilize other pathways of elimination, some, like with acetaminophen, may be deleterious.

IV. PTU-induced ANA specificity

Investigation into the specificity of ANA was performed in order to identify the target autoantigen(s) and to examine possible mechanisms underlying autoantibody formation.

The predominate component of ANA activity is due to anti-native DNA antibodies [4, 19]. Since the induction of these antibodies is rarely seen in drug-induced IMDS and is a hallmark of systemic lupus erythematosus (SLE), we carefully confirmed their presence, using two different assays. A solid-phase enzyme-linked immunosorbent assay (ELISA) was used with highly purified S1-nuclease-treated native double-stranded DNA as the ligand [34]. Additionally, we used the *Crithidia luciliae* immunofluorescent assay which, although less sensitive than ELISA, is essentially an unambiguous assay for nDNA antibodies [35].

The formation of anti-nDNA antibodies in cats with PTU-induced IMDS is highly significant, because it is a hallmark of idiopathic SLE and is rarely reported in drug-induced lupus-like syndromes in humans [36 – 39]. The presence of anti-nDNA antibodies helps eliminate one possible mechanism of this disease. The formation of these antibodies cannot be explained by mechanisms involving PTU which render the DNA structure antigenic, since alterations in the DNA structure would be expected to induce antibodies to the altered DNA, and not to the native form [39, 40].

Unlike most drug-induced ANA, PTU does not appear to induce a significant amount of anti-histone antibodies. However, more like in human patients with SLE, it does induce more than anti-nDNA antibodies. Preliminary radioimmunoprecipitation studies using PTU-induced ANA serum have identified a small 12 – 14 000 dalton protein [4]. This protein may be responsible for the cytoplasmic staining seen in the immunofluorescent ANA tests [19].

It is possible that this autoantibody which reacts with this small mol.-wt. protein is similar to the anti-Sm autoantibody seen exclusively in SLE patients and MRL/*lpr*/*lpr* lupus mice [41 – 43]. The anti-Sm antibody has been shown to recognize a very selected group of RNA-binding proteins found in a nuclear structure called the splicesome. This structure is involved in splicing of heteronuclear RNA into messenger RNA. The seven RNA molecules in the splicesome are called U1 – U7. Seven polypeptides bound to U1 RNA have been characterized by SDS-PAGE, and by Western blot analysis it has been shown that anti-Sm antibodies recognize epitope(s) on the B, B' and D polypeptides [44]. The role which this autoantibody has in the production of SLE is unknown, but its highly selected specificity is almost virtually restricted to these patients. The finding of this antibody in PTU-induced ANA would be enormously exciting, since the reasons for its presence in SLE patients, its association with anti-nDNA antibodies, and its role in the induction of clinical disease are the subject of considerable investigation.

Therefore, PTU-induced ANA cat sera from four cats were tested for the presence of anti-Sm antibodies, using an established ELISA technique [43]. Briefly, the Sm preparation was prepared from rabbit thymus extract (RTE) (Cal BioChem). The RTE was extracted into a 6 M urea/0.1 M Tris-saline buffer to free soluble cellular proteins. These proteins were precipitated with a 30%, followed by a 60% ammonium sulfate solution. The pellet was resuspended in PBS, dialyzed against PBS, and then purified by affinity chromatography. The Sepharose column was bound with a highly purified human IgG anti-Sm antibody (courtesy of Dr. David Pisetsky). The eluted protein contains a number of proteins as determined by SDS-PAGE and Western blot analysis, including the Sm-specific U1 RNA binding polypeptides B, B' and D [42, 44].

Microtiter plates (Immunol II, Dynatech) were coated with 200 μl of the Sm preparation (2.5 μg/ml) in a borate buffer (pH = 8.0). The plates were incubated overnight at 4°C and then blocked with 0.1% gelatin in PBS for 2 h at room temperature. Plates were washed and then incubated at room temperature with a 1 : 100 dilution of ANA and control cat serum. Antibody binding was detected using a peroxidase-labeled affinity-purified anti-cat IgG. The system was developed using 2,2'-azino-di-(3-ethylbenzthiazoline-6-sulfonic acid) (ABTS) substrate and absorbance units reported in O.D. units determined at 414 nm. MRL/*lpr/lpr* mice serum

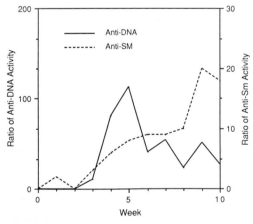

Fig. 4. Plotted is the activity of two autoantibodies in a cat receiving 150 mg per day of PTU. Antibody activity was determined by ELISA as described (see text), and the ratio of anti-DNA and anti-Sm activity by dividing the O.D. value of a 1:100 dilution of the cat's serum by the O.D. value of the negative control used in that day's assay. The negative control was this same cat's serum, prior to administration of PTU. The Y-axis on the right side of the graph is significantly lower than the left, indicating that the anti-DNA activity is the predominate autoantibody response to PTU.

and human serum from an SLE patient (kindly supplied by Dr. David Pisetsky) were used as positive controls and were detected using peroxidase-labeled anti-mouse and anti-human antibody, respectively. Sera collected from cats prior to PTU administration were used as negative controls.

Fig. 4 shows the formation of anti-DNA and anti-Sm antibodies over a 10-week treatment period. The non-concurrent appearance of these two antibodies indicates that they represent separate antibody populations. The appearance of low levels of these anti-Sm antibodies is seen in cats without anti-DNA activity but their activity does appear to be higher in those cats with high anti-DNA activity.

The fine specificity of this antibody population is currently being investigated. It is not known if this PTU-induced autoantibody recognizes the same epitopes on the same polypeptides as is seen in human SLE patients or in the MRL mouse. However, this is the first demonstration of autoantibodies with anti-Sm and anti-native DNA specificities in drug-induced lupus-like disease. The similarities of these two chemically-induced autoantibody populations similar to those seen in SLE patients makes this model even more exciting and potentially very valuable in the investigation into the mechanism of autoantibody formation, and its possible relationship to the pathogenesis of SLE.

V. Conclusion

The prototypic disease of immune disregulation in SLE and drug-induced lupus-like syndromes in man are an example of man acting as his own animal model for an idiopathic disease. However, it lacks some obvious requirements of a good model, and the desire to produce an animal model of drug-induced lupus is strong. The inability to develop a drug-induced lupus-like syndrome in laboratory animals has been frustrating. The exciting primate model of L-canavanine-induced lupus-like syndrome in macaques has been the one exception and offers some important opportunities to study an induced SLE-like disease in an animal genetically close to man [45].

This cat model of a drug-induced IMDS offers an excellent opportunity for dissecting the basic cellular mechanisms involved in immune regulation and self tolerance. It has not escaped my attention that many investigators have shown the antithyroidal drugs to be immunosuppressive in human patients with autoimmune disease (i.e. Graves'), and that adverse effects attributed to many other SH-containing compounds, many of them immune-mediated, have been noted for many of the anti-rheumatic drugs [46, 47]. The explanation for these observations needs a closer, more detailed look at the exact biochemical alterations occurring with these drugs and their relationship to the development of disease.

Therefore, future studies first must include determination of the cellular site of action of PTU. It is known that in rats the drug neither binds to nor is taken up into lymphocytes [9]. However, they are avidly taken up into neutrophilic or monocytic phagocytes [9]. It is fairly clear that, if enzyme inhibition and/or reactive metabolites are involved in the production of this syndrome, then these actions should occur in those cell populations involved in the regulation of antibodies (i.e. macrophages which control presentation of antigens to the T cell).

In vitro metabolism studies in these populations of immune regulatory cells from cats are in progress, and should help focus the questions and thus the experiments regarding the mechanism of autoantibody production.

This is a unique animal model of drug-induced autoantibodies. Induction of anti-nDNA antibodies is a rare event, and to have a model where they are not only produced but are the major autoantibody produced, is very exciting. In addition, the formation of other antibodies directed against cytoplasmic proteins is also unique for any drug-induced autoantibody. The mechanism for induction and their role in the production of clinical disease can now be investigated in an animal genus not genetically prone to the development of immune-mediated diseases.

References

1. Peterson, M. E., Hurvitz, A. I., Leib, M. C., Cavanaugh, P. and Dutton, R. (1984) Propylthiouracil-associated hemolytic anemia, thrombocytopenia, and antinuclear antibodies in cats with hyperthyroidism. J. Am. Vet. Med. Assoc. 184, 806–810.
2. Aucoin, D. P., Peterson, M. E., Hurvitz, A. I., Drayer, D. E., Lahita, R. G., Quimby, F. W. and Reidenberg, M. M. (1985) Propylthiouracil induced immune-mediated disease in the cat. J. Pharmacol. Exp. Ther. 234, 13–18.
3. Aucoin, D. P., Peterson, M. E., Reidenberg, M. M., Drayer, D. E., Lahita, R. L. and Hurvitz, A. I. (1985) Dose-response relationship for propylthiouracil induced immune-mediated disease in cats. Clin. Res. 33, 217A.
4. Aucoin, D. P., Lahita, R. G., Krater, S. M., Peterson, M. E., Drayer, D. E., Hurvitz, A. I. and Reidenberg, M. M. (1985) Preliminary antinuclear antibody characterization in propylthiouracil-induced immune-mediated disease in the cat. Arthritis Rheum. 28(4), S57.
5. Cooper, D. S. (1984) Antithyroid drugs. N. Engl. J. Med. 311, 1353–1362.
6. Peterson, M. E. and Turrel, J. M. (1986) Feline hyperthyroidism. In: R. W. Kirk (Ed.), Current Veterinary Therapy. W. B. Saunders, Philadelphia, PA, pp. 1026–1033.
7. Taurog, A. (1976) The mechanism of action of thioureylene antithyroid drugs. Endocrinology 98, 1031–1046.
8. Anderson, M. R., Curtis, A. L. and Harmon, E. J. (1982) Intact form of myeloperoxidase from normal human neutrophils. Arch. Biochem. Biophys. 214, 273–283.
9. Weetman, A. P., McGregor, A. M. and Hall, R. (1983) Methimazole inhibits thyroid autoantibody production by action on accessory cells. Clin. Immunol. Immunopathol. 28, 39–45.
10. Lindsay, R. H., Aboul-Enein, H. Y., Morel, D. and Bowen, S. (1974) Synthesis and antiperoxidase activity of propylthiouracil and metabolites. J. Pharm. Sci. 63, 1383–1386.
11. Lindsay, R. H., Kelly, K. and Hill, J. B. (1978) Oxidative products of antithyroid drug 6-propyl-2-thiouracil. Alabama J. Med. Sci. 15, 29–41.
12. Lindsay, R. H. and Husley, B. S. (1975) Enzymatic S-methylation of 6-propyl-2-thiouracil and other antithyroid drugs. Biochem. Pharmacol. 24, 463–468.

13. Poulsen, L. L., Hyslop, R. M. and Keigler, D. M. (1974) S-oxidation of thioureylenes catalyzed by a microsomal flavoprotein mixed-function oxidase. Biochem. Pharmacol. 23, 3431 – 3440.

14. Kedderis, G. L. and Richert, D. E. (1985) Loss of rat liver microsomal cytochrome *P450* during methimazole metabolism. Drug Metab. Disp. 13, 58 – 63.

15. Kallenberg, C. G. M., Hoorntje, S. J., Smit, A. J., Weening, J. J., Donker, A. J. M. and Hoedemaeker, T. H. (1982) Antinuclear and antinative DNA antibodies during captopril treatment. Acta Med. Scand. 211, 297 – 300.

16. Reidenberg, M. M., Case, D. B. and Drayer, D. E. (1984) Development of antinuclear antibody in patients treated with high doses of captopril. Arthritis Rheum. 27, 579 – 581.

17. Heel, R. C., Brogden, R. N., Speight, T. M. and Avery, G. S. (1980) Captopril: a preliminary review of pharmacological properties and therapeutic efficacy. Drugs 20, 409 – 452..

18. Peterson, M. E., Kintzer, D. P. and Hurvitz, A. I. (1985) Evaluation of methimazole in the treatment of feline hyperthyroidism. In: Proceedings Am. Coll. Vet. Intern. Med., pp. 128.

19. Aucoin, D. P., Rubin, R. L., Peterson, M. E., Reidenberg, M. M., Drayer, D. E., Hurvitz, A. I. and Lahita, R. L. (1988) Dose-dependent induction of anti-native DNA antibodies by propylthiouracil in cats. Arthritis Rheum. 31, 688 – 693.

20. Peterson, M. E., Aucoin, D. P. and Davis, C. A. (1988) Altered disposition of propylthiouracil in cats with hyperthyroidism. Res. Vet. Sci. 45, 1 – 3.

21. Eichelbaum, M. (1983) Drug metabolism in thyroid disease. In: M. Gibaldi and L. Prescott (Eds.), Handbook of Clinical Pharmacokinetics. AIDS Health Science Press, Balgowkh, Australia, pp. 169 – 181.

22. Woosley, R. L., Drayer, D. E., Reidenberg, M. M., Nies, A., Carr, K. and Oates, J. (1978) Effect of acetylator phenotype on the rate at which procainamide induces antinuclear antibodies and the lupus like syndrome. N. Engl. J. Med. 298, 1157 – 1159.

23. Reidenberg, M. M. and Drayer, D. E. (1978) Aromatic amines and hydrazines, drug acetylation and lupus erythematosus. Human Genet. Suppl. 1, 57 – 63.

24. SAS-NONLIN, SAS Software, Cary, NC.

25. Skellern, G. G. and Steer, S. T. (1981) The metabolism of $[2^{-14}C]$methimazole in the rat. Xenobiotica 11, 627 – 634.

26. Dutton, G. L. (1966) The biosynthesis of glucuronides. In: G. L. Dutton (Ed.), Glucuronic Acid, Free and Combined. Chemistry, Biochemistry, Pharmacology and Medicine. Academic Press, New York, pp. 185 – 299.

27. Baggot, J. D. (1977) Comparative patterns of drug biotransformation. In : J. D. Baggot (Ed.), Principles of Drug Disposition in Domestic Animals: The Basis of Veterinary Clinical Pharmacology. W. B. Saunders Co., Philadelphia, PA, pp. 73 – 94.

28. Keith, R. A., Van Loon, J., Wussow, L. F. and Weinshilboum, R. M. (1983) Thiol methylation pharmacogenetics: heriditability of human erythrocyte thiol methyltransferase activity. Clin. Pharmacol. Ther. 34, 51 – 58.

29. Takuwas, N., Kojima, I. and Orgata, E. (1981) Lupus-like syndrome: a rare complication in thioamide treatment for Graves' disease. Endocrinology (Japan) 28, 663 – 667.

30. Cetina, J. A., Fishbein, E. and Alarcón-Segovia, D. (1972) Antinuclear antibodies and propylthiouracil therapy. J. Am. Med. Assoc. 220, 1012.

31. Amrhein, J. A., Kenny, F. M. and Ross, D. (1970) Granulocytopenia, lupus-like syndrome and other complications of propylthiouracil therapy. J. Pediat. 76, 54 – 63.

32. Oh, B. K., Overveld, G. P. J. and MacFarland, J. C. (1983) Polyarthritis induced by propylthiouracil. Br. J. Rheumatol. 22, 106 – 108.

33. Searles, R. P., Plymate, S. R. and Troup, G. M. (1980) Familial thioamide-induced lupus syndrome in thyrotoxicosis. J. Rheumatol. 8, 498 – 500.

34. Rubin, R. L., Joslin, F. G. and Tan, E. M. (1983) An improved ELISA for anti-nDNA by elimination of interference by anti-histone antibodies. J. Immunol. Methods 63, 359 – 366.

322

35. Aarden, L. A., De Groot, E. R. and Feltkamp, T. E. W. (1975) Immunology of DNA. III. *Crithidia luciliae,* a simple substrate for the determination of anti-dsDNA with the immunofluorescent technique. Ann. NY Acad. Sci. 254, 505 – 515.
36. Weinstein, A. (1980) Drug induced systemic lupus erythematosus. Prog. Clin. Immunol, 4, 1 – 21.
37. Harmon, C. E. and Portanova, J. P. (1982) Drug-induced lupus: clinical and serological studies. Clin. Rheum. Dis. 8, 121 – 135.
38. Tan, E. M. (1982) Autoantibodies to nuclear antigens: their immunobiology and medicine. Adv. Immunol. 33, 167 – 240.
39. Schwartz, R. S. and Stollar, B. D. (1985) Origins of anti-DNA autoantibodies. Clin. Invest. 75, 321 – 327.
40. Stollar, B. D. (1981) The antigenic potential and specificity of nucleic acids, nucleoproteins, and their modified derivatives. Arthritis Rheum. 24, 1010 – 1018.
41. Cohen, P. L. (1985) Anti-Sm autoantibody in MRL mice: analysis of precursor frequency. Cell. Immunol. 96, 448.
42. Forman, M. S., Nakamura, M., Mimori, T., Gelpi, C. and Hardin, J. A. (1985) Detection of antibodies to small nuclear ribonucleoproteins and small cytoplasmic ribonucleoproteins using unlabeled cell extracts. Arthritis Rheum. 28, 1356.
43. Pisetsky, D. S., Hock, S. O., Klatt, C. L., O'Donnell, M. A. and Keene, J. D. (1985) Specificity of idiotypic analysis of a monoclonal anti-Sm antibody with anti-DNA activity. J. Immunol. 135, 4080 – 4086.
44. Pettersson, I., Hinterberger, M., Mimori, T., Gottlieb, E. and Steitz, J. A. (1984) The structure of mammalian small nuclear ribonucleoproteins: identification of multiple protein components reactive with anti-(U1)RNP and anti-Sm antibodies. J. Biol. Chem. 259, 5907 – 5914.
45. Malinow, M. R., Bardana, E. M., Pirofsky, B., Craig, S. and McLaughlin, P. (1982) Systemic lupus erythematosus like syndrome in monkeys fed alfalfa sprouts: role of a nonprotein amino acid. Science 216, 23 – 25.
46. Kendall-Taylor, P. (1984) Are antithyroid drugs immunosuppressive? Br. Med. J. 288, 509 – 510.
47. Jaffe, I. A. (1986) Adverse effects profile of sulfhydryl compounds in man. Am. J. Med. 80, 471 – 476.

M.E. Kammüller, N. Bloksma and W. Seinen (Eds.)
Autoimmunity and Toxicology
© 1989 Elsevier Science Publishers B.V. (Biomedical Division)

Autoimmune reactions induced by dietary antigens with an emphasis on amino acids

13

EMIL J. BARDANA, JR.[a], ANTHONY MONTANARO[a] and M. RENE MALINOW[b]

[a] *Division of Allergy and Clinical Immunology, Oregon Health Sciences University, Portland, OR 97201, USA and* [b] *Oregon Regional Primate Research Center, Beaverton, OR 97006, USA*

I. Introduction

Despite the fact that adverse reactions to foods were well described by Hippocrates (460 – 370 BC) and Galen (131 – 210 AD), there is a paucity of data linking dietary immunogens to the generation of autoimmune disorders. However, there is an increasing recognition that foodstuffs may contain substances that can affect immune regulation, and thus may have the capacity to influence immune homeostasis. Just as in the case with drug-related autoimmune disorders, acetylator phenotype and certain HLA haplotypes may act as predisposing factors in food-induced immune disregulation. Other predisposing factors may include alterations in gastrointestinal function including mucosal permeability, secretory immunity and alterations in bacterial flora. A number of animal models have been described which demonstrate the development of rheumatic disorders following changes in diet. Though many of the early clinical reports linking food and autoimmune disorders were anecdotal in nature, an increasing number of carefully recorded clinical observations has intensified both the interest and level of further investigation in this whole area. This chapter will review evidence related to food-induced immunological reactions. It will focus on studies conducted at our facilities implicating dietary amino acids in the induction of a systemic lupus erythematosus (SLE) like disorder in monkeys.

324

II. Historical review

Suggestions of possible associations with food and the immune system began to appear at the turn of the century. In 1895, Osler expanded Henoch's earlier observations of Henoch-Schönlein purpura by describing cutaneous, abdominal and articular abnormalities [1]. He meticulously reviewed 50 cases from the literature and noted that 32 had presented some form of arthritis. In 1914, he cited several additional cases of Henoch-Schönlein purpura and suggested that dietary protein sensitivity might be pathogenetically important [2]. In the same year, Solis-Cohen reported 27 cases in which painful swelling of the joints occurred at various intervals associated with ingestants [3]. Alexander and Eyermann who reported nine cases of Henoch-Schönlein purpura, felt to have unmistakable evidence of food sensitivity playing a causative role [4, 5].

In 1936, Lewin and Taub reported a young man who had recurrent hydrarthrosis of the knees related to the ingestion of English walnuts [6]. Intradermal injection of homologous serum, followed by oral challenge with walnut resulted in a wheal and flare at the skin test site. Exclusion of this food antigen was associated with disappearance of the recurrent synovitis. A similar observation involving English walnuts was made by Berger in 1939 [7].

Hench and Rosenberg coined the term palindromic rheumatism to characterize fleeting attacks of synovitis which they attributed to ingestants in 16 of 34 patients. They were unable to clearly substantiate this in any of their patients [8]. Two years later Vaughn described 27 cases with recurrent or persistent articular symptoms among a larger group of allergic individuals, in which the arthritic symptoms were attributed to one or more dietary antigens [9]. Zeller reviewed the subject in 1949 and noted that patients with rheumatic disorders had two to three times the incidence of allergic problems when compared to a similar number of controls [10]. He proposed a hypothesis of ingestants contributing to the development of rheumatoid arthritis (RA), but acknowledged that very few rheumatologists gave this theory any credence. Zussman reported similar observations in four patients with recurrent painful joints [11]. The foods implicated in these and other reports of adverse food reactions included wheat, eggs, beef and pork. These early studies of dietary-induced arthropathy were largely based on inadequate data, improper study design and dietary restrictions that produced no consistent abrogation to rheumatic disease [12 – 15].

The last several decades have seen a marked increase in both the quality and quantity of reports linking adverse food reactions to autoimmune rheumatic disorders. In a personal study, Epstein reported that 5 mg of sodium nitrate contained in food, or 0.5 mg of menthol, would provoke attacks of palindromic rheumatism lasting for up to 15 days [16, 17]. The observation of a palindromic course in these patients which indicates the complete absence of signs or symptoms of arthritis between attacks, implies that the stimulus to develop inflammation appears episodically. This pattern may be consistent with ingestants acting as a potential immunogen. Similar observations were made by Williams [18]. While Behcet's syndrome differs pathogenetically from rheumatoid arthritis, it may present with prominent inflammatory arthritis as well as oral and vaginal ulceration. Black walnut ingestion has been associated with clinical flares as well as other cellular immune responses of Behcet's syndrome [19]. Theorell and associates reported a spectrum of vasculitic illnesses associated with dietary ingestants [20].

The first controlled study of food-induced autoimmune disease was carried out by Skoldstam et al. in patients with RA. Five of 15 patients who underwent a period of 7 to 10 days of fasting, benefitted with reduced symptom scores and acute-phase reactants, whereas only one of 10 controls improved [21]. Continuation of a lactovegetarian diet for an additional 9 weeks was without consistent benefit. On the other hand, in a partially controlled study, Stroud reported a definite anti-rheumatic effect with fasting [22].

Dairy products have been the focus of several studies relating to the induction of other autoimmune disorders. In 1972, Carr and his associates found higher levels of antibody to bovine γ-globulin and bovine serum albumin in serum from patients with SLE. It was hypothesized that these commonly ingested proteins could conceivably enter the circulation of certain predisposed individuals, forming potentially pathogenic immune complexes [23]. Parke and Hughes reported an individual with chronic seronegative RA whose symptoms regressed after dietary exclusion of dairy products for 5 weeks. After 8 months of this diet, the patient was challenged with a large meal of milk and cheese. The challenge resulted in a significant flare of symptoms with acute synovitis for 2 weeks [24]. Transient leukocytosis and IgE-specific antibody to milk were observed, though changes in circulating immune complexes were not seen.

III. Immunopathogenesis

1. IMMEDIATE HYPERSENSITIVITY

With the demonstration that IgE played a role in the deposition of circulating immune complexes in experimental serum sickness [25], many investigators sought to find whether individuals with autoimmune disorders were 'hyperresponsive' to a variety of exogenous and endogenous antigens. IgE-mediated activation of tissue mast cells could stimulate the release of vasoactive amines and result in increased vascular permeability and deposition of circulating complexes. The recent elucidations of the late-phase reaction as the inflammatory component of an IgE-mediated reaction further supports its potential role in dietary-induced autoimmunity [26]. Block and his associates were unable to demonstrate any significant differences in skin test reactivity to bacterial and fungal antigens, except for a depressed response

326

to tuberculin in patients with SLE, when compared to a control population [27]. Diminished tuberculin reactivity has also been confirmed by other groups [28]. Interestingly, others have demonstrated significantly diminished responses to several bacterial antigens in patients with SLE [29].

Several investigators have reported peripheral eosinophilia in association with RA [30, 31]. Aside from the fact that vasoactive amines may be involved in this disorder, the significance of the eosinophilia is not understood. Among 57 patients with definite SLE, Becker found no increase in the incidence of atopid dermatitis, rhinitis, asthma or food and drug allergy. Urticaria was found in 28% of these patients with definite SLE compared with 10% in a control group [32]. Forty patients with 'possible' SLE had a significantly higher incidence of allergic rhinitis and drug allergy than controls. Goldman et al. further studied 27 SLE patients for the presence of allergic reactivity and total serum IgE. Compared to controls, SLE patients had significant increases of allergic rhinitis and drug allergy [33]. Total serum IgE levels were not elevated in these patients, irrespective of the very significant hyperimmunoglobulinemia that was observed. Another group of investigators found elevated total IgE both in the serum and synovial fluid of patients with RA [34]. These conflicting data have made it difficult to assess the role of immediate hypersensitivity in these autoimmune disorders.

Specific antinuclear antibodies (ANA) of the IgE class were reported in the sera of patients with SLE [35]. Permin and Wiik reported IgE granulocyte-specific ANAs which correlated with neurotropenia in RA [36]. In this study, the specific IgE ANA was organ-non-specific, and serum levels paralleled disease activity. Permin and associates reported enhanced basophil-mediated histamine release following exposure to deoxyribonucleic acid (DNA), ribonucleic acid (RNA) and aggregated IgG in patients with RA [37]. Similar observations were noted in response to native (double-stranded) deoxyribonucleic acid (dsDNA) in patients with SLE [38].

2. CIRCULATING IMMUNE COMPLEXES

Immune complexes injure tissues through their ability to activate humoral and cellular amplification systems. The nature of disease caused by soluble antigen-antibody complexes is determined by the size, distribution and extent of their localization in tissues. Unfortunately, in the vast majority of cases, the antigenic composition of immune complexes in human disease is unclear. The search for dietary antigens in immune complexes has proved a technically formidable task since the potential number of antigens is vast. In addition, the process of digestion causes many food proteins to undergo considerable modification [39]. Following up on the observations of Carr et al. [23], Paganelli et al. were able to demonstrate small quantities of bovine serum albumin in circulating immune complexes in normal individuals after milk consumption [40]. Despite this, Elkon et al., using several fluid-phase assays, failed to demonstrate any quantitative change in circulating immune complexes following a protein meal in serum from patients with both RA and SLE [41].

3. IgA DEFICIENCY

Since selective IgA deficiency is relatively common and plays a primary role in the gastrointestinal immune response, many potential roles for IgA's association to the etiopathogenesis of autoimmunity have been evaluated. Selective IgA deficiency is the most common primary immunodeficiency disorder and afflicts one out of 400 to 2 000 individuals of European ancestry. Both serum and secretory IgA levels are decreased in most affected individuals, although in some patients with this humoral immunodeficiency, salivary IgA levels are not substantially altered [42]. Secretory IgA deficiency may be an important factor contributing to recurrent infections involving the upper and lower respiratory tracts, gastrointestinal and urinary tracts as well as various allergic disorders. IgG_2 deficiency has also been associated with IgA deficiency, and this combination would very likely be associated with infections with pneumococcus and *Hemophilus influenzae* type B [43]. It is difficult to assess whether such combined immunodeficiencies would create changes in bowel flora as well. On the systemic level, autoimmune diseases, including RA and SLE have been reported in association with IgA deficiency, suggesting more global aberrations in immunoregulation [44 – 47]. It has been hypothesized that a lack of secretory IgA may facilitate gastrointestinal absorption of environmental antigens that have the propensity to induce a systemic immune response against cross-reactive autoantigens. Cunningham-Rundles studied 30 consecutive patients with selective IgA deficiency and found 15 sera with precipitins to cow's milk, all of which additionally had immune complexes demonstrated by Raji cell radioassay [47].

4. GASTROINTESTINAL ABNORMALITIES

There is increasing evidence to suggest that dietary antigens may cross the gastrointestinal barrier, enter the circulation in immunogenic form and potentially act to induce immune complex disease [48]. In addition, abnormalities of the bowel are commonly found in autoimmune disorders [49 – 51]. These functional changes may be associated to abnormal absorption of dietary antigens which in turn could play a role in the immunopathogenesis of these autoaggressive disorders. Individuals with the HLA-B27 haplotype seem strongly predisposed to develop polyarthritis following a variety of enteric infections [52].

The well-recognized relationship between inflammatory bowel disease, inflammatory spondylitis and peripheral arthritis adds further support for the association of altered bowel permeability and immune dysfunction. As well, about 20% of patients with regional enteritis and 10% of those with ulcerative colitis develop peripheral inflammatory arthritis [53, 54]. Clinically, there also appears to be a correlation between flares of inflammatory bowel disease and exacerbation of arthritis in some patients. Ankylosing spondylitis is found in about 4% of patients with inflammatory bowel disease [55], and 50–80% of these patients have an HLA-B27 haplotype [56]. Though some have postulated increased absorption of dietary antigens as a cause of autoimmune disease [57], this relationship has never been directly proven. In this respect, some 20% of patients who have received intestinal bypass operations for obesity develop polyarthritis. A variety of autoimmune features have been associated with this syndrome [58]. Furthermore, when these individuals are reanastomosed, their clinical autoimmune process remits. Though absorption of dietary constituents may play a role in bypass syndromes, changes in bowel flora are believed to be playing the principal role.

IV. Animal models demonstrating nutritional modification of the immune response

Much of our current knowledge relating to the development of SLE has been derived from the murine model. Although the New Zealand Black (NZB) strain of mice regularly develop autoimmune hemolytic anemia and hepatosplenomegaly as part of their lupus complex, nephritis is rare. In contrast, severe lupus nephritis develops uniformly in the progeny of crosses between NZB and New Zealand White (NZW) mice (a strain in which overt lupus never occurs). The (NZB × NZW)F_1 hybrid almost uniformly manifests a severe, proliferative glomerulonephritis with serologic features including LE cells. ANAs, and antibodies to native and denatured DNA and RNA. In recent years, additional strains of murine lupus have been bred and studied.

Using the murine model, considerable experimental evidence has accumulated supporting the profound effect of nutritional status on basic immune status. Protein calorie malnutrition, zinc deficiency, low fat-low calorie diets and general caloric restriction all have been shown to affect immunologic responsiveness. Restriction of dietary protein has been associated with hypogammaglobulinemia, reduction in antibody-forming cells, increased allograft rejection, heightened delayed hypersensitivity and increased lymphokine production in both experimental animals and man [59–61].

Fasting has also been associated with notable changes in immune responsiveness in both experimental animals and in man [62]. Impaired T cell mediated responses and immunodeficiency states have been associated with zinc deficiency in certain animal experiments [63]. As well, reduction of dietary fat [64], phenylalanine or tyrosine [65] and essential fatty acids [66] have all been demonstrated to have beneficial effects on murine lupus. The underlying mechanisms for all these observations are not entirely clear at this time.

Several investigators have noted that $(NZB \times NZW)F_1$ hybrid mice treated with prostaglandin E^1 experienced prolonged survival [67, 68]. Similar observations were made with mice fed a diet rich in eicosapentenoic acid [69]. Such studies suggest that nutritional factors modifying the generation of arachidonic acid-derived prostaglandins and/or leukotrienes might inhibit inflammatory immune responses. Panush has suggested that if such dietary manipulations could be extrapolated to human autoimmune disease they would provide novel, non-toxic and inexpensive therapeutic alternatives to our current therapeutic armamentarium [70].

Several animal experiments have provided insight into the association between a dietary ingestant and an autoimmune disorder. When fed a diet high in fish protein, pigs occasionally develop polyarthritis and subcutaneous nodules which closely resemble RA. In this porcine model the gut flora reveals significantly raised levels of atypical *Clostridium perfringens* with the acute onset of disease [71]. Although some isolated observations of increased *C. perfringens* and its associated serum alpha toxin have been made in human RA, the significance of these findings is yet unclear [72]. Coombs and Oldham fed six old English rabbits 8 ozs. of cow's milk daily for 12 weeks. Three rabbits developed synovitis with an inflammatory joint exudate. Antibodies to milk were demonstrated in these three animals by passive hemagglutination [73].

In addition to the murine model of SLE, the canine model has provided insights into the possibility of microbial influences in SLE. Canine SLE usually manifests an antiglobulin-positive hemolytic anemia, thrombocytopenia, arthritis and glomerulonephritis. Antibodies to ssDNA, native dsRNA and positive LE cell preparations are common. However, antibodies to native dsDNA are very infrequent. Observations in the dog have supported vertical passage of an infectious agent in this model [74].

V. Canavanine-induced SLE in primates

This series of observations originated from a totally serendipitous sequence of experimental observations relating to reductions of plasma cholesterol levels and regression of atherosclerotic lesions by ingestion of alfalfa meal saponins in cholesterol-fed monkeys [75]. The impalatability of these materials for humans prompted further studies with more palatable alfalfa seeds. While ingestion of seeds reduced plasma cholesterol levels in humans [76], and prevented atherosclerosis in rabbits [77], the appearance of pancytopenia and antinuclear antibodies in one human volunteer after prolonged ingestion of alfalfa seeds prompted cessation of human observation [78]. This led to further investigation into the role of alfalfa in the induction of an autoimmune process.

Ten adult female cynomulgus macaques *(Macaca fascicularis)*, obtained in Indonesia and quarantined at the Oregon Regional Primate Center were randomly selected for study. All animals were fed semi-purified diet (SPD) containing casein, sucrose, butter, vitamins, salts and 0.34 mg of cholesterol/cal. Twenty-three percent of calories were provided by protein, 34% by carbohydrate and 43% by fat. After 1 month on this diet, baseline studies were carried out and the animals randomly assigned to two groups of five animals each. One group was maintained on SPD for 9 months and served as controls. The other group was fed SPD which had been modified by the addition of 45% ground alfalfa seed obtained from a commercial supplier (pesticide-free) [79]. The final fat, carbohydrate and protein concentrations of the study diets were identical. Venous blood was drawn from each animal at the beginning of the study, and subsequently at monthly intervals starting 6 months after seeds were added to the diet.

The five control animals maintained on SPD remained healthy during 9 months of observation after which they were released back into the general colony. There were no hematologic or serologic aberrations and their mean plasma cholesterol was 236 ± 16 mg/dl. Two monkeys fed alfalfa seed had hematologic and serologic find-

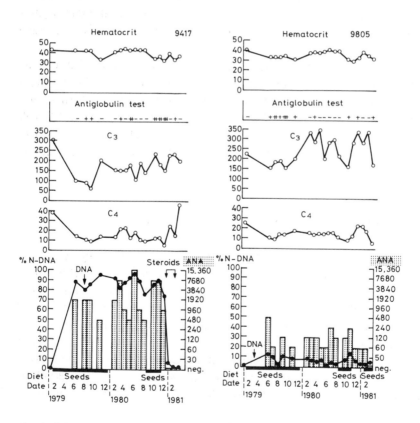

Fig. 1. Schematic representation of hematologic and serologic findings in monkeys (Nos. 9 417 and 9 805) over a 27-month period. (From Bardana et al., 1982 [79], with permission.)

ings which paralleled the control group and they were released from further study after 9 months of observation. The remaining three animals developed signs of a systemic illness characterized by an antiglobulin-positive hemolytic anemia, high titer ANAs (highest titer 1 : 15 360) with a rim pattern and elevated anti-dsDNA binding with variable degrees of serum hypocomplementemia. One animal developed a *Staphylococcus aureus* infection of the scalp and ultimately succumbed to a malarial infection. The two remaining animals survived for 20 months of observation and the hematologic and serologic data from these two animals are schematically summarized in Fig. 1. One animal (No. 9 417) developed florid signs of SLE which were temporally related to alfalfa seed ingestion. Hemolytic anemia, high titer ANA (rim pattern) and the presence of LE cells were associated with very high levels of circulating antibody to dsDNA. Depression of both C3 and C4 components of complement were also noted (Fig. 1). Clinically normal skin revealed granular deposition of IgG and complement at the dermal-epidermal junction when studied by electron

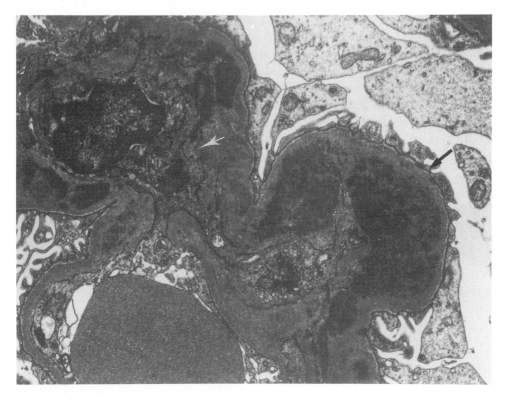

Fig. 2. Electron micrograph, initial kidney biopsy, monkey No. 9 417. Voluminous electron-dense deposits are present in the mesangium (black arrow). Small deposits were also found within some segments of the glomerular basement membrane (white arrow) (× 14 600). (From Bardana et al., 1982 [79], with permission.)

microscopy. Renal histopathology was consistent with an immune complex induced glomerulonephritis (Fig. 2). In addition, an inflammatory arteritis with resultant arterial thrombosis in the tail was felt to be a manifestation of SLE. Both the clinical and serologic manifestations of SLE were exacerbated by a second challenge to alfalfa seeds, and abated considerably with corticosteroid treatment (Fig. 1). At the height of the illness, the animal developed a nephrotic appearance with a subtle macular erythematous rash about the face which cleared promptly with steroid therapy. Patchy alopecia was also evident (Fig. 3).

The withdrawal of alfalfa seeds from the diet of these two animals was associated with a return to normal hematological parameters. Serum complement gradually became normal, but antinuclear ANAs and anti-dsDNA antibodies were noted to persist for 2 years when observations were discontinued [79].

Although the precise nature of the toxic substance causing the autoimmune process was not determined initially, we hypothesized that L-canavanine, the guanidinoxy structural analog of arginine, present in relatively large concentrations in alfalfa seeds, was the likely culprit. It constitutes about 1.5% of the dry weight of alfalfa seeds and alfalfa sprouts [80] and is toxic to many organisms [81], including mammals [82].

Because alfalfa sprouts are consumed on a regular basis by the people, we instituted a larger study of monkeys fed alfalfa sprouts [83]. Twelve adult female cynomulgus macaques were randomly assigned to two groups of six animals each and fed for 7 months SPD (Group 1), or similar food containing 40% (oven-dried) alfalfa sprouts (Group 2). Control animals as well as four of the monkeys ingesting alfalfa sprouts did not exhibit hematologic or serologic abnormalities during the period of observation, except for one monkey in Group 2 that developed an ANA titer of 1 : 240 (homogeneous pattern) but who was clinically well (Table 1) [83].

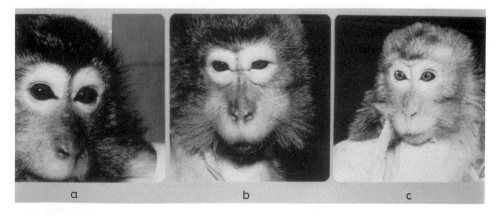

Fig. 3. Monkey No. 9 417 before receiving alfalfa seed (a) and at the height of illness with a nephrotic, puffy facies and rash (b) (not well illustrated in black and white). (c) Monkey No. 9 805 at height of illness with patchy alopecia evident.

TABLE 1

Hematologic and serologic observations in cynomolgus macaques maintained on a diet containing alfalfa sprouts

Group monkey number	Hb (g/dl)	RBC (× 10^6/mm³)	Hct (%)	Direct anti-globulin test	ANA titer (pattern)	dsDNA (% binding)	C3 (mg/dl)	C4 (mg/dl)
Group 1[a] (n = 6)	12.9 ± 0.7	6.53 ± 0.41	40.1 ± 2.3	–	–	0.9 ± 0.3	317 ± 34	28 ± 6
Group 2[b] (n = 4)	13.2 ± 1.3	6.50 ± 0.70	40.0 ± 4.3	–	–[c]	0.8 ± 0.1	280 ± 38	35 ± 5
Group 2[d] No. 10 661	10.8	5.78	32	+	–	0.6	247	30
Group 2[e] No. 10 670	7.5	3.32	23.3	+	1 : 240 (R)	21.9	92	7

Group 1, controlled diet.
Group 2, diet controlled with 40% dried alfalfa sprouts.
[a] Mean ± SD of monthly determinations for 6 months.
[b] Mean ± SD of monthly determinations for 10 months.
[c] One animal on five occasions had ANA titers between 1 : 30 (speckled pattern) and 1 : 240 (homogeneous pattern).
[d] Values after 10 months on diet.
[e] Values after 2 months on diet.

Hb, hemoglobin; RBC, red blood cells (erythrocytes); Hct, hematocrit; ANA, antinuclear antibodies; dsDNA, double-stranded DNA antibodies; C3, C3-complement component; C4, C4-complement component; –, negative; +, positive; R, rim pattern.
(Adapted from Malinow et al. [83], with permission.)

TABLE 2

Hematologic[a] and serologic[b] observations in cynomolgus macaques maintained on a diet containing 1.0% L-canavanine sulfate

Monkey number	Length of diet feeding (weeks)	Hb (g/dl)	RBC (× 10^6/mm^3)	Hct (%)	Direct anti-globulin test	ANA titer (pattern)	Anti-dsDNA (% binding)	C3 (mg/dl)	C4 (mg/dl)
9 880	4	10.8	5.23	32.3	(−) +	(−) −	(0) 2.4	(355) 190	(42) 20
9 704	9	7.9	3.25	23.8	(−) −	(−) 1 : 120 [H]	(0.1) 6.5	(340) 188	(48) 12
10 670	4	5.3	2.13	15.5	(−) +	(−) 1 : 240 [H]	(1.0) 9.2	(324) 72	(29) 7

[a] Lowest values observed. Initial values shown between parentheses.

[b] Most abnormal value observed. Initial values shown between parentheses.

Hb, hemoglobin; RBC, red blood cells (erythrocytes); Hct, hematocrit; ANA, antinuclear antibodies; dsDNA, double-stranded DNA antibodies; C3, C3-complement component; C4, C4-complement component; −, negative; +, positive; H, homogeneous pattern.

(Adapted from Malinow et al. [83], with permission.)

Significant abnormalities appeared in the remaining two animals from Group 2. One monkey (No. 10 661) developed a mild hemolytic anemia after 10 months. Another Group 2 monkey (No. 10 670) developed hematologic and serologic aberrations characteristic of SLE (Table 1) after 2 months including hemolytic anemia, ANAs up to a titer of 1 : 240 (rim pattern), elevated anti dsDNA (22% binding) and hypocomplementemia C3 and C4 [83].

Since an SLE-like syndrome was observed in a select number of monkeys fed alfalfa seeds or sprouts, three animals that had previously developed the syndrome, but who had recovered after being fed Purina Monkey Chow diet were fed 1% L-canavanine sulfate (Sigma) in SPD. The protein content in the diet was decreased to avoid dilution of the foreign amino acid. Blood was drawn weekly for analysis. All three animals became significantly ill (Table 2) [83]. Monkey No. 9 880 developed a mild hemolytic anemia and hypocomplementemia within 4 weeks of starting L-canavanine. Monkey No. 9 704 developed a profound anemia with antinuclear antibodies and hypocomplementemia. This monkey died after 10 weeks of canavanine ingestion. Necropsy showed extensive lobar pneumonia. Monkey No. 10 670 developed hemolytic anemia after 4 weeks on L-canavanine with associated leukocytosis, ANAs, elevated anti-dsDNA antibody, hypocomplementemia, splenomegaly and peripheral adenopathy.

These observations tended to confirm the suspicion that L-canavanine, found in relatively large concentrations in alfalfa seeds and sprouts, was involved in the pathogenesis of the SLE-like syndrome. However, a direct toxic effect of other components within alfalfa seed or sprouts could not be excluded. It was felt that the decrease in blood cholesterol might be an independent effect secondary to saponins present in alfalfa seeds. Although L-canavanine is metabolized to urea and guanidine in rats [84], the proportion remaining intact in monkeys was unknown. This was essential for a better understanding of how canavanine could be operating in the immunopathogenesis of this SLE syndrome. Because of structural analogies, L-canavanine may substitute for arginine in histones and thus affect the interaction with nucleic acids and the functions of the genome [85]. Moreover, arginyl-transfer RNA synthetase reacts with L-canavanine [86], which could then be incorporated into endogenous proteins [87]. The latter could affect synthesis of messenger RNA molecules and disrupt replication, giving rise to abnormal canavanyl proteins and resultant autoantibodies.

In order to clarify whether the L-canavanine in alfalfa seed and sprouts was responsible for the lupus-like syndrome, a group of monkeys were studied while being maintained on SPD or the same SPD containing 45% autoclaved alfalfa seeds. The latter was believed to destroy L-canavanine. The alfalfa seeds were washed 1 h with running water, strained, autoclaved for 3 h at 15 lbs. of pressure and 120°C and dried in an air convection oven at 70°C for 3 h. Some of the seeds were additionally roasted at 170°C for 10 min. Analysis for L-canavanine showed disappearance of the amino acid after 2 h of heating at 100°C (unpublished). After feeding groups of six or seven monkeys autoclaved unroasted or autoclaved roasted seeds for 7 – 12 months with appropriate control groups, no animal was observed to develop hemolytic anemia, or features of an SLE-like syndrome [88]. Plasma cholesterol was lowered significantly in animals fed autoclaved alfalfa seeds as opposed to controls. The data suggested that the factor responsible for inducing autoimmune disease, probably L-canavanine, was destroyed by autoclaving, but the anti-hypercholesterolemic activity was maintained.

Canavanine is one of some 200 non-protein amino acids that are synthesized by higher plants [89]. Using a colorimetric assay, surveys have disclosed that although the occurrence of canavanine is limited to the *Lotoideae* (*Papilionaceae* or *Fabaceae* or currently referred to as the pea tribe) (Table 3), a major subfamily of the Leguminosae, it is the principal free amino acid of numerous legumes some of which are important forage crops, e.g., clover, soybean, alfalfa, etc. [89]. Both Rosenthal [89] and Kuon and Bernhard [90] report canavanine as a constituent of the common onion (*Allium cepa*), a member of the lily family (Table 3) [91]. Since a significant portion of the toxic properties of L-canavanine is destroyed by heating, this may ex-

TABLE 3

Members of the biological families of pea (legume) and lily family

Lily family	Pea (legume) family
Aloe	Acacia
Asparagus	Alfalfa
Chives	Black-eyed pea
Garlic	Fava bean
Leek	Carob bean
Onion	Garbanzo
Sarsaparilla	Common bean
Shallot	kidney
	navy
	pinto
	green (string)
	Jack bean
	Lentil
	Licorice
	Lima bean
	Mesquite
	Pea
	Peanut
	Soybean
	Tamarind
	Tragacanth

(Adapted from Anderson and Sogn, 1984 [91], with permission.)

plain why more individuals are not adversely affected by its toxic properties. However, it is equally possible that adverse outcome may require genetic predisposition as well as significant doses not often encountered by man.

VI. Recent studies on the immunomodulatory role of L-canavanine as well as other dietary factors

1. L-CANAVANINE

In 1984, Prete and her associates presented experimental data which indicated that L-canavanine inhibited in vitro lymphoproliferative responses to mitogens, but not to antigens in normal individuals. Preliminary data in untreated SLE patients indicated that L-canavanine operated at lower concentrations suggesting a heightened sensitivity to this dietary amino acid in lupus modulation [92]. Further studies by this investigator reported the effects of L-canavanine on lymphocyte function in both normal and autoimmune mice [93]. At high doses, in vitro L-canavanine inhibited all DNA synthesis within 24 h. At lower doses, it selectively affected B cell function in the (NZB × NZW)F_1 hybrid. L-canavanine inhibited the incorporation of ^{3}H-thymidine in response to B cell mitogens, as well as pokeweed-induced intracytoplasmic immunoglobulin synthesis. Addition of L-canavanine to the diet resulted in a decrease in the life span of the NZB and the (NZB × NZW)F_1 hybrid mice, and abolished the protective effect of male sex on their survival [93]. The effect was principally on B cells and was felt to carry its effect out by competitively inhibiting the availability of L-arginine, an essential amino acid, to the cells.

In a subsequent series of studies, Prete subjected lymphocytes from normal DBA/2 mice and (NZB × NZW)F_1 hybrid mice to countercurrent distribution and observed that T cells partitioned to one of two major poles. No differences were observed between the two strains of mice. However, when murine lymphocytes were exposed to cationic L-canavanine in vitro, a selective effect was observed on the countercurrent distribution of B cells from (NZB × NZW)F_1 hybrid mice. This was felt to reflect an alteration of surface membrane. The impaired B cell response associated with L-canavanine was isolated to this altered lymphocyte fraction. No such effect was noted on the countercurrent distribution pattern or function of normal murine B cells [94]. It was hypothesized that L-canavanine bound to the cell membrane of predisposed murine B cells, and interfered with their capacity to accept and/or interpret T cell signals with resultant B cell dysfunction and autoantibody production [94]. This important but preliminary work will require further elucidation.

In 1985, Alcocer-Varela et al. [95] studied the effect of L-canavanine sulfate on the in vitro responses of human peripheral blood mononuclear cells. Contrary to the observations of Prete [93], these investigators observed that L-canavanine induced a diminution of mitogenic response to both phytohemagglutinin and concanavalin A, but not to pokeweed mitogen, as determined in both thymidine incorporation and cell cycle studies [95]. As well, L-canavanine abrogated concanavalin A induced suppressor cell function, resulting in increased release of both IgG and DNA-binding activity into supernatants by cells from normal subjects and SLE patients. The inhibitory effects of L-canavanine on the generation of concanavalin A induced suppression varied among individuals. The authors felt that this might explain why not all monkeys fed alfalfa seed did develop the disease [95].

These experimental data relating to L-canavanine-induced murine and primate lupus are both interesting and important, but lack clear-cut associations to human SLE. Our report of a single volunteer ingesting large doses of roasted alfalfa seed to lower plasma cholesterol was certainly an unusual anomaly of diet [78]. However, more than a few individuals, and particularly those with chronic disease, frequently consume a variety of dietary 'health' supplements. Among these products sold in health food stores are alfalfa tablets. In 1983, Roberts et al. reported two individuals with serologically quiescent SLE wo experienced a reactivation of their disease with the ingestion of relatively large doses of alfalfa tablets [96]. Analysis of the tablets revealed the presence of L-canavanine and the patients had no history of exposure to other agents known to induce or reactivate SLE.

2. HYDRAZINE

In 1983 an additional patient with a genetic predisposition to SLE was observed to develop a lupus-like disease secondary to an occupational exposure to hydrazine [97]. Hydrazine occurs naturally in tobacco and tobacco smoke and a number of aromatic hydrazines are present in mushrooms. It is extensively used in the synthesis of plastics, rubber products, herbicides, preservatives, textiles, dyes, and pharmaceuticals. These observations should serve to alert the clinician to explore dietary and environmental exposures carefully in the evaluation of all such patients.

3. RED MEAT AND DAIRY PRODUCTS

Recent studies by Panush and his associates have served to rekindle the interest in dietary-induced autoimmune disorders. These investigators have carried out several prospective, controlled and randomized studies addressing this problem. They have evaluated a prescription diet eliminating red meat, fruit, dairy products, herbs and spices, preservatives, and alcohol for 10 weeks in patients with rheumatoid arthritis. The latter appeared to have no demonstrable benefit when compared to a placebo diet [98]. However, two patients did improve significantly on the experimental diet, and experienced recurrences when deviating from it. Subsequent studies using controlled, double-blind encapsulated challenges showed that certain food antigens could exacerbate symptoms of inflammatory arthritis in selected patients [99 – 101].

Thus far, these investigations do not provide insight regarding the frequency of food sensitivity in patients with RA. Panush et al. estimate that the prevalence was less than 10% of patients based on preliminary studies. This group of investigators has also recently described a dietary-induced experimental inflammatory arthritis in rabbits [102].

4. POLYUNSATURATED FATTY ACIDS AND EICOSAPENTENOIC ACID

Recent epidemiological studies of Inuit people in Greenland have documented a low frequency of coronary vascular disease which has been partly attributed to lower levels of plasma cholesterol and triglycerides and partly to reduced coagulability and viscosity of blood [103]. These benefits appear to be the result of a diet high in marine mammals and fish, and low in dairy products. Marine oils are rich in long-chain polyunsaturated fatty acids, particularly the omega-3 series eicosapentenoic and docosahexenoic acid. The omega-3 marine fatty acids are also of therapeutic interest because of their role in inflammatory pathways, i.e. prostaglandin and leukotriene metabolism are dependent on unsaturated fatty acid precursors in the diet.

In 1985, Kremer et al. [104] reported a double-blind study showing that a diet high in polysaturated fatty acids and eicosapentenoic acid led to improvement in morning stiffness, number of tender joints and grip strength compared with controls who were maintained on an American diet high in saturated fat plus placebo eicosapentenoic acid. These clinical observations were not supported by improvement in laboratory parameters [104]. Additional studies from the same group have demonstrated reduction in leukotriene B_4 levels in patients treated with fish-oil supplement [105]. Statistically significant improvement was seen in fatigue time and number of tender joints during the treatment period compared with the control period, but not within laboratory measurements [105]. Though interesting, these observations must be considered preliminary and in need of further verification [106].

Studies in experimental animals are inconclusive. (NZB $\times$ NZW)F_1 hybrid mice fed a diet rich in eicosapentenoic acid experienced prolonged survival and attenuated glomerular dysfunction [67 – 69]. On the other hand, models of experimental arthritis in the rat have worsened when treated with eicosapentenoic acid [107].

VII. Summary

It is clear that there has been a long-standing interest in the area of dietary-induced autoimmune disease. Early observations suggested a relationship between a variety of food antigens and autoimmune rheumatic disorders. Milk and related dairy products appear to hold a special prominence among the ingestants implicated in these processes. Over the past decade there is mounting evidence that other dietary factors may play an immunopathogenic role. A series of experimental observations demonstrated that a non-protein amino acid, L-canavanine, the guanidinoxy structural analog of L-arginine, which is present in certain Leguminosae, induced an SLE-like syndrome in non-human primates. Additionally, ingestion of alfalfa seeds containing large amounts of L-canavanine was associated with pancytopenia and ANA in one man. It has been shown that L-canavanine can be incorporated into the nascent polypeptide chain of canavanine-free species disrupting critical reactions of RNA and DNA metabolism as well as protein synthesis. The plants in which L-canavanine is likely present are not consumed in large amounts by humans and are likely to be cooked before eaten. Another set of observations have demonstrated that omega-3 marine fatty acids have a significant effect on immune function as well as within inflammatory pathways. Together, all these observations support the hypothesis that dietary factors play an important role in immunomodulation, and may be participating to a greater or lesser degree in some commonly encountered autoimmune processes. Further controlled studies will be required to elucidate these issues in human disorders, and to develop appropriate dietary therapeutic approaches.

References

1. Osler, W. (1895) On the visceral complications of erythema exudativum multiforme. Am. J. Med. Sci. 110, 629 – 646.
2. Osler, W. (1914) The visceral lesions of purpura and allied conditions. Br. Med. J. 1, 517 – 525.
3. Cohen, S. S. (1914) On some angio-neural arthroses commonly mistaken for gout or rheumatism. Am. J. Med. Sci. 147, 228 – 243.
4. Alexander, D. L. and Eyermann, C. H. (1927) Food allergy in Henoch's purpura. Arch. Derm. Syph. (Chic.) 16, 322 – 327.
5. Alexander, D. L. and Eyermann, C. H. (1919) Allergic purpura. J. Am. Med. Assoc. 92, 2092 – 2094.
6. Lewin, P. and Taub, S. J. (1936) Allergic synovitis due to ingestion of English walnuts. J. Am. Med. Assoc. 106, 2144.
7. Berger, H. (1939) Intermittent hydroarthrosis with an allergic basis. J. Am. Med. Assoc. 112, 2402 – 2405.
8. Hench, P. S. and Rosenberg, E. F. (1941) Palindromic rheumatism: A 'new' oft-recurring disease of joints apparently producing no articular residues. Proc. Mayo Clin. 16, 808 – 815.
9. Vaughn, W. T. (1943) Palindromic rheumatism among allergic persons. J. Allergy 14, 256 – 264.
10. Zeller, M. (1949) Rheumatoid arthritis – food allergy as a factor. Ann. Allergy 7, 200 – 239.
11. Zussman, B. M. (1966) Food hypersensitivity simulating rheumatoid arthritis. Southern Med. J. 59, 935 – 939.
12. Turnbull, J. A. (1944) Changes in sensitivity to allergenic foods in arthritis. Am. J. Dig. Dis. 15, 182 – 190.

13. Kaufman, W. (1953) Food-induced allergic musculoskeletal syndromes. Ann. Allergy 11, 197 – 184.
14. Millman, M. (1972) An allergic concept of the etiology of rheumatoid arthritis. Ann. Allergy 30, 135 – 141.
15. Rowe, A. H. and Rowe, A. Jr. (1972) Food Allergy: Its Manifestations and Control and the Elimination Diets. A compendium, C. C. Thomas, Inc., Springfield, IL, pp. 435 – 443.
16. Epstein, S. (1969) Hypersensitivity to sodium nitrate: a major causative factor in a case of palindromic rheumatism. Ann Allergy 27, 343 – 349.
17. Epstein, S. (1970) Sodium nitrate and palindromic rheumatism. Ann. Allergy 28, 187 – 188.
18. Williams, B. (1972) Palindromic rheumatism: a request. Med. J. Aust. 2, 390 – 391.
19. Marquardt, J. L., Spyderman, R. and Oppenheim, J. J. (1973) Depression of lymphocyte transformation and exacerbation of Behcet's syndrome by ingestion of English walnuts. Cell. Immunol. 9, 263 – 272.
20. Theorell, H., Blomback, M. and Kockum, C. (1976) Demonstration of reactivity to airborne food allergens in cutaneous vasculitis by variations in fibrinopeptide A and other blood coagulation, fibrinolysis and complement parameters. Thromb. Haemost. (Stuttgart) 36, 593 – 604.
21. Skoldstam, L., Larsson, L. and Lindström, F. D. (1979) Effects of fasting and lactovegetarian diet on rheumatoid arthritis. Scand. J. Rheumatol. 8, 249 – 255.
22. Stroud, R. M. (1983) The effect of fasting followed by specific food challenge on rheumatoid arthritis. In: B. H. Hahn, F. C. Arnett, T. M. Zizic and M. C. Hochbergd. (Eds.), Current Topics in Rheumatology, Upjohn, Kalamazoo, MI, pp. 145 – 157.
23. Carr, R. I., Wold, R. T. and Farr, R. S. (1972) Antibodies to bovine gamma-globulin (BGG) and the occurrence of a BGG-like substance in systemic lupus erythematosus sera. J. Allergy Clin. Immunol. 50, 18 – 30.
24. Parke, A. L. and Hughes, G. R. V. (1981) Rheumatoid arthritis and food: a case study. Br. Med. J. 282, 2027 – 2029.
25. Cochrane, C. G. and Koffler, D. (1973) Immune complex disease in experimental animals and man. Adv. Immunol. 16, 185 – 264.
26. Kaliner, M. A. (1987) The late-phase reaction and its clinical implications. Hosp. Pract. 22, 73 – 83.
27. Block, S. R., Gibbs, C. B., Stevens, M. B. and Shulman, L. E. (1968) Delayed hypersensitivity in systemic lupus erythematosus. Ann. Rheum. Dis. 27, 311 – 318.
28. Abe, T. and Homma, M. (1971) Immunological reactivity in patients with systemic lupus erythematosus. Humoral antibody and cellular immune responses. Acta Rheumatol. Scand. 17, 35 – 46.
29. Baum, J. and Ziff, M. (1969) Decreased 19S antibody response to bacterial antigens in systemic lupus erythematosus. J. Clin. Invest. 48, 758 – 767.
30. Panush, R. S., Franco, A. E. and Schur, P. H. (1971) Rheumatoid arthritis associated with eosinophilia. Ann. Intern. Med. 75, 199 – 205.
31. Winchester, R. J., Litwin, S. D., Koffler, D. and Kunkel, H. G. (1971) Observations on the eosinophilia of certain patients with rheumatoid arthritis. Arthritis Rheum. 14, 650 – 665.
32. Becker, L. C. (1973) Allergy in systemic lupus erythematosus. Johns Hopkins Med. J. 133, 38 – 44.
33. Goldman, J. A., Klimek, G. A. and Ali, R. (1976) Allergy in systemic lupus erythematosus: IgE levels and reaginic phenomenon. Arthritis Rheum. 19, 669 – 676.
34. Hunder, G. G. and Gleich, G. J. (1974) Immunoglobulin E (IgE) levels in serum and synovial fluid in rheumatoid arthritis. Arthritis Rheum. 17, 955 – 963.
35. Miyawaki, S. and Ritchie, R. F. (1974) Heterogenicity of antinucleolar antibody and IgE antinuclear antibody in patients with systemic rheumatic disease. J. Immunol. 113, 1346 – 1352.
36. Permin, H. and Wiik, A. (1978) The prevalence of IgE antinuclear antibodies in rheumatoid ar-

342

thritis and systemic lupus erythematosus. Acta Pathol. Microbiol. Scand. 86, 245 – 249.

37. Permin, H., Stahlskor, P., Norn, S. and Juhl, F.   (1978)   Basophil histamine release by RNA, DNA and aggregated IgG examined in rheumatoid arthritis and systemic lupus erythematosus. Allergy 33, 15 – 23.

38. Egido, J., Sanchez-Crespo, M., Lahoz, C., Garcia, R., Lopez-Trascasa, M. and Hernando, L. (1980)   Evidence of an immediate hypersensitivity mechanism in systemic lupus erythematosus. Ann. Rheum. Dis. 39, 312 – 317.

39. Pearson, D. J. and Rix, K. J. B.   (1985)   Allergomimetic reactions to food and pseudo-food-allergy. In P. Dukor, P. Kallos, H. D. Schlumberger, and G. B. West (Eds.), Pseudo-allergic Reactions, Involvement of Drugs and Chemicals, Karger, Basel, pp. 59 – 105.

40. Paganelli, R., Levinsky, R. J., Brostoff, J. and Wraith, D. G.   (1979)   Immune coplexes containing food proteins in normal and atopic subjects after oral challenge and effect of sodium cromoglycate on antigen absorption. Lancet 1, 1270 – 1272.

41. Elkon, K. B., Lanham, J. G., Dash, A. C. and Hughes, G. R. V.   (1981)   The effect of a protein meal on three fluid-assays for circulating immune complexes. Clin. Exp. Immunol. 45, 279 – 282.

42. Mestecky, J., Russell, M. W., Jackson, S. and Brown, T. A.   (1986)   The human IgA system: A reassessment. Clin. Immunol. Immunopath. 40, 105 – 114.

43. Oxelius, V., Laurell, A., Lindquist, B., Golebiowska, H., Axelsson, V., Bjorkander, J. and Hanson, L. A.   (1981)   IgG sub-classes in selective IgA deficiency: Importance of IgG_2-IgA deficiency. N. Engl. J. Med. 304, 1476 – 1477.

44. Wells, J. V., Michaeli, D. and Fudenberg, H. H.   (1975)   In: D. Bergsma (Ed.), Birth Defects: Original Article Series, Vol. XI, Sinauer, Sunderland, MA, pp. 144.

45. Barkley, D. O., Hohermuth, H. J., Howard, A., Webster, A. D. B. and Ansell, B. M.   (1979) IgA deficiency in juvenile chronic polyarthritis. J. Rheumatol. 6, 219 – 224.

46. Cameron, J. S., Turner, D. R., Ogg, C. S., Williams, D. G., Lessoff, M. H., Chantler, C. and Liebowitz, S.   (1979)   Systemic lupus with nephritis: a long-term study. Quart. J. Med. 48, 1 – 24.

47. Cunningham-Rundles, C., Brandeis, W. E., Pudifin, D. J., Day, N. K. and Good, R. A.   (1981) Autoimmunity in selective IgA deficiency: relationship to anti-bovine protein antibodies, circulating immune complexes and clinical disease. Clin. Exp. Immunol. 45, 299 – 304.

48. Walker, W. A. and Isselbacher, K. J.   (1974)   Uptake and transport of macromolecules by the intestine. Possible role in clinical disorders. Gastroenterology 67, 531 – 550.

49. Siurala, M., Julkunen, H., Toivenen, S., Pelkonen, R., Saxen, E. and Pitkanen, E.   (1965) Digestive tract in collagen diseases. Acta Med. Scand. 178, 13 – 25.

50. Olhagen, B.   (1975)   On the aetiopathogenesis of rheumatoid arthritis. Ann. Clin. Res. 7, 119 – 128.

51. Hoffman, B. I. and Katz, W. A.   (1980)   The gastrointestinal manifestations of systemic lupus erythematosus: a review of the literature. Semin. Arthritis Rheum. 9, 237 – 247.

52. Bitter, J., Calin, A. and Hughes, G. R. V.   (1979)   Reiter's syndrome. Ann. Rheum. Dis. 38, suppl., 1 – 150.

53. Haslock, I. and Wright, V.   (1973)   The musculoskeletal complications of Crohn's disease. Medicine 52, 217 – 225.

54. Wright, V. and Watkinson, G.   (1965)   The arthritis of ulcerative colitis. Br. Med. J. 2, 670 – 675.

55. Greenstein, A. J., Janowitz, H. D. and Sachar, D. B.   (1976)   The extra intestinal complications of Crohn's disease and of ulcerative colitis: a study of 700 patients. Medicine 55, 401 – 412.

56. Good, A. E.   (1981)   Enteropathic arthritis. In: W. N. Kelley, E. D. Harris, S. Ruddy, and C. B. Sledge (Eds.), Textbook of Rheumatology, W. B. Saunders, Philadelphia and London, pp. 1063 – 1075.

57. Walker, W. A.   (1976)   Host defense mechanisms in the gastrointestinal tract. Pediatrics 57, 901 – 906.

58. Shagrin, J. W., Frame, B. and Duncan, H. (1971) Polyarthritis in obese patients with intestinal bypass. Ann. Intern. Med. 75, 377 – 380.

59. Good, R. A. (1981) Nutrition and immunity. J. Clin. Immunol. 1, 3 – 11.

60. Good, R. A., West, A. and Fernandes, G. (1980) Nutritional modulation of immune response. Fed. Proc. 39, 3048 – 3104.

61. Weindruch, R. and Walford, R. L. (1982) Dietary restriction in mice beginning at 1 year of age: effect on life span and spontaneous cancer incidence. Science 215, 1415 – 1418.

62. Wing, E. J., Barczynski, L. K. and Boehmer, S. M. (1983) Effect of acute nutritional deterioration on immune function in mice. I. Macrophages. Immunology 48, 543 – 550.

63. Fernandes, G., Nair, M., Onoe, K., Tanaka, T., Floyd, R. and Good, R. A. (1979) Impairment of cell-mediated immunity in dietary zinc deficiency in mice. Proc. Natl. Acad. Sci. USA 76, 457 – 461.

64. Fernandes, G., Yunis, E. J., Smith, S. and Good, R. A. (1972) Dietary influences on breeding behavior, hemolytic anemia and longevity in NZB mice. Proc. Soc. Exp. Biol. Med. 139, 1189 – 1196.

65. Dubois, E. L. and Strain, L. (1973) Effect of diet on survival and nephropathy of NZB/NZW hybrid mice. Biochem. Med. 7, 336 – 340.

66. Hurd, E. R., Johnson, J. M., Okita, J. R., MacDonald, P. C., Ziff, M. and Gilliam, J. N. (1981) Prevention of glomerulonephritis and prolonged survival in New Zealand black/New Zealand white F_1 hybrid mice fed an essential fatty acid-deficiency diet. J. Clin. Invest. 67, 476 – 485.

67. Zurier, R. B., Sayadoff, D. M., Torrey, S. B. and Rothfield, N. F. (1977) Prostaglandin E^1 treatment of NZB/NZW mice. Arthritis Rheum. 20, 723 – 728.

68. Kelley, V. E. (1983) Fish oil diet decreases prostaglandin (PGE) production in autoimmune lupus in MRL-lpr mice. Fed. Proc., Abst., 42, 1211.

69. Prickett, J. D., Robinson, D. R. and Steinberg, A. D. (1983) Effects of dietary enrichment with eicosapentoenoic acid upon autoimmune nephritis in female NZB/NZW F_1 mice. Arthritis Rheum. 26, 133 – 139.

70. Panush, R. S. (1986) Delayed reactions to foods, food allergy and rheumatic disease. Ann. Allergy 56, 500 – 503.

71. Mansson, I., Norberg, R., Olhagen, B. and Bjorklund, N. E. (1971) Arthritis in pigs produced by dietary factors. Clin. Exp. Immunol. 9, 677 – 693.

72. Olhagen, B. and Mansson, I. (1968) Intestinal *Clostridium perfringens* in rheumatoid arthritis and other collagen disases. Acta Med. Scand. 184, 395 – 402.

73. Coombs, R. R. A. and Oldham, G. (1981) Early rheumatoid-like joint lesions in rabbits drinking cow's milk. Int. Arch. Allergy Appl. Immunol. 64, 287 – 292.

74. Lewis, R. M., Andre-Schwartz, J. and Harris, G. S. (1983) Canine systemic lupus erythematosus: transmission of serologic abnormalities by cell-free filtrates. J. Clin. Invest. 52, 1893 – 1899.

75. Malinow, M. R., McLaughlin, P., Naito, H. K., Lewis, L. A. and McNulty, W. P. (1978) Effect of alfalfa meal on shrinkage of atherosclerotic plaques during cholesterol findings in monkeys. Atherosclerosis 30, 27 – 35.

76. Malinow, M. R., McLaughlin, P. and Stafford, C. (1980) Alfalfa seeds: effects on cholesterol metabolism. Experientia 36, 562 – 563.

77. Malinow, M. R., McLaughlin, P., Stafford, C., Livingston, A. L. and Kohler, G. O. (1980) Alfalfa saponins and seeds: dietary effects in cholesterol-fed rabbits. Atherosclerosis 37, 433 – 438.

78. Malinow, M. R., Bardana, E. J. and Goodnight, S. H. (1981) Pancytopenia during ingestion of alfalfa seeds. Lancet 1, 615 – 617.

79. Bardana, E. J., Malinow, M. R., Houghton, D. C., McNulty, W. P., Wuepper, K. D., Parker, F. and Pirofsky, B. (1982) Diet-induced systemic lupus erythematosus (SLE) in primates. Am.

J. Kidney Dis. 1, 345 – 352.

80. Bell, E. A. (1960) Canavanine in the leguminosae. Biochem. J. 75, 618 – 620.

81. Rosenthal, G. A. (1981) A mechanism of L-canaline toxicity. Eur. J. Biochem. 114, 301 – 304.

82. Tschiersch, B. (1962) Zur toxischen Wirkung der Jackbohne. Pharmazie 17, 621 – 623.

83. Malinow, M. R., Bardana, E. J., Pirofsky, B. and Craig, S. (1982) Systemic lupus erythematosus-like syndrome in monkeys fed alfalfa sprouts: role of a non-protein amino acid. Science 216, 415 – 417.

84. Reiter, A. J. and Horner, W. H. (1979) Studies on the metabolism of guanidine compounds in mammals. Formation of guanidine and hydroxy-guanidine in the rat. Arch. Biochem. Biophys. 197, 126 – 131.

85. Ackerman, W. N., Cox, D. C. and Dinka, S. (1965) Control of histone and DNA synthesis with canavanine, paronycin and poliovirus. Biochem. Biophys. Res. Commun. 19, 745 – 750.

86. Allende, C. C. and Allende, J. E. (1964) Purification and substrate specificity of arginyl-ribonucleic acid synthetase from rat liver. J. Biol. Chem. 239, 1102 – 1106.

87. Kruse, P. F., White, P. B., Carter, H. A. and McCoy, T. A. (1959) Incorporation of canavanine into protein of Walker carcinosarcoma 256 cells cultured in vitro. Cancer Res. 19, 122 – 128.

88. Malinow, M. R., McLaughlin, P., Bardana, E. J. and Craig, S. (1984) Elimination of toxicity from diets containing alfalfa seeds. Food Chem. Toxicol. 22, 583 – 587.

89. Rosenthal, G. A. (1977) The biological effects and mode of action of L-canavanine, a structural analogue of L-arginine. Quart. Rev. Biol. 52, 155 – 178.

90. Kuon, J. and Bernhard, R. A. (1963) An examination of the free amino acids of the common onion (Allium cepa). J. Food Sci. 28, 298 – 304.

91. Anderson, J. A. and Sogn, D. D. (1984) Adverse reactions to foods. U.S. Dept. of Health Hum. Serv., NIH Publ. No. 84 – 2442, July, 1984, pp. 1 – 220.

92. Boniske, C. and Prete, P. (1984) L-canavanine, dietary immune modulator. Fed. Proc. 43, 781, Abst.

93. Prete, P. E. (1985) Effects of L-canavanine on immune function in normal and autoimmune mice: disordered B cell function by a dietary amino acid in the immunoregulation of autoimmune disease. Can. J. Physiol. Pharmacol. 63, 843 – 854.

94. Prete, P. E. (1986) Membrane surface properties of lymphocytes of normal DBA/2 and autoimmune NZB/NZW F_1 hybrid mice: effects of L-canavanine and a proposed mechanism for diet-induced autoimmune disease. Can. J. Physiol. Pharmacol. 64, 1189 – 1196.

95. Alcocer-Varela, J., Iglesias, A., Llorente, L. and Alarcon-Segovia, D. (1985) Effects of L-canavanine on T cells may explain the induction of systemic lupus erythematosus by alfalfa. Arthritis Rheum. 28, 52 – 57.

96. Roberts, J. L. and Hayashi, J. A. (1983) Exacerbation of SLE associated with alfalfa ingestion. N. Engl. J. Med. 380, 1361.

97. Reidenberg, M. M., Durant, P. J., Harris, R. A., deBoccardo, G., Lahita, R. and Stenzel., K. H. (1983) Lupus erythematosus-like disease due to hydrazine. Am. J. Med. 75, 365 – 369.

98. Panush, R. S., Carter, R. L., Katz, P., Kowsari, B., Longley, S. and Finnie, S. (1983) Diet therapy for rheumatoid arthritis. Arthritis Rheum. 26, 462 – 471.

99. Panush, R. S. (1986) Food-induced ('allergic') arthritis. 1. Inflammatory arthritis exacerbated by milk. Arthritis Rheum. 29, 220 – 226.

100. Panush, R. S., Corman, L., Longley, S., Webster, E., Endo, L., Brown, D., Delafuente, J., Searle, M., Hammack, S. and Nauman, J. (1986) Food-induced arthritis, clinical and serologic studies. Arthritis Rheum. 29, Suppl. 90, Abstr. No. D46.

101. Panush, R. S., Corman, L. and Webster, E. M. (1986) Food-induced ('allergic') arthritis. Clinical and serologic studies. Arthritis Rheum. 29, Suppl. 90, 33.

102. Panush, R. S., Webster, E., Endo, L., Searle, M., Hammack, S. and Woodard, J. C. (1986)

Food-induced (allergic) arthritis. A unique new model of inflammatory synovitis in rabbits. Arthritis Rheum. 29, Suppl. 90, Abstr. No. 347.

103. Bang, H. O., Dyerberg, J. and Nielsen, A. B. (1971) Plasma lipid and lipoprotein pattern in Greenlandic West-coast Eskimos. Lancet 1, 1143 – 1146.

104. Kremer, J. M., Bigauoette, J., Michalek, A. V., Timchalk, M.A., Lininger, L., Rynes, R. I., Huyck, C. and Zieminskij, T. (1985) Effects of manipulation of dietary fatty acids on clinical manifestations of rheumatoid arthritis. Lancet I, 1984 – 1987.

105. Kremer, J. M., Jubiz, W., Michalek, A. V., Rynes, R. I., Bartholomew, L. E. Bigaouette, J., Timchalk,, M., Beeler, D. and Lininger, L. (1987) Fish-oil fatty acid supplementation in active rheumatoid arthritis. Ann. Intern. Med. 106, 497 – 502.

106. Anonymous (1987) Fish oils in rheumatoid arthritis. Lancet 2, 720 – 721.

107. Prickett, J. D., Trentham, D. E. and Robinson, D. R. (1984) Dietary fish-oil augments the induction of arthritis in rats immunized with type II collagen. J. Immunol. 132, 725 – 729.

M.E. Kammüller, N. Bloksma and W. Seinen (Eds.)
Autoimmunity and Toxicology
© 1989 Elsevier Science Publishers B.V. (Biomedical Division)

Autoimmune reactions induced by metals

14

PHILIPPE DRUET, LUCETTE PELLETIER, JÉRÔME ROSSERT, ELVIRA DRUET, FRANÇOIS HIRSCH and CATHERINE SAPIN

INSERM U 28, Hôpital Broussais, 96, rue Didot, 75674 Paris Cedex 14, France

I. Introduction

Several metals are known to induce immunologically mediated manifestations, whether autoimmune or not, in humans. Gold is one of the most widely used compounds in the treatment of rheumatoid arthritis. In genetically predisposed patients gold salts may induce skin rash, fever, cytopenia or proteinuria. Mercury was also used in the past as a drug and is still present as an active compound or as a preservative in several ointments or skin-lightening creams. This metal is responsible for hypersensitivity reactions and proteinuria. Such manifestations have also been reported in industrial or laboratory workers exposed to mercury. Other metals such as platinum or beryllium are responsible for immune-mediated pulmonary manifestations. Finally, it is also possible, although unproven, that various pollutants including metals, could play a role in the appearance of so-called primary autoimmune manifestations. Experimental models are therefore of interest because they allow: (a) to confirm the ability of a compound to induce adverse immunologic manifestations, (b) to evaluate the basic role of genetic factors since several species or strains may be tested, and (c) to elucidate the mechanisms responsible for immunotoxic manifestations.

Mechanisms are indeed still badly understood in the human situation. It is usually considered [1] that a toxic agent may induce adverse immunologic effects, because: (a) it binds to self-constituents and triggers an anti-hapten immune response, (b) hapten-modified autoantigens may lead to a true autoimmune response restricted to the autoantigens, or (c) it disregulates the immune system, resulting in the appearance of more generalized autoimmune manifestations.

In this review we will first describe findings reported in the mercury model which has been the more thoroughly studied. Experiments using gold salts and other metals will be then reported.

II. Mercury-induced autoimmunity

1. MERCURY-INDUCED AUTOIMMUNITY IN BROWN-NORWAY RATS

(a) Description of the disease

Mercuric chloride when injected subcutaneously thrice weekly at a dose of 0.1 mg/per 100 g body weight induces highly reproducible autoimmune disorders in Brown-Norway (BN) rats (Table 1) with a biphasic autoimmune glomerulonephritis [2 – 4]. One week after the first injection of $HgCl_2$, circulating autoantibodies to glomerular basement membrane (GBM) are detectable using various assays [4, 5] and found deposited along the GBM by direct immunofluorescence (Fig. 1a) at the end of the second week [3]. The antibody titer reaches a peak during the 2nd and 3rd week and then spontaneously decreases although $HgCl_2$ injections are con-

TABEL 1

$HgCl_2$-induced autoimmunity in Brown-Norway rats

---

1. Lymphoproliferation (number of T helper and B cells increased in the spleen and lymph nodes)

2. Hyperimmunoglobulinemia (mainly IgE)

3. Autoantibody production (anti-single-stranded DNA, anti-glomerular basement membrane, natural antibodies, etc.)

4. Production of antibodies to exogenous antigens (TNP, sheep red blood cells)

5. T-dependent autoimmune glomerulonephritis (anti-glomerular basement membrane and immune complex mediated)

6. Mechanisms of induction:
    induction of autoreactive T cells, including anti-Ia (MHC Class II) T cells;
    T-dependent polyclonal activation of T cells;
    transfer of autoimmunity with autoreactive T cells

7. Spontaneous autoregulation:
    role for T suppressor cells and for auto-anti-idiotypic antibodies

8. Susceptibility is genetically controlled

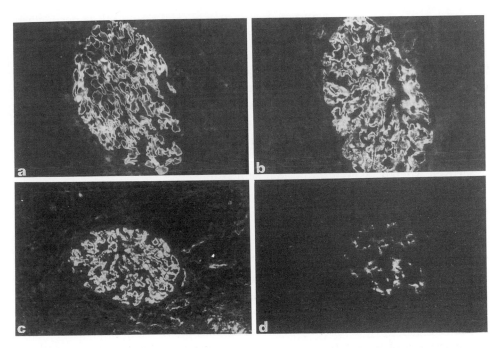

Fig. 1. Kidney cryostat sections stained with a fluoresceinated anti-rat IgG antiserum. (a) Brown-Norway rat 2 weeks after the first injection of HgCl₂. Note the linear pattern of fixation of the conjugate. Capillary lumina are expanded due to the presence of fibrin plugs. (b) Brown-Norway rat at time of sacrifice. The pattern of fixation is more granular. (c) Typical membranous glomerulopathy in a Wistar-Furth rat and, (d) mesangial granular deposits in a BD IX rat at time of sacrifice.

tinued. Anti-GBM antibodies have been found to recognize laminin, procollagen IV [4], proteoglycan and entactin [6]. Kidney-bound antibodies have the same specificities [6]. Concomitantly, urinary protein excretion increases, often associated with the nephrotic syndrome, without renal failure [3]. At that time a moderate glomerular monocytic influx is observed without crescentic nephritis [7]. Later on, sometimes from the 3rd week and continually at the end of the 2nd month, an immune complex type nephritis (Fig. 1b) is superadded to the anti-GBM nephritis [3]. Granular IgG deposits are seen along the glomerular capillary wall as subepithelial electron-dense deposits but also in the mesangial areas and in the vessel walls (Fig. 1b). Circulating immune complexes are detected using various assays, but their participation in glomerular immunoglobulin deposition as well as their composition is unknown [4]. Rats may die during the anti-GBM phase of the disease, probably as a consequence of intravascular coagulation [8].

Other interesting autoimmune manifestations are noted along with the autoimmune glomerulonephritis. Rats exhibit a striking enlargement of spleen and lymph nodes, and this lymphoproliferation has been shown to be mainly due to proliferation of B cells and T helper cells [9]. Total serum immunoglobulin level is increased

[10]; all isotypes are affected [9] but the increase in total serum IgE is particularly prominent [11]. Finally other autoantibodies with specificity for DNA [12], collagen type II, and thyroglobulin (M.C. Lockwood, personal communication) are produced. Furthermore, these rats develop mucositis and a Sjögren-like syndrome [13]. Most of these autoimmune symptoms are transient.

The autoimmune glomerulonephritis is also observed when $HgCl_2$ is given intravenously, orally or intratracheally [14]. Similar kidney lesions were seen using methyl-mercury or various pharmaceutical ointments and solutions containing organic mercury. It should be noted that the latter products were very effective when applied on wounds or even on normal skin [15].

(b) Genetic control of susceptibility

Interestingly, other strains of rats such as Lewis (LEW) rats do not develop autoimmune disorders even when high doses of $HgCl_2$ (0.4 mg instead of 0.1) are used. The resistance of LEW rats is not due to the absence of GBM antigen in that strain since antibodies eluted from kidneys obtained from $HgCl_2$-injected BN rats bind in vitro to normal LEW kidneys [16]. Moreover, anti-GBM antibodies produced by the susceptible (LEW × BN)F_1 hybrids are found deposited on a LEW kidney previously transplanted into these rats [17]. Furthermore, LEW rats irradiated and reconstituted with bone-marrow cells from the susceptible (LEW × BN)F_1 hybrids develop some degree of autoimmunity when injected with $HgCl_2$ [18]. These findings already suggest that $HgCl_2$ acts on lymphocytes and has different effects depending upon the strain tested. This prompted us to study the susceptibility of segregants obtained between BN and LEW rats [16, 19, 20]. Their RT1 haplotype at the major histocompatibility complex (MHC), which is the rat equivalent of the human HLA complex, has also been determined. BN rats bear the $RT1^n$ haplotype and LEW rats the $RT1^l$. It could thus be demonstrated that susceptibility to the autoimmune glomerulonephritis was inherited as an autosomal and dominant trait and that about three genes were involved in the genetic control of susceptibility to anti-GBM antibody-mediated nephritis [16]. One of these genes has been found to be RT1-linked. More recent results have shown that the RT1-linked gene was localized in the RT1-B region (equivalent of the DR region in humans) which encodes for class II molecules [20]. The RT1-linked gene(s) seem to be even more important in controlling susceptibility to the immune complex type nephritis [19]. It is of interest in that respect, that susceptibility to gold-induced membranous nephropathy is increased in DR3-positive patients [21] and that the incidence of HLA-DR2 is very high (relative risk = 36) in patients with anti-GBM antibody-mediated nephritis [22]. Susceptibility to polyclonal serum IgE increase in the mercury model is also genetically determined and depends upon four genes, one of which is again RT1-linked [23].

(c) Mechanisms of induction of autoimmunity

Since HgCl$_2$-injected BN rats exhibit multiple autoimmune abnormalities, this suggested that the toxic agent could act, at least in part, by disregulating the immune system. This hypothesis was strengthened when it was found that the number of spontaneous anti-sheep red blood cells and anti-TNP plaque-forming cells obtained from the spleen of diseased rats was significantly increased [12]. It was furthermore observed that BN rat spleen cells, when exposed in vitro to non-toxic amounts of HgCl$_2$ generated an increased number of such plaque-forming cells, when compared to control spleen cells. T cells were required for this phenomenon to occur [12]. All these findings strongly supported that HgCl$_2$ initiated a T-dependent polyclonal activation of B cells. Fusion experiments in this model allowed to obtain numerous monoclonal auto-antibodies (anti-GBM, anti-DNA, anti-mitochondria, etc.) and natural antibodies which also confirmed that several clones were affected [24, 25].

More recently, co-culture experiments were performed leading to the conclusion that lymphocytes from BN rats injected with HgCl$_2$ were able to stimulate normal syngeneic lymphocytes [26, 27]. The subsets involved were further analysed and the conclusion of these studies was that HgCl$_2$ was responsible for an abnormal T helper cell cooperation requiring the presence of normal Ia (MHC class II)-positive cells. The most likely explanation is that mercury induces autoreactive T helper cells, probably anti-Ia, which then stimulate Ia-bearing B cells [27]. Using limiting dilution analysis, it has been possible to demonstrate that at least two different autoreactive T helper cells were induced (or expanded) by HgCl$_2$. The first one, observed from day 4 is stimulated by T helper cells exposed to HgCl$_2$; the second one, found from day 6, recognized Ia-positive cells, presumably B cells [27b]. The exact specificity of these autoreactive T cells will only be known when T cell lines or clones will be available. The precise mechanism of induction of such autoreactive T cells remains also to be determined.

The relevance of the just described in vitro phenomenon to the pathogenesis of mercury-induced autoimmune disease was shown by the following in vivo experiments. (a) Injection of irradiated T cells from HgCl$_2$-injected BN rats into the footpad of normal syngeneic recipients caused popliteal lymph node enlargement. Indeed the number of cells in the draining popliteal lymph nodes was increased and proliferating cells were mainly helper T cells (presumably autoreactive) and B cells [26, 27]. (b) In a second set of experiments, T cell deprived BN rats were used. They were obtained in two ways: firstly, the nude mutation was transferred on BN rats (BN *rnu/rnu*) and, secondly, BN'B' rats (BN rats thymectomized, irradiated and reconstituted with foetal liver cells) were constructed. These rats did not develop the mercury-induced autoimmune disease when injected with HgCl$_2$, while anti-GBM antibodies and the autoimmune glomerulonephritis were again observed when these rats were replenished with T cells and exposed to HgCl$_2$ [28]. This demonstrates that T cells are required. (c) Transfer experiments have recently been performed which show clearly the role of autoreactive T cells in the appearance of autoimmunity in this model [29]. T cells from BN rats injected with $HgCl_2$ (T Hg) were transferred into normal BN rats that did not receive $HgCl_2$. Such a transfer resulted in a weak anti-GBM antibody response in the recipient. Interestingly, a 10-fold increase in the number of $OX8^+$ (suppressor/cytotoxic) T cells was observed in the recipient, while the number of $OX8^+$ T cells did not increase significantly in $HgCl_2$-injected BN rats [9]. This suggested that $OX8^+$ cells proliferated in response to transfer of T Hg cells. For that reason T Hg cells were then transferred into normal BN rats previously treated with the OX8 monoclonal antibody. These rats developed a full-blown disease with anti-GBM antibodies, typical glomerular linear IgG deposits, heavy proteinuria and a marked increase in total serum IgE level. Transfer of B cells from $HgCl_2$-injected rats into normal BN rats, either OX8-treated or not, had no effect. These experiments show that autoreactive T cells play a crucial role in this model; they also suggest that $HgCl_2$ could interfere with T suppressor cells in $HgCl_2$-injected rats.

The reason why BN rats do develop preferentially anti-GBM antibodies is of theoretical interest when considering the susceptibility of HLA-DR2-positive patients [22]. It is quite striking that BN rats are prone to the development of such antibodies under several circumstances, for example following immunization with heterologous [30] or homologous [31] GBM. (LEW × BN)F_1 hybrids also produce anti-GBM antibodies during chronic graft-versus-host (GVH) disease, probably due to stimulation of F_1 B cells by parental T cells [32]. Similarities between the mercury model and the GVH model are impressive. An excess of T help is probably furnished in both situations: parental T cells stimulate allogeneic Ia-bearing B cells during GVH [33] and autoreactive T cells stimulate self Ia-bearing cells in the mercury model [26 – 29]. Another explanation would be that $HgCl_2$ 'modifies' Ia determinants then recognized as allogeneic Ia determinants, but our data do not support this thesis.

(d) Autoregulation of mercury-induced autoimmunity

As described above, most of the autoimmune abnormalities observed in $HgCl_2$-injected BN rats as a consequence of polyclonal activation, progressively disappear spontaneously. The mechanisms responsible for this autoregulation have been studied by Lockwood et al. [34, 35]. They have shown that the anti-GBM antibody response was partially inhibited by transferring spleen cells from convalescent BN rats into naive BN rats before injection of $HgCl_2$. This inhibition was no longer observed when suppressor T cells ($OX8^+$) had been previously removed from the cells transferred [34]. These data fit very well with the observation that injections of small amounts of $HgCl_2$ in BN rats prevent the typical disease when high doses of $HgCl_2$ are subsequently administered. They are also in agreement with the fact that the number of suppressor T cells increases slightly in the spleen and in the lymph nodes after day 15, while, concomitantly, the number of T helper cells and B cells decreases [9]. The mechanisms for this spontaneous autoregulation are still obscure as well as is the specificity of suppressor T cells. There is, however, some evidence that anti-idiotypic antibodies are involved. Chalopin et al. [35] have indeed developed in that model a plaque-forming cell assay using sheep red blood cells coated with GBM. The peak of the anti-GBM response using this assay occurred at day 9. The authors observed that the serum of some convalescent $HgCl_2$-injected BN rats was able to inhibit the GBM-specific plaque-forming capability of cells collected at day 9. Although this phenomenom could be related to the presence of free circulating antigen or to immune complexes containing GBM antigens, the authors' demonstration support a role for auto-anti-idiotypic antibodies. However, such antibodies, either in a free or complexed form have not been yet demonstrated to the best of our knowledge.

In conclusion, mercury appears to first induce autoreactive T cells leading to autoantibody production. This polyclonal activation is then abrogated due to the emergence of suppressor T cells and/or of auto-anti-idiotypic antibodies.

2. EFFECTS OF $HgCl_2$ IN LEWIS RATS

As mentioned above, LEW rats do not develop autoimmunity even when injected with high $HgCl_2$ doses. The resistance of LEW rats could be due to the development of suppressor T cells.

Recent experiments have indeed shown that $HgCl_2$ prefentially induces non-specific, active, suppressor T cells in that strain (Table 2). The number of OX8$^+$ (suppressor/cytotoxic) T cells increases in the spleen and in the lymph nodes from day 7, reaching a peak around day 15 [36]. All the T cell functions tested [36] were

TABLE 2

$HgCl_2$-induced immunosuppression in Lewis rats

1. Increase in the number of OX8$^+$ (suppressor/cytotoxic) T cells in the spleen and lymph nodes

2. Depression of T cell functions (mitogen responsiveness, mixed lymphocyte reaction, local graft-versus-host reaction)

3. Absence of autoimmune disorder

4. Suppression of antibody-mediated (Heymann's nephritis) and cell-mediated (experimental autoimmune encephalomyelitis) autoimmunity

5. Mechanisms:
   induction of active non-specific suppressor T cells;
   role for autoreactive T cells (?)

inhibited or depressed (responsiveness to phytohemagglutinin and Concanavalin A, and to alloantigens as well as local GVH reaction). This immunosuppressive effect of HgCl$_2$ is due to activated OX8$^+$ T cells, since lymph node cells and OX8$^+$ cells from HgCl$_2$-injected LEW rats are able to inhibit the proliferative response of normal LEW rats lymph node cells to alloantigens [36]. Our findings suggested that, in contrast to observations in BN rats, HgCl$_2$ suppressed the onset of autoimmune responses in LEW rats. Interestingly, LEW rats are highly susceptible to several autoimmune diseases such as Heymann's nephritis, an antibody-mediated disease, or experimental allergic encephalomyelitis (EAE), a T cell mediated process. It was observed that LEW rats previously injected with HgCl$_2$ had a depressed antibody response to the gp330 antigen responsible for Heymann's nephritis when compared to normal LEW rats [37]. Consequently, glomerular immune deposits were absent or weak in those rats receiving HgCl$_2$ and they did not develop proteinuria [37]. Similarly, clinical EAE in HgCl$_2$-injected rats was significantly attenuated when compared to normal rats. The responsiveness of T cells to basic protein (BP) was inhibited [38]. This depression of T cell responsiveness was not due to a defect at the level of T helper cells or antigen-presenting cells, because proliferation of isolated (W3/25$^+$) T cells from BP-immunized LEW rats was not influenced by treatment with HgCl$_2$ in vivo. Furthermore, OX8$^+$ T cells from HgCl$_2$-treated rats were able to inhibit the proliferative response of lymphocytes from LEW rats immunized with BP.

Taken together, these data demonstrate that HgCl$_2$ induces an active immunosuppression in LEW rats, and that the same agent which induces autoimmunity in BN rats is able to inhibit autoimmune diseases in LEW rats. Whatever the exact mechanism of action of HgCl$_2$, it is interesting to observe that several agents such as D-penicillamine, rifampicin or captopril which may induce autoimmune nephritis [39 – 41] are also able to induce immunosuppression [42 – 44]. Whether the differential responses are genetically controlled is not known.

3. AUTOIMMUNE GLOMERULONEPHRITIS IN OTHER STRAINS OF RATS

The response of several other strains [45] of rats receiving HgCl$_2$ as described for BN rats is listed in Table 3. All the strains with the RT1^l haplotype that were tested, were found to be resistant. Rats with the u haplotype had a somewhat different response. Although most of them were resistant, a percentage among Wistar-Furth rats developed a typical membranous nephropathy (Fig. 1c), a finding reminiscent of our early report in outbred Wistar rats. The specificity of the antibodies in these rats is still unknown. Findings in rats with the u haplotype suggest that, at variance with results obtained in BN rats, the genetic control of susceptibility in Wistar-Furth rats does not depend so tightly upon MHC-linked genes.

Several other strains of rats with other RT1 haplotypes (a, b, c, d, f, k, s) have also been tested [45, 46]. None of them developed anti-GBM antibodies but they all

TABLE 3

HgCl$_2$-induced autoimmunity in various strains of rats

Strain	RT1 haplotype	Autoimmune nephritis	ANA
BN	n	anti-GBM nephritis and ICGN	+
LEW	l	absent	−
(BN × LEW)F$_1$	n/l	anti-GBM nephritis and ICGN	NT
AS, BS, F$_{344}$	l	absent	−
LOU, WAG	u	absent	−
Wistar Furth	u	membranous glomerulonephritis	−
PVG/c	c	ICGN	+
AUG	c	ICGN	−
DA	a	ICGN	+
AVN	a	ICGN	−
BD V	d	ICGN	+
BD IX	d	ICGN	NT
BUF	b	ICGN	+
OKA	k	ICGN	−
AS2	f	ICGN	−
LEW.1N	n	ICGN	NT
ACI.1N	n	ICGN	NT
BN.1L	l	absent	NT
(LEW.1N × BN.1L)F$_1$	l/n	anti-GBM nephritis and ICGN	NT
AUG.1N	n	anti-GBM nephritis and ICGN	NT

ANA, anti-nuclear antibodies; GBM, glomerular basement membrane; ICGN, immune complex type nephritis, refers to the presence of granular IgG deposits along the capillary loop but also in mesangial areas and in vessel walls. NT, not tested.

exhibited an immune complex type nephritis with granular IgG deposits along the GBM, in mesangial areas, and in the wall of vessels (Fig. 1d). Several of them had circulating anti-single-stranded DNA antibodies which, in PVG/c rats, could be eluted from the kidney suggesting that they were involved in immune complex formation [45]. However, the exact composition of granular deposits is not known nor the mechanism of formation of these deposits. The mechanisms of action of HgCl$_2$ has been studied by Weening et al. [47], who found that, in PVG/c rats, the T suppressor function was inhibited. Several congenic and recombinant rats have been recently tested allowing to define more precisely the respective roles of MHC-linked genes and that of background genes [20]. Several facts emerge from these studies.

(a) Anti-GBM antibodies have only been found until now in rats with the n haplotype. They are, for example, absent in BN-1L (RT1^l) congenic rats. But, genes present in the background of BN rats are also important since congenic LEW.1N or ACI.1N (RT1^n) rats did not develop anti-GBM antibodies. However, genes which are important for the anti-GBM antibody response to occur are also present in other strains because AUG.1N (RT1^n) rats do develop linear IgG deposits while AUG rats do not.

(b) We also used recombinant rats with the n allele at the RT1-B subregion, which is the equivalent of the I-A subregion in mice, encoding for Ia molecules. These rats (ACI-WRC) do develop only granular IgG deposits following HgCl$_2$ injections but, interestingly, linear IgG deposits and circulating anti-GBM antibodies were observed when these rats were crossed with BN.1L rats. Our experiments, therefore, show that the region encoding for class II molecules within the MHC is important in the control of anti-GBM antibody production.

4. MERCURY-INDUCED NEPHRITIS IN OTHER SPECIES

Mercury-induced nephritis has also been described in rabbits and mice (Table 4). Roman-Franco et al. [48] have described in rabbits a disease quite similar to that seen in BN rats. They develop linear glomerular IgG deposits that were characterized as anti-GBM antibodies. Granular IgG deposits were also observed in a situation quite similar to that seen in BN rats. These authors have performed autoradiographic studies in this model; mercury could not be detected in the GBM, suggesting that mercury was not a part of the deposited material.

We initially tested the susceptibility of seven different strains of mice, because it would have been more convenient for genetic analysis of susceptibility. Unfortunately none of the strains tested produced anti-GBM antibodies. Other groups [49, 50] have found that BALB/c mice developed mesangial IgG deposits when injected with HgCl$_2$. Robinson et al. [51, 52] found that several strains of mice also produce antinuclear antibodies. It has been shown that MHC-linked genes played a major role [51 – 53] and that H-2^s mice were the most susceptible. Three groups

TABLE 4

HgCl$_2$-induced autoimmunity in other species

Species	Strain	H-2 haplotype	Autoimmune nephritis	ANA
Rabbit			anti-GBM nephritis and ICGN	+
Mouse	C3H.NB	H-2^p	mesangial GN	NT
	BALB/c	H-2^d	mesangial GN membranous GN	–
	DBA/2	H-2^d	resistance	–
	A.SW	H-2^s	IC-mediated GN	+

ANA, anti-nuclear antibodies; GBM, glomerular basement membrane; ICGN immune complex glomerulonephritis; NT, not tested.

of mice: high responders, low responders and resistant were defined [52]. High responder mice also exhibited glomerular IgG deposits [53] and it has recently been shown that $HgCl_2$ induced in the susceptible A.SW strain (H-2^s) a strong activation of B cell with an increase in total serum IgG and IgE levels. By contrast DBA/2 mice (H-2^d) were resistant. Finally, Fleuren et al. [54] could obtain subepithelial deposits in BALB/c mice injected with $HgCl_2$. These mice produced anti-gp330 antibodies and developed proteinuria.

III. Other metals

Several other metals have been used to induce experimental immunologically mediated diseases. It must be stressed, however, that it is not clear whether the manifestations observed are truly autoimmune. In addition, the mechanisms at play have not been always elucidated. Nagi et al. [55] have shown that a membranous glomerulonephritis occurs as a consequence of gold thiomalate administration in Wistar rats. It was suggested that binding of gold to brush border antigens would induce an immune response towards this antigen which is also expressed on glomerular visceral epithelial cells. However, such a mechanism remains to be proven. More recently it has been observed that BN as well as PVG/c rats receiving gold salts develop anti-nuclear antibodies and glomerular deposits of immunoglobulins [56]. Mice with the H-2^s haplotype such as A.SW mice also produce anti-nuclear antibodies following gold administration [52].

Other metals such as beryllium, zirconium, lead, nickel or zinc are known to induce contact hypersensitivity in humans as well as in animals. It is quite tempting to speculate that these manifestations are a consequence of a delayed-type hypersensitivity towards the hapten bound to autoantigen or towards the modified antigen. It is interesting to mention to that point, that hypersensitivity reactions following $HgCl_2$ applications have been described by Polak et al. [57] in guinea pigs. These authors could demonstrate that susceptibility was genetically controlled. However, it is also possible that these metals are able to induce autoimmune manifestations. Warner and Lawrence [58, 59] have indeed shown that Pb^{2+}, Ni^{2+} and Zn^{2+} are able to stimulate murine lymphocyte proliferation [58]. They also demonstrated, using murine splenocytes, that these metals induce cell cycle progression and suggested that metal-induced proliferation requires the recognition of class II molecules by T cells. There are, therefore, many similarities with the mercury model exposed above.

IV. Conclusion

Experimental models of autoimmune disorders induced by metals are of great interest for several reasons. (1) They may confirm the potential toxicity of a given agent; (2) They provide considerable information concerning the mechanisms at play in such situations. It is interesting that in several circumstances metals induce a B cell hyperactivity, at least in susceptible species or strains. It appears also that autoreactive T cells which recognize class II molecules (either native or modified) play a crucial role in the induction of B cell hyperactivity; (3) The study of the mechanisms involved in such models may be very important for a better understanding of physiologic and pathologic autoimmunity.

References

1. Allison, A. C. (1977) Autoimmune diseases: concepts of pathogenesis and control. In: N. Talal (Ed.), Autoimmunity, Genetic, Immunology, Virology and Clinical Aspects, Academic Press, New York, San Francisco, London, pp. 91 – 139.
2. Sapin, C., Druet, E. and Druet, P. (1977) Induction of anti-glomerular basement membrane antibodies in the Brown-Norway rat by mercuric chloride. Clin. Exp. Immunol. 28, 173 – 179.
3. Druet, P., Druet, E., Potdevin, F. and Sapin, C. (1978) Immune type glomerulonephritis induced by $HgCl_2$ in the Brown Norway rat by mercuric chloride. Ann. Immunol. (Paris) 129C, 777 – 792.
4. Bellon, B., Capron, M., Druet, E., Verroust, P., Vial, M. C., Sapin, C., Girard, J. F., Foidart, J. M., Mahieu, P. and Druet, P. (1982) Mercuric chloride induced auto-immune disease in Brown-Norway rats: sequential search for antibasement membrane antibodies and circulating immune complexes. Eur. J. Clin. Invest. 12, 127 – 133.
5. Druet, E., Mahieu, P., Foidart, J. M. and Druet P. (1982) Magnetic solid-phase enzyme immunoassay for the detection of anti-glomerular basement membrane antibodies. J. Immunol. Methods. 48, 149 – 157.
6. Fukatsu, A., Brentjens, J., Killen, P., Kleinman, H., Martin, G. and Andres, G. (1987) Glomerular immune deposits in rats injected with mercuric chloride ($HgCl_2$). Kidney Int. 31, 320.
7. Hinglais, N., Druet, P., Grossetete, J., Sapin, C. and Bariety, J. (1979) Ultrastructural study of nephritis induced in Brown-Norway rats by mercuric chloride. Lab. Invest. 41, 150 – 159.
8. Michaud, A., Sapin, C., Leca, G., Aiach, M. and Druet, P. (1983) Involvement of hemostasis during an autoimmune glomerulonephritis induced by mercuric chloride in Brown-Norway rats. Thromb. Res. 33, 77 – 78.
9. Pelletier, L., Pasquier, R., Vial, M. C., Mandet, C., Nochy, D., Bazin, H. and Druet, P. (1988) $HgCl_2$ induces T and B cells to proliferate and differentiate in BN rats. Clin. Exp. Immunol., 71, 336 – 342.
10. Pusey, D. C., Bowman, C., Peters, D. K. and Lockwood, C. M. (1983) Effects of cyclophosphamide on autoantibody synthesis in the Brown-Norway rat. Clin. Exp. Immunol. 54, 697 – 704.
11. Prouvost-Danon, A., Abadie, A., Sapin, C., Bazin, H. and Druet, P. (1981) Induction of IgE synthesis and potentiation of anti-ovalbumin IgE antibody response by $HgCl_2$ in the rat. J. Immunol. 126, 699 – 702.
12. Hirsch, F., Couderc, J., Sapin, C., Fournie, G. and Druet, P. (1982) Polyclonal effect of $HgCl_2$ in the rat, its possible role in an experimental autoimmune disease. Eur. J. Immunol., 12, 620 – 625.
13. Prummel, B., Aten, J., Bosman, C., Van der Wal, A. M., Hoedemaeker, Ph. J. and Weening, J. J. (1985) Modulation by cyclosporin A (CyA) of toxin-induced autoimmune reactions and glomerulonephritis in the Brown-Norway (BN) rat. Kidney Int. 28, 696.

14. Bernaudin, J. F., Druet, E., Druet, P. and Masse, P. (1981) Inhalation or ingestion of organic or inorganic mercurials produces autoimmune disease in rats. Clin. Immunol. Immunopathol. 20, 129 – 135.

15. Druet, P., Teychenne, P., Mandet, C., Bascou, C. and Druet, E. (1981) Immune type glomerulonephritis induced in the Brown-Norway rat with mercury containing pharmaceutical products. Nephron 28, 145 – 148.

16. Druet, E., Sapin, C., Gunther, E., Feingold, N. and Druet, P. (1977) Mercuric chloride induced anti-glomerular basement membrane antibodies in the rat. Genetic control. Eur. J. Immunol. 7, 348 – 351.

17. Druet, E., Houssin, D. and Druet, P. (1983) Mercuric chloride nephritis depends on host rather than kidney strain. Clin. Immunol. Immunopathol. 29, 141 – 145.

18. Sapin, C., Druet, P. and Mandet, C. (1980) Induction of susceptibility to $HgCl_2$ immune glomerulonephritis in the Lewis rat by immunocompetent cells from susceptible F_1 hybrids. Eur. J. Immunol. 10, 371 – 374.

19. Sapin, C., Mandet, C., Druet, E., Gunther, E. and Druet, P. (1982) Immune complex type disease induced by $HgCl_2$ in the Brown-Norway rat. Genetic control of susceptibility. Clin. Exp. Immunol. 48, 700 – 704.

20. Sapin, C., Mandet, C., Guttmann, R.D., Druet, P. and Gill, T. J. (1987) Polyclonal activation induced by mercuric chloride ($HgCl_2$). Role of RT1-linked gene(s). Transplant. Proc. 19, 3194 – 3195.

21. Wooley, P. H., Griffin, J., Panayi, G., Batchelor, J. R., Welsh, K. I. and Gibson, T. J. (1980) HLA-DR antigens and toxic reaction to sodium aurothiomalate and D-penicillamine in patients with rheumatoid arthritis. New Engl. J. Med. 303, 300 – 302.

22. Rees, A. J., Peters, D. K., Amos, N., Welsh, K. I. and Batchelor, J. R. (1984) The influence of HLA-linked genes on the severity of anti-GBM antibody-mediated nephritis. Kidney Int. 26, 444 – 450.

23. Sapin, C., Hirsch, F., Delaporte, J. P., Bazin, H. and Druet P. (1984) Polyclonal IgE increase after $HgCl_2$ injections in BN and LEW rats. A genetic analysis. Immunogenetics 20, 227 – 236.

24. Hirsch, F., Kuhn, J., Vial, M. C., Ventura, M., Fournie, G., Sapin, C. and Druet, P. (1986) Autoimmunity induced by $HgCl_2$ in Brown-Norway rats. I. Production of monoclonal antibodies. J. Immunol. 136, 3272 – 3276.

25. Lymberi, P., Hirsch, F., Kuhn, J., Ternynck, T., Druet, P. and Avrameas, S. (1986) Autoimmunity induced by $HgCl_2$ in Brown-Norway rats. II. Monoclonal antibodies sharing specificities and idiotypes with mouse natural monoclonal antibodies. J. Immunol. 136, 3277 – 3281.

26. Pelletier, L., Pasquier, R., Hirsch, F., Sapin, C. and Druet, P. (1985) In vivo self reactivity of mononuclear cells to T cells and macrophages exposed to $HgCl_2$. Eur. J. Immunol. 15, 460 – 465.

27. Pelletier, L., Pasquier, R., Hirsch, F., Sapin, C. and Druet, P. (1986) Induction of autoreactive T cells in mercury-induced autoimmune disease. In vitro demonstration. J. Immunol. 137, 2548 – 2554.

27b. Rossert, J., Pelletier, L., Pasquier, R. and Druet, P. Autoreactive T cells in mercury-induced autoimmunity. Demonstration by limiting dilution analysis. Eur. J. Immunol., in press.

28. Pelletier, L., Pasquier, R., Vial, M. C., Mandet, C., Moutier, R. and Salomon, J. C. (1987) Mercury-induced autoimmune glomerulonephritis. Requirement for T cells. Nephrol. Dial. Transplant. 1, 211 – 218.

29. Pelletier, L., Pasquier, R., Rossert, J., Vial, M. C. and Druet, P. (1988) Autoreactive T cells in mercury-induced autoimmunity. Ability to induce the autoimmune disease. J. Immunol., 140, 750 – 754.

30. Stuffers-Heimann, M., Gunther, E. and Van Es, L. A. (1979) Induction of autoimmunity to antigens of the glomerular basement membrane in inbred Brown-Norway rats. Immunology, 36, 759 – 767.

31. Pusey, C. D., Sinico, R. A. and Lockwood, C. M. (1985) Antiglomerular basement membrane (GBM) autoantibody synthesis induced by homologous GBM alone in the Brown-Norway rat. Eur. J. Clin. Invest. 15, A45.

32. Hoedemaeker, Ph, J., Fleuren, G. J. and Weening, J. J. (1984) Etiologic factors in immunologically mediated glomerulonephritis. In: R. R. Robinson (Ed.), Nephrology, Springer-Verlag, New York, Berlin, Heidelberg, Tokyo, pp. 540 – 549.

33. Gleichmann, E., Pals, S. T., Rolink, A. G., Radaszkiewicz, T. and Gleichmann, H. (1984) Graft-versus-host reactions. Clues to the etiopathology of a spectrum of immunological diseases. Immunol. Today 5, 324 – 332.

34. Bowman, C., Mason, D. W., Pusey, C. D. and Lockwood, C. M. (1984) Autoregulation of antibody synthesis in mercuric chloride nephritis in the Brown-Norway rat. I. A role for T suppressor cells. Eur. J. Immunol. 14, 464 – 470.

35. Chalopin, J. M. and Lockwood, C. M. (1984) Autoregulation of autoantibody synthesis in mercuric chloride nephritis in the Brown-Norway rat. II. Presence of antigen-augmentable plaque-forming cells in the spleen is associated with humoral factors behaving as auto-anti-idiotypic antibodies. Eur. J. Immunol. 14, 470 – 475.

36. Pelletier, L., Pasquier, R., Rossert, J. and Druet, P. (1987) $HgCl_2$ induces non specific immunosuppression in LEW rats. Eur. J. Immunol. 17, 49 – 54.

37. Pelletier, L., Ronco, P., Pasquier, R., Verroust, P., Bariety, J. and Druet, P. (1987) $HgCl_2$ inhibits the development of Heymann nephritis in Lewis rats. Kidney Int. 32, 227 – 232.

38. Pelletier, L., Rossert, J., Pasquier, R., Villarroya, H., Belair, M. F., Vial, M. C., Oriol, R. and Druet, P. (1988) Effect of $HgCl_2$ on experimental allergic encephalomyelitis in Lewis rats. $HgCl_2$-induced down-modulation of the disease. Eur. J. Immunol., 18, 243 – 247.

39. Fillastre, J. P., Druet, P. and Mery, J. Ph. (1988) Drug-induced glomerulonephritis. In: J. S. Cameron and R. J. Glassock (Eds.), The Nephrotic Syndrome, Marcel Dekker Inc., New York, pp. 697 – 744.

40. Hoorntje, S. J., Weening, J. J., The, T. H., Kallenberg, C. G. M., Donker, A. J. M. and Hoedemaeker, Ph. J. (1980) Immune complex glomerulopathy in patients treated with captopril. Lancet 1, 1212 – 1214.

41. Kleinknecht, D., Kanfer, A., Morel-Maroger, L. and Mery, J. Ph. (1978) Immunologically mediated drug-induced acute interstitial nephritis. In: G. M. Berlyne and S. Thomas (Eds.), Contributions to Nephrology, Vol. 10, Karger, Basel, pp. 42 – 52.

42. Delfraissy, J. F., Galanaud, P., Balavoine, J. F., Wallon, C. and Dormont, J. (1984) Captopril and immune regulation. Kidney Int., 25, 925 – 929.

43. Lipsky, P. E. (1984) Immunosuppression by D-penicillamine in vitro. Inhibition of human T lymphocyte proliferation by copper or ceruloplasmin-dependent generation of hydrogen peroxide and protection by monocyte. J. Clin. Invest. 73, 53 – 65.

44. Sanders, W. E. (1976) Diagnosis and treatment. Drugs five years later Rifampicin. Ann. Intern. Med. 85, 82 – 86.

45. Druet, E., Sapin, C., Fournie, G., Mandet, C., Gunther, E. and Druet, P. (1982) Genetic control of susceptibility to mercury-induced immune nephritis in various strains of rat. Clin. Immunol. Immunopathol. 25, 203 – 211.

46. Weening, J. J., Fleuren, G. J. and Hoedemaeker, P. J. (1978) Demonstration of antinuclear antibodies in mercuric chloride-induced glomerulopathy in the rat. Lab. Invest. 39, 405 – 411.

47. Weening, J. J., Hoedemaeker, Ph.J. and Bakker, W. W. (1981) Immunoregulation and antinuclear antibodies in mercury-induced glomerulopathy in the rat. Clin. Exp. Immunol. 45, 64 – 71.

48. Roman-Franco, A. A., Turiello, M., Albini, B., Ossi, E., Milgrom, F. and Andres, G. A. (1978) Anti-basement membrane antibodies and antigen-antibody complexes in rabbits injected with mercuric chloride. Clin. Immunol. Immunopathol. 9, 464 – 481.

49. Albini, B., Glurich, I. and Andres, G. A.   (1982)   Mercuric chloride-induced immunologically mediated diseases in experimental animals. In: G. A. Porter (Ed.), Nephrotoxic Mechanisms of Drugs and Environmental Toxins, Plenum Press, New York, pp. 413 – 423.

50. Hultman, P. and Enestrom, S.   (1987)   The induction of immune complex deposits in mice by per oral and parenteral administration of mercuric chloride: strain dependent susceptibility. Clin. Exp. Immunol. 67, 283 – 292.

51. Robinson, C. J. G., Abraham, A. A. and Balazs, T.   (1984)   Induction of anti-nuclear antibodies by mercuric chloride in mice. Clin. Exp. Immunol. 58, 300 – 306.

52. Robinson, C. J. G., Balazs, T. and Egorov, I. K.   (1986)   Mercuric chloride, gold sodium thiomalate and D-penicillamine-induced antinuclear antibodies in mice. Toxicol. Appl. Pharmacol. 86, 159 – 169.

53. Pietsch, P., Allmeroth, M., Gleichmann, E. and Vohr, H. W.   (1987)   Increased synthesis of IgE, but not IgM, in strains of mice susceptible to $HgCl_2$. Immunobiology, in press.

54. Fleuren, G. J., De Heer, E., Van Burgers, J., Osnabrugge, C. and Hoedemaeker, Ph. J.   (1985) Mercuric chloride-induced glomerulopathy in Balb/c mice. Kidney Int. 28, 702.

55. Nagi, A. H., Alexander, F. and Barabas, A. Z.   (1971)   Gold nephropathy in rats. Light and electron microscopic studies. Exp. Molecul. Pathol. 15, 354 – 362.

56. Balazs, T., Robinson, C. and Abraham, A.   (1986)   Drug-induced autoimmunity in rats. Sixth International Congress of Immunology. Toronto 5, 43.

57. Polak, L., Barnes, J. M. and Turk, J. L.   (1968)   The genetic control of contact sensitization by inorganic metal compounds in guinea-pigs. Immunology 14, 707 – 711.

58. Warner, G. L. and Lawrence, D. A.   (1986)   Stimulation of murine lymphocyte responses by cations. Cell. Immunol. 101, 425 – 439.

59. Warner, G. L. and Lawrence, D. A.   (1986)   Cell surface and cell cycle analysis of metal-induced murine T cell proliferation. Eur. J. Immunol. 16, 1337 – 1342.

M.E. Kammüller, N. Bloksma and W. Seinen (Eds.)
Autoimmunity and Toxicology
© *1989 Elsevier Science Publishers B.V. (Biomedical Division)*

Testing the sensitization of T cells to chemicals. From murine graft-versus-host (GVH) reactions to chemical-induced GVH-like immunological diseases

15

ERNST GLEICHMANN[a], HANS-WERNER VOHR[a], CLIVE STRINGER[a], JAN NUYENS[b] and HELGA GLEICHMANN[c]

[a]*Division of Immunology, Medical Institute of Environmental Hygiene at the University of Düsseldorf, Auf'm Hennekamp 50, D-4000 Düsseldorf 1, FRG,* [b]*Central Laboratory of The Netherlands Red Cross Blood Transfusion Service, Plesmanlaan 125, NL-1066 CX Amsterdam, The Netherlands and* [c]*Diabetes Research Institute at the University of Düsseldorf, Auf'm Hennekamp 65, D-4000 Düsseldorf 1, FRG*

I. Introduction

This chapter will start with a brief review of the immunopathological alterations inducible by the GVH reaction in mice. Then we will examine experimental evidence for the hypothesis that certain adverse immunological side effects of drugs may be caused by a GVH-like pathogenic mechanism; to a major extent this part reviews our data obtained with the popliteal lymph node assay (PLNA) in mice. Some recent variations of this assay will be described which make the PLNA a useful tool for assessing the immunogenic and/or immunostimulatory capacity of small chemicals and other xenobiotics during the preclinical test phase. Finally, we will report recent advances in establishing a mouse model for the autoimmunizing and IgE-enhancing effects of mercuric chloride ($HgCl_2$).

II. The parent → F₁ hybrid GVH reaction: a model for diseases caused by chemical modification of cell-surface molecules

1. EXPERIMENTAL DESIGN

The GVH reaction was induced by injection of parental strain T lymphocytes into, otherwise untreated, adult F₁ hybrid recipients. For genetic reasons, the grafted cells are tolerated and not rejected by the semi-allogeneic F₁ host (Fig. 1). The injected T lymphocytes, however, recognize the allogeneic (genetically foreign) histocompatibility molecules which the F₁ host has inherited from the other paren-

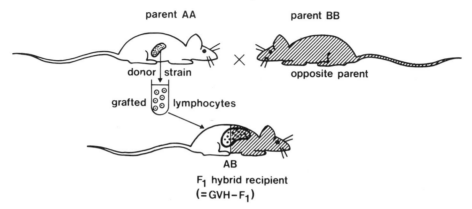

Fig. 1. Scheme of induction of GVH reactions using a parent into F₁ hybrid combination. The histocompatibility antigens of both parental strains are expressed in the heterozygous F₁ hybrid. For this reason the parental strain cells are not recognized as foreign. In contrast, T lymphocytes of the parental donor strain AA injected into the F₁ host AB recognize the histocompatibility antigens inherited from the opposite parental strain BB as foreign and react against them. (Reproduced from Am. J. Clin. Pathol. (1979) 72, 708–723, with kind permission of J. B. Lippincott Company, Philadelphia.)

tal strain. The ensuing response of the donor T cells, the GVH reaction, results in the development of various immunopathological lesions. For optimal induction of GVH disease, a strong histoincompatibility must exist in the recipient; in non-irradiated F₁ mice, which have intact immunologic control mechanisms, this histoincompatibility must be at the H-2 locus, the murine major histocompatibility complex (MHC).

2. SPECTRUM OF GVH REACTION-INDUCED IMMUNOLOGICAL DISORDERS

Fig. 2, A, shows the spectrum of pathological alterations which can be induced by GVH reaction. The majority of these alterations has been observed as sequelae of GVH reaction in both human and laboratory animals. Two basic forms of GVH reaction-induced pathological lesions can be distinguished: a stimulatory GVH reaction and a suppressive (or hypoplastic) GVH reaction. Stimulatory pathological signs are shown in the middle and on the left-hand side of Fig. 2, A. They include a persistent lymphoid hyperplasia of mainly B lymphocytes, resulting in hypergammaglobulinemia and the formation of autoantibodies characteristic of systemic

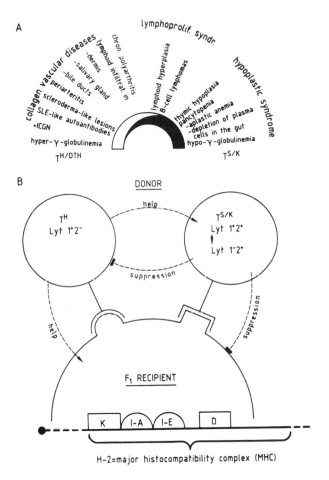

Fig. 2. Spectrum and concept of cellular pathogenesis of immunological disorders resulting from GVH reactions in F_1 mice. Not listed here is toxic epidermal necrolysis or Lyell's disease, which is a serious GVH complication in species other than mouse, such as hamster and man. (A) Spectrum of pathological lesions that may develop in GVH F_1 mice. (B) Concept of the basic cellular and MHC requirements for induction of stimulatory (middle and right) and suppressive (right) GVH lesions, respectively. According to contemporary nomenclature, the donor T_h cell is a $CD4^+8^-$ cell and the $T_{s/k}$ cell is a $CD4^-8^+$ cell [19a]. The F_1 cell (depicted at the bottom) represents stimulator/target cells situated at various anatomical sites. Preferential target cells in the GVH reaction are the ubiquitous antigen-presenting cells, B lymphocytes, and hemopoietic cells. (Reproduced from Immunol. Today (1984) 5, 324–332, with kind permission of Elsevier North-Holland.)

lupus erythematosus (SLE), such as antibodies against nuclear antigens (ANA), double-stranded DNA (dsDNA), erythrocytes, and thymocytes [1 – 7]. In addition, stimulatory GVH lesions include a severe immune-complex glomerulonephritis [8]. The SLE-like GVH lesions may occur together with characteristic signs of other collagen vascular diseases or non-organ-specific autoimmune diseases, such as arteritis [2, 9, 10], chronic progressive polyarthritis [10], Sjögren- and scleroderma-like lesions, and liver changes resembling sclerosing cholangitis [9, 10]. Usually, stimulatory GVH lesions present themselves as chronic GVH disease which can last for more than a year.

Suppressive or hypoplastic GVH reaction induced lesions are shown on the right hand side of Fig. 2, A. Clinically, they manifest themselves as acute GVH disease, which is often fatal. The suppressive GVH lesions consist of a severe hypoplasia of the lympho-hemopoietic compartment leading to aplastic anemia and hypogammaglobulinemia [5 – 7, 11, 12].

3. SUBSETS OF ALLOREACTIVE T LYMPHOCYTES INDUCE EITHER STIMULATORY OF SUPPRESSIVE GVH DISEASE SYNDROMES

In rodents as well as in man, there are two major subsets of functionally different T lymphocytes, T helper (T_h) and T killer (T_k) cells. A third type, the T suppressor (T_s) cell, has been less well defined and seems to be heterogeneous. In several experimental systems, including the GVH reaction, T_s cells share several features with T_k cells. In fact, it could not be dissected whether the effector T cells causing the pancytopenia of acute GVH disease were T_k cells or abnormally activated T_s cells [11, 13, 14], therefore, we shall refer to them in the context of GVH reaction as $T_{s/k}$ cells.

The rules that govern T cell alloreactivity have been well established by many studies, most of which were performed in vitro. There is general agreement that alloreactive T_h cells react preferentially and most vigorously towards incompatible class II MHC molecules, whereas T_k cells react preferentially against incompatible class I molecules. In the murine GVH model, several experimental approaches established that functionally different subsets of alloreactive donor T cells cause the different forms of GVH disease shown in Fig. 2, A [4, 5, 15]. Based on the results of these experiments, a general concept of the cellular pathogenesis of GVH reaction induced diseases has emerged, as illustrated in Fig. 2, B. When the donor T_h cells are activated by allogeneic class II MHC structures of the F_1 recipient, and if there is no concomitant reaction by class I reactive $T_{s/k}$ cells, persistent lymphoid hyperplasia, hypergammaglobulinemia and SLE-like GVH disease develop [4 – 6]. Whether class II reactive donor T_h cells alone also trigger the GVH-associated malignant lymphomas [16 – 18] and signs of collagen vascular disease, such as chronic progressive polyarthritis, Sjögren- and scleroderma-like disease, has not been formally established. The effector T cells causing suppressive pathological

GVH lesions are class I reactive $T_{s/k}$ cells. Optimal activation of $T_{s/k}$ effector cells, however, requires initial help, probably in the form of interleukin-2, from class II MHC-reactive donor T_h cells (Fig. 2, B) [5–7, 11, 12, 19].

4. MECHANISM OF AUTOANTIBODY FORMATION DURING GVH REACTION

It has been unequivocally established that B lymphocytes with the capacity to produce autoantibodies, at least to certain self antigens such as DNA, exist in healthy individuals [20]. Normally, these potentially autoreactive B cells are silent, or produce only small amounts of autoantibody of the IgM isotype. Upon adequate activation by T_h cells, these autoreactive B cells clones expand and switch to the production of large amounts of IgG antibodies which have a high average affinity.

During GVH reaction, alloreactive donor T_h cells provide help, i.e., various interleukins, such as IL-2 and IL-4, to the F_1 B cells. This type of help is indiscriminate because all F_1 B cells are semi-allogeneic and can thus receive allohelp. Nevertheless, the resulting B cell stimulation is a highly selective one; only those clones of autoreactive B cells are activated to produce large amounts of IgG autoantibodies characteristic of SLE [2, 3, 21]. Autoreactive B cells capable of producing antibodies to organ-specific self antigens are not activated during GVH reaction. The type of T-B cell cooperation operating in GVH reactions is also termed noncognate T-B cooperation because the antigen to which the B cell reacts is not recognized by the cooperating T_h cell which is an allohelper T cell reacting against the allogeneic class II MHC structures.

There are two hypotheses to explain this preferential production of non-organ-specific autoantibodies. The first hypothesis states that this is due to the characteristics of the non-organ-specific self antigens involved, such as DNA [2, 3, 14, 21]. In other words, this hypothesis postulates that, in addition to T cell help, autoreactive B cells need another signal which is provided by self antigen. Therefore, structural features and the concentration of available self antigen play a selective role. There is solid experimental evidence that in a GVH reaction those B cells are preferentially triggered to which the antigen is presented in the form of repeating identical epitopes on a rigid backbone. If the *same* epitopes are presented to the B cells on a *globular* protein the B cells receive an inadequate signal. Certain self antigens, such as DNA, appear to have adequate structural features to provide that signal to the corresponding autoreactive B cells, whereas globular self antigens, such as thyroglobulin and insulin, appear less able to do so [2, 3, 14, 21]. The second possible explanation holds that autoreactive B cells with specificity for certain self antigens, such as DNA, occur at a much higher frequency than others. It should be emphasized that these two explanations are by no means mutually exclusive.

III. Can GVH reaction-like immunological disorders be induced by modified self?

1. CONCEPT OF PATHOGENESIS

It has been well established that the principles that govern T cell alloreactivity also apply to the physiological reactions of T cells. In an autologous system, T_h cells recognize foreign antigen together with the individual's own class II MHC structures, while T_k cells recognize foreign antigen together with the individual's own class I MHC structures. Therefore, the basic principles established for T cell alloreactivity in GVH reaction might also operate in the cellular pathogenesis of GVH-like diseases that develop after exposure to a foreign etiologic agent. GVH-like cellular interactions might be stimulated in autologous (and syngeneic) systems provided that cell-surface determinants of hemopoietic cells, such as B cells and/or antigen-presenting cells, can be modified by a given etiologic agent. Evidence for this concept stems from the observation that B lymphocytes that were experimentally rendered 'foreign' by covalent coupling of trinitrophenol (TNP) to their membrane, elicited a GVH-like reaction in vivo by normal syngeneic T_h cells and, as a consequence, showed an enhanced production of IgG antibodies [22].

Certain exogenous chemicals might directly alter MHC class II structures on such target cells. Conceivably, certain chemicals might bind to certain class II MHC structures better than others. Indirect evidence for a preferential interaction of certain drugs with certain HLA class I molecules has been obtained by Claas and Van Rood [23]. These authors incubated human peripheral blood leucocytes with high concentrations of various drugs in vitro prior to addition of HLA class I specific antibodies and they demonstrated consistent patterns of a selective blocking of HLA-specific antibody reactions by certain drugs.

In the experiment of Ptak et al. [22] mentioned above, murine B cells were rendered 'foreign' by TNBSA (trinitrobenzene sulfonic acid), a chemical that covalently binds to proteins. Whether other chemicals, such as drugs, spontaneously bind to the membrane of lymphoid cells in vivo, and thus render them 'foreign', is largely unknown. Some indirect evidence that this may happen has been obtained from studies on the sensitization to penicillin in humans [24] and D-penicillamine (D-pen) in mice (see below, Section IV.2. in this chapter). While drugs are not usually constructed to spontaneously bind in a covalent fashion to proteins, such as MHC molecules, certain drug metabolites might do so [25, 26]. On the other hand, it is perhaps not even necessary that a chemical agent binds covalently to MHC structures in order to render them 'foreign'. Conceivably, strong non-covalent bonds might be sufficient.

In any case, altered MHC structures would trigger reactions by autologous T cells comparable to the reactions of parental strain T cells towards the allogeneic MHC molecules on F_1 recipient cells (Fig. 2, B). Thus, autologous (or syngeneic) T_h cells might be preferentially activated if a foreign antigen X is recognized in association with class II MHC determinants. In contrast, T_k cells might be preferentially activated if the same foreign antigen X is recognized in association with class I MHC determinants. Depending on the T cell subpopulation activated, stimulatory or suppressive pathological symptoms may develop, as shown in Fig. 2, A.

2. DRUGS INDUCING GVH REACTION-LIKE LESIONS AS AN ADVERSE IMMUNOLOGICAL SIDE EFFECT

Several drugs are known to cause numerous pathological symptoms within the broad spectrum of GVH-like conditions shown in Fig. 2, A. For example, the anti-epileptic drug diphenylhydantoin (DPH, phenytoin, dilantin) has been reported to cause hypergammaglobulinemia, drug-induced SLE, arthritis, dermatitis, toxic epidermal necrolysis, B cell lymphomas, aplastic anemia, and hypogam-maglobulinemia [17, 27 – 29]. Furthermore, immune complex glomerulonephritis and lymphadenopathy, features of drug-induced SLE, or thrombocytopenia and granulocytopenia developed during therapy with the anti-rheumatic drug D-pen [30] or with captopril, an anti-hypertensive drug.

In view of the striking similarity of the immunopathological lesions induced by GVH reaction and those induced by drugs, such as DPH, experiments were undertaken to investigate whether the injection of such drugs into mice caused GVH-like reactions by autologous T cells.

IV. Murine T cell reactions to a variety of different chemicals

Originally, the PLNA was developed to measure T cell alloreactivity in the GVH reaction [31 – 34]. Then, one of us extended application of the PLNA to measure the T cell dependent immune response to the anti-epileptic drug DPH [35, 36]. Subsequently, the PLNA was used to measure immune responses to a variety of other chemical compounds [37   41]. The PLNA is described in Fig. 3.

1. MURINE T CELL REACTIONS TO DIPHENYLHYDANTOIN (DPH) DETECTED BY THE PLNA

When a single injection of 1 mg of DPH was administered s.c. into one hind foot-pad, a significant PLN weight increase ensued, which peaked about 1 week later and had reverted back to normal by 3 weeks. This PLN reaction was T cell dependent because only the euthymic + /nu recipients mounted a response, whereas their congenitally athymic counterparts failed to do so [35]. The peak of PLN weight increase induced by DPH coincided with maximal outburst of proliferation, as determined by the uptake of [^{3}H]thymidine by the draining PLN. This determination of cell

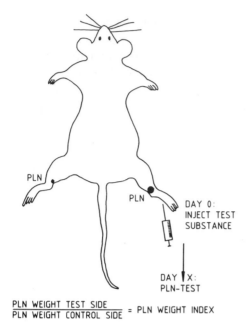

PLN

PLN

DAY 0:
INJECT TEST
SUBSTANCE

DAY X:
PLN-TEST

$$\frac{\text{PLN WEIGHT TEST SIDE}}{\text{PLN WEIGHT CONTROL SIDE}} = \text{PLN WEIGHT INDEX}$$

Fig. 3. Scheme of the popliteal lymph node assay (PLNA) in rodents. The test compound is injected sub-cutaneously (s.c.) without adjuvant into one hind footpad of a test animal. The contralateral side is left untreated or inoculated with the solvent of the test compound and thus serves as an internal control. Days thereafter an ensuing immune reaction can be assessed by removing the PLNs and determining either the PLN weight index, the number of cells in the PLNs, or ^{3}H-thymidine incorporation in the PLNs.

proliferation in the PLN was a more sensitive method than determination of the PLN *weight* index. Recruitment into the draining PLN of circulating lymphocytes, as determined by trapping in the PLN of ^{51}Cr-labelled lymphocytes, contributed much less to the PLN enlargement than did lymphocyte proliferation within the PLN [36].

Histologically, a diffuse infiltration of the PLN parenchyma with mononuclear cells was seen 6 days after injection of DPH, followed by development of germinal centers between day 8 and 10. By that time, numerous lymphoid cells and im-munoblasts were present in the paracortical areas, and plasma cells and their precur-sors occurred in the medulla. By serological criteria and immuno-peroxidase stain-ing it was shown that the percentage of the B cell derived population was increased, whereas the relative proportion of T cells was decreased. Functional studies using the protein A plaque-forming cell assay demonstrated a tremendous increase of T cell dependent IgM- and, especially, IgG-secreting cells. Adult thymectomy of pro-spective recipient mice significantly amplified their PLN reaction to DPH and great-ly facilitated the activation of Ig-secreting cells in the draining PLN [36]. This, and other observations [35], suggest that in normal mice the lymphadenopathy (PLN enlargement) and T cell dependent B cell activation are rapidly down regulated by specific $T_{s/k}$ cells. It is conceivable, however, that in certain individuals the process of DPH-induced T cell dependent proliferation and functional activation of B cells is not rapidly down regulated, but persists for weeks or months. In such cases, it might lead to the GVH-like lymphomagenesis and autoimmunization observed in patients treated with DPH [36].

The stimulatory effects caused by DPH cannot be attributed to a direct mitogenic effect on lymphocytes. Studies with lymphocytes cultured in vitro showed that DPH induced proliferation in cultures of some patients sensitized to the drug but did not act non-specifically, i.e. as a mitogen [28]. Similarly, DPH failed to induce proliferation when added to cultures of normal murine lymphocytes. Furthermore, the lack of lymphoproliferation and B cell activation observed in T cell deprived recipients of DPH also excluded the possibility that DPH acts as a polyclonal B cell stimulator [36]. By using radiolabelled DPH it was shown that DPH exhibits an affinity for cells; when murine spleen cells, pre-incubated with DPH in vitro, were inoculated s.c. into the footpads of syngeneic mice, they induced a significant PLN enlargement [35].

DPH has two chemical properties that might enable it to induce the T cell dependent lymphadenopathy. Because DPH belongs to the class of lipid-soluble drugs [42], it might be incorporated into the lipid bilayer of cell membranes and, thus, create new membrane determinants. Alternatively, arene oxide metabolites of DPH might be involved in the DPH-induced lymphadenopathy. In studies on the metabolism of DPH, it has been found that biotransformation of DPH by cytochrome *P450* to its monophenolic and dihydriol metabolites involves the formation of highly reactive arene oxide intermediates [43]. It is conceivable that DPH, after association with the cell membrane of lymphocytes and/or macrophages, may be oxidized by these cells as they too possess the cytochrome *P450* system. Covalent binding of the arene oxide metabolite to membrane constituents of lymphoid cells would render them 'non-self', thus providing stable structures able to stimulate autologous T cells. The finding that injection of hydantoin only, i.e. a compound lacking the two phenyl groups, failed to induce any PLN response, supports the assumption that the PLN reactions to DPH are caused by the phenyl groups or the highly reactive arene oxide intermediates of DPH [36]. Further evidence in favor of this possibility was obtained by Kammüller et al. [41] who showed that substitution of the hydantoin ring by only one phenyl group sufficed to render the compound immunogenic in the PLNA.

Interestingly, injection of $1 - 2$ mg of phenobarbital failed to induce PLN reactions. Phenobarbital was chosen for comparison because it is chemically and pharmacologically related to DPH, but not known to cause significant immunopathological lesions or allergic reactions in man. It is assumed that phenobarbital, which is water-soluble, is unable to interact with lymphoid cells in the same manner as the hydrophobic compound DPH and thus fails to produce 'non-self' structures capable of stimulating autologous T cells [36].

2. MURINE T CELL REACTIONS TO D-PEN DETECTED BY IN VITRO STUDIES AND BY THE PLNA

In man, the anti-rheumatic drug D-pen causes a variety of adverse immunological side-effects, which include a lupus-like syndrome, immune complex glomerulonephritis, Sjögren's disease, lymphadenopathy, IgA deficiency, and various cytopenias [44, 45]. Some of these alterations are known to be associated with certain HLA phenotypes ([46 – 48] and Emery and Panayi, this volume). The similarities between the pathological alterations induced by D-pen, as mentioned above, and those induced by a GVH reaction has led to the hypothesis that these D-pen induced alterations may have a GVH-like pathogenesis as well [14]. This would require that D-pen binds to autologous lymphoid and/or antigen-presenting cells and, as a membrane-bound epitope, elicits specific T cell reactions. This possibility is supported by several pieces of indirect evidence reviewed below.

(a) In vitro re-stimulation of specific T cells primed to D-pen in vivo

In these experiments, mice were primed with D-pen in vivo and the secondary response of specific T cells was measured in a proliferative assay in vitro. Priming was achieved by injecting either free D-pen or, more effectively, D-pen in complete Freund's adjuvant at the base of the tail. After 7 – 9 days, the draining lymph node cells (responder cells) were specifically re-stimulated in vitro with syngeneic spleen cells that had been pre-incubated with D-pen for 20 – 22 h and then washed. The thiol (-SH)group of D-pen was required for generating effective stimulator cells in vitro; this was deduced from the observation that D-pen disulfide, which does not have free thiol groups, failed to generate specific stimulator cells for D-pen primed responder T cells. Whereas spleen cells pre-incubated with D-pen proved to be good stimulator cells, thymocytes and mouse erythrocytes after having been pre-incubated with D-pen, completely failed to induce stimulation. This and additional circumstantial evidence [37] suggests that the drug was associated with certain surface structures specific to macrophages and/or dendritic cells, possibliy class II MHC molecules [49]. The proliferating responder cells had the phenotype of T_h cells (Thy-l$^+$, Lyt-l$^+$2$^-$); these T_h cells were highly specific for spleen cells pre-incubated with D-pen, and they were even capable of distinguishing between the two stereoisomers D-pen and L-pen. The splenic T cells of recipient mice were effectively primed by intravenous injection of syngeneic spleen cells pre-incubated with D-pen, but not by injection of free D-pen. Taken together, these findings indicate that D-pen spontaneously haptenates appropriate stimulator cells and, thus, serves as an epitope for specific T cells [49].

In man, the drug D-pen is administered orally. Therefore, the question was asked if orally administered D-pen could haptenate peritoneal macrophages of recipient mice and prime their specific T cells. For this purpose, D-pen was given in the drinking water at a dose of $5-7$ mg/kg of mice for periods ranging from 1 to 10 weeks. Peritoneal macrophages or adherent spleen cells obtained from such mice, and control mice, were used as stimulator cells without an additional pre-incubation with the drug in vitro. Cells prepared from the mesenteric lymph nodes or Peyer's patches served as responder cells. The results of these experiments indicate that orally administered D-pen can, indeed, haptenate the recipient's macrophages and prime their T cells (Vogeler et al., unpublished results). It should be noted, however, that the oral dose of D-pen per kg body weight used in these experiments exceeds the maximal dosage used in man by a factor of about 12.

(b) Specific T cell responses to D-pen detected by the PLNA

Mice of various inbred strains were injected s.c. into one hind footpad with 1 mg of D-pen without adjuvant, and the PLN weight assay was performed [37]. The peak of the primary PLN response was obtained between day 7 and 10. Again, measuring the cell proliferation in the draining PLN, as determined by incorporation of ^{3}H-thymidine, proved to be a more sensitive parameter than measuring the PLN weight. Recruitment of lymphocytes from the circulation, as determined by trapping of ^{51}Cr-labelled syngeneic lymphocytes in the draining PLN, also contributed to the PLN enlargement, but was significantly less important than lymphocyte proliferation in the PLN.

The failure to induce PLN enlargement in congenitally athymic nude mice demonstrated that the PLN reaction to D-pen is a T cell dependent process. Histologically, a diffuse infiltration of the PLN parenchyma with mononuclear cells was seen on day 6 after the injection of D-pen. This was followed by the formation of germinal centers and an increase in complement-receptor positive lymphocytes, indicating B cell activation [37]. These changes were quite similar to those caused by DPH [35, 36] and a local GVHR [32 – 34].

Presumably the initial event in the PLN enlargement induced by D-pen consists of an activation of D-pen specific T cells, which recognize the drug attached to certain surface structures of macrophages and/or dendritic cells. Four pieces of experimental evidence indirectly support this hypothesis. First, binding studies with ^{14}C-D-pen have shown that the drug accumulates in the murine macrophage population, where it is preferentially bound to the plasma membrane [50]. Second, D-pen pretreated, 18-h non-adherent spleen cells, a population enriched for macrophages [51, 52], induced PLN enlargement after injection into the footpad. In contrast, D-pen pretreated 2 h-non-adherent cells, a population containing mainly lymphocytes, failed to cause PLN enlargement [37]. Third, binding studies, in vitro, have shown that D-pen selectively blocks the interaction of IgG_1 with the IgG_1 Fc receptor on peritoneal macrophages of guinea pigs [53]. Fourth, only D-pen modified spleen cells, and not free D-pen, added to cultures of D-pen primed lymph node cells were able to specifically re-stimulate T_h cells in vitro [49]. Taken together, the immune response to D-pen appears to be similar to those of classical haptens, such as TNP [54 – 57]. Cell-bound TNP was shown to elicit a GVH-like 'allogeneic' effect on syngeneic B cells in vitro [57] and in vivo [22], and the B cell activation seen in the draining PLN after D-pen injection may have a similar cellular basis. If true, the observed B cell activation would be a *non-specific* consequence of the *specific* reaction of T helper cells toward cell-bound D-pen.

For induction of a PLN response to D-pen, the stereoisomer L-pen, and the dimer D-pen disulfide, it was mandatory that the compounds were administered in ionized form, i.e. at low pH [37].

PLN reactivity to D-pen is controlled by at least two loci, one mapping to the I-region, probably I-A, the other(s) to the non-H-2 background [37]. This finding is consistent with our concept that specific T_h cells react to cell-bound D-pen and thus trigger a general B cell activation. If persistent, such a general B cell activation might result in a SLE-like autoantibody formation [14, 49]. Animal models for some of the GVH-like pathological alterations induced by D-pen have been developed by using susceptible strains of rat [58] and mouse [59].

In man, an additional factor accounting for an increased genetic risk to develop immunological side effects under D-pen therapy appears to be a poor sulfoxidation of the drug [60]. Other factors that might be involved in the development of D-pen induced autoimmunity, at least in experimental animals, are the extent of D-pen ionisation and the initial dosage administered. Hurtenbach et al. [37] observed that an initial injection of a low dosage of D-pen induced a state of specific unresponsiveness to a subsequent challenge with an immunogenic dose of the drug. Similarly, whereas Brown Norway rats that were given a daily dosage of 20 – 50 mg D-pen orally over a period of several months developed dermatitis, antinuclear autoantibodies, circulating immune complexes, and IgG deposits along the glomerular basement membrane of the kidney; those rats initially receiving only 5 mg of D-pen per day and subsequently 20 and 50 mg, did not develop the disease [58]. Whether or not this interesting observation is related to the T cell dependent immunity to D-pen studied by Nagata et al. [49] and Hurtenbach et al. [37], remains to be elucidated.

The PLN reaction to D-pen proved to be antigen specific, since D-pen primed mice exhibited an enhanced reaction when boostered with a suboptimal dose of D-pen, but not when boostered with an unrelated drug, DPH. This was the first report of a specific secondary immune reaction detected by means of the PLNA; it established that the PLNA can, indeed, serve as a test system in vivo to measure specific immune responses to simple chemicals administered without adjuvant [37].

3. MURINE T CELL REACTIONS TO STREPTOZOTOCIN DETECTED BY THE PLNA

Streptozotocin (STZ, 2-deoxy-2-(3'-methyl-3'-nitrosourea)-D-glucopyranose) is a naturally occurring compound isolated from *Streptomyces achromogenes*. STZ is widely used as diabetogen in experimental animals. Under certain experimental conditions, repeated low-dose injections of STZ into mice can induce hyperglycemia, and it is generally accepted that immunological reactions participate in the induction of this abnormality. However, the mechanism(s) underlying the immunological reactions involved in the induction of hyperglycemia remain to be elucidated. By using the PLNA, it has recently been demonstrated that STZ can act as an epitope for

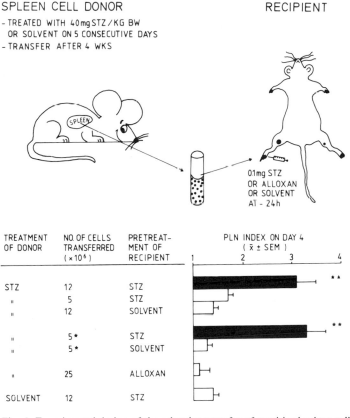

Fig. 4. Experimental design of the adoptive transfer of sensitized spleen cells, and mean values ± SEM of the ratios of PLN weights obtained. Spleen cells of BALB/c donor mice, which had received i.p. injections of either streptozotocin (STZ) or the solvent of STZ, were inoculated s.c. into one hind footpad of syngeneic mice. The recipients had received an s.c. injection of either a subimmunogenic dose (0.1 mg) of STZ, alloxan, or solvent into the same footpad at 24 h before the cell transfer. Groups of seven mice each were used as recipient. *, enriched for T cells; **, $p < 0.005$ versus controls. (Reproduced from Klinkhammer et al., 1988 [38], with kind permission from the American Diabetes Association, Inc.)

T cells [38]. A single injection of STZ induced an immunological reaction in the draining PLN, as determined by significant increase in weight, cell number, and ^{3}H-thymidine uptake. For this reaction to occur T lymphocytes were required. Furthermore, it was shown, that STZ-primed mice developed an enhanced secondary PLN response upon challenge with STZ.

Repeated low-dose i.p. injections of STZ primed the splenic T cells of recipient mice. This was shown by using the adoptive transfer PLNA depicted in Fig. 4. The donors of STZ-primed splenic T cells were sensitized by five repeated i.p. injections of low doses of STZ; thereafter, these mice were left untreated for 3 weeks. Upon transfer to syngeneic mice the T cells induced a specific PLN enlargement in the recipient, provided the recipient had received an s.c. injection of a small dose of STZ a few hours before cell transfer. Neither the transferred T cells, nor the small dose of STZ, given alone, were able to induce PLN enlargement in the recipient. The necessity to pretreat the prospective recipients with the sensitizing compound prior to the adoptive cell transfer suggests that binding of STZ to cells of the recipient, possibly Langerhans cells, is a prerequisite to detect specific reactions by the sensitized donor T cells [38]. More recent experiments indicate that STZ is a potent agent in inducing the expression of class II MHC molecules (Klinkhammer and H. Gleichmann, unpublished results).

4. PLNA RESPONSES TO OTHER DRUGS

In addition to the compounds discussed in the preceding sections, several other chemicals were tested for immunogenicity in the PLNA. A survey of all the compounds and results obtained by our group is given in Table 1. Kammüller et al. [41] have recently reported their results obtained with a great variety of other compounds tested in the PLNA.

5. THE MURINE PLN REACTION TO QUARTZ (SiO$_2$)

Quartz, the etiologic agent of silicosis, was injected s.c. into one hind footpad at a dose of 2.5 mg. This single injection induced a progressive PLN enlargement up to day 180, the last time-point tested. By that time the weight increase of the draining PLN had reached values of up to 200 times of that of the contralateral PLN (Stark, Hilscher, Gleichmann et al., manuscript in preparation). Quartz was also exceptional in that the lymph node enlargement induced did not require presence of T lymphocytes [62]; this is compatible with the notion that quartz is not an antigen. Quartz is known to act on macrophages selectively. It is phagocytosed by these cells and, before killing them, it activates the macrophages to release factors which secondarily activate lymphocytes. Quartz is not degradable and cannot be eliminated from the body. Once quartz crystals have killed the first generation of macrophages through the abrasive action of their sharp edges, they are taken up by

TABLE 1

Chemicals that have been screened by the PLN weight assay in mice; survey of results obtained by Gleichmann and colleagues[a]

Compound tested	Maximal PLN weight index obtained[b]
A. Drugs	
captopril	+
enalapril	+ +
D-penicillamine	+ +
gold sodium thiomalate	±
hydralazine	−
isoniazid	−
α-methyldopa	−
phenobarbital	−
phenytoin (diphenylhydantoin, dilantin)	+ +
procainamide	−
streptozotocin	+ +
B. Other compounds	
cadmium chloride ($CdCl_3$)	+
gold chloride ($AuCl_3$)	+ +
lead acetate ($(CH_3COO)_2Pb \cdot 3H_2O$)	−
mercuric chloride ($HgCl_3$)	+
methylmercury (CH_3HgCl)	+
quartz (SiO_2)	+ +

[a] For detailed information, see [35 – 39, 61].
[b] − denotes index < 1.3;
  ± denotes index between 1.5 and 2.0;
  + denotes index between 2.0 and 4.0;
  + + denotes index > 4.0.

a second generation of macrophages − which in turn are then activated, killed, and so on [63]. Thus, in the case of quartz the PLNA reflects non-specific, immunostimulatory properties of the test compound.

6. EVALUATION OF THE PLNA AS A TEST PREDICTING THE IMMUNOSTIMULATORY AND/OR SENSITIZING POTENTIAL OF XENOBIOTICS

Currently, the most frequently used method for assessing the immunogenicity of new chemicals, if immunogenicity is tested at all, is the Magnusson Kligman test which assesses the potential of a compound to induce contact dermatitis in the guinea pig. Although well standardized, this test has a number of limitations:

378

(1) While the skin is a relevant target organ in immunotoxicology and allergy, topical administration to the skin is not the only and not the most frequent route of exposure to chemicals in man.

(2) In order to be a contact sensitizer, a chemical must bind to Langerhans cells in the skin and thus be presented to circulating T cells. It is known, however, that a number of soluble xenobiotics do not fulfil this requirement because they readily penetrate the skin, so that sensitization is only manifest in the lymphoid organs, such as the lymph nodes and spleen, but not in the skin.

(3) Testing for contact dermatitis involves subjective scoring of the lesion.

(4) Testing for contact dermatitis does not readily provide access to the sensitised lymphocytes which are needed for advanced immunological and toxicological studies.

(5) Compared with the guinea pig, the rat and mouse are relatively insensitive species with respect to contact hypersensitivity, but those two species are most frequently used in toxicology and immunology.

The PLNA in laboratory rodents may overcome some of these limitations. Its essential features can be summarised as follows:

(1) There is no anatomic variation in either the localisation or the number of PLN in one hind leg; thus, preparation of the PLN is a simple and reliable procedure.

(2) To elicit a primary or secondary PLN reaction, the test compound is administered as a single injection without adjuvant.

(3) In the same animal, the contralateral PLN provides an internal control.

(4) Measurement of the PLN weight is an *objective* parameter, and not liable to subjective readings by different investigators. The same is true for other parameters that can be used in conjunction with the PLN weight assay, such as determination of the cell number in the PLN, ^{3}H-thymidine uptake by the PLN, and analysis of PLN cells by flow immunocytometry. As we propose use of the PLNA in conjunction with toxicological studies, it is worthwhile mentioning that in the rat the values of PLN indices usually are higher than in the mouse.

(5) It should be emphasized that by no means all the compounds tested in the PLNA were able to induce a primary PLN reaction [35, 41; Table 1]. Therefore, the PLNA is suited to compare the immunogenicity and/or immunostimulatory effect of closely related chemical compounds and thus establish structure-activity relationships [36, 40, 41].

In untreated mice, the PLN weight index ranges from about 0.8 to about 1.2; indices above 1.5 suggest and those above 2.0 indicate an immunological reaction to the test compound. During the primary PLN response to small chemicals or conventional antigens, the maximal response in the mouse very rarely exceeds a PLN weight index of 10. However, determination of cell number in, and ^{3}H-thymidine uptake by the PLN, are more sensitive methods so that the corresponding PLN indices calculated from such determinations are higher than the PLN weight index. The primary PLN response to most immunogenic chemicals tested peaked within the first 10 days after injection and returned back to normal by week 3 to 4; exceptions from this rule were seen with high dosages of heavy metals, such as $HgCl_2$ [39], and, in particular, with quartz (SiO_2) (see Section IV.5. in this chapter).

Quartz also proved to be exceptional in that the PLN response to this agent did not require presence of T lymphocytes. By contrast, in all other instances where this was tested, the PLN response to xenobiotics was T cell dependent [35 – 38, 40, 41]. Furthermore, whenever this was tested the PLN response to small chemicals proved to be antigen-specific. Specificity was proven by the fact that primed mice showed an enhanced PLN response following a second injection of the same compound, but not following injection of a structurally related compound [37, 38].

Like other tests, the PLNA has a number of shortcomings, too. These can be summarized as follows:

(1) Only material capable of passing through a small hypodermic needle can be tested by the PLNA; water-insoluble material cannot or can only be tested with difficulty. When such material can be solubilized in solvents, such as DMSO, controls assessing the immunogenic and/or immunostimulatory effect of the solvent have to be performed [40, 41].

(2) There may be 'false' negative reactions. Out of a variety of different drugs known to have adverse immunological side effects in man most induced a primary PLN enlargement. Exceptions included such notorious autoimmunizing agents as hydralazine and procainamide (Table 1). The reasons for these 'false' negative results are not known. There is a general impression that the immunogenic and/or immunostimulatory effects of chemical compounds, as detected by the PLNA, increase with their lipophilicity [41]. Moreover, as with D-pen, the pH of solvent can influence the immunogenicity of a drug screened by the PLNA [37]. It is also possible, however, that hydralazine and procainamide cause drug-induced SLE by mechanisms other than sensitization of specific T_h cells (cf. chapters by Sim, Hein and Weber, and Rubin, in this volume).

(3) Detecting the immunogenic and/or immunostimulatory property of a given chemical in the PLNA does not necessarily predict, of course, that this material will induce clinically relevant immunological side effects in humans exposed to that chemical. A positive PLN reaction merely indicates that the compound tested may provide a risk with respect to such side effects. Considering the complexity of immunologic and pharmacologic processes involved in chemical-induced immunopathological disorders, no conclusions can be drawn on the basis of one set of data alone, and additional immunological tests have to be performed in such cases.

Injection of chemicals into hind footpad is admittedly an artificial maneuver. In real life, most chemicals are taken up via other routes, for example, orally, respiratory or parenterally, so that the mesenteric and mediastinal lymph nodes and the spleen, respectively, are the candidate lymphoid organs that would harbor sensitized T lymphocytes. Trying to detect such T cells by specific re-stimulation with the test compound in a proliferation assay in vitro is technically demanding and much too often unsuccessful. It is of great practical importance, therefore, to have a relatively simple test system in which mesenteric, mediastinal or splenic T lymphocytes from rodents, which have received a chemical in the context of *conventional* toxicity testing, can be assayed for possible sensitization to that chemical. Such a test system has recently been developed in the form of an *adoptive transfer system* that employs the PLNA as the final indicator system (Fig. 4).

The transfer experiment employing the PLNA showed that memory T cells from the spleen of a donor mouse, which had been sensitized to a drug by multiple i.p. injections several weeks previously, can specifically be re-stimulated to trigger a secondary PLN response in the recipient [38]. It should be emphasized here that the spleens of the donor animals, which harbored the specifically sensitized T cells, were inconspicuous by histopathological criteria. Thus, these sensitized T cells would have gone undetected by the 'extented histopathology program', which has recently been recommended for use in immunotoxicology; they reacted vigorously, however, upon re-encounter with the sensitizing chemical.

The optimal conditions for this adoptive transfer system need to be worked out. It should be tested, for instance, if the chemical will also be recognized by the transferred memory T cells when it is administered to the prospective recipient via the route and at a dosage that represents a more realistic exposure to that chemical, rather than injected into the footpad along with the donor T cells. This should allow measurement of T cell reactions to immunologically relevant metabolites, provided these reach the circulation. In our experience, measuring specific T cell responses to simple chemicals by *in vivo* tests, such as the PLNA, has a much greater chance of succeeding than trying to do so by specific (re)stimulation of T cells *in vitro* using the same chemicals, e.g. DPH, D-pen, and STZ. A major problem of T cell proliferation tests performed *in vitro* seems to be the proper presentation of the chemical, or its relevant metabolite, to the T cells.

In conclusion, the PLNA is a rapid and objective, but also adaptable method for assessing the immunogenicity and/or immunostimulatory effect of xenobiotics in the pre-clinical phase. It can detect specific T cell responses to test compounds and, in this respect, is superior to both histopathological examination of lymphoid tissues and assessment of specific T cell responses in vitro. In addition, the PLNA can detect non-specific, T cell independent responses to immunologic response modifiers, such as quartz, which is immunostimulatory without being an antigen. Finally, by using an adoptive transfer system, the PLNA also lends itself to answer the question of whether T cells of animals that have undergone a repeated exposure regime in routine toxicology are primed by that chemical or a metabolite.

In our view, efforts should be undertaken to determine if, indeed, the PLNA is of general use for routine testing in immunotoxicology. Such efforts should include (1) standardization of the PLNA, (2) comparison with related assays, in particular the Magnusson Kligman test, (3) further evaluation of the adoptive transfer protocol using compounds other than STZ and using known metabolites of such test compounds, and (4) validation of the PLNA. Clearly, this task surpasses the capacity of a single laboratory. Therefore, a collective effort by several laboratories should be sponsored by the responsible agencies in order to achieve this goal.

V. Autoimmunizing and IgE-enhancing effects of $HgCl_2$ in mice

In contrast to the autoimmunizing side effects of drugs which are well documented, very little is known about the autoimmunizing potential of occupational and environmental chemicals. A possible exception to this is mercury (Hg). Hg compounds have been shown to cause an SLE-like autoimmune syndrome as well as a marked increase in IgE formation in several rodent species, as shown in Table 2. A prominent feature of the Hg-induced autoimmune syndrome in rodents is glomerulonephritis, and at least this disease has also been documented in humans exposed to mercurials (also shown in Table 2). As far as the IgE-enhancing effect of Hg is concerned, a striking increase in IgE production has been noted when peripheral blood lymphocytes obtained from normal human donors were cultured in the presence of both pokeweed mitogen and $HgCl_2$ [64]. The case reports of Hg-induced glomerulonephritis in man were made in cases of Hg poisoning or exposure to Hg as a constituent of drugs or cosmetic preparations. In all these cases, people were exposed over a relatively short period of time to high concentrations of Hg. While it is unknown whether or not the concentrations of Hg existing at the workplace and in the environment constitute a risk with regard to immunopathology, it is noteworthy that the immunopathological signs inducible by Hg are not confined to certain Hg compounds or routes of administration of such compounds [65, 66]. Furthermore, the dosages of $HgCl_2$ that induce autoimmune disease and enhanced IgE formation in rodents are clearly below the dose range in which general toxicity is observed in these species ([67]; Stiller-Winkler et al., unpublished results).

Following the pioneering studies of Philippe Druet and coworkers in Paris, and of the group of Hoedemaker, Weening, and Fleuren in The Netherlands, who performed experiments in the rat ([67, 71, 73] and Druet et al., this volume), several groups have recently started to establish mouse models of Hg-induced autoimmunity and enhanced IgE formation. The mouse is more advantageous for such studies since, in this species, the immunology, genetics, and molecular biology are more fully understood than in the rat. A survey of the results obtained by administration of Hg compounds to rats and mice is given in Table 2. As can been seen from this Table, most of the immunopathological signs inducible by Hg compounds in the rat have also been induced by Hg administration to mice. As in the rat, strong genetic factors, coded for by both MHC and non-MHC loci, determine the susceptibility and resistance of mice to the immunopathological effects of $HgCl_2$ [59]. Studies of

TABLE 2

Survey of autoimmune and other immunopathological symptoms induced by exposure to mercury compounds of humans and genetically susceptible strains of rat and mouse, respectively

Species studied	Mercury compounds studied	Route of application	Pathological symptom induced	Selected references
Man	Various Hg-containing drugs and ointments	Oral, percutaneous, and various routes of injection	Membraneous glomerulonephritis with granular IgG deposits in the mesangium and at the glomerular basement membrane	[68, 69]
			Contact dermatitits and other forms of dermatitis	[70]
			Enhanced IgE formation in vitro	[64]
Rat	$HgCl_2$, CH_3HgCl, Hg-containing drugs and ointments	Respiratory, intraperitoneal, oral, percutaneous, subcutaneous	Lymphadenopathy, splenomegaly	[66, 67, 71]
			Lymphocytic infiltration of salivary glands and intestinal mucosa	[72]
			Intravascular blood coagulation	[67]
			IgG autoantibodies against the glomerular basement membrane	[67, 71]
			Membranous glomerulonephritis with granular IgG deposits in the mesangium and at the glomerular basement membrane	[67, 71, 73]
			IgG deposits in the walls of blood vessels	[67, 71]
			IgG autoantibodies to various nuclear antigens and other autoantibodies	[73]
			Polyclonal B cell stimulation	[67, 71]

TABLE 2 *(continued)*

Species studied	Mercury compounds studied	Route of application	Pathological symptom induced	Selected references
			Extreme increase in total serum IgE and, if antigen is administered simultaneously, formation of specific IgE antibodies	[67, 71]
Mouse	$HgCl_2$, methyl- $-Hg^+$	Oral, intramuscular, subcutaneous	Lymphadenopathy	[39, 74]
			Membranous glomerulonephritis with deposits of IgG, especially IgG_1, in the mesangium and capillary walls	[75 – 80]
			IgG deposits in the walls of blood vessels	[75, 77, 78]
			Increased Ig-producing cells in the spleen	[81]
			Increase in serum IgG, especially IgG_1	[78, 81]
			Increased serum IgE	[81]
			IgG antinuclear and antinucleolar autoantibodies	[59, 77, 79, 80, 82]

the cellular pathogenesis of $HgCl_2$-induced immunopathology in mice, however, are not advanced as far as in the rat.

In the rat, all the immunopathological phenomena inducible by $HgCl_2$ are T cell dependent because they failed to develop in $HgCl_2$-treated athymic animals [83], and, as far as studied, this is also the case in mice [39]. It has been noted that the pathological alterations of $HgCl_2$-induced autoimmunity resemble those of chronic GVH disease [14, 71]. This analogy can also be extended to the enhancement of IgE production because F_1 hybrid mice undergoing chronic GVH disease also show an increased IgE concentration in their serum (Pietsch and Vohr, unpublished). As outlined above, chronic GVH disease is caused by an excessive activation of T_h cells which, secondarily, activate other immune cells, in particular B cells; the latter then produce antibodies, especially SLE-like autoantibodies of the IgG-isotype [14].

In HgCl$_2$-induced autoimmunity, too, there is an excessive activation T$_h$ cells [71]. This suggests that there is a common final pathway leading to SLE-like autoimmunity and enhanced IgE production in both chronic GVH disease and Hg-induced autoimmunity.

The mechanism, however by which T$_h$ cells are activated by exposure to Hg might differ from that operating during the GVH reaction. In chronic GVH disease, the number of T$_h$ cells activated is restricted to those donor T$_h$ cell clones that possess specific receptors for the F$_1$ recipient's allogeneic histocompatibility antigens. HgCl$_2$, by contrast, appears to activate T$_h$ cells in a non-specific mitogen-like fashion [84]. This generalized activation of T$_h$ cells appears to include activation of autoreactive T$_h$ cells [85]. Conceivably, HgCl$_2$ activates the expression of immunoregulatory genes, such as that of interleukin-4. Interleukin-4 is a product of T$_h$ cells that induce B cells to switch from the production of IgM and IgG$_3$ to that of IgG$_1$ and IgE. On the other hand, however, it is worth mentioning that HgCl$_2$, when applied to the skin, is a potent contact sensitizer [70, 86], which implies that it generates epitopes that are recognized by specific T cells. Hence, Hg^{2+} might activate T$_h$ cells by two different mechanisms, a non-specific mechanism and a specific one initiated by Hg^{2+}-induced epitopes on lymphoid and/or antigen-presenting cells.

Mice carrying the H-2^s haplotype, such as A.SW, B10.S, and SJL, are highly susceptible to the autoimmunizing and IgE-enhancing effect of HgCl$_2$ [59, 77, 79 – 82]. Within the H-2 complex, class II loci, most likely I-A$_\alpha$A$_\beta$, are decisive [59, 87]. Thus, induction by HgCl$_2$ of antinucleolar autoantibodies clearly depends on the presence of permissive MHC class II molecules. This strongly suggests that, as in the rat, reactions of specific T$_h$ cells are involved in the pathogenesis. At the present time it is unclear, however, what these T$_h$ cells recognize. One possibility is that the permissive MHC class II molecules on lymphoid cells are directly altered by Hg^{2+} ions; this possibility is reminiscent of contact dermatitis and, if it occurs, would result in GVH-like reactions of T$_h$ cells. Another possibility is that HgCl$_2$ alters the self antigens to which autoantibodies are produced, notably the autoantigens present in the nucleolus. While at the time being there is no evidence favoring the latter possibility, characterization of the relevant nucleolar antigen has considerably progressed. It is a small ribonucleoprotein, termed U3 snRNP, which has a size of 36 kDa and a pI of 8.6 [88, 89]. Strains of mice, such as NZB/W, which spontaneously develop non-organ-specific autoimmune syndromes, only very rarely produce antinucleolar autoantibodies. Interestingly, however, U3 snRNP is also recognized by IgG autoantibodies present in patients with idiopathic scleroderma. At least in the scleroderma-like syndrome developing in HgCl$_2$-treated SJL mice, antinucleolar autoantibodies are also pathogenetically relevant because they are responsible for the glomerulonephritis seen in these mice [77].

VI. Conclusions

Adverse immunological reactions to drugs, both autoimmune and allergic, are well-documented, frequent and often serious events in humans. The pathogenesis of these disorders is poorly understood, however. Immunological theory and available experimental evidence favors the notion that many of these reactions are initiated by specific T lymphocytes towards the drug, or a metabolite, bound to the cell surface. The work reviewed in this chapter focuses on the spectrum of GVH-like immunological diseases caused by chemicals. The experimental evidence supporting the concept of GVH-like pathogenesis has been reviewed here. Apart from specific T cell reactions towards cell-bound chemicals, certain chemicals appear to activate T_h cells by different mechanisms, such as the mitogen-like activity of $HgCl_2$. From an analytical point of view, studying chemical-induced immunopathological diseases is a fascinating subject, because chemicals with selective immunological effects can be used as probes for both the immune system and the frequently obscure pathogenesis of immunological diseases.

It is desirable that new chemicals be tested for potential immunogenicity before they are marketed. From a practical point of view, the PLNA, which was extensively reviewed in this chapter, might offer a number of advantages over other tests currently in use. A newly developed *adoptive transfer system using the PLNA* appears to be especially promising for detecting specific T cells that have been primed to a given compound during the course of routine toxicological testing of that compound. As we pointed out, this test needs validation before it can be recommended for use in routine (immuno)toxicology. Collective efforts by several laboratories should be undertaken to achieve this goal, and this endeavour should be supported by responsible agencies.

Acknowledgements

This study was supported in parts by Grant No. 422-4001-01VM86 149 from the Federal Ministry of Research and Technology, Bonn, a grant from the Krupp Foundation, Essen, and Grant No. G1 131/1-1 from the Deutsche Forschungsgemeinschaft, Bonn, FRG.

References

1. Gleichmann, E. and Gleichmann, H. (1976) Diseases caused by reactions of T-lymphocytes to incompatible structures of the major histocompatibility complex. I. Autoimmune hemolytic anemia. Eur. J. Immunol. 6, 899–906.
2. Gleichmann, E., Van Elven, E. H. and Van der Veen, J. P. W. (1982) A systemic lupus erythematosus (SLE)-like disease in mice induced by abnormal T-B-cell cooperation. Preferential

formation of autoantibodies characteristic of SLE. Eur. J. Immunol. 12, 152 – 158.

3. Van Rappard-Van der Veen, F. M., Kiesel, U., Poels, L., Schuler, W., Melief, C. J. M., Landegent, J. and Gleichmann, E.   (1984)   Further evidence against random polyclonal antibody formation in mice with lupus-like graft-versus-host disease. J. Immunol. 132, 1814 – 1820.

4. Van Rappard-Van der Veen, F. M., Rolink, A. G. and Gleichmann, E.   (1982)   Diseases caused by reactions of T lymphocytes towards incompatible structures of the major histocompatibility complex. VI. Autoantibodies characteristic of systemic lupus erythematosus induced by abnormal T-B-cell cooperation across I-E. J. Exp. Med. 155, 1555 – 1560.

5. Rolink, A. G., Pals, S. T. and Gleichmann, E.   (1983)   Allosuppressor- and allohelper-T cells in acute and chronic graft-versus-host disease. II. F_1 recipients carrying mutations at H-2K and/or I-A. J. Exp. Med. 157, 755 – 771.

6. Rolink, A. G. and Gleichmann, E.   (1983)   Allosuppressor- and allohelper-T cells in acute and chronic graft-versus-host diseases. III. Different Lyt subsets of donor T cells induce different pathological syndromes. J. Exp. Med. 158, 546 – 558.

7. Pals, S. T., Radszkiewicz, T. and Gleichmann, E.   (1984)   Allosuppressor- and allohelper-T cells in acute and chronic graft-versus-host disease. IV. Activation of donor allosuppressor cells is confined to acute GVHD. J. Immunol. 132, 1669 – 1678.

8. Rolink, A. G., Gleichmann, H. and Gleichmann, E.   (1983)   Diseases caused by reactions of T lymphocytes to incompatible structures of the major histocompatibility complex. VII. Immune-complex glomerulonephritis. J. Immunol. 130, 209 – 215.

9. Van Rappard-Van der Veen, F.M., Radaszkiewicz, T., Terraneo, L. and Gleichmann, E.   (1983)   Attempts at standardization of lupus-like graft-versus-host disease: inadvertent repopulation by DBA/2 spleen cells of H-2-different non-irradiated F_1 mice. J. Immunol. 130, 2693 – 2701.

10. Pals, S. T., Radaszkiewicz, T., Roozendaal, L. and Gleichmann, E.   (1985)   Chronic progressive polyarthritis and other symptoms of collagen vascular disease induced graft-versus-host reaction. J. Immunol. 134, 1475 – 1482.

11. Rolink, A. G., Radaszkiewicz, T., Pals, S. T., Van der Meer, W. and Gleichmann, E.   (1982)   Allosuppressor- and allohelper-T cells in acute and chronic graft-versus-host disease. I. Alloreactive suppressor cells rather than killer T cells appear to be the decisive effector cells in lethal graft-versus-host disease. J. Exp. Med. 155, 1501 – 1522.

12. Pals, S. T., Gleichmann, H. and Gleichmann, E.   (1984)   Allosuppressor- and allohelper-T cells in acute and chronic graft-versus-host disease. V. F_1 mice with secondary chronic GVHD contain F_1-reactive allohelper but no allosuppressor T cells. J. Exp. Med. 159, 508 – 523.

13. Van Elven, E. H., Rolink, A. G., Van der Veen, F. and Gleichmann, E.   (1981)   Capacity of genetically different T lymphocytes to induce lethal graft-versus-host disease correlates with their capacity to generate suppression but not with their capacity to generate anti-F_1 Killer cells. A non-H-2 locus determines the inability to induce lethal graft-versus-host disease. J. Exp. Med. 153, 1474 – 1488.

14. Gleichmann, E., Pals, S. T., Rolink, A. G., Radaszkiewicz, T. and Gleichmann, H.   (1984)   Graft-versus-host reactions: clues to the etiopathology of a spectrum of immunological diseases. Immunol. Today 5, 324 – 332.

15. Rolink, A. G., Van der Meer, W. G. K., Melief, C. J. M. and Gleichmann, E.   (1983)   Intra-H-2 requirements for the induction of maximal positive and negative allogeneic effects in vitro. Eur. J. Immunol. 13, 191 – 197.

16. Gleichmann, E., Gleichmann, H. and Wilke, W.   (1976)   Autoimmunization and lymphomagenesis in parent → F_1 combinations differing at the major histocompatibility complex: model for spontaneous disease caused by altered self-antigens? Transplant. Rev. 31, 156 – 224.

17. Gleichmann, E., Van Elven, F. and Gleichmann, H.   (1979)   Immunoblastic lymphadenopathy, systemic lupus erythematosus and related disorders. Possible pathogenetic pathways. Am. J. Clin. Pathol. 72, 708 – 723.

18. Pals, S. T., Zijlstra, M., Radaszkiewicz, T., Quint, W., Cuypers, T., Schoenmakers, H. J., Melief, C. J. M., Berns, A. and Gleichmann, E. (1986) Immunological induction of malignant lymphoma: graft-versus-host reaction-induced-B-cell lymphomas contain reintegrations of several types of murine leukemia virus sequences. J. Immunol. 136, 331–339.

19. Kimura, M., Van Rappard-Van der Veen, F. M. and Gleichmann, E. (1986) Requirement of H-2-subregion differences for graft-versus-host autoimmunity in mice: superiority of the differences at Class-II H-2 antigens (I-A/I-E). Clin. Exp. Immunol. 65, 542–552.

19a. Via, C. S. and Schearer, G. M. (1988) T cell interactions in auto-immunity: insights from a murine model of graft-versus-host disease. Immunol. Today 9, 207–213.

20. Dighiero, G., Lymberi, P., Mazie, J.-C., Rouyre, S., Butler-Browne, G. S., Whalen, R. G. and Avrameas, S. (1983) Murine hybridomas secreting natural monoclonal antibodies reacting with self-antigens. J. Immunol. 131, 2267–2272.

21. Kuppers, R. C., Suiter, T., Gleichmann, E. and Rose, N. R. (1988) The induction of organ-specific antibodies during the graft-versus-host reaction. Eur. J. Immunol. 18, 161–166.

22. Ptak, W., Rewicka, M. and Marcinkiewicz, J. (1984) Induction of 'allogeneic effect'-like reaction by syngeneic TNP-modified lymphoid cells. Immunobiology 166, 368–381.

23. Claas, F. H. J. and Van Rood, J. J. (1985) The interaction of drugs and endogenous substances with HLA class-I antigens. Prog. Allergy 36, 135–150.

24. De Weck, A. L. (1983) Penicillins and cephalosporins, In: A. L. De Weck and J. O. Bundgaard (Eds.), Handbook of Experimental Pharmacology, Vol. 63: Allergic Reactions to Drugs, Springer, Berlin, pp. 423–482.

25. Beaune, P. H., Dansette, P. M., Mansuy, D., Kiffel, L., Finck, M., Amar, C., Leroux, J. P. and Homberg, J. C. (1987) Human anti-endoplasmic reticulum autoantibodies appearing in a drug-induced hepatitis are directed against a human liver cytochrome P-450 that hydroxylates the drug. Proc. Natl. Acad. Sci. USA 84, 551–555.

26. Merk, H., Schneider, R. and Scholl, P. (1988) Lymphocyte stimulation by drug-modified microsomes. In: R. W. Estabrook, E. Lindenlaub, F. Oesch and A. L. de Weck (Eds.), Toxicological and Immunological Aspects of Drug Metabolism and Environmental Chemicals, Symposia Medica Hoechst, Vol. 22, Schattauer, Stuttgart/New York, in press.

27. Gleichmann, E. and Gleichmann, H. (1976) Graft-versus-host reaction: a pathogenetic principle for the development of drug allergy, autoimmunity, and malignant lymphoma in non-chimeric individuals. Hypothesis. Z. Krebsforsch. 85, 91–109.

28. Shelby, H. J., Rothman, S. J. and Buckley, R. H. (1980) Phenytoin hypersensitivity. J. Allergy Clin. Immunol. 66, 166–172.

29. Rosenthal, C. J., Noguera, C. A., Coppola, A. and Kapelner, S. N. (1982) Pseudolymphoma with mycosis fungoides manifestations, hyperresponsiveness to diphenylhydantoin, and lymphocyte disregulation. Cancer 49, 2305–2314.

30. Jaffe, I. A. (1979) Penicillamine in rheumatoid arthritis: clinical pharmacology and biochemical properties. Scand. J. Rheumatol., Suppl. 28, 58–64.

31. Emeson, E. E. and Thursh, D. R. (1973) Mechanism of graft-versus-host-induced lymphadenopathy in mice. J. Exp. Med. 137, 1293–1302.

32. Piguet, P. F., Dewey, H. K. and Vasalli, P. (1975) Study of the cells proliferating in parent versus F_1 hybrid mixed lymphocyte culture. J. Exp. Med. 141, 775–787.

33. Piguet, P. F., Dewey, H. K. and Vasalli, P. (1977) Origin and nature of the cells participating in the popliteal graft-versus-host reaction in mouse and rat. Cell Immunol. 31, 242–254.

34. Rolstad, B. (1976) The host component of the graft-versus-host reaction. A study on the popliteal LN reaction in the rat. Transplantation 21, 117–123.

35. Gleichmann, H. (1981) Studies on the mechanism of drug sensitization: T cell dependent popliteal lymph node reaction to diphenylhydantoin. Clin. Immunol. Immunopathol. 18, 203–211.

388

36. Gleichmann, H., Pals, S. T. and Radaszkiewicz, T. (1983) T cell dependent B-cell proliferation and activation induced by administration of the drug-diphenylhydantoin to mice. Hematol. Oncol. 1, 165 – 176.

37. Hurtenbach, U., Gleichmann, H., Nagata, N. and Gleichmann, E. (1987) Immunity to D-penicillamine: genetic, cellular, and chemical requirements for induction of popliteal lymph node enlargement in the mouse. J. Immunol. 139, 411 – 416.

38. Klinkhammer, C., Popowa, P. and Gleichmann, H. (1988) Specific immunity to the diabetogen streptozotocin: cellular requirements for induction of lymphoproliferation. Diabetes 37, 74 – 80.

39. Stiller-Winkler, R., Radaszkiewicz, T. and Gleichmann, E. (1988) Immunpathological signs in mice treated with mercury compounds. I. Identification by the popliteal lymph node assay of responder and nonresponder strains. Int. J. Immunopharmacol. 10, 475 – 484.

40. Kammüller, M. E., Penninks, A. H., De Bakker, J. M., Thomas, C., Bloksma, N. and Seinen, W. (1987) An experimental approach to chemically induced systemic (auto)-immune alterations: the Spanish toxic oil syndrome as an example. In: B. A. Fowler (Ed.), Mechanisms of Cell Injury: implications for Human Health, J. Wiley and Sons Ltd., New York, Chichester, Brisbane, pp. 175 – 192.

41. Kammüller, M. E. and Seinen, W. (1988) Structural requirements for hydantoins and 2-thiohydantoins to induce lymphoproliferative popliteal lymph node reactions in the mouse. Int. J. Immunopharmacol., in press.

42. Seeman, P. (1972) The membrane actions of anesthetics and tranquilizers. Pharmacol. Rev. 24, 584 – 655.

43. Dudley, K. H. (1980) Phenytoin metabolism. In: Th.M. Hassell, M. C. Johnston and K. H. Dudley (Eds.), Phenytoin-induced Teratology and Gingival Pathology, Raven Press, pp. 13 – 24.

44. Feltkamp, T. E. W., Ed. (1979) Fundamental studies on penicillamine for rheumatoid diseases. Scand. J. Rheumatol., Suppl. 28, 13 – 20.

45. Zilko, P. J. and Dawkins, R. L. (1982) D-Penicillamine-immunogenetics of effects and side effects. In: R. L. Dawkins, F. T. Christiansen and P. J. Zilko (Eds.), Immunogenetics in Rheumatology, Musculoskeletal Disease and D-Penicillamine, Excerpta Medica, Amsterdam, pp. 280 – 375.

46. Dequeker, J., Van Wanghe, P. and Verdickt, W. (1984) A systemic survey of HLA-A, B, C and D antigens and drug toxicity in rheumatoid arthritis. J. Rheumatol. 11, 282 – 289.

47. Chalmers, A., Thompson, D., Stein, H. E., Reid, G. and Patterson, A. C. (1982) Systemic lupus erythematosus during penicillamine therapy for rheumatoid arthritis. Ann. Intern. Med. 97, 659 – 663.

48. Kolb, H., Toyka, K. and Gleichmann, E., (1987) Histocompatibility antigens and chemical reactivity in autoimmunity. Immunol. Today 8, 3 – 6.

49. Nagata, N., Hurtenbach, U. and Gleichmann, E. (1986) Specific sensitization of Lyt 1^+2^- T cells to spleen cells modified by the drug D-penicillamine or a stereoisomer. J. Immunol. 136, 136 – 142.

50. Binderup, L. and Arrigoni-Martelli, E. (1979) ^{14}C-D-Penicillamine: uptake and distribution in rat lymphocytes and macrophages. Biochem. Pharmacol. 28, 189 – 192.

51. Sunshine, G. H., Katz, D. R. and Feldmann, M. (1980) Dendritic cells induce T cell proliferation to synthetic antigens under Ir gene control. J. Exp. Med. 152, 1817 – 1822.

52. Steinman, R. M., Kaplan, G., Witmer, M. D. and Cohen, Z. A. (1979) Identification of a novel cell type in peripheral organs of mice. V. Purification of spleen dendritic cells, new surface markers, and maintenance in vitro. J. Exp. Med. 149, 1 – 16.

53. Alexander, M. D. and Carrick, B. M. (1983) Selective action of D-penicillamine on guinea pig peritoneal macrophage Fc gamma receptors for homologous monomeric IgG_1. Immunol. Lett. 6, 219 – 222.

54. Martinez-Alonso, C., Coutinho, A., Bernabe, R. R., Augustin, A., Haas, W. and Pohlit, H.

(1980) Hapten-specific helper T cells. I. Collaboration with B cells to which the hapten has been directly coupled. Eur. J. Immunol. 10, 403 – 410.

55. Miller, S. D., Wetzig, R. P. and Claman, H. N.   (1979)   The induction of cell-mediated immunity and tolerance with protein antigens coupled to syngeneic lymphoid cells. J. Exp. Med. 149, 758 – 773.

56. Polisson, R. P., Fujiwara, H. and Shearer, G. M.   (1980)   H-2 linked genetic control of priming for secondary cytotoxic responses to autologous cells modified with low concentrations of trinitrobenzene sulfonate. J. Immunol. 124, 349 – 354.

57. Eastman, A. Y. and Lawrence, D. A.   (1982)   TNP-modified syngeneic cells enhance immunoregulatory T cell activities similar to allogeneic effects. J. Immunol. 128, 926 – 931.

58. Donker, A. J., Venuto, R. C., Vladutiu, A. O., Brentjens, J. R. and Andres, G. A.   (1984)   Effects of prolonged administration of D-penicillamine or captopril in various strains of rats. Brown Norway rats treated with D-penicillamine develop autoantibodies, circulating immune complexes, and disseminated intravascular coagulation. Clin. Immunol. Immunopathol. 30, 142 – 155.

59. Robinson, C. H. G., Balazs, T. and Egorov, I. K.   (1986)   Mercuric chloride-, gold sodium thiomalate-, and D-penicillamine-induced antinuclear antibodies in mice. Toxicol. Appl. Pharmacol. 86, 159 – 169.

60. Panayi, G. S., Huston, G., Shah, R. R., Mitchell, S. C., Idle, J. R. L. and Waring, R. H.   (1983)   Deficient sulphoxidation status and D-penicillamine. Lancet 1, 414.

61. Gleichmann, H. and Klinkhammer, C.   (1988)   Predictive tests in immune reactions to drugs. In: R. W. Estabrook, E. Lindenlaub, F. Oesch and A. L. de Weck (Eds.), Toxicological and Immunological Aspects of Drug Metabolism and Environmental Chemicals, Symposia Medica Hoechst, Vol. 22, Schattauer, Stuttgart/New York, in press.

62. Zaidi, S. H., Hilscher, B., Hilscher, W., Brassel, D. and Grover, R.   (1979)   Vergleichende morphometrische und autoradiographische Untersuchungen quarzinduzierter Läsionen bei nu/nu-Mäusen und Kontrollmäusen. Ergebnisse von Untersuchungen auf dem Gebiet der Staub und Silikosebekämpfung im Steinkohlenbergbau. Verlag Glückauf, Essen, 12, 187 – 192.

63. Davis, G. S.   (1986)   The pathogenesis of silicosis. State of the art. Chest 89, 166S – 169S.

64. Kimata, H. Shinomiya, K. and Mikawa, H.   (1983)   Selective enhancement of human IgE production in vitro by synergy of pokeweed mitogen and mercuric chloride. Clin. Exp. Immunol. 53, 183 – 191.

65. Druet, P., Teychenne, P., Mandet, C., Bascou, C. and Druet, E.   (1981)   Immune-type glomerulonephritis induced in the Brown-Norway rat with mercury-containing pharmaceutical products. Nephron 28, 145 – 148.

66. Bernaudin, J. F., Druet, E., Druet, P. and Masse, R.   (1981)   Inhalation or ingestion of organic or inorganic mercurials produces auto-immune disease in rats. Clin. Immunol. Immunopathol. 20, 129 – 135.

67. Druet, P., Sapin, C., Druet, E. and Hirsch, F.   (1983)   Genetic control of mercury-induced immune response in the rat. In: G. A. Porter (Ed.), Nephrotoxic Mechanisms of Drugs and Environmental Toxins, Plenum Medical Book Company, New York/London, pp. 425 – 435.

68. Fillastre, J. P., Mery, J. P., Morel-Maroger, L., Kanfer, A. and Goden, M.   (1984)   Drug-induced glomerulonephritis. In: K. Solez, and A. Whelton (Eds.), Acute Renal Failure, M. Dekker, New York, Basel. pp. 389 – 407.

69. Tubbs, R. R., Gephardt, G. N., Mahon, J. T., Pohl, M. C., Vidt, D. G., Barenberg, S. A. and Valenzuela, R.   (1982)   Membranous glomerulonephritis associated with industrial mercury exposure. Study of pathogenetic mechanisms. Am. J. Clin. Pathol. 77, 409 – 413.

70. Taugner, M. and Schütz, R.   (1966)   Beitrag zur Quecksilber-Allergie. Dermatologica 133, 245 – 261.

71. Druet, P., Hirsch, F., Pelletier, L., Druet, E., Baran, D. and Sapin, C.   (1987)   Mechanisms of chemical-induced glomerulonephritis. In: B. A. Fowler (Ed.), Mechanisms of Cell Injury, Implica-

tions for Human Health, Wiley and Sons Ltd., New York, Chichester, Brisbane, pp. 153 – 173.

72. Aten, J. and Weening, J. (1987) In: H. Kolb, K. V. Toyka and E. Gleichmann (Eds.), Histocompatibility antigens and chemical reactivity in autoimmunity (Workshop report). Immunol. Today 8, 3 – 6.

73. Weening, J. J., Hoedemaeker, J. and Bakker, W. W. (1981) Immunoregulation and antinuclear antibodies in mercury-induced glomerulopathy in the rat. Clin. Exp. Immunol. 45, 64 – 71.

74. Stiller-Winkler, R., Michelmann, I. and Gleichmann, E. (1986) Genetic differences in the susceptibility of mouse strains to $CdCl_2$ respectively $HgCl_2$ detected by the popliteal lymph node assay (PLNA), Naunyn-Schmiedeberg's Arch. Pharmacol. Suppl. 334, 171.

75. Albini, B., Glurich, I. and Anders, G. A. (1983) Mercuric chloride-induced immunologically mediated diseases in experimental animals. In: G.A. Porter (Ed.), Nephrotoxic Mechanisms of Drugs and Environmental Toxins, Plenum Medical Books Comp., New York/London, pp. 413 – 423.

76. Fleuren, G. J., De Heer, E., Burgers, J. V., Osnabrugge, C. and Hoedemaeker, P. J. (1985) Mercuric chloride-induced autoimmune glomerulopathy in BALB/c mice. Kidney Int. 28, 702, Abstract.

77. Hultman, P. and Eneström, S. (1988) Mercury induced antinuclear antibodies in mice: characterization and correlation with renal immune complex deposits. Clin. Exp. Immunol. 71, 269 – 274.

78. Hultman, P. and Eneström, S. (1987) The induction of immune complex deposits in mice by peroral and parenteral administration of mercuric chloride: strain dependent susceptibility. Clin. Exp. Immunol. 67, 283 – 292.

79. Mirtschewa, A., Hallmann, B., Stark, M. and Gleichmann, E. (1986) Genetic differences in the induction of murine autoimmunity by respectively $HgCl_2$, gold sodium thiomalate (GST) and D-penicillamine. Naunyn-Schmiedeberg's Arch. Pharmacol. Suppl. 334, 172.

80. Mirtschewa, J., Nürnberger, W., Hallmann, B., Stiller-Winkler, R. and Gleichmann, E. (1987) Genetically determined susceptibility of mice to $HgCl_2$-induced antinuclear antibodies (ANA) and glomerulonephritis. Immunobiology 175, 323 – 324.

81. Pietsch, P., Allmeroth, M., Gleichmann, E. and Vohr, H. W. (1987) Increased synthesis of IgE, but not IgM, in strains of mice susceptible to $HgCl_2$. Immunobiology 175, 324.

82. Robinson, C. J. G., Abraham, A. A. and Balazs, T. (1984) Induction of anti-nuclear antibodies by mercuric chloride in mice. Clin. Exp. Immunol. 58, 300 – 306.

83. Pelletier, L., Pasquier, R., Vial, M. C., Mandet, C., Moutier, R., Salomon, J. C. and Druet, P. (1987) Mercury-induced autoimmune glomerulonephritis: requirements for T-cells. Nephrol. Dial. Transplant. 1, 211 – 218.

84. Reardon, C. L. and Lucas, D. O. (1987) Heavy-metal mitogenesis: Zn^{++} and Hg^{++} induce cellular cytotoxicity and interferon production in murine T lymphocytes. Immunobiology 175, 455 – 469.

85. Pelletier, L., Pasquier, R., Hirsch, F., Sapin, C. and Druet, P. (1986) Autoreactive T cells in mercury-induced autoimmune disease: in vitro demonstration. J. Immunol. 137, 2548 – 2554.

86. Polak, L., Barnes, J. M. and Turk, J. L. (1986) The genetic control of contact sensitization to inorganic metal compounds in guinea-pigs. Immunology 14, 707 – 711.

87. Gleichmann, E., Kavka, M., Stiller-Winkler, R. and Mirtschewa, J. (1988) Susceptibility to $HgCl_2$-induced antinucleolar autoantibodies (ANo1A) is determined by I-A, and concomitant expression of I-E seems to dampen it. Immunobiology, Abstract 178, 137.

88. Tessars, G., Reuter, R., Vohr, H. W., Gleichmann, E. and Lührmann, R. (1988) Mercuric chloride induces autoantibodies against U3 small nuclear ribonucleoprotein in susceptible mice. Immunobiology, Abstract 178, 149.

89. Reuter, R., Tessars, G., Vohr, H. W., Gleichmann, E. and Lührmann, R. (1988) Mercuric chloride induces autoantibodies against U3 small nuclear ribonucleoprotein in susceptible mice. Proc. Natl. Acad. Sci. USA, in press.

M.E. Kammüller, N. Bloksma and W. Seinen (Eds.)
Autoimmunity and Toxicology
© 1989 Elsevier Science Publishers B.V. (Biomedical Division)

The pathology of diphenylhydantoin-induced lymphoproliferative reactions in animals

16

GERHARD R.F. KRUEGER

Immunopathology Section, Pathology Institute, University of Cologne, D-5000 Cologne 41, FRG

I. Introduction

The drug 5,5-diphenylhydantoin (DPH; phenytoin; dilantin) was introduced into medicine in 1938 for the treatment of convulsive disorders [1, 2]. It is chemically related to the barbiturates, but exerts antiepileptic activities without general central nervous system (CNS) depression. The pharmacological effect is felt to be caused by stabilization of the threshold of neuronal excitability by promoting sodium efflux through activating the sodium pump in the cytoplasmic membrane [3]. Sodium extrusion is coupled to simultaneous calcium and potassium ion exchange and to hydrolysis of adenosine triphosphate (ATP). The latter releases high energy to be used for various cellular synthetic processes. Metabolic and synthetic pathways in general are regulated by changes in enzyme activities which are in part controlled by the intracellular calcium ion pool. In nerve cells, for instance, calcium ions function as second messenger in the initiation of neurotransmitter secretion [4].

This effect of DPH should by no means be specific for nerve cells but may also be seen in other tissues [5], since metabolic processes preceding cell activation resemble those in immunocompetent cells following the binding of antigens or of lectins to surface receptors [6]. Since attachment to the lymphocyte membrane of DPH as a hapten has been shown [7 – 9], stimulation and functional activation of lymphoid tissues by this drug must be expected, provided it will reach these tissues in effective doses. Binding of DPH to the lymphocyte membrane is probably non-specific through hydrophobic forces [10]. It may result in functional changes of the cell secondary to blocking of certain membrane receptors [11]. According to Babcock's cock's experiments with cats and rats [12], DPH is concentrated in salivary glands. Thus, through a secretion and reabsorption mechanism, effective DPH doses should be reached at least in lymph nodes draining the oropharynx and the gastrointestinal tract. The effect of DPH on cells, however, appears more complicated than being just a mechanism of transmembrane activation. Intracellularly, the drug will exert inhibitory influences on the production of cyclic adenosine phosphate (AMP) and on calcium-dependent activation of protein kinases [13]. DPH apparently interferes with calcium mobilization from intracellular reservoirs such as lysosome-like granules. Since phosphorylation of membrane proteins in lymphocytes through calcium-dependent protein phosphokinases is an essential step in lymphocyte activation following antigen binding, DPH may interfere as well with an effective cellular response to antigenic substances.

It exceeds the task of this chapter to further detail the molecular pharmacology of DPH action. The brief outline given yet may explain, why DPH belongs to the group of drugs in which atypical lymphoid reactions may be expected. It essentially can cause conditions of persistent immunostimulation and immunosuppression which have been identified before as being an important co-factor in the pathogenesis of malignant lymphomas [14, 15].

II. Clinical side effects in man

Toxic reactions following prolonged administration of DPH or related substances are usually mild and generally do not lead to discontinuation of therapy (side effects of acute overdose will not be discussed in this chapter). Most common in up to 40% of the patients on DPH for epilepsy is hyperplasia of the gums [16].

Occasional additional side effects, probably independent of immune disregulation, are hemorrhagic necrosis at the site of intramuscular injection, anorexia, vomiting and nausea, ataxia, hyperactive reflexes, nystagmus, mydriasis, blurring of vision, and head aches, keratosis of skin and hirsutism, cholestatic hepatosis, megaloblastic anemia, and eventually teratogenic effects [3, 17].

There is an accumulating number of publications, however, relating side effects of DPH therapy to its influence on the immune system.

1. IMMUNOSUPPRESSIVE EFFECTS OF DIPHENYLHYDANTOIN

B lymphocyte immunodeficiencies are among the most frequently documented defects complicating chronic DPH administration. Specifically, B lymphocytopenia in the peripheral blood was observed with decreased IgA and IgG, partially also low IgM, and persistent IgE increase [18–24]. In vitro studies suggest a direct effect of the drug on the B lymphocyte [25]. Since DPH apparently blocks the CD4 receptor of T helper cells [11], one wonders whether deficient IgG and IgA antibody production is additionally compromized by loss of T helper cell function. Further adding to this disturbance in antibody production and T cell help is an increased DPH-induced T suppressor cell activity [26, 27].

Concanavalin A (ConA) stimulation of lymphocytes in vitro is inhibited by DPH, yet this effect is abolished when macrophages are added to the culture [28]. Interestingly, this depressive effect is apparently restricted to DNA synthesis, while RNA and protein synthesis remain unaffected [29]. Stimulation of lymphocyte from patients on DPH treatment and of DNA synthesis by ConA and phytohemagglutin (PHA) [30, 31] is not inhibited, which in consideration of results of *in vitro* studies might be consistent with a regulatory influence of macrophages. However, DPH is added to tissue culture cells generally in significant larger doses than blood levels would be in patients.

Among other cell populations inhibited by DPH are natural killer cells and killer cells whose response is significantly repressed [32]. In the hematopoietic bone marrow, DPH causes a selective loss of stem cells in S-phase which can be restored by administration of thymic epithelial factors [33]. This observation suggests that the thymus is probably another primary target for DPH, since comparable depletion of hematopoietic stem cells occurs after thymectomy [34, 35].

Thus, there appears to exist a complex immunologic disregulation in patients on chronic DPH therapy involving functional defects of B and T lymphocytes, natural killer cells and killer cells, as well as probably thymic epithelial cells. We are currently far from conclusively explaining such defects, especially since they do not uniformly occur in all patients. The initially described IgG and IgA deficiency associated with increased IgE constitutes a condition which makes one expect allergic reactions.

2. ALLERGIC AND AUTOIMMUNE REACTIONS FOLLOWING DPH TREATMENT

As theoretically expected from the haptenic nature of the compound and from observed immunoglobulin imbalances, allergic and autoimmune reactions are not infrequent in patients on DPH therapy. They are listed in Table 1.

Comprehensive experimental studies as to the pathogenesis of such reactions were done by Gleichmann and associates [36, 37]. They are summarized in another chapter of this book [38] and will not be discussed here.

In essence, however, certain autoimmune diseases with their basic immunologic disregulation predispose patients for later development of malignant lymphomas [39].

TABLE 1

Allergic and autoimmune reactions following diphenylhydantoin therapy in man

Cardiovascular system
  hypersensitivity myocarditis
  hypersensitivity vasculitis
  serum sickness like syndrome

Respiratory system
  pleural effusions
  interstitial pneumonitis

Gastrointestinal system
  hepatitis, granulomatous mononucleosis-like

Urogenital system
  lupus glomerulonephritis (with or without systemic lupus erythematosus and antinuclear antibodies)
  nephrotic syndrome

Hematopoietic system
  allergic thrombocytopenia with purpura
  autoimmune anemia with anti-erythrocyte antibodies
  pure red cell aplasia
  anti-lymphocyte antibodies

Integument
  morbilliform rash
  erythema multiforme
  lupus dermatitis
  exfoliative dermatitis
  Stevens-Johnson syndrome
  toxic epidermal necrolysis

In addition multiple other pathologies probably unrelated to allergy (ref. to R.H. Riddel (1982) Pathology of Drug-Induced and Toxic Diseases, Churchill Livingstone, New York.)

3. ATYPICAL LYMPHOPROLIFERATION AND MALIGNANT LYMPHOMAS FOLLOWING DPH TREATMENT

Since Chiari's first description in 1951 of dilantin lymphadenopathy resembling Hodgkin's disease [40], similar reports were published at regular intervals [41 – 51]. The lesions observed included infectious mononucleosis-like syndromes, pseudo-lymphomas, immunoblastic lymphadenopathy and true malignant lymphomas (Hodgkin's and non-Hodgkin's lymphomas). Anthony [52] reported of a ten times increased incidence of lymphomas in epileptics on hydantoin therapy, yet the tumors were not further classified. Li and collaborators [53] calculated the lymphoma incidence in such patients even as being 1.6% (as compared to 12 per 100 000 for Hodgkin's and non-Hodgkin's lymphomas in the comparable population without DPH therapy). A study by Rausing [54] in Swedish patients of Malmö showed an apparent predominance of immunoblastic lymphomas.

Thus, the risk to develop atypical lymphoproliferation and malignant lymphomas appears significantly increased in patients on DPH treatment. Publications of quite different histological types of lymphomas in such patients suggest no simple carcinogenic action of DPH but rather a progression to malignancy following a combined carcinogenic, co-carcinogenic, and possibly genetic influence. Because of this stepwise development of malignant lymphomas, no clear-cut latent period can be given. Vice versa also unknown is the minimal dose or duration of DPH administered and causing lymphomas. If one attempts to conclude from the results of mouse experiments, it took at least 2 – 4 months of DPH treatment to obtain atypical lymphoproliferation or malignant lymphomas even in susceptible strains [67]. This would equal about 5 – 15 man years. Since we are discussing a selective human population (epileptics) without adequate controls (non-epileptics on chronic DPH treatment), genetic predispositions for atypical lymphoproliferation can not be excluded. In fact, HLA A2-linked IgA deficiency was observed in these patients preceding DPH treatment [55, 56], and IgA deficiency in other patients is associated with a higher risk of autoimmune disease and malignant lymphomas [6, 57]. On the other hand, chromosomal aberrations and sister chromatid exchange are apparently induced by DPH [58 – 61], indicating a direct effect of the drug on the genetic apparatus.

Whatever the pathogenetic effects of DPH are during the course of lymphoma development, they will probably be elucidated by detailed experimental studies rather than by collected case histories in man.

III. Experimental lymphoma induction by diphenylhydantoin

Two main experimental approaches were followed independently over the years: Gleichmann's group, stimulated by early experiments on dilantin effects on lymphoid tissues [62], investigated in detail DPH-induced lesions in mice that may relate to endogenous graft-versus-host reaction [36, 63]; their studies are summarized in another chapter of this book [38]. Our group administered DPH to mice in search for an experimental model to induce Hodgkin's disease (in reference to Chiari's first observation in man [40]). We did not obtain Hodgkin's lymphomas in any of the experiments, yet observed an enhanced incidence of other types of lymphomas which will be described here.

1. EXPERIMENTAL DESIGN

Three strains of mice were selected according to spontaneous lymphoma incidence and to their resistance to develop lymphomas upon induction: C3Hf (H-2^k; resistant), C57BL (H-2^b; not resistant, but low spontaneous incidence), and SJL/J (H-2^s; not resistant, high spontaneous incidence). The dosage of DPH was chosen on the basis of an initial experiment [62] and resembled a medium dose used for human treatment (Group II). In addition, one tenth of this dose was administered (Group I) as well as two high dose regimens for estimating acute toxicity (Groups IV and V). The latter were based on reports of experiments in rats which supposedly will tolerate five times the maximum dose for mice [64]. All mice were kept on a liquid diet containing the drug to guarantee a continuous uptake and steady blood levels. The diet consisted of a commercial chocolate drink for humans (Metrecal® Dutch chocolate flavor, USA) according to Dunn [65]. In the final chronic experiments for lymphoma induction, a medium DPH dose (6 mg/100 g mouse) was given representing ten times the usual dose for man. Administered and actually consumed doses as calculated from measured uptake of Metrecal® are given in Table 2.

Complete autopsies were done at regular intervals with detailed light- and electron microscopic studies of lymphoid tissues and immunotyping of selected lymphomas.

Immunological pilot studies served for evaluating the state of immune reactivity of mice and for controlling the eventual haptenic nature of DPH [62, 66, 69].

TABLE 2

Metrecal® consumption and diphenylhydantoin dose

Group Nr.	Mouse strain	Metrecal intake (ml/day)	DPH dose added (mg/ml Metrecal)	DPH dose consumed (mg/100 g mouse/day)	DPH dose total/mouse[a] (mg)
A. Acute experiment					
I	C57BL	12.6	0.06	0.06	4.55
II	C57BL	12.6	0.6	0.6	45.44
III	C57BL	11.8	6.0	5.8	415.7
IV	C57BL	5.0	25.0	23.5	273.9
V	C57BL	4.3	50.0	36.1	342.5
B. Chronic experiment					
VI	C3Hf	13.0	6.0	4.88	204.96
VII	C57BL	10.2	6.0	3.84	162.24
VIII	SJL/J	11.8	6.0	4.44	189.81

[a] As of the 168th day of the experiment.

2. GROSS PATHOLOGIC CHANGES

C3Hf mice, resistant for lymphoma induction, showed a slow and mild enlargement of lymph nodes, spleen, and Peyer's patches with a splenic weight of about 260 mg at 6 months. The color and overall shape of these organs remained unchanged throughout the course of the experiment, and no lymphoma development was noted.

C57BL mice instead developed lymphoreticular atrophy involving primarily thymus and lymph nodes after initial organ enlargement at about 6 – 8 weeks. Atrophy was noted at about 4 months in groups on a medium dose (Group III). Mice on high doses of DPH (Groups IV and V) were markedly starved (body weight between 10 and 16 gram as compared to 21 to 23 gram) and showed neurologic symptoms such as slow and atactic movement, abnormal postures, and seizures upon minimal stimulation such as by noise. These mice started to die 14 days after initiation of treatment and did not survive until lymphomas may have developed. Lymphomatous enlargement of thymuses was observed in C57BL mice on medium dose DPH from 8 months on, while lymph nodes were usually still atrophic. Systemic malignant lymphomas were present in 12% of the DPH-treated mice at 12 months and later as compared to a spontaneous lymphoma incidence of 4% by 18 months of age.

Lymph nodes and spleen in SJL/J mice were markedly enlarged by 6 months of treatment while the thymus was normal in size or smaller; the average splenic weight was 380 g, increasing subsequently to about 510 g. A quarter of the DPH-treated SJL/J mice developed lymphomatous enlargement of their thymuses and lymph nodes by 4 – 8 months, while in 75% of these mice spleen and lymph nodes were enlarged by lymphoma at 6 – 8 months. A similar incidence of splenic and lymph node lymphoma is observed in untreated SJL/J mice by 8 – 12 months.

3. LIGHT MICROSCOPY

Control mice on Metrecal® alone did not show significant changes in lymphoid tissues.

In lymph node, spleen, and Peyer's patches of low dose DPH-treated mice, a marked follicular hyperplasia was noted associated with increased numbers in immunoblasts in the paracortex and extensive diffuse histiocytosis (Fig. 1). Cellular activation was evident by enlargement of nucleoli, nuclei and of the entire cell (Fig. 2). The thymus remained essentially unchanged. No lymphomas occurred in these experimental groups (I and II).

Mice on high dose DPH treatment (Groups IV and V) had initially a similar hyperplastic response of lymphoid tissues, yet obviously more extensively. Germinal centers exhibited a loss of basophilic cells and paracortical immunoblasts were abundant. The histiocytic response progressed to form small granulomas resembling

398

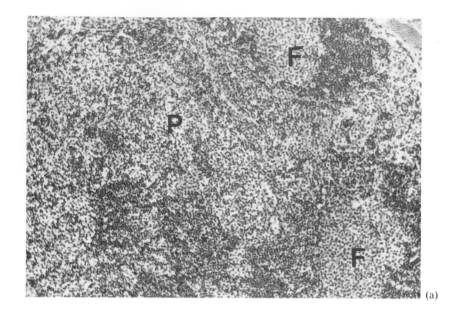

(a)

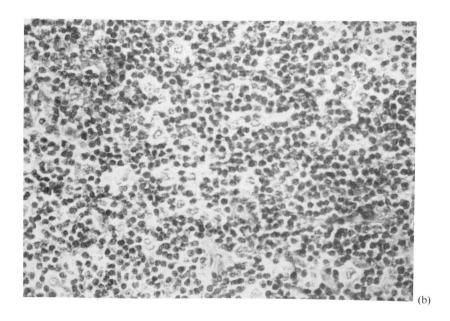

(b)

Fig. 1. Follicular hyperplasia and paracortical histiocytosis in lymph node after medium dose of DPH in Metrecal®. (a) Overview; F, follicle; P, paracortex (H & E, × 150). (b) Larger magnification of paracortex with histiocytosis (H & E, × 375).

to some extent the Potter lesion (Fig. 3; [70]). Abundant masses of large immature plasma cells and pyroninophilic blasts populated the medullary cords. Disseminated nuclear debris laden macrophages indicated enhanced lymphocyte turnover. Thymuses in these mice were severely atrophic with cortices almost completely depleted of small lymphocytes. Occasional foci of pyroninophilic lymphoid cells were noted in the bone marrow. Mice in this group did not survive the expected la-

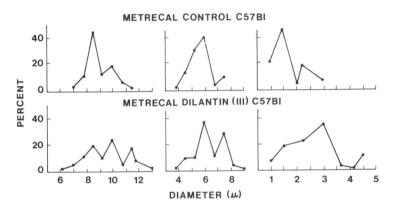

Fig. 2. Cell measurements of paracortical lympho-histiocytic cells after medium-dose DPH treatment. Left to right: cell diameter, nuclear diameter, nucleolar diameter. Note increase in large cell populations with prominent nucleoli.

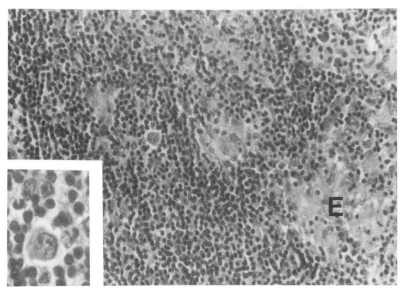

Fig. 3. Potter lesion in SJL/J lymph node after DPH feeding at medium dose. Foci of epithelioid cells (E) and occasional giant cells remind of so-called Lennert's lymphoma in man (H & E, × 150: inset × 375).

400

tent period for lymphoma development. They died prematurely of starvation because severe neurologic symptoms kept them from adequate feeding.

Most conclusive results with regard to eventual lymphoma development gave C57BL and SJL/J mice on intermediate dose DPH therapy (i.e. Group III with ten times the average dose for human patients).

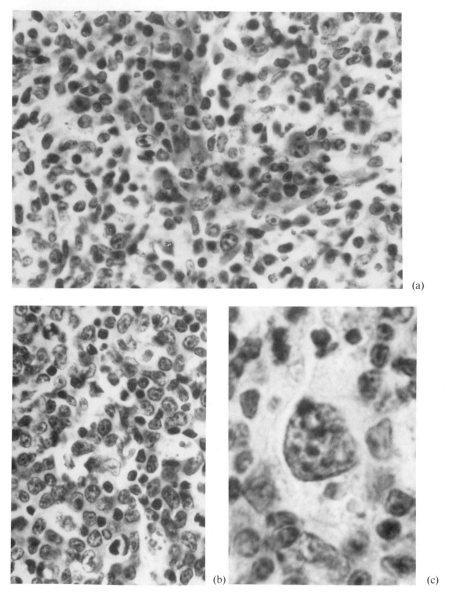

(a)

(b)

(c)

Fig. 4. Marked paracortical atrophy of C57BL lymph node post DPH treatment. (a) prominent loss of small lymphocytes (H & E, × 375); (b) focal lymphoblastic transformation (H & E, × 375); (c) occasional atypical giant cells (H & E, × 1000).

Aside from initially enhanced lymphoid hyperplasia, a progressive loss of small lymphocytes was noted from paracortical T zones of lymph nodes and from the thymic cortex (Fig. 4) starting at about 4 months of DPH feeding. Lesions were most obvious in lymph nodes draining salivary glands. Foci of pyroninophilic lymphoid cells occurred in the subcapsular region of the atrophic thymic cortex, more frequently in C57BL mice than in SJL/J mice (Fig. 5). In 12% of the C57BL mice and in 25% of the SJL/J mice these foci became confluent to replace the entire thymic lymphocyte population by 8 and 5 months, respectively, with progression to systemic lymphoblastic lymphoma thereafter (Figs. 6, 7). SJL/J mice, in addition, showed foci of fibrosis and aggregates of histiocytes in lymph nodes after 2 months of DPH feeding. Histologically identical lymphomas occurred in 4% of untreated C57BL mice after long latent periods of 18 months, which corresponds to the expected spontaneous incidence of such tumors in this strain. Untreated SJL/J mice, however, did not develop lymphoblastic lymphomas but suffered from reticulum cell sarcoma type B of Dunn beyond the age of 8 months; this represents the common lymphoid tumor in this strain of mouse afflicting about 90% of the mice by the age of 13 months [71].

Malignant lymphoblastic lymphomas following DPH treatment in both, C57BL and SJL/J mice were characterized by an enlarging peak of aneuploid cells in cell sorter studies (Fig. 8).

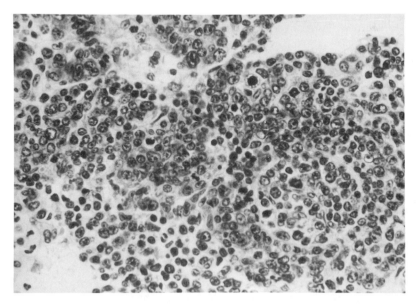

Fig. 5. Focal accumulations of lymphoblasts in the subcapsular cortex of the atrophic thymus in a C57BL mouse on DPH diet, medium dose (H & E, × 375).

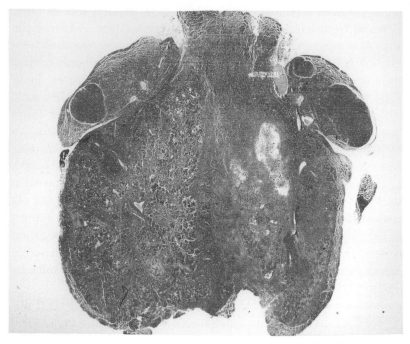

Fig. 6. Thymic lymphoma in SJL/J mouse after 4 months of DPH feeding. The upper part of the photo shows involvement of the mediastinum and of mediastinal lymph nodes (H & E, × 8).

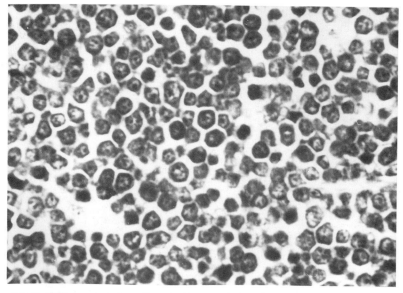

Fig. 7. Diffuse population of lymphoblasts replacing the normal thymic cell population in DPH-induced thymic lymphoma of C57BL mouse (H & E, × 600).

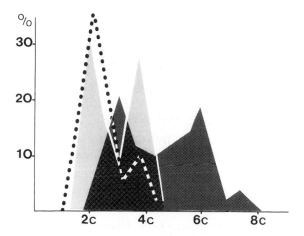

Fig. 8. Ploidy of lymphocytes in untreated control mice (dotted line), in antigen-stimulated mice (lightly shadowed area), and in DPH fed mice with lymphoma (dark area). Note peak of aneuploid cells in DPH-treated mice, while antigen stimulation alone increases the number in tetraploid cells (cell sorter study after ethidium bromide staining).

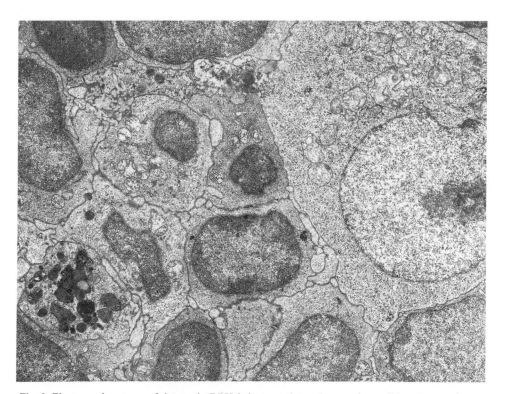

Fig. 9. Electron microscopy of thymus in DPH fed mouse shows decrease in small lymphocytes in cortex with signs of degeneration (left lower corner) and increase in large pale cells (right side) ($\times$ 3 000).

4. ULTRASTRUCTURAL STUDIES

Grossly atrophic prelymphomatous thymuses showed decreased numbers of small lymphocytes with increase in large pale lymphoid cells, reticular epithelial cells, and interdigitating reticulum cells (Fig. 9). This early change was followed by degenerative changes in reticular epithelial cells ('dark cells') (Fig. 15) and by progressive proliferation of large lymphoid cells. Finally, the organ was entirely replaced by lymphoblasts which, however, showed a certain polymorphism. The overall development of changes resembled the ones described in Moloney virus induced thymic lymphomas in the mouse [72]. There was no substantial difference between C57BL and SJL/J mice. In lymph nodes, prelymphomatous lesions were characterized by decreasing numbers of small lymphocytes in the paracortical T zone with accumulation of histiocytes and foci of immature plasma cells. Histiocytes frequently had pronounced phagocytic vacuoles with various kinds of debris, and both, histiocytes and lymphoid cells showed signs of degeneration including loss of mitochondrial cristae with swelling, vacuolization and myelin figures (Fig. 10). There were foci of collagenous fibrosis in paracortical regions especially of SJL/J

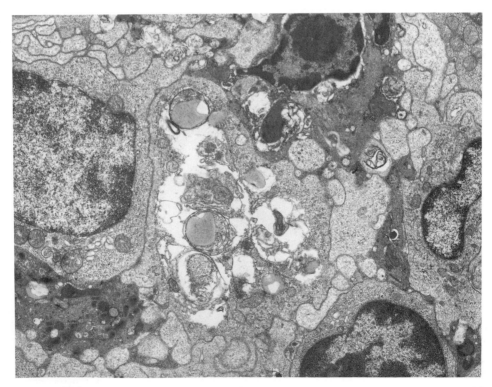

Fig. 10. Lymph node paracortex shows degenerative changes in lymphocytes, histiocytes (center) and in interdigitating reticulum cells (dark areas in upper right and lower left) ($\times$ 4 000).

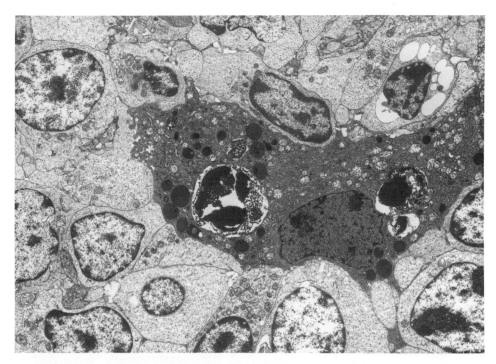

Fig. 11. Degenerating reticular epithelial cell ('dark cell') in the thymus after DPH treatment (× 4 000).

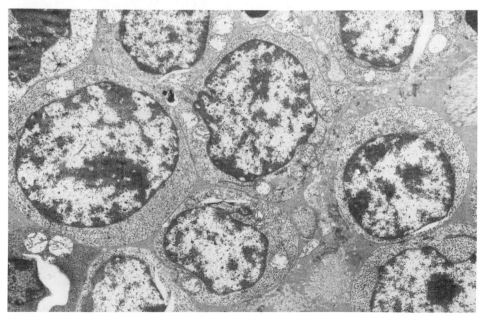

Fig. 12. Diffuse lymphoblast proliferation in thymus of DPH-treated C57BL mouse (6 mg/100 g mouse DPH for 8 months) (× 2 000).

mice. Subsequently, starting apparently in the paracortex, a mixed population of polymorphic lymphoblasts and dark degenerating cells predominated (Fig. 11). The degenerating cells were primarily histiocytes and interdigitating reticulum cells, yet also lymphoblasts exhibited similar changes. Occasionally large multinucleated giant cells were seen as well as residual plasma cells.

The predominant tumor cell at the lymphoma stage was a large lymphoblast with round or ovoid regular nuclei, clear or slightly peripherally clumped chromatin and a single prominent nucleolus. The cytoplasm with abundant polyribosomes contained scarce endoplasmic reticulum and few polarized mitochondria (Fig. 12). In addition, degenerative changes were seen in lymphoblasts-like myelin figures, mitochondrial swelling and disruption, and widening of the perinuclear cisterna. Vesicles or clear cytoplasmic foci without surrounding membrane sometimes contained ribosome-like material and electrondense whorles. Bundles of delicate fibrils were arranged in the perinuclear cytoplasm. Dense laminar-lamellar structures were noted in some lymphoma cells (Fig. 13), yet no virus particles in tumor cells of the original lymphoma tissue could be observed. When tumor cells were grown in culture, however, many intracisternal A particles and type C virsuses were seen (Figs. 14, 15).

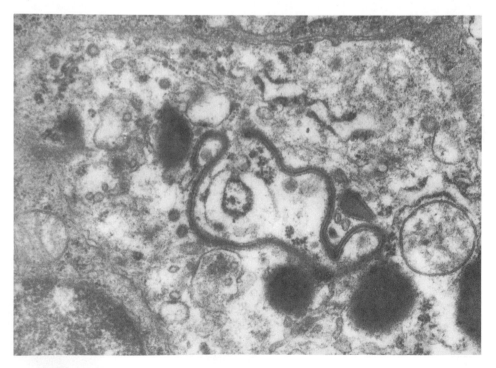

Fig. 13. Unusual trilaminar lamellar or tubular structure in cytoplasm of thymic lymphoma cell. Similar structures were described in mouse mesenchymal tumors and were thought to be virus-related ($\times$ 31 500) (C57BL mouse treated like in Fig. 12).

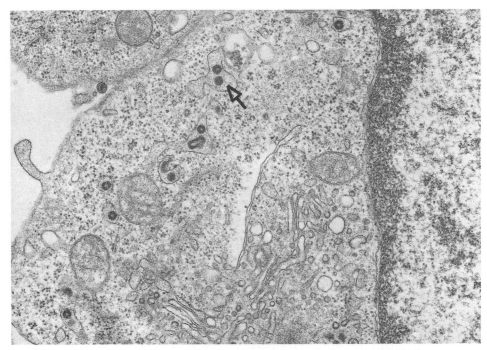

Fig. 14. Tumor lymphoblast with intracisternal type A particles (arrow; × 30 000) (C57BL mouse treated like in Fig. 12).

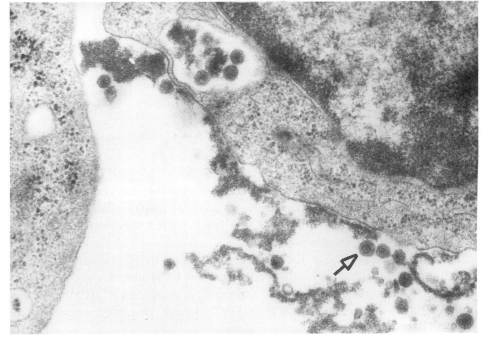

Fig. 15. Tumor lymphoblast in tissue culture with extracellular type C particles (arrow; × 35 000) (C57BL mouse treated like in Fig. 12).

5. IMMUNOCYTOLOGICAL LYMPHOMA TYPING

Lymphoblastic lymphomas in DPH-treated C57BL and SJL/J mice were both T cell lymphomas similar to spontaneous lymphomas occurring in untreated C57BL mice. Spontaneous reticulum cell sarcomas type B in SJL/J mice instead were primarily B cell lymphomas with a few exceptions of probably histiocytic nature.

6. IMMUNOLOGICAL STUDIES

Early histologic reactions of lymphoid tissues in DPH-fed mice of all groups and strains were representative for changes following antigenic stimulation [73]. When C57BL mice were sensitized by DPH skin drops, 25% of the mice exhibited reactions upon challenge suggestive of delayed hypersensitivity [62]. The reaction was considerably weaker and less frequent in C3Hf mice (SJL/J mice not being tested). Suspension of DPH in turpentine for sensitization increased frequency and extent of the skin reaction. In addition, control mice and DPH-fed mice were immunized with unrelated antigens (C57BL mice received two weekly i. p. injections of 0.25 ml of a 10% solution of bovine serum albumin (BSA, powder of fraction V, Pentex Kankakee, USA) and one booster injection 2 weeks later. Another group of C57BL mice was sensitized by two subcutaneous injections of complete Freund's adjuvant 2 weeks apart). Untreated control mice had antibody titers against BSA varying from 1 : 64 to 1 : 512 with a medium titer of 1 : 256 (passive microhemagglutination), while mice on a DPH diet had titers of 1 : 8 to 1 : 512 with a medium of 1 : 128.

Footpad testing with 0.01 ml Tuberkulin 'GT' Hoechst (strength 100) was indicative for delayed type hypersensitivity in 80% of untreated controls and in none of the DPH-fed mice [66].

IV. Summary of results and Discussion

Results of presented experimental studies allow following statements:

1. Malignant lymphomas are observed following DPH feeding in mice susceptible to such tumors (C57BL); their incidence as compared to spontaneous lymphoma development is three times increased, the latent period significantly reduced (8 months instead of 18 months).

2. Mice with a high rate of spontaneous lymphomas (SJL/J) develop malignant lymphomas at a significantly earlier date when on DPH diet.

3. Mice with a natural resistance for lymphoma development (C3Hf) do not show any malignant lymphomas after DPH feeding (although these mice can be sensitized by DPH like the other two strains).

4. Histological and immunological types of lymphomas observed after DPH ad-

ministration in C57BL mice (moderate susceptibility) compare well with those developing spontaneously at older age.

5. Malignant lymphomas occurring in SJL/J mice (high susceptibility) after DPH therapy differ histologically and immunologically from spontaneous lymphomas in this strain (lymphoblastic T cell lymphomas versus reticulum cell sarcoma type B of Dunn, i.e. B cell lymphoma). Spontaneous lymphomas, however, do also appear at a slightly earlier date when DPH is administered.

6. Lymphoblastic lymphomas in both C57BL and SJL/J mice with DPH feeding contain considerable amounts of murine oncorna viruses (C-type particles) which become overt, at least in tissue culture of lymphoma cells.

7. Preceding lymphoma development in both strains on DPH is an atrophy of the thymus and of thymus-dependent parts of lymphoid tissues (paracortical T zones), associated with signs of rapid cell turnover and reactive phagocytosis. It is in these regions where first foci of (probably regenerative) lymphoblasts occur. This atrophy correlates well with decreased cell-mediated immunity of the mice while depression of humoral immunity is not significant.

'Regenerative' lymphoblastic foci in the thymus grow out to form malignant lymphomas while reticular epithelial cells (essential for maturation of thymic lymphocytes) degenerate. This phenomenon resembles changes observed in oncorna virus induced lymphoma development in mice [72].

8. DPH was shown to attach to the surface of lymphocytes [11, 10] and to stimulate the immune system of mice. Stimulation may be a response to DPH as hapten or a response to DPH-induced changes in lymphocyte antigenicity eliciting an endogenous graft-versus-host reaction [36, 38]. In addition, the substance interferes with regulatory cellular immune reactions thus depressing cell-mediated immunity and T cell help-dependent specific antibody production (anamnestic immune response). Such combined immunostimulation and immunosuppression was identified in various other models of lymphoma induction as characteristic prelymphomatous immune disregulation [14, 15].

In essence, it appears that DPH — not being necessarily carcinogenic per se — creates a state of immune disregulation which renders the host more susceptible to malignant transformation possibly by other additional influences. The combination of DPH-related antigenic stimulation, toxic damage of lymphoid cells, and defective immune responsiveness in DPH-fed mice will initiate regenerative cell proliferation in the lymphoid system. Thus, the pool of immature proliferating cells labile for oncogenic transformation is increasing. Similarities in our mouse model with changes in virus-induced mouse lymphomas provide suggestive evidence that the ultimate malignant transformation of lymphocytes may be brought about by reactivated endogenous oncorna viruses. The obvious genetic resistance to DPH-related lymphomagenesis (e.g. in C3Hf mice) concurs with this assumption.

DPH treatment of human epileptic patients produces many morphologic and immunologic changes similar to those described in the mouse. The essential immune disturbance rendering such patients susceptible to lymphoma development may thus be quite similar too. Whatever the ultimate oncogenic stimulus is, initiating malignant transformation in man still needs to be elucidated.

References

1. Merritt, H. H. and Putnam, T. J. (1938) Sodium diphenyl hydantoinate in treatment of convulsive disorders. J. Am. Med. Assoc. 111, 1068 – 1073.
2. Merritt, H. H. and Putnam, T. J. (1939) Sodium diphenyl hydantoinate in treatment of convulsive disorders: toxic symptoms and their prevention. Arch. Neurol. Psychiat. 42, 1053 – 1058.
3. Goodman, L. S. and Gilman, A. (1983) The Pharmacological Basis of Therapeutics, Macmillan, London, pp. 207 – 213.
4. Alberts, B., Bray, D., Lewis, J., Raff, M., Roberts, K. and Watson, J. D. (1983) Molecular Biology of the Cell. Garland, New York.
5. Woodbury, D. M. (1955) Effects of diphenylhydantoin on electrolytes and radiosodium turnover in brain and other tissues of normal, hyponatremic and postictal rats. J. Pharmacol. Exp. Ther. 115, 74 – 95.
6. Krueger, G. R. F. (1985) Klinische Immunpathologie. Kohlhammer, Stuttgart.
7. Bluming, A., Homer, S. and Khiroya, R. (1975) Selective diphenylhydantoin-induced suppression of lymphocyte reactivity in vivo. J. Lab. Clin. Med. 88, 417 – 422.
8. Coope, R. and Burrows, R. G. R. (1940) Treatment of epilepsy with sodium diphenyl hydantoinate. Lancet I, 490.
9. Lehr, H. A. and Raisbeck, A. P. (1985) Ungerechtfertigter Ausschluß von Spendernieren nach Phenytoin-Behandlung? Dtsch. Med. Wschr. 47, 1834 – 1835.
10. Gleichmann, H. (1981) Studies on the mechanism of drug sensitization: T-cell-dependent popliteal lymph node reaction to diphenylhydantoin. Clin. Immunol. Immunopathol. 18, 203 – 211.
11. Zimmer, J. P., Lehr, H. A., Kornhuber, M. E., Breitig, D., Montagnier, L. and Gietzen, K. (1986) Diphenylhydantoin (DPH) blocks HIV receptor on T-lymphocyte surface. Blut 53, 447 – 450.
12. Babcock, J. R. (1964) Gingival hyperplasia and dilantin content of saliva: a pilot study. J. Am. Dent. Assoc. 68, 195 – 198.
13. Sugaya, E., Kishi, K. and Onozuka, M. (1985) Inhibitory effect of phenytoin on intracellular cyclic nucleotide and calcium changes during pentylenetetrazole-induced bursting activity in snail neurons. Brain Res. 341, 313 – 319.
14. Krueger, G., Berard, C. W. and Malmgren, R. A. (1971) Malignant lymphomas and plasmacytosis in mice under prolonged immunosuppression and persistent antigenic stimulation. Transplantation 11, 138 – 144.
15. Krueger, G. (1972) Chronic immunosuppression and lymphomagenesis in man and mice. Natl. Cancer Inst. Monogr. 35, 118 – 125.
16. Livingstone, A. and Livingstone, H. L. (1969) Diphenyl hydantoin gingival hyperplasia. Am. J. Dent. C. 117, 165 – 170.
17. Riddell, R. H. (1982) Pathology of Drug-induced and Toxic Diseases. Churchill Livingstone, New York.
18. Guerra, I. C., Fawcett, W. A., IV, Redmon, A. H., Lawrence E. C., Rosenblatt, H. M. and Shearer, W. T. (1986) Permanent intrinsic B cell immunodeficiency caused by phenytoin

hypersensitivity. J. Allergy Clin. Immunol. 77, 603 – 608.

19. Sorrell, T. C., Forbes, I. J., Burness, F. R. and Rischbieth, R. H. C. (1971) Depression of immunological function in patients treated with phenytoin. Lancet II, 1233 – 1235.

20. Andersen, P. and Mosekilde, L. (1977) Immunoglobulin levels and autoantibodies in epileptics on long-term anticonvulsant therapy. Acta Med. Scand. 201, 69 – 74.

21. Grob, P. J. and Herold, G. E. (1972) Immunological abnormalities and hydantoins. Br. Med. J. 2, 561 – 563.

22. MacKinney, A. A. and Booker, H. E. (1972) Diphenylhydantoin effects on human lymphocytes in vitro and in vivo. Arch. Int. Med. 129, 988 – 992.

23. Blanco, A., Palencia, R., Solis, P., Arranz, E. and Sanchez Villares, E. (1986) Transient phenytoin induced IgA deficiency and permanent IgE increase. Allergol. Immunopathol. 14, 535 – 538.

24. Talesnik, E., Rivero, S. and Gonzales, B. (1985) Alteraciones de los niveles de immunoglobulinas séricas inducidas por fenitoína en niños epilépticos. Rev. Chilena Pediat. 56, 76 – 80.

25. Wangel, A. G., Avrilommi, H. and Jokinen, I. (1985) The effect of phenytoin in vitro on normal human mononuclear cells and on human lymphoblastoid B cell lines of different Ig isotype specificities. Immunobiology 170, 232 – 238.

26. Dosch, H. M., Jason, J. and Gelfand, E. W. (1982) Transient antibody deficiency and abnormal T-suppressor cells induced by phenytoin. N. Engl. J. Med. 306, 406 – 409.

27. Levo, Y., Markowitz, O. and Trainin, N. (1975) Hydantoin immunosuppression and carcinogenesis. Clin. Exp. Immunol. 19, 521 – 527.

28. Dahllöf, G., Otteskog, P. and Modéer, T. (1986) Phenytoin potentiates accessory cell dependent DNA synthesis in human lymphocytes in vitro. Scand. J. Dent. Res. 94, 202 – 207.

29. Mackinney, A. A., Vyas, R. and Lee, S. S. (1975) The effect of parahydroxylation of diphenylhydantoin on metaphase accumulation. Proc. Soc. Exp. Biol. Med. 149, 371 – 375.

30. Thatcher, N., War, H. H., Swindell, R., Wilkinson, P. M. and Crowther, D. (1982) Effects of diphenylhydantoin on killer cell activity and other immunological functions. Int. J. Immunopharmacol. 4, 167 – 174.

31. Gabourel, J. D., Davies, G. H., Bardana, E. J. and Ratzlaff, N. A. (1982) Phenytoin influence on human lymphocyte mitogen response: prospective study of epileptic and non-epileptic patients. Epilepsia 23, 367 – 376.

32. Margaretten, N. C., Hincks, J. R., Warren R. P. and Coulombe, R. A., Jr. (1987) Effects of phenytoin and carbamazepine on human natural killer cell activity and genotoxicity in vitro. Toxicol. Appl. Pharmacol. 87, 10 – 17.

33. Tucker, A. N., Hong, L., Boorman, G. A. and Luster M. I. (1986) Alterations in bone marrow cell cycle kinetics by diphenylhydantoin and folate deficiency are restored by thymic peptides. Thymus 8, 121 – 127.

34. Zipori, D. and Trainin, N. (1975) The role of thymus humoral factor in the proliferation of bone marrow CFU-S from thymectomized mice. Exp. Hematol. 3, 389 – 398.

35. Lepault, F., Dardenne, M. and Frindel, E. (1979) Restoration by serum thymic factor of colony-forming units (CFU-S) entry into DNA synthesis in thymectomized mice after T-dependent antigen treatment. Eur. J. Immunol. 9, 661 – 664.

36. Gleichmann, E. and Gleichmann, H. (1976) Graft-versus-host reaction: a pathogenetic principle for the development of drug allergy, autoimmunity, and malignant lymphoma in non-chimeric individuals. Hypothesis. Z. Krebsforsch. 85, 91 – 109.

37. Gleichmann, E., Van Elven, F. and Gleichmann, H. (1979) Immunoblastic lymphadenopathy, systemic lupus erythematosus and related disorders. Am. J. Clin. Pathol. 72, 708 – 723.

38. Gleichmann, E., Vohr, H.-W., Stringer, C., Nuyens, J. and Gleichmann, H. (1989) Testing the sensitization of T cells to chemicals. From murine graft-versus-host (GVH) reactions to chemical-induced GVH-like immunological diseases. In: M. E. Kammüller, N. Bloksma and W. Seinen

412

(Eds.), Autoimmunity and Toxicology. Immune Disregulation Induced by Drugs and Chemicals, Elsevier Science Publ., Amsterdam this volume, Chapter 15.

39. Talal, N. and Bunim J. J. (1964) The development of malignant lymphoma in the course of Sjögren's syndrome. Am. J. Med. 36, 529 – 540.

40. Chiari, H. (1951) Über das feingewebliche Bild der bei Mesantoinbehandlung zu beobachtenden Lymphknotenschwellung. Wien. Klin. Wschr. 63, 77 – 81.

41. Saltzstein, S. L. and Ackerman, L. V. (1959) Lymphadenopathy induced by anticonvulsant drugs and mimicking clinically and pathologically malignant lymphoma. Cancer 12, 164 – 182.

42. Schreiber, M. M. and McGregor, J. G. (1968) Pseudolymphomas syndrome. A sensitivity to anticonvulsant drugs. Arch. Dermatol. 97, 297 – 300.

43. Butler, J. J. (1969) Non-neoplastic lesions of lymph nodes in man to be differentiated from lymphomas. Natl. Cancer Inst. Monogr. 32, 233 – 255.

44. Beil, E. and Prechtel, K. (1973) Malignes Lymphom oder Hydantoin Lymphadenopathie? Münch. Med. Wschr. 115, 2033 – 2039.

45. Lukes, R. J. and Tindle, B. (1975) Immunoblastic lymphadenopathy: a hyperimmune entity resembling Hodgkin's disease. N. Engl. J. Med. 292, 1 – 8.

46. Pereira, A., Cervantes, F. and Rozman, C. (1985) Anemia macrocitica por deficit de acido folico y linfome no hodgkiniano asociados de la ingesto prolongata de difenilhidantoina. Med. Clin. (Barc.) 85, 503 – 510.

47. Rubinstein, N., Weinrauch, L. and Matzner, Y. (1985) Generalized pruritus as a presenting symptom of phenytoin-induced Hodgkin's disease. Int. J. Dermatol. 24, 54 – 55.

48. Rubinstein, I., Langevitz, P. and Shibi, G. (1985) Isolated malignant lymphoma of the jejunum and long-term diphenylhydantoin therapy. Oncology 42, 104 – 106.

49. Gyte, G. M. L., Richmond, J. E., Williams, J. R. B. and Atwood, J. L. (1985) Hairy cell leukemia occurring during phenytoin (diphenylhydantoin) treatment. Scand. J. Haematol. 35, 358 – 362.

50. Gams, R. A., Neal, J. A. and Conrad, F. G. (1968) Hydantoin-induced pseudolymphoma. Ann. Intern. Med. 9, 557 – 568.

51. Hyman, G. W. and Sommers, S. C. (1966) The development of Hodgkin's disease and lymphoma during anticonvulsant therapy. Blood 28, 416 – 427.

52. Anthoni, J. J. (1970) Malignant lymphoma associated with hydantoin drugs. Arch. Neurol. 22, 450 – 454.

53. Li, F. P., Willard, D. R., Goodman, R. and Vawter, G. (1975) Malignant lymphoma after diphenylhydantoin (dilantin) therapy. Cancer 36, 1359 – 1362.

54. Rausing, A. (1978) Hydantoin-induced lymphadenopathies and lymphomas. Rec. Results Cancer Res. 64, 263 – 264.

55. Fontana, A., Joller, H., Skvaril, F. and Grob, P. J. (1978) Immunological abnormalities and HLA antigen frequencies in IgA deficient patients with epilepsy. J. Neurol. Neurosurg. Psychiat. 41, 593 – 597.

56. Shakir, R. A., Behan, P. O., Dick, H. and Lambie, D. G. (1978) Metabolism of immunoglobulin A, lymphocyte function and histocompatibility antigens in patients on anticonvulsants. J. Neurol. Neurosurg. Psychiat. 41, 307 – 311.

57. Harris, O. D., Cooke, W. T. and Thompson, H. (1967) Malignancy in adult celiac disease and idiopathic steatorrhoea. Am. J. Med. 42, 899 – 912.

58. Herha, J. and Obe, G. (1977) Chromosomal damage in patients with epilepsy: possible mutagenic properties of longterm antiepileptic drug treatment. In: J. K. Penry (Ed.), Epilepsy, Eighth International Symposium, Raven Press, New York, pp. 87 – 94.

59. Kulkarni, P. S., Mondkar, V. P., Sonawalla, A. B. and Ambani, L. M. (1984) Chromosomal studies of peripheral blood from epileptic patients treated with phenobarbital and/or phenylhydantoin. Food Chem. Toxicol. 22, 1009 – 1012.

60. De Oca-Luna, R. M., Leal-Garza, C. H., Baca-Sevilla, S. and Garza-Chapa, R. (1984) The effect of diphenylhydantoin on the frequency of micronuclei in bone marrow polychromatic erythrocytes of mice. Mutat. Res. 141, 183 – 187.

61. Maurya, A. K. and Goyle, S. (1985) Mutagenic potential of anticonvulsant diphenylhydantoin (DPH) on human lymphocytes in vitro. Methods Find. Exp. Clin. Pharmacol. 7, 109 – 112.

62. Krueger, G. (1970) Effect of dilantin in mice. I. Changes in the lymphoreticular tissue after acute exposure. Virchow's Arch. Abt. A, Pathol. Anat. 349, 297 – 311.

63. Gleichmann, H. (1980) Mechanism of sensitization to diphenylhydantoin, a drug known to cause autoimmunity and lymphadenopathy. Proc. Dutch Fed. Meeting Vol. 21, 141, Nijmegen.

64. Gruhzit, O. M. (1939) Sodium diphenyl hydantoinate: pharmacologic and histopathologic studies. Arch. Pathol. 28, 761 – 762.

65. Dunn, T. B. (1969) Cancer of the uterine cervix in mice fed a liquid diet containing an antifertility drug. J. Natl. Cancer Inst. 43, 671 – 692.

66. Krueger, G., Harris, D. and Sussman, E. (1972) Effect of dilantin in mice. II. Lymphoreticular tissue atypia and neoplasia after chronic exposure. Z. Krebsforsch. 78, 290 – 302.

67. Krueger, G. and Bedoya, V. A. (1978) Hydantoin-induced lymphadenopathies and lymphomas: experimental studies in mice. Rec. Results Cancer Res. 64, 265 – 270.

68. Bedoya, V. and Krueger, G. (1978) Ultrastructural studies on hydantoin induced lymphomas in mice. Z. Krebsforsch. 91, 195 – 204.

69. Krueger, G. and Meyer, E. M. (1982) Classification of malignant lymphomas of the mouse using morphological, immunological and cytochemical methods: a working proposal. Cancer Res. Clin. Oncol. 104, 41 – 52.

70. Potter, J. S., Victor, J. and Ward, M. A. (1943) Histologic changes preceding spontaneous lymphatic leukemia in mice. Am. J. Pathol. 19, 239 – 253.

71. Dunn, T. B. and Deringer, M. K. (1986) Reticulum cell neoplasm, type B, or the 'Hodgkin's-like lesion' of the mouse. J. Natl. Cancer Inst. 40, 771 821.

72. Heine, U. I., Krueger, G., Karpinski, A., Munoz, R. and Krueber, M. B. (1983) Quantitative light and electron microscopic changes in thymic reticular epithelial cells during moloneyvirus induced lymphoma development. J. Cancer Res. Clin. Oncol. 106, 102 – 111.

73. Syrjänen, K. J. (1982) The lymph nodes: reactions to experimental and human tumors. Exp. Pathol. Suppl. 8, 1 – 123.

M.E. Kammüller, N. Bloksma and W. Seinen (Eds.)
Autoimmunity and Toxicology
© 1989 Elsevier Science Publishers B.V. (Biomedical Division)

Immune-endocrine interactions and autoimmune diseases

S. ANSAR AHMED and N. TALAL

Clinical Immunology Section, Audie L. Murphy Memorial Veterans Hospital, and the Department of Medicine, The University of Texas Health Science Center at San Antonio, TX 78284, USA

I. General introduction

It is now widely recognized that gonadal hormones have a profound effect on the immune system in addition to their actions promoting the development and the differentiation of sexual characteristics. Indeed, sex hormones have a more general role in biology and they interact with receptors on a variety of widely diverse tissues including the central nervous system, the macrophage-monocyte system, the immune system and other endocrine systems [1, 2]. The complex interactions of sex hormones with the immune system, particularly as it relates to autoimmune diseases, is discussed in this chapter.

Studying the interaction of naturally occurring sex steroids with the cells of the immune system is important because of the following reasons: (1) sex hormones interact and influence the immune system at all stages of life to maintain immune homeostasis. Sex hormones may be employed as endogenous tools to delineate the complex ontogenetic events occurring in lymphocytes; (2) sex hormones influence the onset, development and course of autoimmune diseases. Sex hormones, following their interaction with specific steroid receptor proteins, may be used to investigate the molecular pathways by which activated or suppressed genes are involved in autoimmune processes; and (3) modified sex hormone analogues and an-

Address correspondence to: S. Ansar Ahmed, DVM, PhD, Department of Medicine, Division of Clinical Immunology, The University of Texas Health Science Center, 7703 Floyd Curl Drive, San Antonio, TX 78284, USA.

tagonists may be exploited therapeutically in the development of a new approach towards the treatment of autoimmune diseases.

The field of immunoendocrinology is relatively in its 'infancy' and much information must be gathered in all the above areas.

II. Sex hormones and autoimmune diseases

A salient feature of almost all autoimmune disorders is their preferential occurrence in females [1 – 10]. For example, the female to male susceptibility ratio of systemic lupus erythematosus (SLE) and rheumatic arthritis (RA) is 9 – 13 to 1 and 2 – 4 to 1, respectively [4, 5]. Sjögren's syndrome also occurs ten times more frequently in women than in men [1]. A similar preferential female susceptibility occurs in myasthenia gravis [6], idiopathic adrenal insufficiency (autoimmune adrenal disease) [7], scleroderma [8], multiple sclerosis [9] and autoimmune diabetes mellitus [10]. The female to male susceptibility ratio in these diseases is 2 – 5 : 1. Furthermore, independent survey studies of normal population revealed that there is a higher prevalence of autoantibodies in women than age-matched men [11].

Analogous to these clinical observations, normal women have better immune capabilities than men [1, 2]. This includes a more efficient response to a variety of antigens, higher levels of immunoglobulin levels, better cell-mediated immunity and reduced incidence of various tumors [1]. The better survival rate of women compared to men may also be explained, in part, by more efficient immune mechanisms to combat infectious diseases. Despite these compelling observations, acceptance of a role for sex factors in autoimmune diseases was slow in coming. Although the precise reasons for this skewed sex susceptibility pattern to autoimmune diseases is not precisely known, it is becoming increasingly apparent that this phenomenon may be the consequence of sex hormonal action, particularly in SLE. The occurrence of autoimmune diseases (e.g. SLE) in Klinefelter's syndrome, a genetically determined disease (XXY) characterized by sex hormonal abnormalities, small testes and genitalia and gynecomastia, is strongly suggestive of this possibility [12]. SLE patients of both sexes, as well as those with Klinefelter's syndrome, have an abnormal metabolism of estrogen resulting in excess production of 16-α-hydroxyesterone and estriol metabolites, which can induce a chronic hyperestrogenic state [12, 13]. Female SLE patients also have increased oxidation of testosterone at C-17 and have lowered levels of testosterone, dehydroepiandrosterone and dehydroepiandrosterone sulfate [14]. Further, male RA patients have decreased concentrations of serum testosterone and dehydroepiandrosterone providing evidence for sex hormonal involvement in this disease [15]. The course of many autoimmune diseases, particularly SLE and RA, is modulated during menarche or pregnancy or ingestion of estrogen-containing oral contraceptives [16 – 26].

Taken together, these data suggest that a combination of increased levels of 'immunostimulatory' estrogen or its products, coupled with reduced levels of 'immunosuppressive' androgens, may influence the onset or course of autoimmune diseases.

Analogous to the human situation, a similar sex-related susceptibility to autoimmune diseases is also evident in many experimental models of autoimmune disease [1]. These experimental models have provided excellent opportunities to study the contribution of sex factors to disease initiation, progression and treatment. (NZB × NZW)F_1 or B/W mice have served as a classical model for lupus, as they exhibit striking similarities with the human diseases. For instance, female B/W mice develop autoantibodies, immune complex glomerulonephritis, proteinuria and die many months earlier than males [27, 29]. A similar sex-related expression of SLE and RA-like diseases occurring spontaneously has also been noted in other strains including (NZB × SJL/J)F_1, MRL/n, MRL/*lpr,* PN and (NZB × DBA/2)F_1 [1, 2].

Sex hormone mediated direct effects on the pathogenesis of many experimental animal models of autoimmune disease have been demonstrated. For example, prepubertal orchidectomy or estrogen or progesterone treatment of B/W mice results in enhanced mortality and an earlier development of immune abnormalities compared to controls [27 – 29]. In contrast, various male hormones suppress the disease [27 – 31]. Autoimmune thyroiditis in rats induced by thymectomy and irradiation (Tx-X) occurs at least 4 – 6 times more frequently in females than males [32 – 35]. Females also have higher levels of autoantibodies to thyroglobulin and more severe tissue lesions. The disease is markedly modulated by sex hormones [33 – 35]. Male LEW/N rats are relatively resistant to the induction of polyarthritis following injection of peptidoglycan-polysaccharide fragments of streptococci [36]. Collagen-induced arthritis in rats, susceptible DA (RTI^{avi}) and resistant BN (RTI^n), can be induced in female hybrids compared with males, again suggesting sex hormone involvement [37]. Prepubertal orchidectomy or estrogen administration, however, renders these males susceptible to disease induction.

The development of autoantibodies to the acetylcholine receptor (AchR) in mice immunized with AchR in complete Freund's adjuvant can also be altered by sex hormones. Male sex hormone administration retards the genesis of autoantibodies to AchR [38]. Spontaneous autoimmune hemolytic anemia, which develops in NZB mice, although not in a female-predominant fashion, can be modulated by sex hormones. Testosterone and dehydroepiandrosterone (DHEA) reduced autoantibodies [39]. Autoimmune hemolytic anemia, inducible in mice by xenogeneic erythrocyte immunization, can be abrogated or delayed by testosterone administration [40].

Autoimmune-prone B/W mice, in addition to lupus, also develop a Sjögren's syndrome-like disease. The salient feature of lesions is mononuclear cellular infiltration in the submandibular salivary glands [41]. Nandrolone decanoate had both beneficial prophylactic and therapeutic effects on established disease [42, 43]. Other steroids, ethylestranol (progestational anabolic steroid with minimal virilizing effects), and lynestrenol (progestational effects with no androgenic or little estrogenic activities) were shown to reduce Sjögren's syndrome as well as lupus occurring in B/W mice [44].

In summary, the predominance of autoimmune diseases in females in general can be explained as a consequence of the effect of sex hormones. In general, male hormones are beneficial while female hormones are detrimental. Importantly, male sex hormones have been successfully employed to treat experimental autoimmune diseases such as murine lupus and autoimmune thyroiditis in rats [45]. However, it must be pointed out that female hormones at pharmacologic doses have been beneficial in certain autoimmune diseases [46, 47].

III. Sex hormone-influenced cellular events: targets and mechanisms of action

Experimental animals have been used almost exclusively to understand the mechanism by which sex hormones act on the immune system. However, despite elaborate work in several laboratories, these mechanisms are still poorly understood. Furthermore, recent evidence reveals additional complexities because of the involvement of various body systems [1]. It is now known that sex hormones act on several organ systems in addition to the classical reproductive system and reproduction-related tissues [48]. These include the pituitary and other endocrine glands, various parts of the brain, and the immune system itself. All these systems are known to interact directly or indirectly. In particular, evidence is rapidly accumulating to suggest that the central nervous system and the immune system interact intimately. The reader is referred to reviews for more detail [49, 50]. In brief, it appears that the brain and pituitary can influence immunoregulation (1) via innervation of the lymphoid organs, and (2) by the release of various neuroendocrine peptides (e.g. ACTH and endorphine). Receptors for these ligands may be regulated by the hypothalamus analogous to pituitary cells. Immune cells have been envisaged as 'free floating' nerve cells and collectively as a mobile brain [49]. Thus, three major systems act both independently and interdependently, namely, (1) sex hormones and immune system, (2) sex hormones and CNS, and (3) CNS and the immune system. We have postulated that interactions of sex hormones, the immune system and the brain serve many functions including immune homeostasis ultimately facilitating species survival [48]. Obviously, sex hormones can affect the immune system through multiple pathways, both direct and indirect [1, 2].

Even within the immune system, sex hormones act on several lymphatic organs. However, the thymus appears to be the main lymphoid organ through which sex hormones mediate their effects. Administration of sex hormones to animals brings about atrophy of the thymus, while prepubertal orchidectomy of normal animals results in hyperplasia [1]. This hyperplasia of the thymus is due to quantitative but not qualitative alterations in thymocyte subpopulations.

Sex hormones induce the thymus gland to release immunoregulatory thymic factors. The action of sex hormones via the thymus is suggested by studies in which simultaneous thymectomy and orchidectomy abolished immunopotentiation observed after orchidectomy alone [51]. In B/W mice, the thymus must be present to demonstrate some of the effects of gonadectomy. Furthermore, in the absence of the thymus, administration of estrogen to normal mice does not alter colony-forming units (multipotential stem cells) [52]. Sex steroid receptors have been demonstrated on thymic tissue in a number of species [1, 53], thus indirectly suggesting that immunoregulation by sex steroids may be mediated via the thymus gland. These receptors may be present both on thymic epithelial/reticular cells and perhaps also on thymic lymphocytes. It has been difficult to demonstrate the latter, due to the very low affinity and/or number of these receptors and the use of whole thymocyte populations instead of sex hormone sensitive thymocytes [54, 55].

The gonadal function in turn is influenced by the thymus. Congenital athymic mice or neonatal thymectomized mice have ovarian and other reproductive abnormalities [56]. Administration of thymic hormones modulates the levels of sex hormones by regulating the release of LH from the pituitary [57, 58]. It appears that immunoregulation is in part dependent upon the finely synchronized action of several organs including the thymus, gonads and pituitary [59]. Studies have also shown that sex hormonal effects can be demonstrated even in the absence of the thymus. These include: (1) the marked modulation of autoimmune thyroiditis by sex hormones in thymectomized animals [34] and the immunological alterations in neonatally thymectomized mice [55]; (2) chronic administration of estrogen results in bone marrow hypocellularity and osteopetrosis and, therefore, estrogen may reduce the efflux of lymphocytes from bone marrow to the thymus; (3) sex hormone receptors have been found in the reticular tissues of lymph nodes and the spleen suggesting that sex hormones may act directly on these cells; (4) in birds, the B cell producing bursa is the main target organ for sex hormones. Incubation of fertilized ovarian eggs in testosterone solution brings about a chemical bursectomy in addition to the atrophy of the thymus.

The effects of sex hormones have also been studied at the cellular and molecular level. That sex hormones act on T cells is suggested by the modulation of T cell dependent responses. In our series of experiments, we observed that manipulation of testosterone levels by orchidectomy or testosterone administration markedly alters specific in vitro lymphocyte proliferative responses to the T-dependent antigen, purified protein derivative (PPD) [60]. Similarly, T-dependent mitogen response to concanavalin A (ConA) is modulated by sex hormones [60]. Estrogens also affect T cells. We measured the activity of ornithine decarboxylase (ODC), an early enzyme in polyamine synthesis which correlates with DNA and RNA synthesis, in lymphocytes from estrogen- and sham-treated mice. Splenic lymphocytes from these mice were stimulated, with ConA and the ODC activity measured subsequently. We found that estrogen-treated mice had reduced ODC activity compared to controls (Ansar Ahmed, Talal, and Fischbach, in preparation). Estrogens suppressed experimental demyelinating disease [46] and autoimmune thyroiditis [47] which are presumably T cell mediated.

Bone marrow T cells from B/W mice bearing the enzyme 21-α-hydroxysteroid dehydrogenase are sensitive to the effects of testosterone, again suggesting an action on T cells [61]. Autoimmune mice have decreased interleukin-2 (IL-2) levels which are produced by T cells [62]. The production of this lymphokine can be modulated by sex hormones. For example, administration of male sex hormones to autoimmune mice normalized and maintained IL-2 levels [62].

Suppressor T cells are relatively more susceptible to sex hormone action. Sex differences have been noted between male and female B/W mice in the genesis of antigen-specific suppressor cells to rat red cells [63]. Male mice generate these suppressor cells while female mice are unable to generate them. Similarly, the development of autoimmune thyroiditis in thymectomized and irradiated animals can be prevented more effectively by the transfer of lymphocytes (suppressor) from normal males compared to age-matched females [64]. We and others have demonstrated that the Ly-2$^+$ cell subpopulation (CD8) in mice, which is believed to have suppressor/cytotoxic function, is altered by sex hormones [65, 66]. The sex hormone induced changes in immune responses to foreign antigens have been attributed to manipulation of suppressor cells by sex hormones [67].

The belief that suppressor cells are susceptible to sex hormone modulation gained further support from human studies. For example, OKT-8 (CD8) positive lymphocytes which have suppressor/cytotoxic function have estrogen receptors [68]. The addition of estradiol to human peripheral blood lymphocytes in pokeweed mitogen stimulated cultures greatly enhanced B cell differentiation [69], an effect attributed to the inhibition of suppressor cell activity by estradiol.

Sex hormones also modulate autoantibody levels, thus suggesting that B cells are targets of sex hormones. In general, male hormones reduce while female hormones, particularly estrogen, enhance autoantibodies. Autoantibodies to bromelain-treated mouse red blood cells (Br-MRBC) are produced largely by Ly-1$^+$ B cells and are modulated by sex hormones. We found that these autoantibody plaque forming cells (APFC) in spleen, peritoneal cavity and bone-marrow cells are increased in female autoimmune as well as normal mice (Table 1) (Ansar Ahmed, Dauphinee, Montoya and Talal, submitted). Estrogen administration to orchidectomized normal males further increased this response (Table 2). The precise mechanisms by which estrogen induces B cell hyperactivity is not clear and is the subject of current investigations in our laboratories.

Non-lymphoid cells in the lymphoid organs are also important targets of sex hormone action. For example, chemical bursectomy induced by the immersion of fertile eggs in testosterone solution primarily affects the bursal epithelial cells and not the lymphoid cells, thus indirectly affecting B cells. Similarly, thymic epithelium and reticular (stromal) tissues are rich in sex steroid receptors. Thus, sex hormones may act on these cells and alter the thymic microenvironment and thus affect differentiation, maturation and migration of lymphoid cells. A recent report describes that thymic epithelial cultures have shown that these cells release immunoregulatory factors in response to estrogen [70]. Furthermore, sex hormones may act on thymic stromal cells to influence the number of Ia-positive cells or the function of Ia molecules.

Macrophages-monocytes are considered another target for sex hormones. Estrogens enhance macrophage phagocytic activity [71], bring about cytostasis of malignant cells, and the secretion of plasminogen activators. Estrogens stimulate the reticuloendothelial cells [72, 73], the number of circulating monocytes [74], and the division of Kupffer cells [75]. Estrogens also enhance clearance of immunoglobulin-G-coated erythrocytes [76]. Peritoneal and alveolar macrophages themselves can

TABLE 1

Autoantibodies to bromelain-treated mouse erythrocytes and Ly-1[+] B cells in NZW mice

Sex	Br-MRBC[a] (per million)	Ly-1[+] B cells[b] (% positive)
Male	67	7
Female	982	8

[a] Spleen cells (fresh) from 12-months old NZW mice were assayed for autoantibody plaque-forming cells (APFC) by a hemolytic plaque assay using bromelain-treated mouse red blood cells (Br-MRBC).
[b] Ly-1[+] B cells were enumerated by dual color FACS analysis.

TABLE 2

Estrogen increases the autoantibody plaque-forming cells (APFC) to bromelain-treated mouse erythrocytes (Br-ME) in normal male C57BL/6J mice

Hormone treatment	Br-ME APFC (per million)
(1) Sham orchidectomized + sham implant	32
(2) Orchidectomized + sham implant	20
(3) Orchidectomized + estrogen	178

4-weeks old C57BL/6J were prepubertally orchidectomized or sham operated and subcutaneously implanted with 0.5 cm of silastic implant containing estrogen for 3 months. Lymphocytes from spleens were isolated to determine APFC to Br-MRBC.

convert testosterone to 5α-reduced metabolites which can, in turn, influence the activity of the cell [77].

Certain areas of the brain and pituitary are highly responsive to sex hormones. For example, neurons in the ventro-medial nucleus of the hypothalamus, which markedly influence immune responses, are enriched in sex hormone receptors. Although lacking in evidence, these neurons which bear receptors for sex hormones may be the same ones influencing immune responses. Thus, it is conceivable that sex hormones may act via these cells and affect autoimmune diseases indirectly.

Natural killer (NK) cells are important cells participating in spontaneous cytotoxicity against a variety of malignant and virus-infected cells. Natural killer cell activity in the spleen is reduced in autoimmune mice [78]. Estrogens reduce splenic NK cell activity in normal as well as in autoimmune mice [79]. The mechanism of action is not precisely understood. Several possibilities exist. First, estrogens bring about occlusion of the bone marrow cavity of long bones, thus severely diminishing the precursors of NK cells. Estrogen may reduce the production of T cell lymphokines, such as γ-interferon or IL-2, which promote NK cell activity. Finally, estrogen may affect the suppressor cells regulating NK cell activity, although this possibility remains unproven.

IV. Sex steroid receptors

Following intensive studies in reproductive tissues, it is now believed that sex hormones act on their target tissues by initially interacting with specific receptor proteins to form a steroid-receptor complex [81]. This steroid-receptor complex is thought to acquire increased binding affinity for nuclear acceptor sites to modulate the transcription of specific genes [81]. Hormones can be viewed as agents which 'activate' receptor proteins to become DNA regulatory molecules.

In general, it has been difficult to demonstrate estrogen receptor (ER) (measured by ligand binding techniques) in lymphocytes perhaps because of low capacity (i.e. number). Additionally, only a selected population may possess these receptors as differential sensitivity to estrogen among lymphocytes is apparent. Therefore, the use of whole lymphocyte populations may mask the expression of receptors in a small yet significant population of lymphocyte subset. Specific sex steroid binding proteins have been reported in the thymus of normal rats, mice and guinea pigs, and in the spleens of mice, by biochemical and autoradiographic techniques [82, 83]. Localization of ^{3}H-estrogen has been demonstrated in supporting connective tissues of the baboon spleen but not in the red pulp or lymphocytes. In yet other studies, these estrogen binding receptor proteins have also been demonstrated in human mononuclear cells, splenic lymphocytes and thymocytes [84]. Further, nuclear uptake and retention of ^{3}H-estrogen has been reported in lymphocytes of germinal centers and in the connective tissue capsules of the guinea pig lymph nodes

[82]. These receptors have been detected in human thymomas and leukemic cells [85]. Further, by employing a modified binding assay, ER have been found in CD8 (suppressor/cytotoxic) but not in CD4 (helper/inducer) human lymphocytes [68]. However, in most cases the binding by estrogen receptor was low.

V. Summary

Sex hormones, as we now know, act on multiple organs and multiple cells [1, 2]. The thymus appears to be one of the primary targets. Sex hormones may quantitatively or qualitatively affect thymocytes by direct action or via thymic epithelium. Thymic epithelial Ia-positive cells may release certain immunoregulatory factors and modify the thymic microenvironment, thereby modulating differentiation, maturation and migration of cells. Thymic hormones released following sex hormone stimulation may interact with the pituitary to produce products regulating intrathymic events. T cells appear to be comparatively sensitive to sex hormonal action. Alterations in these cells by sex hormones may be one way to influence autoimmunity.

Sex hormones have complex but extremely important influences on the immune system. Their effects must be envisioned in a broader context, which we have termed 'neuroimmunoendocrinology', involving at least three major systems, the immune system, the endocrine system and the neuroendocrine system. Neuroimmunoendocrinology, although a new field, has begun to make significant contributions to immunobiology.

Understanding basic mechanisms underlying the effects of sex hormones on the immune system is vital, as these hormones influence many immunologically mediated disorders such as autoimmune diseases and possibly neoplastic conditions. Molecular biological technology should elicit new information with regards to the identification of sex hormone sensitive lymphocytes, and functional changes induced by sex hormones. Any information on the altered regulation of transcriptional molecules from this series of experiments would significantly contribute to our knowledge of autoimmune processes and be helpful in understanding the pathogenesis of autoimmune diseases. Hopefully, this will lead to newer and more effective means of treating patients. Further, the development of newer estrogen antagonists or male hormone analogues with minimal side effects may prove to be beneficial therapeutically.

Acknowledgements

We wish to thank the expert secretarial assistance of Marian Langston and Ann Kirkland. These studies were supported in part by the NIH Multiple Arthritis Center and the General Medical Council of the Veterans Administration.

References

1. Ansar Ahmed, S., Penhale, W. J. and Talal, N. (1985) Sex hormones, immune responses and autoimmune diseases: mechanism of sex hormone action. Am. J. Pathol. 121, 531 – 551.

2. Ansar Ahmed, S. and Talal N. (1988) Sex steroids, sex steroid receptors and autoimmune diseases. In: P. S. Sheridan, K. Blum and M. C. Trachtenberg (Eds.), Steroid Receptors and Disease: Cancer, Autoimmune, Bone and Circulatory Disorders, Marcel Dekker Inc., New York, Basel, pp. 289 – 316.

3. Doniach, D. and Roitt, I. M. (1976) Autoimmune thyroid disease. In: Textbook of Immunopathology, Vol. II, Grune and Stratton, New York, pp. 715.

4. Dubois, E. L. (1974) Lupus erythematosus. In: E. L. DuBois (Ed.), Lupus Erythematosus, University of Southern California Press, Los Angeles, pp. 340.

5. Glynn, L. E. and Holborrow, E. J. (Eds.), (1965) Rheumatoid arthritis. In: Autoimmunity and Disease, Blackwell, Oxford, pp. 132.

6. Schwab, R. S. and Leland, C. C. (1953) Sex and age in myasthenia gravis as critical factors in incidence and remission. J. Am. Med. Assoc. 153, 1270 – 1273.

7. Kahn, C. R. and Flier, J. S. (1980) Immunologic aspect of endocrine disease. In: C. W. Parker (Ed.), Clinical Immunology, W. B. Saunders, Philadelphia, pp. 815.

8. Harris, E. D., Jr. (1982) Scleroderma. In: J. B. Wyngarden and L. H. Smith (Eds.), Cecil Textbook of Medicine, W. B. Saunders, Philadelphia, pp. 1857.

9. Cook, R. D. (1981) Multiple sclerosis: is the domestic cat involved? Med. Hypotheses 7, 147 – 154.

10. Chapel, H. and Haeney M. (Eds.) (1984) Essentials of Clinical Immunology, Blackwell Scientific Publications, Oxford, pp. 267.

11. Khangure, M. S., Dingle, P. R., Stephenson, J., Bird, T., Hall, R. and Evered, D. C. (1977) A long term followup of patients with autoimmune thyroid disease. Clin. Endocrinol. 6, 41 – 48.

12. Stern, R., Fishman, J., Brushman, H. and Kunkel, H. G. (1977) Systemic lupus erythematosus associated with Klinefelter's syndrome. Arthritis Rheum. 20, 18 – 22.

13. Lahita, R. G., Bradlow, H. L., Kunkel, H. G. and Fishman, J. (1979) Alterations of estrogen metabolism in systemic lupus erythematosus. Arthritis Rheum. 22, 1195 – 1198.

14. Lahita, R. G., Bradlow, L., Grinzler, E., Pang, S. and New M. (1987) Low plasma androgens in women with systemic lupus erythematosus. Arthritis Rheum. 30, 241 – 248.

15. Cutolo, M., Balleari, E., Accardo, S., Samanta, E., Cimmino, M. A., Quisti, M., Monochesi, M. and Lomeo, A. (1984) Preliminary results of androgen level testing in men with rheumatoid arthritis. Arthritis Rheum. 327, 958 – 959 (Letter).

16. Smolen, J. S. and Steinberg, A. D. (1949) Systemic lupus erythematosus and pregnancy. Clinical, immunological and theoretical aspects. In: N. Gleicher (Ed.), Reproductive Immunology, Liss, New York, pp. 283.

17. Hench, P. A. (1949) The potential reversibility of rheumatoid arthritis. Mayo Clin. Proc. 24, 167 – 178.

18. Lorz, H. M. and Frumin, A. M. (1961) Spontaneous remission in chronic idiopathic thrombocytopenic purpura during pregnancy. Obstet. Gynecol. 17, 362 – 363.

19. Amino, N., Miyai, K. and Yamamoto, T. (1977) Transient recurrence of hyperthyroidism after delivery in Graves' disease. J. Clin. Endocrinol. Metab. 44, 130 – 136.

20. Gutierrez, G., Dagnini, R. and Mintz, G. (1984) Polymyositis/dermatomyositis and pregnancy. Arthritis Rheum. 27, 291 – 294.

21. Amino, N., Miyai, K., Kuro, R., Tanizawa, O., Azukizawa, M., Takei, S., Tanaka, F., Nishi, K., Kahwashima, M. and Kumahara, Y. (1977) Transient postpartum hypothyroidism: fourteen cases with autoimmune thyroiditis. Ann. Intern. Med. 87, 155 – 159.

22. Chapel, T. A. and Burns, R. E. (1971) Oral contraceptives and exacerbations of lupus erythematosus. Am. J. Obstet. Gynecol. 110, 366 – 369.

23. McKenna, C. H., Weiman, K. C. and Schulman, L. E. (1969) Oral contraceptives, rheumatic diseases, and autoantibodies. Arthritis Rheum. 12, 313 – 314 (Abstract).

24. Schleicher, E. M. (1968) LE cells after oral contraceptives. Lancet 1, 821 – 822.

25. Spiera, H. and Plotz, C. M. (1969) Rheumatic symptoms and oral contraceptives. Lancet 1, 571 – 572.

26. Garovich, M., Agudelo, C. and Pisko, E. (1980) Oral contraceptives and systemic lupus erythematosus. Arthritis Rheum. 23, 1396 – 1398.

27. Roubinian, J. R., Talal, N., Greenspan, J. S., Goodman, J. R. and Siiteri, K. (1978) Effect of castration and sex hormone treatment survival, anti-nucleic acid antibodies and glomerulonephritis in NZB × NZW F1 mice. J. Exp. Med. 147, 1568 – 1583.

28. Roubinian, J. R., Papoian, R. and Talal, N. (1977) Androgenic hormones modulate autoantibody responses and improved survival in murine lupus. J. Clin. Invest. 59, 1066 – 1070.

29. Steinberg, A. D., Melez, K. A., Raveche, E. S., Reeves, J. P., Boegel, W. A., Smathers, P. A., Taurog, J. D., Weinlein, L. and Duvic, M. (1979) Approach to the study of the role of sex hormones in autoimmunity. Arthritis Rheum. 22, 1170 – 1176.

30. Verheul, H. A. M., Stimson, W. H., Hollander, F. C. D. and Schuurs, A. H. W. M. (1981) The effects of nondrolone, testosterone and their decanoate esters on murine lupus. Clin. Exp. Immunol. 44, 11 – 17.

31. Lucas, J. A., Ansar Ahmed, S., Casey, M. L. and MacDonald, P. C. (1985) The prevention of autoantibody formation and prolonged survival in NZB/NZW F1 mice fed dehydroisoandrosterone. J. Clin. Invest. 75, 2091 – 2093.

32. Ansar Ahmed, S. and Penhale W. J. (1980) The role of sex steroids in autoimmune thyroiditis. In: J. L. Preud'Homme and V. A. L. Hawken (Eds.), 4th International Congress of Immunology, Paris Abstract, Academic Press, Paris, p. 14.3.02.

33. Penhale, W. J. and Ansar Ahmed S. (1981) The effect of gonadectomy on the sex-related expression of autoimmune thyroiditis in thymectomized and irradiated rats. Am. J. Reprod. Immunol. 1, 326 – 330.

34. Ansar Ahmed, S. and Penhale, W. J. (1982) The influence of testosterone on the development of autoimmune thyroiditis in thymectomized and irradiated rats. Clin. Exp. Immunol. 48, 367 – 374.

35. Ansar Ahmed, S., Young, P. R. and Penhale, W. J. (1983) The effects of female sex steroids on the development of autoimmune thyroiditis in thymectomized and irradiated rats. Clin. Exp. Immunol. 54, 351 – 358.

36. Allen, J. B., Blatter, D., Calandrea, G. B. and Wilder, R. L. (1983) Sex hormonal effects on the severity of streptococcal cell wall-induced polyarthritis in the rat. Arthritis Rheum. 26, 560 – 565.

37. Griffiths, M. E. and DeWitt, C. W. (1984) Modulation of collagen-induced arthritis in rats by non-RT1-linked genes. J. Immunol. 133, 3043 – 3046.

38. Talal, N., Dauphinee, M. J., Ansar Ahmed, S. and Christadoss, P. (1983) Sex factors in immunity and autoimmunity. In: Y. Yamamura and T. Tada (Eds.), Progress in Immunology, Vol. V., Academic Press, pp. 1589.

39. Steinberg, A. D., Smathers, P. A. and Boegel, W. B. (1980) Effects of sex hormones on autoantibody production by NZB mice and modification by environmental factors. Clin. Immunol. Immunopathol. 17, 562 – 572.

40. Milich, D. R. and Gershwin, M. E. (1981) Murine autoimmune hemolytic anemia via xenogeneic erythrocyte immunization. III. Differences of sex. Clin. Immunol. Immunopathol. 18, 1 – 11.

41. Kessler, H. S. (1968) A laboratory model for Sjögren's syndrome. Am. J. Pathol. 52, 671 – 685.

426

42. Schot, L. P. C., Verheul, H. A. M. and Schuurs, A. H. W. N. (1984) Effect of nandrolone decanoate on Sjögren's syndrome like disorders in NZB/NZW mice. Clin. Exp. Immunol. 57, 571 – 574.
43. Verheul, H. A. M., Schot, L. P. C. and Schuurs, A. H. W. N. (1986) Therapeutic effects of nandrolone decanoate, tibolone, lynsternol and ethylesternol on Sjögren's syndrome-like disorders in NZB/W mice. Clin. Exp. Immunol. 64, 243 – 248.
44. Roubinian, J. R., Talal, N., Greenspan, J. S., Goodman, J. R. and Siiteri, P. K. (1979) Delayed androgen treatment prolongs survival in murine lupus. J. Clin. Invest. 63, 902 – 911.
45. Ansar Ahmed, S., Young, P. R. and Penhale, W. J. (1986) Beneficial effect of testosterone in the treatment of chronic autoimmune thyroiditis in rats. J. Immunol. 136, 143 – 147.
46. Arnason, B. G. and Richman, D. P. (1969) Effect of oral contraceptives on experimental demyelinating disease. Arch. Neurol. 21, 103 – 106.
47. Kappas, A., Jones, H. E. H. and Roitt, I. M. (1963) Effects of steroid sex hormones on immunological phenomenon. Nature 198, 902.
48. Ansar Ahmed, S. and Talal, N. (1985) The survival value of non-clonic target sites for sex hormone action in the immune and central nervous system. Clin. Immunol. Newslett. 6, 97 – 99.
49. Blalock, J. E. and Smith, E. M. (1985) The immune system: our mobile brain? Immunol. Today 6, 115 – 142.
50. Goetzl, E. S. (Ed.) (1985) In: Proceedings of a Conference on Neuroimmunomodulator of Immunity and Hypersensitivity. J. Immunol. 135, 7395 – 8615.
51. Eidinger, D. and Garrett, T. J. (1972) Studies of the regulatory effects of sex hormones on antibody formation and stem cell differentiation. J. Exp. Med. 136, 1098 – 1116.
52. Luster, M. I., Boorman, G. A., Kovach, K. S., Dieter, M. P. and Hong, L. (1984) Mechanism of estrogen-induced myelotoxicity. Int. J. Immunopharmacol. 6, 287 – 297.
53. Grossman, C. J., Sholiton, L. J. and Helmsworth, J. A. (1983) Characteristics of the cytoplasmic and nuclear dihydrostestosterone receptors of human thymic tissues. Steroids 42, 11 – 22.
54. Ansar Ahmed, S., Dauphinee, M. J. and Talal, N. (1985) Effects of short term administration of sex hormones on normal and autoimmune mice. J. Immunol. 134, 204 – 210.
55. Kalland, T. J. (1980) Alterations of antibody response in female mice after neonatal exposure to diethylstilbestrol. J. Immunol. 24, 194 – 198.
56. Nishizuka, Y. and Sakakura, Y. (1971) Ovarian dysgenesis induced by neonatal thymectomy in the mouse. Endocrinology 89, 886 – 893.
57. Rebar, R. W., Mujake, A., Low, T. L. K. and Goldstein, A. L. (1981) Thymosin stimulates secretion of luteinizing hormone-releasing factor. Science 214, 669 – 671.
58. Michael, S. D., Taguchi, O., Nishizuka, Y., McClure, J. E., Goldstein, A. L. and Barkley, M. S. (1983) The effect of neonatal thymectomy on early follicular loss and circulating levels of cortisone, progesterone, estradiol and thymosin αl. In: N. Schwartz and M. Hunzicker-Dunn (Eds.), Dynamics of Ovarian Function, Raven Press, New York, pp. 279.
59. Grossman, C. J. (1984) Regulation of the immune system by sex steroids. Endocrinol. Rev. 5, 435 – 454.
60. Ansar Ahmed, S., Talal, N. and Christadoss, P. (1987) Genetic control of testosterone-induced immune suppression cell. Cell Immunol. 104, 91 – 98.
61. Weinstein, Y. and Berkovich, Z. (1981) Testosterone effect on bone marrow, thymus and suppressor T cells in the NZB × NZW F1 mice: it's relevance to autoimmunity. J. Immunol. 128, 998 – 1002.
62. Talal, N., Dauphinee, M. J. and Wofsy, D. (1981) Interleukin-2 deficiency, genes and systemic lupus erythematosus. Arthritis Rheum. 127, 2483.
63. Cooke, A. and Hutchings, P. (1980) Sex differences in the regulation of experimentally induced autoantibodies in (NZB × NZW) F1 mice. Immunology 41, 819 – 823.

64. Ansar Ahmed, S. and Penhale, W. J. (1988) Modulation of lymphoid cell equilibria by sex hormones. Unpublished.

65. Novotny, E. A., Raveche, E. S., Sharrow, S., Ottinger, M. and Steinberg, A. D. (1983) Analysis of thymocyte subpopulations following treatment with sex hormones. Clin. Immunol. Immunopathol. 28, 205 – 217.

66. Bruley-Rosset, M., Dardenne, M. and Schuurs, A. (1985) Functional and quantitative changes of immune cells of aging NZB mice treated with nandralone deconate. Clin. Exp. Immunol. 62, 630638.

67. Brick, J. E., Wilson, D. A. and Walker, S. E. (1985) Hormonal modulation of responses to thymic independent and thymic-dependent antigens in autoimmune NZB/W mice. J. Immunol. 136, 3693 – 3698.

68. Cohen, J. H. M., Daniel, L., Cordier, G., Saez, S. and Revillard, J. P. (1983) Sex steroid receptors in peripheral T cells. J. Immunol. 131, 2767 – 2771.

69. Paavonen, T., Anderson, L. C. and Adlercreutz, H. (1981) Sex hormone regulation of in vitro immune responses. J. Exp. Med. 154, 1935 – 1945.

70. Luster, M. I., Hayes, H. T., Korach, K., Tucker, A. N., Dean, J. H., Greenlee, W. F. and Boorman, G. A. (1984) Estrogen immunosuppression is regulated through estrogenic responses in the thymus. J. Immunol. 133, 11 – 116.

71. Vernon Roberts, B. (1969) The effects of steroid hormones on macrophage activity. Int. Rev. Cytol. 25, 131 – 159.

72. Kelly, L. S., Brown, B. A. and Dobson, E. L. (1962) Cell division and phagocytic activity in liver reticuloendothelial cells. Proc. Soc. Exp. Biol. Med. 110c, 555 – 559.

73. Dean, J. H., Laver, L. D., Murrey, M. J., Luster, M. I., Neptum, D. and Adams, D. O. (1986) Functions of mononuclear phagocytes in mice exposed to diethylstilbestrol: a model of aberrant macrophage development. Cell Immunol. 102, 315 – 322.

74. Boorman, G. A., Luster, M. I., Dean, J. H. and Wilson, R. E. (1980) The effect of adult exposure of diethylstilbestrol in the mouse and macrophage function and numbers. J. Reticuloendothelial Soc. 28, 547 – 559.

75. Diesselhoff-Dulk, M. M. C., Crofton, R. W. and Van Furth, R. (1979) Origin and kinetics of Kupffer cells during an acute inflammatory response. Immunology 37, 7 – 14.

76. Friedman, D., Netl, F. and Schreiber, A. D. (1985) Effect of estradiol and steroid analogues on the clearance of immunoglobulin G-coated erythrocytes. J. Clin. Invest. 75, 162 – 167.

77. Lofthus, R., Marthinsen, A. B. L. and Eik-Nes, K. B. (1984) Metabolism of testosterone to 17-β-hydroxy-5α-androstone-3-one and 5 α-androstanc-3α, 17-β-diol in alveolar macrophages from rat lung. J. Steroid Biochem. 20, 1243 – 1246.

78. Li-Zhen, P., Dauphinee, M. J., Ansar Ahmed, S. and Talal, N. (1986) Altered natural killer and natural cytotoxic cellular activities in lpr mice. Scand. J. Immunol. 23, 415 – 423.

79. Talal, N. (1985) Interferons and natural killer cells in rheumatic diseases. In: S. Gupta and N. Talal (Eds.), Immunology of Rheumatic Diseases, Plenum Publ., New York, pp. 141 – 163.

80. Cole, R. K., Kite, J. H. and Witebsky, W. (1968) Hereditary autoimmune thyroiditis in the fowl. Science 160, 1357 – 1358.

81. Yamamoto, K. R. (1985) Steroid receptors regulated transcription of specific genes and gene networks. Annu. Rev. Genet. 19, 209 – 252.

82. Stumpf, W. E. and Sar, M. (1976) Autoradiographic localization of estrogen, androgen, progestin and glucocorticosteroid in 'target tissues' and 'non-target tissues'. In: J. R. Pasqualine, Jr. (Ed.), Receptor and Mechanism of Action of Steroid Hormones, Marcel Dekker, New York and Basle, pp. 41.

83. Sasson, S. and Mayer, M. (1981) Effect of androgenic steroids on rat thymus and thymocyte suspension. J. Steroid Biochem. 14, 509 – 513.

84. Danel, L., Sovweine, G., Monier, J. C. and Saez, S. (1983) Specific estrogen binding sites in human lymphoid cells and thymic cells. J. Steroid Biochem. 18, 559 – 562.

85. Ranelleti, F. P., Carmigani, M., Marchetti, P., Natoli, C. and Jacobelli, S. (1979) Estrogen binding by neoplastic human thymus cytosols. Eur. J. Cancer 16, 951 – 953.

M.E. Kammüller, N. Bloksma and W. Seinen (Eds.)
Autoimmunity and Toxicology
© 1989 Elsevier Science Publishers B.V. (Biomedical Division)

Toxicity of purine metabolites for human lymphoid cells: mechanisms and disease associations

18

B.J.M. ZEGERS, J.G.M. SCHARENBERG and G.T. RIJKERS

Department of Immunology, University Hospital for Children and Youth 'Het Wilhelmina Kinderziekenhuis', P.O. Box 18009, 3501 CA Utrecht, The Netherlands

I. Introduction

The present knowledge on the toxicity of some naturally occurring purine metabolites for cells of the lymphoid system originates primarily from the discovery in the seventies of an association between congenital deficiency of two consecutively acting enzymes in the purine metabolic pathway and two distinct immune deficiency syndromes. The first association, described in 1972 by Dr. E.R. Giblett and her colleague pediatricians [1], concerned deficiency of the purine enzyme adenosine deaminase occurring in two unrelated children suffering from a severe combined immune deficiency disease (SCID). Three years later, deficiency of purine nucleoside phosphorylase (PNP) deficiency was described in a patient with a selective cellular immune deficiency, again by Dr. Giblett [2]. In the years thereafter additional patients were found, and the initial hypothesis that a causal association did exist between these purine enzyme deficiencies and the associated immune deficiency syndromes became firmly founded [3, 4]. Subsequently, mechanistic models became available which explained why these enzyme deficiencies are primarily expressed in the lymphoid system. As far as adenosine deaminase (ADA) deficiency is concerned the metabolite deoxyadenosine (dAdo) which together with adenosine (Ado) accumulates in the body fluids in this condition, appeared to be toxic for the lymphoid cells. In PNP deficiency high levels of guanosine (Guo), deoxyguanosine (dGuo), inosine and deoxyinosine are found in the body fluids and among these dGuo appeared to have a detrimental effect on T lymphocyte function. Accordingly, a toxic effect of accumulated metabolites rather than a deficiency appeared to be the basis for the defective lymphocyte function in ADA or PNP deficiency [5].

The model studies aimed to unravel the selective effect of ADA and PNP deficiency on lymphocyte development and function not only disclosed clues to the underlying mechanism(s) but also drew attention to the intimate relationship between purine metabolism and lymphocyte development and function. With respect to the latter it was suggested that deoxynucleosides play a role in the physiology of intrathymic T cell differentiation by regulating cell death and cell survival [6]. Moreover, the model studies resulted in the development and use of anti-cancer drugs with more or less selective effects on lymphocytes.

This chapter will describe the toxic effects of purine metabolites on human lymphoid cells not only under the conditions of either ADA or PNP deficiency but also under normal conditions, i.e. the presence of active ADA or PNP. Emphasis will be given to the purine metabolites Ado, dAdo, Guo and dGuo, and to the biochemical mechanisms which cause the toxic effects. Clinical consequences and disease associations will be included.

II. Purine metabolism in man

Biosynthesis of purine and pyrimidine nucleotides takes place by either de novo synthesis from simple compounds and by salvage of purine and pyrimidine bases, originating from the diet or from the breakdown of nucleotides derived from RNA and DNA (Fig. 1). Carbondioxide and amino acids are the precursors of the de novo purine biosynthesis, and via several steps ultimately inosine monophosphate (IMP) is formed. Adenine- and guanine-nucleotides (AMP and GMP) are derived from IMP by amination and by oxidation and amination, respectively.

The salvage pathway can occur by two mechanisms, i.e. on the one hand the phosphoribosylation of the purine bases guanine and hypoxanthine by hypoxanthine guanine phosphoribosyl transferase (HGPRT) and alternatively, phosphorylation of purine nucleosides and purine deoxynucleosides (Fig. 1). IMP and GMP as well as their deoxyribonucleotides are converted in their corresponding nucleosides by purine 5'-nucleotidase (5'-NT); the same enzyme can convert AMP to adenosine. Guanosine and inosine and their deoxyribonucleosides are converted to guanine and hypoxanthine by the enzyme purine nucleoside phosphorylase. In case of adenosine and deoxyadenosine the enzyme adenosine deaminase converts both nucleosides to inosine and deoxyinosine.

Part of the purine/pyrimidine pathway comprises the reduction of ribonucleoside diphosphates into deoxyribonucleotides by ribonucleotide reductase. This regulatory pathway provides in a balanced rate the deoxyribonucleoside triphosphates, the precursors of DNA (Fig. 2).

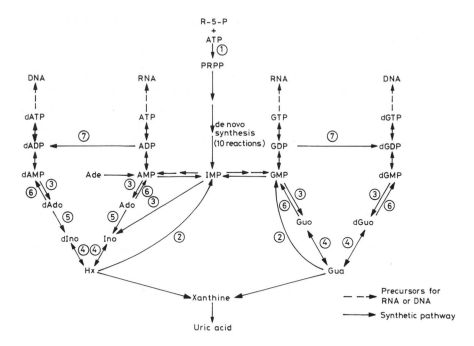

Fig. 1. Scheme of metabolic pathways for biosynthesis of purine nucleotides and deoxyribonucleotides. 1, phosphoribosyl pyrophosphate synthetase; 2, hypoxanthine guanine phosphoribosyl transferase; 3, 5′ nucleotidase; 4, purine nucleoside phosphorylase; 5, adenosine deaminase; 6, kinase, 7, ribonucleotide reductase.

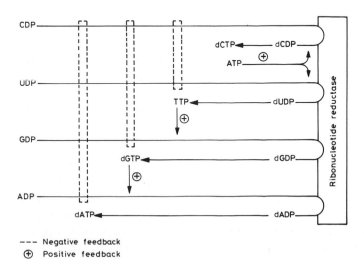

Fig. 2. Regulation of the reduction of purine and pyrimidine nucleotides to deoxyribonucleotides.

III. Toxicity of purine metabolites for human lymphoid cells in purine enzyme deficient conditions

The conditions of ADA deficiency and PNP deficiency each result in characteristic excretion patterns of purine metabolites. ADA-deficient patients excrete Ado and dAdo in the range of $30 - 600$ nmoles/mg creatinine. In plasma levels of $0.5 - 6.0$ μmol/l are found [7]. PNP-deficient patients excrete Guo, dGuo, inosine and deoxyinosine in the range of $7 - 16$ μmoles/mg creatinine; the plasma contains levels of $3 - 15$ μmol/l [8]. It should be mentioned that in normal individuals purine metabolites are below 0.1 μmol/l in serum and below 4 μmoles/mg creatinine in urine.

It is to be expected that the local concentrations of the purine metabolites as e.g. in the interstitial fluids is much higher, however, no results on that matter are available as yet. As mentioned earlier dAdo in ADA deficiency and dGuo in PNP deficiency are thought to be the primary toxic substances for the lymphoid system. This view is strongly determined by the observation that lymphocytes, unlike most other tissues, phosphorylate deoxynucleosides into dXMP, which is further converted to dXTP. It has indeed been shown that in ADA deficiency elevated dATP levels are present in lymphocytes and erythrocytes [9]; in PNP-deficient patients elevated dGTP levels are found in these cells [10]. Both dATP and dGTP are potent inhibitors of ribonucleotide reductase, the enzyme which catalyzes the reduction of nucleoside diphosphates to the respective deoxynucleoside diphosphates (Fig. 2). Inhibition of ribonucleotide reductase results e.g. in a deficiency of the DNA precursor deoxycytidinetriphosphate (dCTP) which leads to impairment of DNA synthesis and inhibition of cell proliferation [5, 11].

Two other mechanisms have been postulated to explain ADA deficiency, i.e. cyclic AMP mediated modulation of immune function and Ado- or dAdo-mediated increase of S-adenosylhomocysteine. Examples of processes which are inhibited by elevated levels of cAMP are lymphocyte proliferation, lymphocyte mobility and lymphocyte-mediated cytotoxicity [12]. Increases of S-adenosylhomocysteine under ADA-deficient conditions are based on the fact that the enzyme S-adenosylhomocysteine hydrolase which converts S-adenosylhomocysteine into Ado and homocysteine can be inactivated by accumulated Ado. Besides Ado, also dAdo and other Ado analogues cause an irreversible inactivation of S-adenosylhomocysteine hydrolase [13]. S-adenosylhomocysteine hydrolase activity apparently only has evolved in a cell that possesses ADA activity [14]. Methylation reactions correlate with the ratio of intracellular S-adenosylmethionine/S-adenosylhomocysteine, and accumulation of the latter leads to a decrease of this ratio and inhibition of methylation reactions. Methylation reactions are required for a number of cellular processes such as chemotaxis, cytotoxicity and capping and redistribution of membrane determinants. Recently it has been reported that dAdo is also toxic to resting, i.e. non-activated ADA-deficient lymphocytes. The latter observation implies that there is also a dAdo-mediated effect on lymphocytes which is independent of the inhibition of ribonucleotide reductase (see the next paragraph).

In PNP deficiency, ribonucleotide reductase inhibiton by dGTP is as yet the generally accepted model in the dGuo-mediated toxicity of the lymphoid cells, and no additional mechanisms are known.

IV. Toxicity of deoxyadenosine in model studies

The mechanism of dAdo-induced toxicity is mostly studied in in vitro model systems. To that end (partial) ADA-deficient lymphoblastoid cell lines and continuously growing mouse T cell lymphosarcoma cells have been used. In addition, normal peripheral blood lymphocytes may be used which can be rendered ADA deficient by pretreatment with deoxycoformycin (dCF), an irreversible inhibitor of ADA [16]. For the sake of completeness it should be mentioned that in lymphocytes with a normal activity of ADA no effect of dAdo on cell proliferation is demonstrable.

The fate of dAdo within a cell is primarily dependent on the activity of ADA by virtue of its low K_m of about 7 mM. When ADA is deficient or adequately inhibited by dCF, dAdo will be phosphorylated into dAMP by deoxyadenosine- or deoxycytidine kinase ($K_m \sim 400$ mM). Deoxynucleoside kinases are present chiefly in cells of the lymphoid system. The activity as found in thymocytes is higher than in peripheral blood T cells and B cells.

Addition of dAdo to cultures of human peripheral blood lymphocytes pretreated with dCF and stimulated with mitogens or to cultures of lymphoblastoid ADA-deficient T and B cell lines, induces inhibition of cell growth [17–20]. In dCF-treated mouse T lymphosarcoma (S49) cells it has been demonstrated unequivocally that dAdo can only exert its growth inhibitory effect when it is transported into the cell and phosphorylated to accumulate as dATP [21]. In general, human T lymphoblastoid cell lines are more sensitive to dAdo than human B cell lines [19]. This phenomenon may be explained in two ways: T lymphoblasts show higher deoxyadenosine phosphorylating activities than B blasts, and the rate in which deoxynucleotides are degraded is less in T lymphoblasts than in B lymphoblasts, because the latter show higher 5′-NT activity [20]. DeoxyATP accumulation appears to be of prime importance in mediating the toxic effect since it inhibits ribonucleotide reductase activity. Hence a depletion of deoxyribonucleotides and in particular of dCTP will occur which causes impairment of cell proliferation. Addition of deoxycytidine and thymidine can at least partially overcome dAdo (i.e. dATP)-mediated inhibition of ADA-deficient and ADA-inhibited lymphoid cells [17]. This observation is in agreement with the ribonucleotide reductase inhibition hypothesis and implies that the effects of dAdo become manifest in the S-phase of the cell cycle.

In addition to the dATP-mediated inhibition of DNA synthesis, other mechanisms of dAdo-mediated toxicity are known, which comprise interference with events of T lymphocyte activation preceding DNA synthesis. These events concern a block in the G_0-G_1 phase of the cell cycle accompanied by inhibition of RNA synthesis, interleukin-2 production and interleukin-2 receptor expression [22 – 25]. More recently, evidence has been presented that under ADA-deficient conditions membrane phospholipid turnover and resulting Ca^{2+} mobilisation in T cells is affected as well (Table 1) [26]. Evidence is accumulating that the effect of dAdo on early events of B cell activation is less pronounced than in T cells.

Next to effects of dAdo exerted and expressed during the process of lymphocyte activation, dAdo is also highly toxic to dCF-treated resting, i.e. non-dividing, peripheral blood lymphocytes. Addition of dAdo causes the accumulation of single-strand DNA breaks, most probably by accumulation of dATP. This induces an imbalance in intracellular deoxynucleotides which leads to a delay in the DNA repair process. As a result, poly ADP ribosylation of nuclear proteins is stimulated, which leads to consumption of NAD. As a consequence, the ability to generate ATP becomes impaired which ultimately induces cell death [27]. These events can happen in a period of 24 to 48 h. Resting human B lymphocytes pretreated with dCF appear to be less sensitive to dAdo than T lymphocytes.

TABLE 1

Effects of deoxyadenosine (dAdo) and deoxyguanosine (dGuo) on T cell activation events

	dAdo		dGuo	
	ADA$^+$	ADA$^-$	PNP$^+$	PNP$^-$
Mitogen-receptor(s) interaction	−	−	−	−
Membrane phospholipid turnover	−	+	−	−
Ca^{2+}-mobilisation	−	+	−	−
Interleukin-2 receptor expression	−	+	−	−
Interleukin-2 production	−	+	−	−
Cell proliferation	−	+	+	+

Sequence of events during T cell activation (for which interference of purine metabolites is studied) are placed in chronological order; a minus (−) indicates no effect of the metabolite, a plus (+) indicates interference.

V. Toxicity of adenosine

Adenosine is a purine nucleoside with a spectrum of biological functions among which the regulation of coronary blood flow. Relevant in the context of this chapter is the role of Ado in regulation of the immune response. Ado conveys transmembrane signals via cell surface receptors. These Ado receptors have been classified as high-affinity inhibitory (A1) and low-affinity stimulatory (A2) receptors. Interaction of Ado with A2 receptors leads to activation of adenylate cyclase and an increase of cyclic AMP (cAMP). The effects of Ado on cells of the immune system (lymphocytes, monocytes and granulocytes) are thought to be mediated through the latter pathway. As far as lymphocytes are concerned, Ado may inhibit the in vitro proliferative response of lymphocytes and also interleukin-2 production. Moreover, Ado affects lymphocyte-mediated cytotoxicity. The activity of ADA, does not appear to play a role in determining the functional effect of Ado through the pathway of adenylase cyclase on lymphocytes [28].

Recently, Ado has been found to play a role in the function of regulatory G-protein. G-proteins constitute the link between 'ligand-receptor'-mediated cell activation and the subsequent events needed for cellular responses. Binding of GTP initiates activation of the G-protein; hydrolysis of GTP by GTPase into GDP and Pi initiates deactivation. This regulatory GTPase, which determines the 'activation state' of the G-protein, itself is under endogenous control of reversible ADP ribosylation. Ado interferes with the latter process and therefore indirectly has an effect on the activation state of G-proteins [29]. The significance of this observation on the ultimate effects of Ado on lymphocyte functions is as yet not clear. Bacterial toxins like cholera toxin irreversibly ADP ribosylate the GTPase which leads to its inactivation.

VI. Toxicity of dGuo and Guo

The fate of dGuo or Guo within a cell is primarily dependent of the activity of PNP which has a K_m of about 50 μM. When PNP is deficient or inhibited the (deoxy)nucleosides will be phosphorylated by (deoxy)kinases. At present, a number of inhibitors of PNP are available: 8NH$_2$-guanosine (8NH$_2$Guo) is a competitive inhibitor of the enzyme (K_i 1.4 μM) [30] and more recently other inhibitors have been described like 8-NH$_2$-9-benzylguanine (K_i 0.2 μM) and 8-NH$_2$-9-(2-thienylmethyl)guanine (K_i 0.067 μM) [31].

The toxicity of dGuo has been studied with PNP-deficient human T and B lymphoblastoid cell lines. The results showed that T cell proliferation is sensitive to dGuo whereas B cells are relatively resistant. Deoxycytidine (dCyd) protects PNP-deficient T cell lines to dGuo-mediated inhibition by competing for phosphorylation by dCyd-kinase [17]. Martin and coworkers [32] elegantly showed the involvement of ribonucleotide reductase and intracellular dGTP accumulation in an experimental model of PNP-deficient mouse lymphoma T cells which were highly sensitive to dGuo. A secondary mutant of these cells with an altered ribonucleotide reductase appeared to be resistant to dGuo despite accumulation of dGTP [33].

Studies with normal peripheral blood lymphocytes pretreated with $8NH_2Guo$ showed that dGuo in a dose-dependent fashion inhibits mitogen- or antigen-induced T cell proliferation [34]. Inhibition of cell proliferation is accompanied by intracellular dGTP accumulation and can be prevented by simultaneous addition of dCyd. PNP-deficient, i.e. $8NH_2Guo$-treated peripheral blood B lymphocytes, are resistant to the effect of dGuo since purified B lymphocytes do respond to B cell growth and differentiation factors in the presence of $8NH_2Guo$ and dGuo [35].

Normal peripheral T cells and B cells not treated with a PNP inhibitor are sensitive to dGuo and also to Guo. The inhibition of cell proliferation mediated by dGuo is associated in both cell types with intracellular accumulation of dGTP and of GTP. dCyd prevents dGTP increase in T and B cells, however, cell proliferation is not restored. A causal role for GTP in mediating the inhibition of the in vitro proliferation of PNP^+ T and B lymphocytes is strongly suggested by the observation that cells deficient in hypoxanthine guanine phosphoribyl transferase are resistant against the toxic effect of Guo [36]. This result indicates that a product beyond HGPRT, presumably GTP, is responsible for the toxic effect of Guo.

Unlike dAdo, dGuo and Guo have no effects on mitogen-induced interleukin-2 production and interleukin-2 receptor expression of either PNP^+ T cells or $8NH_2Guo$-treated T cells. dGuo- or Guo-treated T cells which express interleukin-2 receptors do not proliferate, even when recombinant interleukin-2 is added to the cultures [25]. This finding implies that the process of T cell activation up to the appearance of interleukin-2 receptors is insensitive to dGuo in either PNP^+ and PNP^- lymphocytes. In the latter cells a next step of cell activation, i.e. DNA synthesis, is hampered by accumulation of intracellular dGTP which inhibits ribonucleotide reductase operating in the S-phase of the cell cycle. The mechanism of GTP-mediated inhibition of T cell proliferation as observed in PNP^+ lymphocytes is unexplained, however, it should be investigated whether regulatory G-proteins involved in signal transduction following interaction of interleukin-2 with its receptor act as a possible target for GTP.

Contrary to dAdo, dGuo has no toxic effect on non-dividing peripheral blood lymphocytes either PNP deficient or not.

VII. Disease associations

The various pathways by which dAdo and Ado under ADA-deficient conditions can affect lymphoid cell function imply that the clinical result is the net-effect of several concurrent mechanisms. In ADA-deficient patients both the cellular and the humoral immunity is severely affected. Some patients do have residual B lymphocytes in the lymphoid organs and blood reflecting the relative resistance of ADA$^-$ B cells to accumulated dATP as compared to ADA$^-$ T cells. The severe defect in lymphopoiesis in ADA$^-$ SCID patients may well relate to the downregulatory effect of dAdo on interleukin-2 receptor expression and hence of T cell proliferation. This assumption implies a role for dAdo already at the level of T cell generation and maturation in the thymus. Patients with ADA deficiency have distinct defects of other cells and tissues as well. The most notable defect is the aberrant growth of developing cartilage, a phenomenon which in some patients even leads to short-limbed dwarfism [37].

In experimental animals daily injection or continuous infusion of dCF induced reduced spleen and thymus weights and decreased numbers of circulating lymphocytes. In addition, the in vitro proliferative responses to T and B cell mitogens of spleen cells from dCF-treated animals are decreased, and in vivo antibody production is impaired as well [38, 39]. Abrogation of dCF administration leads to a rapid restoration of ADA activity and a gradual normalization of lymphocyte functions. In man, inhibition of ADA by dCF has been applied in the treatment of leukemias and lymphomas of the T cell lineage. This procedure induces lysis of malignant lymphoblasts and lysis of normal T cells as well. Killing of T lymphoblasts is mediated by dATP. In some patients in vivo inhibition of ADA is shown to be effective; however, serious side effects may occur like renal failure.

As far as Ado is concerned, the main effects in ADA deficiency are an increase in cyclic AMP of lymphocytes and interference with the enzyme S-adenosylhomocysteine hydrolase (see page 432). However, as mentioned earlier, Ado is believed to act as a modifier of the physiologic immune response as well. A possible role for Ado and its analogues in modifying unwanted immune responses might be envisaged in the future.

In PNP deficiency no other mechanism than dGuo-mediated inhibition of T lymphocyte proliferation by accumulated dGTP is known as yet. B lymphocytes of PNP-deficient patients hardly are sensitive to accumulated dGTP. These characteristics mark PNP deficiency as an immune deficiency syndrome with selective defects in the T lymphocyte compartment based on the impairment of proliferation dependent functions of the T cells. This statement is in agreement with the fact that T helper cell function, which is, at least partially, proliferation-independent, is intact in these patients. Contrary to ADA deficiency, patients with PNP deficiency frequently show auto-immune-like diseases and autoimmune phenomena [4]. It is tempting to relate these findings to an imbalance in the T cell regulatory control of B cell function and consequently to an impairment of T suppressor cell function. The latter is a proliferation-dependent phenomenon which easily might be the target for dGTP-mediated toxicity. Experimental evidence for the interference of dGuo with the induction of T suppressor effector cells came from a number of studies, performed both in vitro and in vivo.

In vitro studies showed that micromolar concentrations of dGuo inhibit the in vitro induction of antigen-specific suppressor cell function, whereas T helper cell function and proliferation and differentiation of precursor B lymphocytes into IgM antibody forming cells are resistant to dGuo [40]. Furthermore, it was found that daily in vivo administration of dGuo to mice abrogated the in vivo development of T suppressor effector cells operative in delayed type hypersensitivity reactions and in antibody formation [41, 42]. Finally, the administration of dGuo to lethally irradiated and bone marrow reconstituted mice leads to an increased incidence of transient homogeneous immunoglobulins in their sera [43]. Although all of these studies point to an effect of dGuo on the development and function of T suppressor cells, it must be noted that the enzyme PNP is normally present. Therefore, these studies can not be regarded as models for PNP deficiency. At least the mechanism of interference of dGuo with T suppressor cell generation will be different: in normal cells GTP-mediated toxicity will occur and in the condition of PNP deficiency dGTP-mediated toxicity takes place.

In patients with PNP deficiency, central nervous system dysfunction is common as reflected in spasticity of the extremities and the trunk [3, 4, 44]. A direct role for dGuo or Guo in these abnormalities is not evident.

VIII. Final comments and Conclusions

The unraveling of the biochemical mechanisms underlying the immune deficiency syndromes occurring in ADA and PNP deficiency has disclosed the intimate and selective relationship between deoxynucleoside metabolism and cells of the lymphoid system. Apart from the effect of dAdo and dGuo on lymphocyte development and function in the enzyme-deficient patients, attention has been drawn to the regulatory role of deoxynucleosides in normal physiologic T cell development in the thymus.

Furthermore, anti-cancer drugs have been developed in recent years which, like dAdo and dGuo have more or less selective effects on lymphocytes. Lymphocyte specificity can be envisaged because deoxynucleoside kinases, responsible for phosphorylation of purine(-analogues) almost selectively occur in lymphocytes.

It should be mentioned that the spectrum of effects of purine metabolites on lymphoid cells also encompasses positive regulatory effects. Most notably guanosine derivatives, like 8-mercaptoguanosine, have been described to potentiate e.g. antibody production [45, 46]. The exact working mechanism is not known, but probably activated B cells are target for these compounds.

It can be concluded that purine metabolites started out 15 years ago as being linked to a state of immunodeficiency in rare enzyme-deficient patients. Now, both naturally occurring and 'man-made' purine metabolites have a much wider scope: e.g. the emerging regulatory role of purine metabolites in signal transduction pathways may turn out to have a major impact on our understanding of the development, physiology and pathology of cells of the immune system.

References

1. Giblett, E. R., Anderson, J. E., Cohen, F., Pollara, B. and Meuwissen, H. J. (1972) Adenosine deaminase deficiency in two patients with selectively impaired cellular immunity. Lancet 2, 1067 – 1069.
2. Giblett, E. R., Ammann, A. J., Wara, D. W., Sandman, R. and Diamond, L. K. (1975) Nucleoside phosphorylase deficiency in a child with severely impaired cellular immunity. Lancet 2, 1010 – 1013.
3. Stoop, J. W., Zegers, B. J. M., Hendrickx, G. F. M., Siegenbeek van Heukelom, L. H., Staal, G. E. J., De Bree, P. K., Wadman, S. K. and Ballieux, R. E. (1977) Purine nucleoside phosphorylase deficiency associated with selective cellular immunodeficiency. N. Engl. J. Med. 296, 651 – 655.
4. Enzyme Defects and Immune Dysfunction (1979) Ciba Symposium No. 68, Excerpta Medica, Amsterdam, Oxford, New York, pp. 1 – 289.
5. Martin, D. W. and Gelfand, E. W. (1981) Biochemistry of diseases of immuno development. Annu. Rev. Biochem. 50, 845 – 877.
6. Ma, D. D. F., Sylwestrowicz, T. A., Janossy, G. and Hoffbrand, A. V. (1983) The role of purine metabolic enzymes and terminal deoxynucleotidyl transferase in intrathymic T-cell differentiation. Immunol. Today 4, 65 – 68.
7. Hirschhorn, R., Roegner-Maniscalco, V. and Kuritsky, L. (1981) Bone marrow transplantation only partially restores purine metabolites to normal in adenosine deaminase deficient patients. J. Clin. Invest. 68, 1387 – 1393.
8. Wadman, S. K., De Bree, P. K., Van Gennip, A. H., Stoop, J. W., Zegers, B. J. M., Staal, G. E. J. and Siegenbeek van Heukelom, L. H. (1977) Urinary purines in a patient with a severely defective T cell immunity and a purine nucleoside phosphorylase deficiency. In: M. M. Müller, E. Kaiser and J. E. Seegmiller (Eds.), Purine Metabolism in Man: Regulation of Pathways and Enzyme Defects, Vol. II, Plenum Press, New York, pp. 471 – 476.
9. Bluestein, H. G., Willis, R. C., Thompson, L. F., Matsumoto, S. and Seegmiller, J. E. (1978) Accumulation of deoxyribonucleotides as a possible mediator of immunosuppression in hereditary deficiency of adenosine deaminase. Trans. Assoc. Am. Phys. 91, 394 – 402.
10. Cohen, A., Gudas, L. J., Ammann, A. J., Staal, G. E. J. and Martin, D. W., Jr. (1978) Deoxyguanosine triphosphate as a possible toxic metabolite in the immunodeficiency associated with purine nucleoside phosphorylase deficiency. J. Clin. Invest. 61, 1405 – 1409.
11. Reichard, P. (1978) From deoxynucleotides to DNA synthesis. Fed. Proc. 37, 9 – 14.
12. Bourne, H. R., Lichtenstein, L. M., Melmon, K. L., Henney, C. S., Weinstein, Y. and Shearer, G. M. (1974) Modulation of inflammation and immunity by cyclic AMP. Science 184, 19 – 24.
13. Hershfield, M. S. and Kredich, N. M. (1978) S-adenosylhomocysteine hydrolase is an adenosine binding protein: a target for adenosine toxicity. Science, 202, 757 – 760.
14. Hershfield, M. S., Kurtzberg, J., Aiyar, V. N., Joo Suh, E. and Schiff, R. (1985) Abnormalities in S-adenosylhomocysteine hydrolysis, ATP catabolism, and lymphoid differentiation in adenosine deaminase deficiency. In: G. L. Tritsch (Ed.), Adenosine Deaminase in Disorders of Purine Metabolism and in Immune Deficiency, Vol. 451, Ann. NY Acad. Sci., pp. 78 – 86.
15. Seto, S., Carrera, C. J., Kubota, M., Wasson, D. B. and Carson, D. A. (1985) Mechanism of deoxyadenosine and 2′-chlorodeoxyadenosine toxicity to nondividing human lymphocytes. J. Clin. Invest. 75, 377 – 383.

16. Agarwal, R. P., Spector, T. and Parks, R. E. (1977) Tight-binding inhibition of adenosine deaminase by various inhibitors. Biochem. Pharmacol. 26, 359 – 367.
17. Mitchell, B. S., Mejias, E., Daddona, P. E. and Kelley, W. N. (1978) Purinogenic immunodeficiency diseases: selective toxicity of deoxyribonucleosides for T cells. Proc. Natl. Acad. Sci. USA, 75, 5011 – 5014.
18. Hirschhorn, R., Bajaj, S., Borkowsky, W., Kowalski, A., Hong, R., Rubinstein, A. and Papageorgiou, P. (1979) Differential inhibition of adenosine deaminase deficient peripheral blood lymphocytes and lymphoid cell lines by deoxyadenosine and adenosine. Cell. Immunol. 42, 418 – 423.
19. Carson, D. A., Kaye, J. and Seegmiller, J. E. (1978) Differential sensitivity of human leukemic T cell lines and B cell lines to growth inhibition by deoxyadenosine. J. Immunol. 121, 1726 – 1731.
20. Carson, D. A., Kaye, J., Matsumoto, S., Seegmiller, J. E. and Thompson, L. (1979) Biochemical basis for the enhanced toxicity of deoxyribonucleosides toward malignant human T cell lines. Proc. Natl. Acad. Sci. USA 76, 2430 – 2433.
21. Ullman, B., Gudas, L. J., Cohen, A., Martin, D. W., Jr. (1978) Deoxyadenosine metabolism and cytotoxicity in cultured mouse T lymphoma cells: a model for immunodeficiency disease. Cell 14, 365 – 375.
22. Redelman, D., Bluestein, H. G., Cohen, A. H., Depper, J. M. and Wormsley, S. (1984) Deoxyadenosine (AdR) inhibition of newly activated lymphocytes: blockade at the G_0-G_1 interface. J. Immunol. 132, 2030 – 2038.
23. Thuillier, L., Garreau, F. and Cartier, P. (1981) Inability of immunocompetent thymocytes to produce T-cell growth factor under adenosine deaminase deficiency conditions. Cell. Immunol. 63, 81 – 90.
24. Ruers, T. J. M., Buurman, W. A. and Van der Linden, C. J. (1987) 2′ Deoxycoformycin and deoxyadenosine affect IL-2 production and IL-2 receptor expression on human T cells. J. Immunol. 138, 116 – 122.
25. Scharenberg, J. G. M., Rijkers, G. T., Toebes, E. A. H., Staal, G. E. J. and Zegers, B. J. M. (1988) Expression of deoxyadenosine and deoxyguanosine toxicity at different stages of lymphocyte activation. Scand. J. Immunol. 28, 87 – 93.
26. Scharenberg, J. G. M., Rijkers, G. T., Akkerman, J. W., Staal, G. E. J. and Zegers, B. J. M. (1988) Interference of deoxyadenosine with early events of T cell activation. In: J. Vossen and C. Griscelli (Eds.), Progress in Immunodeficiency Research and Therapy, Vol. II, Elsevier Science Publ., Amsterdam, pp. 9 – 12.
27. Seto, S., Carrera, C. J., Wasson, D. B. and Carson, D. A. (1986) Inhibition of DNA repair by deoxyadenosine in resting human lymphocytes. J. Immunol. 136, 2839 – 2843.
28. Kammer, G. M. (1987) Adenosine: emerging role as an immunomodifying agent. J. Lab. Clin. Med. 110, 255 – 256.
29. Jacquemin, C., Thibout, H., Lambert, B. and Corrèze, C. (1986) Endogenous ADP-ribosylation of G_s subunit and autonomous regulation of adenylate cyclase. Nature, 323, 182 – 184.
30. Stoeckler, J. D., Cambor, C., Kuhns, V., Chu, S.-H. and Parks, R. E., Jr. (1982) Inhibitors of purine nucleoside phosphorylase. Biochem. Pharmacol. 31, 163 – 171.
31. Sircar, J. C., Kostlan, C. R., Pinter, G. W., Suto, M. J., Bobovski, Th. P., Capiris, Th., Schwender, Ch. F., Dong, M. K., Scott, M. E., Bennett, M. K., Kossarek, L. M. and Gilbertsen, R. B. (1987) 8-Amino-9-substituted guanines: potent purine nucleoside phosphorylase (PNP) inhibitors. Agents Actions 21, 253 – 256.
32. Gudas, L. J., Ullman, B., Cohen, A. and Martin, D. W. Jr. (1978) Deoxyguanosine toxicity in a mouse T lymphoma: relation to purine nucleoside phosphorylase-associated immune dysfunction. Cell 14, 531 – 538.
33. Ullman, B., Gudas, L. J., Clift, S. M. and Martin, D. W., Jr. (1979) Isolation and characteriza-

tion of purine-nucleoside phosphorylase-deficient T lymphoma cells and secondary mutants with altered ribonucleotide reductase: genetic model for immunodeficiency disease. Proc. Natl. Acad. Sci. USA 76, 1074 – 1078.

34. Spaapen, L. J. M., Rijkers, G. T., Staal, G. E. J., Rijksen, G., Wadman, S. K., Stoop, J. W. and Zegers, B. J. M. (1984) The effect of deoxyguanosine on human lymphocyte function. I. Analysis of the interference with lymphocyte proliferation in vitro. J. Immunol. 132, 2311 – 2317.

35. Scharenberg, J. G. M., Spaapen, L. J. M., Rijkers, G. T., Duran, M., Staal, G. E. J. and Zegers, B. J. M. (1986) Functional and mechanistic studies on the toxicity of deoxyguanosine for the in vitro proliferation and differentiation of human peripheral blood B lymphocytes. Eur. J. Immunol. 16, 381 – 387.

36. Spaapen, L. J. M., Rijkers, G. T., Staal, G. E. J., Rijksen, G., Wadman, S. K., Stoop, J. W. and Zegers, B. J. M. (1984) The effect of deoxyguanosine on human lymphocyte function. II. Analysis of the interference with B lymphocyte differentiation in vitro. J. Immunol. 132, 2318 – 2323.

37. Meuwissen, H. J., Pollara, B. and Pickering, R. J. (1975) Combined immunodeficiency disease associated with adenosine deaminase deficiency. J. Pediat. 86, 169 – 181.

38. Sordillo, E. M., Ikehara, S., Good, R. A. and Trotta, P. P. (1981) Immunosuppression by 2′-deoxycoformycin: studies on the mode of administration. Cell. Immunol. 63, 259 – 271.

39. Luebke, R. W., Lawson, L. D., Rogers, R. R., Riddle, M. M., Rowe, D. G. and Smialowicz, R. J. (1987) Selective immunotoxic effects in mice treated with the adenosine deaminase inhibitor 2′-deoxycoformycin. Immunopharmacology 13, 25 – 37.

40. Gelfand, E. W., Lee, J. J. and Dosch, H. M. (1979) Selective toxicity of purine deoxynucleosides for human lymphocyte growth and function. Proc. Natl. Acad. Sci USA 76, 1998 – 2002.

41. Lelchuk, R., Cooke, A. and Playfair, J. H. L. (1982) Differential sensitivity to 2′-deoxyguanosine of antigen-specific and non-specific suppressor T cells in delayed hypersensitivity. Cell. Immunol. 72, 202 – 207.

42. Dosch, H. M., Mansour, A., Cohen, A., Shore, A. and Gelfand, E. W. (1980) Inhibition of suppressor T cell development following deoxyguanosine administration. Nature 285, 494.

43. Van den Akker, Th. W., Gillen, A. P., Bril, H., Benner, R. and Radl, J. (1983) Increased incidence of transient homogeneous immunoglobulins in irradiated and reconstituted C57BL/KaLwRij mice treated with 2′-deoxyguanosine. Clin. Exp. Immunol. 54, 411 – 417.

44. Polmar, S. H. (1980) Metabolic aspects of immunodeficiency disease. Sem. Hematol. 17, 30 – 43.

45. Goodman, M. G. and Weigle, W. O. (1983) Manifold amplification of in vivo immunity in normal and immunodeficient mice by ribonucleosides derivatized at C8 of guanine. Proc. Natl. Acad. Sci USA 80, 3452 – 3456.

46. Rijkers, G. T., Dollekamp, E. G. and Zegers, B. J. M. (1988) 8-Mercaptoguanosine overcomes unresponsiveness of human neonatal B cells to polysaccharide antigens. J. Immunol. 141, 2313 – 2316.

M.E. Kammüller, N. Bloksma and W. Seinen (Eds.)
Autoimmunity and Toxicology
© *1989 Elsevier Science Publishers B.V. (Biomedical Division)*

Toxicological considerations on immune disregulation induced by drugs and chemicals

19

M.E. KAMMÜLLER*, N. BLOKSMA and W. SEINEN

Department of Basic Veterinary Sciences, Section of Immunotoxicology, Faculty of Veterinary Sciences, University of Utrecht, Yalelaan 2, NL-3508 TD Utrecht, The Netherlands

* *Present address: Drug Safety Assessment-Toxicology, Sandoz Ltd., CH-4002 Basle, Switzerland*

I. Scope

Low molecular weight (LMW) drugs and chemicals are among the best documented environmental agents that induce or exacerbate systemic autoimmune diseases (AD) in man (see several chapters of this volume; [1, 2]). Moreover, the compounds are chemically well defined, in contrast to, for instance, the molecular structures of viral or bacterial pathogens that have been associated with induction of AD.

Despite this advantage, knowledge of the causal mechanisms of chemical-induced AD is incomplete or hypothetical. A major reason is that effects appear difficult to reproduce in experimental animals (see introductory chapter). This problem becomes apparent in routine toxicology, because the ability of drugs like practolol, zimeldine and nomifensine to induce AD(-like) side effects in man was not revealed prior to their introduction onto the market, while the severity of these effects has led to their withdrawal (see Chapter 7 by Kristofferson and Nilsson; [3, 4]). The lack of convenient and validated animal models also hampers the investigation of structure-activity relationships.

Although currently no clear-cut experimental approaches can be given or recommended for use in routine toxicology, this chapter will attempt to point to some reasons for the apparent unpredictability of these disorders. Also strategies which may lead to a better predictability of the potential of chemicals to induce immune disregulation and clinically manifest systemic AD will be dealt with.

II. Protocol toxicology

1. LIKELY REASONS FOR THE UNPREDICTABILITY OF IMMUNE DISREGULATION IN TOXICOLOGY

The aim of protocol toxicology is to evaluate the qualitative and quantitative aspects of toxic effects of chemicals using various standardized test systems. Routes and duration of exposure, and reactions to chemicals are mimicked as closely as possible in non-human organisms in order to obtain an optimal prediction of a chemical's risk for man [5].

Rats are the most often used experimental animals, and these are usually derived from an outbred population to reflect the heterogeneity of the human population. Protocol toxicological investigations encompass usually 4-week dose-range finding experiments, 90-day studies and 1- and 2-year studies with $10-50$ male and female animals per dose. Screening for adverse immunologic effects is usually confined to morphological examination of lymphoid organs.

The conditions chosen for routine toxicological screening are for various reasons not optimal for detection of the immune disregulating potential of chemicals. (1) The number of animals per group is very small in view of the low incidence of drug- and chemical-induced AD in man, making the statistical chance to find an animal with morphological evidence of immunological alterations very small. (2) Risk assessment in toxicology is based on linear dose-effect relationships, while immunological effects are frequently only apparent over a narrow range of doses. Therefore, the finding of immunological abnormalities in a single animal at a particular dose, is likely to be considered as a statistical outlier. (3) The animals are not 'selected' for an increased susceptibility to develop autoimmune phenomenons in response to chemicals. Half of the animals tested in routine toxicological studies are male which according to findings in man and animals are generally far more resistant to induction of such effects than female animals. In addition, the use of random-bred animals implies that genetically determined factors associated with a predisposition to drug-induced AD in man, e.g. particular major histocompatibility complex (MHC) haplotypes [6], polymorphisms of drug metabolism (see Chapters 6 and 9, by Emery and Panayi, and Hein and Weber; [7]) and complement deficiencies (see Chapter 10 by Sim), are not predominant. (4) Weight and morphology of lymphoid organs are not always sufficient for detection of chemical-induced immune disregulation (see Chapter 16 by Krueger). The determinations represent a snapshot, while symptoms of AD such as systemic lupus erythematosus (SLE) may show a pattern of active and remittent disease in man. Further, transfer experiments have shown that morphologically normal spleens of mice exposed to streptozotocin contain drug-sensitized T lymphocytes (see Chapter 15 by Gleichmann et al.). (5) Range-finding experiments and 90-day experiments may be too short to reveal induction of AD-like symptoms by various chemicals.

2. POSSIBLE IMPROVEMENTS

Although the experimental set-up of routine toxicological investigations is not particularly suited for detection of a chemical's potential to induce AD, some implementations seem feasible without significant changes or extension of test batteries [8]. Extended morphological examination of lymphoid organs after acute, subchronic as well as chronic exposure may improve detection. Especially in the subchronic and chronic studies alertness for possible immune-mediated organ lesions should be increased. In the interpretation of the results it should be realized that hyperplastic or atrophic changes of lymphoid organs in even one or a few animals of a random population may be indicative of the autoimmunity-inducing potential of the compound under investigation, as pointed out above. In addition to morphological examinations, measurements of some immunologically relevant serum parameters could give important information. Parameters may comprise levels of total immunoglobulin of various classes, immune complexes, some commonly observed autoantibodies, e.g. antinuclear (ANA) and anti-single-stranded DNA (denatured; ssDNA) autoantibodies, and total hemolytic complement (CH_{50}). Measurement of the parameters at suitably chosen intervals especially during subchronic and chronic exposure may obviate the snapshot nature of the morphology and will give a reflection of humoral immune function in time. Although measurement of antibody levels may give an indirect indication of T cell function, a more direct parameter of T cell function is desirable, but not easily obtained. Recent findings, however, have indicated that changes of urinary pterin levels parallel all kinds of T cell mediated immune processes in man (see Section III.1.b. in this chapter). Whereas such a parameter would fit very well in routine toxicological procedures, extensive basic studies need still to be done to prove and validate the reliability of pterin determination in this respect in experimental animals.

In case that routine toxicological studies reveal any alteration of the immunological parameters, further studies should be recommended, especially if the compound under investigation bears structural resemblance to compounds with a documented potential to induce AD in man. Explicit demonstration of the AD-inducing potential of a given compound, however, is problematic in routine toxicological studies. Admittedly, clinical manifest AD can be induced by LMW compounds in animals (see Chapters 12, 13 and 14, by Aucoin, Bardana et al. and Druet et al.), but induction seems highly dependent on the combination of the agent and the animal species or strain used. More generally indicative models are urgently needed. Recently started and other approaches to meet this problem will be addressed in the next section.

III. Experimental strategies

The polyetiological nature of chemically-induced AD asks for a polyfactorial investigative approach. It is the concerted action of individual factors and the
chemical that somehow defines whether or not AD ensues. The relative contribution
of endogenous and exogenous factors in the induction of disease can vary and seems
to be complementary, as elegantly evidenced by Hang et al. [9] in different mouse
strains. Because of the integrated nature of the immune system, crucial information
relevant to these systemic disorders is primarily to be expected from *in vivo* animal
studies [8, 10, 11]. *In vitro* studies may gain importance in the delineation of
mechanisms. Therefore, one aim of research should be directed at identification of
host factors that facilitate induction of AD and dissection of the basic mechanisms
leading to disease. Secondly, the particular properties of compounds that are
responsible for induction of AD should be analyzed by structure-activity relationship studies using assays that measure immunologic, pharmacologic, and metabolic
properties as well as chemical reactivity. Ideally, this may also improve the
understanding of the mechanisms by which chemicals interact with biological
systems.

1. ANIMAL-RELATED APPROACHES

An economically and practically relevant question concerning screening studies is
whether actual evidence of an agent's ability to induce manifest AD has to be obtained, or whether short-term assays with non-autoimmune endpoints can give sufficiently reliable data in this respect. Because the fundamental mechanisms underlying
chemical-induced AD are far from understood, both short- and long-term assays
should be investigated in experimental immunotoxicology.

(a) Short-term assays

There is ample evidence that activation of autologous T cells by chemical-modified,
i.e. haptenated, self-antigens can lead to autoantibody formation (see Chapters 3
and 15, by Allison, and Gleichmann et al.). Regarding this, H. and E. Gleichmann
and coworkers have pointed at the similarity with autoimmunity induced by graft-
versus-host (GVH) reactions. In these reactions donor T cells are initially activated
by allogeneic MHC class II molecules of the host. They, therefore, introduced the
popliteal lymph node (PLN) assay, originally developed for quantitation of GVH
activity of lymphocytes, for the study of chemical-induced autoimmunity. Injection
of 5,5-diphenylhydantoin and D-penicillamine without adjuvant into the footpad of
mice was shown to induce a T cell dependent weight increase that could be morphologically characterized by early T cell activation followed by proliferation and
maturation of B cells (see Chapter 15 by Gleichmann et al.; [12 – 14]). Maturation

was confirmed by demonstration of increased numbers of IgM- and especially IgG-secreting cells [13]. All effects observed were very similar to those induced during a local GVH reaction in the PLN. Study of the kinetics and morphology of diphenylhydantoin- and nitrofurantoin-induced PLN reactions has verified the resemblance with a local GVH reaction and showed that the PLN reactions could be clearly distinguished from those induced by sheep red blood cells, the B cell mitogen lipopolysaccharide and the contact sensitizer dinitrochlorobenzene [13a]. Immunogenetic studies in mice with diphenylhydantoin and D-penicillamine have indicated that the extent of PLN enlargement is controlled by MHC (H-2) as well as non-MHC genes, but that complete non-responder strains were scarce [13a, 14]). Further, the PLN assay appeared able to discriminate between structurally closely related compounds, as shown for chemical congeners of D-penicillamine [14], diphenylhydantoin [15, 16] and zimeldine (Thomas et al., in preparation). For zimeldine congeners also a distinction between immunological and pharmacological activity could be made.

Recent screening of a wide variety of drugs and chemicals in the PLN assay revealed a remarkable positive correlation with their potential to cause systemic AD and local contact dermatitis in man and a relatively low incidence of false-negatives (see Chapter 15 by Gleichmann et al.; [13a]). The virtual elimination of pharmacokinetic factors inherent to the assay and/or the limited possibility for local metabolic conversion may account for the false-negatives. Whereas this may be partially solved by use of metabolites in the assay, the indirect PLN assay, based on specific challenge of animals after transfer of syngeneic splenocytes of chronically exposed animals into the footpad (see Chapter 15) may largely, if not completely obviate this problem. In spite of the apparent versatile usefulness of the PLN assay, however, extensive validation of the assay is as yet needed and should have high priority in order to assess the immunotoxicological relevance of this short-term assay.

(b) Long-term experiments

Because the development of AD in man and animals usually requires persistent immune disregulation for a prolonged period of time (months, years), long-term experiments seem to be most suited for the study of drug-induced AD. However, the choice of appropriate parameters which could reflect the immune disregulation, and selection of susceptible species or strains, present a problem.

Detection of immune disregulation. Whereas proliferation and differentiation of autoreactive lymphocytes are a prerequisite for development of AD [17], they are also concomitants of well-controlled specific immune responses to exogenous antigens. Therefore, determination of autoantibodies and autoreactive T cells per se usually yields no conclusive evidence for assessment of AD. This is also evident from data on humoral and/or cellular abnormalities in patients with clinically well-documented SLE. There is not always a clear-cut correlation between the abnormalities and disease activity, although abnormal serologic profiles, e.g. high levels of autoantibodies with various specificities, immune complexes, low complement levels and other alterations, are closely associated with active SLE [18]. Thus, data do not provide clear indications for the choice of parameters to be used in the study of chemical-induced SLE. Things are even more complicated, because it is still a matter of debate whether abnormal serological manifestations are a primary cause or a consequence of active AD [19, 20]. Nevertheless, it should be realized that a change induced by a LMW compound in any immunologically relevant in vivo parameter will have an indicative function of immune disregulating potential, since LMW compounds in general have to be considered as non-immunogenic of themselves and since they should be immunologically inactive. Already for these reasons measurement of serum parameters as indicated in Section II.2. of this chapter is useful. Increases of IgM autoantibodies during exposure are difficult to interpret in this respect, but strong evidence for AD-inducing potential will be obtained when a conversion to IgG antibodies is observed. This may be inferred from studies on murine models of spontaneous SLE in which a switch from IgM to IgG autoantibodies could be associated with development of overt disease [9, 17]. Also data on drug-induced SLE in man point in this direction. Antinuclear antibodies in patients with procainamide-induced SLE appeared to be of the IgG class, whereas IgM antinuclear antibodies were predominant in asymptomatic users of the drug (see Chapter 4 by Rubin; [19]). Further, the relatively low incidence of chlorpromazine-induced SLE has been related to its preferential induction of IgM antinuclear antibodies [21].

Routine methods predicting cell-mediated AD are virtually lacking. As already referred to before, determination of urinary pterin excretion may be a promising approach to assess T cell activation in a non-invasive manner [22, 23]. Elevated urinary neopterin levels in humans have been demonstrated in patients suffering from various conditions of disordered immunity, such as GVH reactions, rheumatoid arthritis, acquired immune deficiency syndrome (AIDS), and other disorders [22 – 24]. The increased neopterin excretion could be related to production of interleukin-2 and interferon-γ [25, 26], being relatively unique secretion products of activated T cells. Both products were found to cause an intracellular accumulation of neopterin in human macrophages while secretion was found in response to interferon-γ [25, 26]. Non-T-cell-derived interferon-α was shown to have similar effects but only at non-physiological levels. Alterations of pterin excretion in the urine may, therefore, indirectly reflect T cell activation at some site in the body. Although data on pterin biosynthesis and metabolism in experimental animals and their relationship with an activated T cell mediated immune function are still scarce [25, 26], we have recently found that urinary biopterin excretion levels in mice are alternately elevated and suppressed during GVH reactions as well as during oral exposure to some drugs with documented potential to induce AD in humans [13a]. Obviously, basic investigations and validation are needed, but monitoring of urinary pterin excretion may become a valuable asset in immunotoxicological research, especially because it could allow a long-term non-invasive follow-up of immunological effects.

Genetic background. As particular MHC haplotypes and metabolic polymorphisms were found to be predisposing factors for development of AD in man, the use of animals without a particular predisposition to AD might explain the failure to detect overt AD in inbred rodents during exposure to well-known inducers of human AD. Despite the absence of signs of AD in long-term experiments, strain-dependent variations of autoantibody responses could be observed, indicating that genetic predisposition in this respect is also apparent in rodents (see introductory chapter). Ample and firm evidence for a role of the MHC in chemical-induced autoantibody formation and autoimmune glomerulonephritis has been obtained with mercuric chloride in inbred rats (see Chapter 14 by Druet et al.). Studies addressing the role of metabolic polymorphisms in chemically induced autoantibody formation and AD have as far as known not yet been performed, but a link between altered metabolism of propylthiouracil and its ability to induce AD in randomly bred cats has been found (see Chapter 12 by Aucoin). Hyperthyroid cats, having a much shorter elimination half-life of the drug than normal cats, were found to be far more resistant to development of SLE-like disease.

As pointed out earlier [27], it may prove to be worthwhile in preclinical screening of new compounds to make use of various genetically well-defined inbred strains. By using species or strains with increased susceptibility to develop systemic AD, the potential of drugs and chemicals to induce autoimmune reactions might be recognized at an early stage. Transfer of accelerator genes such as *lpr* or *gld*, which enhance progression of AD, into strains of mice with different backgrounds (see introductory chapter; [9]), could allow a better dissection of the relative importance of the genetic background in interaction with environmental agents.

2. CHEMICAL-RELATED APPROACHES

In order to assess the significance of drug- and chemical-induced immune disregulation in a biologically relevant manner, it is of importance to attempt to elucidate and define the toxicological targets [8, 10, 11]. Several ways by which LMW compounds may provoke AD are conceivable, and evidence for and against some mechanisms have been reviewed in this volume. These different mechanisms are mutually not exclusive. In view of the complexity and the interrelatedness of immune functions, the following listing of possible targets is certainly not exhaustive, but may give some access to the field from a toxicological perspective.

(a) Chemical reactivity of parent compounds

One of the most extensively discussed mechanisms with regard to drug-induced lymphoproliferative reactions concerns the haptenic nature of LMW compounds. An excellent review addressing drug disposition related to drug allergies has recently appeared [28]. In a number of ways LMW drugs and chemicals may interact with body consituents such as proteins and thereby become antigenic or immunogenic determinants themselves. This may give rise to compound-specific antibodies, such as detected in drug-specific allergies (e.g. penicillin allergies). On the other hand particular proteins on cell membranes which could be chemically modified, such as MHC determinants, or proteins recognized in association with MHC determinants, may lead to the allogeneic effect, and if persistent, to immune derangements such as AD (see Chapters 3 and 15, by Allison, and Gleichmann et al.; [29, 30]). In drug-induced AD usually no compound-specific antibodies can be detected. Association with MHC class I determinants has been shown for penicillin [31] and for chlorpromazine [32]. Further investigations in this field may possibly lead to a better distinction between the basic mechanisms which lead to drug-induced allergic and/or autoimmune-like symptoms, as well as to a better knowledge of other factors (e.g. particular MHC haplotypes) which may co-determine the outcome of the immune response.

Reactive compounds may interact directly with nucleophilic groups ($-NH_2$, $-SH$, $-OH$) of body proteins. For example, D-penicillamine has a free carboxyl group, a free sulfhydryl group, and a free amino group, and may react with macromolecules in several different manners, thereby altering self-constituents [28]. Furthermore, the potential of p-nitrobenzyl compounds to induce skin sensitization has been shown to correlate with their chemical reactivity as well as lipophilicity [33]. Isothiocyanates and isocyanates provide another class of compounds which readily react with nucleophilic groups on proteins [34, 35] or amino sugars [36] under physiological conditions, and are well-documented inducers of adverse local [37, 38] or systemic immunological reactions [39].

Specific components involved in immune regulation such as the complement system may be inhibited in vitro by covalent binding of nucleophilic compounds such as procainamide, hydralazine and D-penicillamine (see Chapter 10 by Sim).

Reactive chemicals may not only covalently bind to cell membrane structures and elicit immunologic reactions, but also to DNA constituents, for instance to guanosine, as extensively studied in the field of mutagenesis [40]. Interestingly, antiguanosine antibodies have been reported as a marker for procainamide-induced SLE [41].

Another interesting aspect is that a number of drugs and chemicals, especially cationic amphiphilic amines, may be significantly retained by endothelial cells in the lungs [42]. Concentration is considered to occur by binding to the highly negatively charged endothelial cell membranes. Because damage to the vascular system appears to play an important role in the pathogenesis of AD, study of chemically induced vascular endothelial changes may yield clues with regard to possible targets of autoimmunity-inducing drugs (see below).

Cationic amphiphilic drugs including chlorpromazine can also interact with polar phospholipids, thereby interfering with phospholipid metabolism which may result in phospholipidosis [43], and enhanced de novo synthesis of phosphatidylinositol in lymphocytes [44]. Whether these phenomenons are related to the finding of antibodies to membrane constituents, notably phospholipids (anti-cardiolipin; anticoagulants) as found in patients with idiopathic SLE and related AD [45, 46], as well as in patients with procainamide- and chlorpromazine-induced autoantibodies and/or SLE [46], is currently unclear.

It should be realized that bioavailability as determined by the vehicle may influence chemical reactivity of LMW compounds after oral exposure. Compounds dissolved in aqueous media are more readily taken up by the blood circulation, whereas agents in an oil matrix are more likely to be conveyed by chylomicrons to the lymph.

(b) Metabolism

The immunomodulating potential of LMW compounds may also be attributed to reactive metabolites. It has been shown that slow acetylators of procainamide, hydralazine and sulfonamides have an increased chance to develop adverse systemic immunological disorders, and particular reactive metabolites have been implicated in the pathogenesis (see Chapters 9 and 4, by Hein and Weber, and Rubin; [7]). Polymorphisms of drug metabolism may not only result in slower elimination of the parent compound or its metabolites, but also in formation of particular metabolites due to stereoselective metabolism (see Section III.3. of introductory chapter; [47, 48]).

Regarding the crucial role of metabolites in the development of AD giving attention to the hepatic metabolism is obvious, but a role of locally generated metabolites should be considered as well. For instance, endothelial cells are not only capable of accumulating drugs as mentioned above, but also of intracellular metabolic conversion [42]. This may result in the local formation of high concentrations of reactive metabolites. Their covalent binding may either cause direct endothelium damage and so evoke local non-specific inflammation, or trigger immunologically specific reactions to endothelium (see below).

Transglutaminases, enzymes which mediate for example covalent cross-linking between glutamine and lysine residues, have been proposed to mediate autoimmune reactions induced by primary amines such as hydralazine or isoniazid [49 – 51]. These enzymes can easily substitute LMW primary amines for the lysine moiety of the reaction [49]. Thereby, these LMW drugs can be covalently bound to plasma and nuclear proteins such as histones.

(c) Immunotoxicologically relevant targets

There are ample data suggesting that upregulation of MHC class II expression in particular organs is related to the induction of autoimmune reactions (see Chapter 3 by Allison; [52]). Among others, interferons and tumor necrosis factor-α were found to mediate this upregulation (see Chapter 3 [52, 53]), and indeed raised blood levels of interferons have been observed in human and murine AD [53]. Tumor necrosis factor-α was recently found to be a mediator of the pathological lesions in GVH disease [54]. Conceivably, the ability of a LMW compound to induce such interleukins may contribute to its AD-inducing potential. Antiviral pyrimidinone derivatives may represent an example. These compounds are potent interferon inducers [55, 56] and one derivative was found to produce a dose-dependent lymphoid hyperplasia, elevation of serum IgG levels and adjuvant-like arthritis in rats after oral administration during 14 days [57]. As follow-up it would be interesting to study the disease-inducing potential of derivatives in relation to their capacity to induce interferons.

Primary or secondary damage to the vascular system plays a role in the pathogenesis of various idiopathic and chemical-induced AD [2, 58 – 60]. Endothelium is likely to be involved in these diseases not only in the effector phase but also in the induction phase. Endothelial cells are ubiquitous in the body, lining both blood and lymph vessels, and thus guarantee a large contact area with immunocompetent lymphoid cells and endothelium. Further, vascular endothelium is one of the few non-immunological tissues that constitutively expresses MHC class II determinants and can produce interleukin-1. It therefore fulfills all requirements for the initiation of T cell-mediated immune responses [61]. It may be speculated that the combined presence of MHC class II molecules and chemically altered self-components on endothelium as a consequence of the above mentioned ability of LMW to bind to the cells, may cause T helper cell activation. Because T helper cells play a central, initiating role in both cellular and antibody-mediated immune responses, chronic T cell activation may eventually lead to destruction of the endothelium itself by cellular or humoral effector mechanisms, as in some forms of vasculitis. Additionally, T cell activation in this way may result in SLE-like AD mediated by the allogeneic effect (see Chapters 3 and 15, by Allison, and Gleichmann et al.).

Impaired function of the mononuclear phagocyte system may lead to a decreased immune complex clearance and contribute to the pathogenesis of AD. Chemicals interfering with this system may therefore superimpose AD. In this context it is interesting to note that the drug methimazole was shown to interfere with antigen handling by macrophages [62]. Other data indicated that diphenylhydantoin impaired macrophage function as judged by depressed polyvinyl pyrrolidone clearance [63]. Although both drugs are documented inducers of vasculitis and other features of systemic AD, assessment of the significance of this mechanism in the pathogenesis of drug-induced AD needs further study.

Secretory IgA at mucosal gastrointestinal surfaces is known to interfere with the binding and uptake of microorganisms and food constituents, and IgA deficiency has been related to enhanced immune responsiveness to food-born antigens [64]. This has been proposed to be one of the mechanisms by which IgA deficiency would lead to an enhanced chance to develop systemic AD [65]. In this context it is interesting to mention that drugs like diphenylhydantoin [66] and D-penicillamine [67] have been shown to induce IgA deficiency, but the relation between this phenomenon and their ability to induce systemic AD has not been proven.

IV. Conclusions

Explicit demonstration of the AD-inducing potential of a given compound in routine toxicology, as currently practiced, will remain problematic. New approaches like the PLN assay and the monitoring of urinary pterins seem promising indicators of a chemical's potential to induce immune disregulation, but validation is still required. Analysis of the relative contribution of environmental chemical and individual factors in the etiology and pathogenesis of AD is needed for proper risk assessment, and asks for a multifactorial investigative approach. Further identification of genetically determined host factors that facilitate development of AD in man should have high priority. These include immunologic and metabolic factors. The use of highly defined inbred animals harboring analogous factors may yield animal models of chemical AD that allow fundamental mechanistic studies. Chemical-related approaches should attempt to correlate biological activity of drugs and chemicals to molecular structure in a qualitative or quantitative way. Biological activity should be assessed by using assays that measure immunologic, pharmacologic, and metabolic properties as well as chemical reactivity. Structure-activity relationship studies may identify the crucial (combinations of) chemical structures required for the induction of AD, and may also improve the understanding of the mechanisms by which chemicals interact with immunological systems. This approach may allow development of safer drugs as well as identification of natural or artificial LMW compounds in the human diet and the (occupational) environment as potential triggers of AD and other kinds of immune disregulation.

References

1. Dubois, E. L. and Wallace, D. J. (1987) Drugs that exacerbate and induce systemic lupus erythematosus: In: D. J. Wallace and E. L. Dubois (Eds.), Dubois' Lupus Erythematosus, 3rd Edn., Lea and Febiger, Philadelphia, pp. 450–469.
2. Zürcher, K. and Krebs, A. (1980) Cutaneous side effects of systemic drugs. A commentated synopsis of today's drugs, Karger, Basel, pp. 165–191.

3. Amos, H. E. (1983) Drugs acting on the cardiovascular system. In: A.L. De Weck and H. Bund-gaard (Eds.), Allergic Reactions to Drugs, Springer Verlag, Berlin, pp. 391 – 422.

4. Anonymous (1986) Withdrawal of nomifensine. Lancet i, 281.

5. Henschler, D. (1987) Concepts for risk assessment and animal-human extrapolation – a tox-icologist's view. In: B.A. Fowler (Ed.), Mechanisms of Cell Injury: Implications for Human Health, Dahlem Konferenzen, John Wiley and Sons, Chichester, pp. 267 – 280.

6. Welsh, K. I. and Black, C. M. (1985) Genetic aspects of the acquired connective tissue diseases. Sem. Dermatol. 4, 152 – 163.

7. Shear, N. H., Spielberg, S. P., Grant, D. M., Tang, B. K. and Kalow, W. (1986) Differences in metabolism of sulfonamides predisposing to idiosyncratic toxicity. Ann. Intern. Med. 105, 179 – 184.

8. Zbinden, L. C. (1987) A toxicologist's view of immunotoxicology. In: A. Berlin, J. Dean, M. H. Draper, E. M. B. Smith and F. Spreafico (Eds.), Immunotoxicology, Martinus Nijhoff Publ., Dordrecht, pp. 1 – 11.

9. Hang, L., Aguado, M. T., Dixon, F. J. and Theofilopoulos, A. N. (1985) Induction of severe autoimmune disease in normal mice by simultaneous action of multiple immunostimulators. J. Exp. Med. 161, 423 – 428.

10. Immunotoxicology. Synopsis, conclusions and recommendations (1987). In: A. Berlin, J. Dean, M. H. Draper, E. M. B. Smith and F. Spreafico (Eds.), Immunotoxicology, Martinus Nijhoff Publishers, Dordrecht, pp. XI – XXVII.

11. Shoham, J. (1985) Specific safety problems of inappropriate immune responses to im-munostimulating agents. Trends Pharmacol. Sci. 6, 178 – 182.

12. Gleichmann, H. (1981) Studies on the mechanism of drug sensitization: T-cell-dependent popliteal lymph node reaction to diphenylhydantoin. Clin. Immunol. Immunopathol. 18, 203 – 211.

13. Gleichmann, H., Pals, S. T. and Radaszkiewicz, T. (1983) T-cell-dependent B-cell proliferation and activation by administration of the drug diphenylhydantoin to mice. Hematol. Oncol. 1, 165 – 176.

13a. Kammüller, M. E. (1988) A toxicological approach to chemical-induced autoimmunity. PhD Thesis, University of Utrecht, Utrecht, The Netherlands.

14. Hurtenbach, U., Gleichmann, H., Nagata, N. and Gleichmann, E. (1987) Immunity to D-penicillamine: genetic, cellular and chemical requirements for induction of popliteal lymph node enlargement in the mouse. J. Immunol. 139, 411 – 416.

15. Kammüller, M. E., Penninks, A. H., De Bakker, J. M., Thomas, C., Bloksma, N. and Seinen, W. (1987) An experimental approach to chemically induced systemic (auto)immune alterations: Spanish toxic oil syndrome as an example. In: B. A. Fowler (Ed.), Mechanisms of Cell Injury: Im-plications for Human Health, Dahlem Konferenzen, John Wiley and Sons, Chichester, pp. 175 – 192.

16. Kammüller, M. E. and Seinen, W. (1988) Structural requirements for hydantoins and 2-thiohydantoins to induce lymphoproliferative popliteal lymph node reactions in the mouse. Int. J. Immunopharmacol., in press.

17. Theofilopoulos, A. N., Prud'homme, G. J. and Dixon, F. J. (1985) Autoimmune aspects of systemic lupus erythematosus. Concepts Immunopathol. 1, 190 – 218.

18. Dubois, E. L. and Wallace, D. J. (1987) Clinical and laboratory manifestations of systemic lupus erythematosus. In: D. J. Wallace and E. L. Dubois (Eds.), Dubois' Lupus Erythematosus, 3rd Edn., Lea and Febiger, Philadelphia, pp. 317 – 449.

19. Tan, E. M., Chan, E. K. L., Sullivan, K. F. and Rubin, R. L. (1988) Antinuclear antibodies (ANAs): diagnostically specific immune markers and clues toward the understanding of systemic autoimmunity. Clin. Immunol. Immunopathol. 47, 121 – 141.

20. Lachmann, P. J. and Walport, M. J. (1987) Deficiency of the effector mechanisms of the im-

mune response and autoimmunity. In: Autoimmunity and Autoimmune Disease (Ciba Foundation Symposium No. 129), John Wiley and Sons, Chichester, pp. 149 – 171.

21. Canoso, R. T. and De Oliveira, R. M. (1986) Characterization and antigenic specificity of chlorpromazine-induced antinuclear antibodies. J. Lab. Clin. Med. 108, 213 – 216.

22. Editorial. (1988) Neopterins in clincal medicine. Lancet i, 509 – 511.

23. Fuchs, D., Hausen, A., Reibnegger, G., Werner, E. R., Dierich, M. P., Wachter, H. (1988) Neopterin as marker for activated cell-mediated immunity: application in HIV infection. Immunol. Today 9, 150 – 155.

24. Dhont, J. L., Walter, M. P., Bauters, F. and Jouet, J. P. (1988) Biopterin and organ transplantation. Lancet i, 1109.

25. Schoedon, G., Troppmair, J., Fontana, A., Huber, C., Curtius, H. C. and Niederwieser, A. (1987) Biosynthesis and metabolism of pterins in peripheral blood mononuclear cells and leukemia lines of man and mouse. Eur. J. Biochem. 166, 303 – 310.

26. Ziegler, I. (1985) Synthesis and interferon-gamma-controlled release of pteridines during activation of human peripheral blood mononuclear cells. Biochem. Biophys., Res. Comm., 132, 404 – 411.

27. Festing, M. F. W. (1987) Genetic factors in toxicology: implications for toxicological screening. CRC Crit. Rev. Toxicol. 18, 1 – 26.

28. Park, B. K., Coleman, J. W. and Kitteringham, N. R. (1987) Drug disposition and drug hypersensitivity. Biochem. Pharmacol. 36, 581 – 590.

29. Eastman, A. Y. and Lawrence, D. A. (1982) TNP-modified syngeneic cells enchance immunoregulatory T cell activities similar to allogeneic effects. J. Immunol. 128, 926 – 931.

30. Ptak, W., Rewicka, M. and Marcinkiewicz, J. (1984) Induction of 'allogeneic effect'-like reaction by syngeneic TNP-modified lymphoid cells. Immunobiology, 166, 368 – 381.

31. Claas, F. H. J. and Van Rood, J. J. (1985) The interaction of drugs and endogenous substances with HLA class-I antigens. Prog. Allergy 36, 135 – 150.

32. Smeraldi, E. and Scorza-Smeraldi, R. (1976) Interference between anti-HLA antibodies and chlorpromazine. Nature 260, 532 – 533.

33. Roberts, D. W., Goodwin, B. F. J., Williams, D. L., Jones, K., Johnson, A. W. and Alderson, J. C. E. (1983) Correlations between skin sensitization potential and chemical reactivity for p-nitrophenyl compounds. Food Chem. Toxicol. 21, 811 – 813.

34. Brown, W. E., Green, A. H., Cedel, T. E. and Cairns, J. (1987) Biochemistry of protein-isocyanate interactions: a comparison of the effects of aryl vs. alkyl isocyanates. Environ. Health Perspect. 72, 5 – 11.

35. Ted Tse, C. S. and Pesce, A. J. (1979) Chemical characterization of isocyanate-protein conjugates. Toxicol. Appl. Pharmacol. 51, 39 – 46.

36. Scott, J. E. (1970) The reactions of isothiocyanates with 2-amino sugars: electrophoresis in borate and tungstate buffers, and spectroscopy of the products. Carbohydr. Res. 14, 389 – 404.

37. Fregert, S., Truslon, L. and Zimerson, E. (1982) Contact allergic reactions to diphenylthiourea and phenylisothiocyanate in PVC adhesive tape. Contact Dermatitis 8, 38 – 42.

38. Furue, M. and Tamaki, K. (1985) Induction and suppression of contact sensitivity to fluorescein isothiocyanate (FITC). J. Invest. Dermatol. 85, 139 – 142.

39. Jennings, G. H. and Gower, N. D. (1963) Thrombocytopenic purpura in toluene di-isocyanate workers. Lancet i, 406 – 408.

40. Hemminki, K. and Randerath, K. (1987) Detection of genetic interaction of chemicals by biochemical methods: determination of DNA and protein adducts. In: B. A. Fowler (Ed.), Mechanisms of Cell Injury: Implications for Human Health, Dahlem Konferenzen, John Wiley and Sons, Chichester, pp. 209 – 227.

41. Weisbart, R. H., Yee, W. S., Colburn, K. K., Whang, S. H., Heng, M. K. and Boucek, J. (1986) Antiguanosine antibodies: a new marker for procainamide-induced systemic lupus erythematosus. Ann. Intern. Med. 104, 310 – 313.

42. Camus, P. and Jeannin, L. (1984) The diseased lung and drugs. Arch. Toxicol. Suppl. 7, 66–87.

43. Lüllmann-Rauch, R. (1979) Drug-induced lysosomal storage disorders. In: J. T. Dingle, P. J. Jacques and I. H. Shaw (Eds.), Lysosomes in Applied Biology and Therapeutics, North-Holland Publishing Co., Amsterdam, pp. 49–130.

44. Allan, D. and Michell, R. H. (1975) Enhanced synthesis de novo of phosphatidylinositol in lymphocytes treated with cationic amphiphilic drugs. Biochem. J. 148, 471–478.

45. Janoff, A. S. and Rauch, J. (1986) The structural specificity of anti-phospholipid antibodies in autoimmune disease. Chem. Phys. Lipids 40, 315–332.

46. Quismorio, F. P. (1987) Other serologic abnormalities in systemic lupus erythematosus. In: D. J. Walace and E. L. Dubois (Eds.), Dubois' Lupus Erythemasosus, 3rd Edn., Lea and Febiger, Philadelphia, pp. 244–261.

47. Caldwell, J., Winter, S. M. and Hutt, A. J. (1988) The pharmacological and toxicological significance of the stereochemistry of drug disposition. Xenobiotica 18, Suppl. 1, 59–70.

48. Smith, R. L. (1988) The role of metabolism and disposition studies in the safety assessment of pharmaceuticals. Xenobiotica 18, Suppl. 1, 89–96.

49. Lorand, L. and Conrad, S. M. (1984) Transglutaminases. Mol. Cell. Biochem. 58, 9–35.

50. Buxman, M. M. (1979) The role of enzymatic coupling of drugs to proteins in induction of drug specific antibodies. J. Invest. Dermatol. 73, 256–258.

51. Schopf, R. E., Hanauske-Abel, H. M., Tschank, G., Schulte-Wissermann, H. and Günzler, V. (1985) Effects of hydrazyl group containing drugs on leucocyte functions: an immunoregulatory model for the hydralazine-induced lupus-like syndrome. J. Immunopharmacol. 7, 385–401.

52. Feldmann, M. (1987) Regulation of HLA class II expression and its role in autoimmune disease. In: Autoimmunity and Autoimmune Disease (Ciba Foundation Symposium No. 129), John Wiley and Sons, Chichester, pp. 88–108.

53. Revel, M. and Schattner, A. (1987) Interferons: cytokines in autoimmunity. In: Autoimmunity and Autoimmune Disease (Ciba Foundation Symposium No. 129), John Wiley and Sons, Chichester, pp. 223–233.

54. Piguet, P. F., Grau, G. E., Allet, B. and Vassalli, P. (1987) Tumor necrosis factor/cachectin is an effector of skin and gut lesions of the acute graft-vs.-host disease. J. Exp. Med. 166, 1280–1289.

55. Fast, P. E., Hatfield, C. A., Sun, E. L. and Stringfellow, D. A. (1982) Polyclonal B-cell activation and stimulation of specific antibody responses by 5-halopyrimidinones with antiviral and antineoplastic activity. J. Biol. Resp. Modif. 1, 199–215.

56. Wierenga, W., Skulnick, H. I., Stringfellow, D. A., Weed, S. D., Renis, H. E. and Eidson, E. E. (1980) 5-Substituted 2-amino-6-phenyl-4(3H)-pyrimidinones. Antiviral and interferon-inducing agents. J. Med. Chem. 23, 237–239.

57. Gray, J. E., Larsen, E. R., Fast, P. E. and Hamilton, R. D. (1985) Orally induced adjuvant-like arthritis in the rat. Toxicol. Pathol. 133, 266–275.

58. Fauci, A. S., Haynes, B. F. and Katz, P. (1978) The spectrum of vasculitis. Clinical, pathologic, immunologic, and therapeutic considerations. Ann. Intern. Med. 89 (part 1), 660–676.

59. Fleischmajer, R., Perlish, J. S. and Duncan, M. (1983) Scleroderma. A model for fibrosis (editorial). Arch. Dermatol. 119, 957–962.

60. Toxic Epidemic Syndrome Study Group (1982) Toxic epidemic syndrome, Spain, 1981. Lancet ii, 697–702.

61. Wagner, C. R., Vetto, R. M. and Burger, D. R. (1984) The mechanism of antigen presentation by endothelial cells. Immunobiology 168, 453–469.

62. Weetman, A. P., McGregor, A. M. and Hall, R. (1983) Methimazole inhibits thyroid autoantibody production by action on accessory cells. Clin. Immunol. Immunopathol. 28, 39–45.

63. Seager, J., Coovadia, H. M. and Soothill, J. F. (1978) Reduced immunoglobulin concentration

and impaired macrophage function in mice due to diphenylhydantoin. Clin. Exp. Immunol. 33, 437 – 440.

64. Underdown, B. J. and Schiff, J. M.   (1986)   Immunoglobulin A: strategic defense initiative at the mucosal surface. Annu. Rev. Immunol. 4, 389 – 417.

65. Cunningham-Rundles, C., Brandeis, W. E., Pudifin, D. J., Day, N. K. and Good, R. A. (1981)   Autoimmunity in selective IgA deficiency: relationship to anti-bovine protein antibodies, circulating immune complexes and clinical disease. Clin. Exp. Immunol. 45, 299 – 304.

66. Shakir, R. A., Behan, P. O., Dick, H. and Lambie, D. G.   (1978)   Metabolism of immunoglobulin A, lymphocyte function, and histocompatibility antigens in patients on anticonvulsants. J. Neurol. Neurosurg. Psychiat. 41, 307 – 311.

67. Hjalmarson, O., Hanson, L. A. and Nilsson, L. A.   (1977)   IgA deficiency during D-penicillamine treatment. Br. Med. J. 1, 549.

Subject index